Attachment Theory and Research in Clinical Work with Adults

edited by
Joseph H. Obegi
Ety Berant

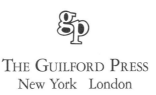

THE GUILFORD PRESS
New York   London

Printed in the United States of America

This book is printed on acid-free paper.

Last digit is print number: 9 8 7 6 5 4 3 2

Library of Congress Cataloging-in-Publication Data

Attachment theory and research in clinical work with adults / edited by Joseph H. Obegi
and Ety Berant.
    p. ; cm.
Includes bibliographical references and index.
ISBN 978-1-59385-998-5 (hardcover : alk. paper)
ISBN 978-1-60623-928-5 (paperback : alk. paper)
1. Attachment behavior. 2. Psychotherapy. I. Obegi, Joseph H. II. Berant, Ety.
[DNLM: 1. Object Attachment. 2. Adult. 3. Psychoanalytic Therapy—methods.
WM 460.5.O2 A88338 2009]
    RC455.4.A84A92   2009
    616.85'88—dc22

                                                          2008037459

Attachment Theory and Research
in Clinical Work with Adults

To our partners, Amy and Michael

About the Editors

Joseph H. Obegi, PsyD, is a clinical psychologist in private practice in Davis, California. Previously a lecturer at the California School of Professional Psychology at Alliant International University in San Diego, he taught courses in psychotherapy, chemical dependency, and professional ethics. Dr. Obegi's recent research has focused on attachment to therapists and the validity of adult attachment scales in clinical populations.

Ety Berant, PhD, is on the faculty of the Department of Psychology at Bar-Ilan University, Ramat-Gan, Israel, and has served as the chairperson of the graduate clinical track. She is also a senior clinical psychologist and has practiced and supervised psychotherapy and personality assessment for nearly two decades. Dr. Berant is the chairperson of the Israeli Rorschach Society. Her research interests include attachment styles in adulthood, personality assessment, and therapeutic processes.

Contributors

Leslie Atkinson, PhD, Department of Psychology, Ryerson University, Toronto, Ontario, Canada

Ety Berant, PhD, Department of Psychology, Bar-Ilan University, Ramat-Gan, Israel

Jude Cassidy, PhD, Department of Psychology, University of Maryland, College Park, Maryland

Rebecca J. Cobb, PhD, Department of Psychology, Simon Fraser University, Burnaby, British Columbia, Canada

Katherine Daly, PhD, Department of Psychology, University of Florida, Gainesville, Florida

Joanne Davila, PhD, Department of Psychology, Stony Brook University, Stony Brook, New York

Morris Eagle, PhD, Derner Institute of Advanced Psychological Studies, Adelphi University, Garden City, New York

Barry A. Farber, PhD, Department of Counseling and Clinical Psychology, Columbia University Teachers College, New York, New York

Paul Florsheim, PhD, School of Social Welfare, University of Wisconsin–Milwaukee, Milwaukee, Wisconsin

R. Chris Fraley, PhD, Department of Psychology, University of Illinois at Urbana–Champaign, Champaign, Illinois

Jeremy Holmes, MD, FRCPsych, University of Exeter, Exeter, Devon, United Kingdom

Susan M. Johnson, EdD, Ottawa Couple and Family Institute, University of Ottawa, Ottawa, Ontario, Canada

Elliot L. Jurist, PhD, Department of Clinical Psychology, Graduate School and University Center, City University of New York, New York, New York

Kristen M. Kelly, PhD, Department of Psychology, The Pennsylvania State University, University Park, Pennsylvania

Kenneth N. Levy, PhD, Department of Psychology, The Pennsylvania State University, University Park, Pennsylvania

Frederick G. Lopez, PhD, Counseling Psychology Program, University of Houston, Houston, Texas

Brent Mallinckrodt, PhD, Department of Psychology, University of Tennessee, Knoxville, Tennessee

Laura McArthur, MS, Department of Psychology, University of Utah, Salt Lake City, Utah

Carolina McBride, PhD, Department of Psychiatry, University of Toronto, Toronto, Ontario, Canada

Kevin B. Meehan, PhD, Department of Psychology, Long Island University, Brooklyn, New York

Jesse A. Metzger, MS, Department of Counseling and Clinical Psychology, Columbia University Teachers College, New York, New York

Mario Mikulincer, PhD, New School of Psychology, Interdisciplinary Center, Herzliya, Israel

Judith Kay Nelson, PhD, The Sanville Institute for Clinical Social Work and Psychotherapy, Berkeley, California

Joseph H. Obegi, PsyD, private practice, Davis, California

Robert L. Phillips, MA, LPC, Connection Clinic, Portland, Oregon

Phillip R. Shaver, PhD, Department of Psychology, University of California, Davis, Davis, California

Rami Tolmacz, PhD, Department of Psychology, Bar-Ilan University, Ramat-Gan, Israel

Chia-Chih D. C. Wang, PhD, Department of Counseling and Educational Psychology, University of Missouri, Kansas City, Missouri

David L. Wolitzky, PhD, Department of Psychology, New York University, New York, New York

Contents

PART III. CLINICAL UTILITY

PART IV. INTEGRATION WITH CLINICAL APPROACHES

PART V. FUTURE DIRECTIONS

Attachment Theory and Research
in Clinical Work with Adults

1

Introduction

Joseph H. Obegi
Ety Berant

Clinicians interested in learning about and applying attachment theory and research to their work with adult clients have a daunting task before them. Because the attachment literature is voluminous and spans over 40 years, the obvious question is this: Where should they begin? Until the late 1990s, becoming acquainted with attachment theory required tackling Bowlby's trilogy (1969/1982, 1973, 1980) and Ainsworth and colleagues' "green book" (Ainsworth, Blehar, Waters, & Wall, 1978) to get a sense of the theory's landscape, and then sifting through research studies, special issues of journals, and edited volumes to get an up-to-date picture. Both the theory and the research have become considerably more accessible following the publications of the *Handbook of Attachment* (Cassidy & Shaver, 1999), *Attachment in Adulthood* (Mikulincer & Shaver, 2007), and several other major volumes by prominent attachment researchers (e.g., Sroufe, Egeland, Carlson, & Collins, 2005; Grossmann, Grossmann, & Waters, 2005). Still, clinicians must scour all these sources for the occasional contributions that address attachment theory's implications for adult psychotherapy. More often than not, these contributions are either tantalizingly brief, narrowly focused on connections to a single clinical school, or lopsided in their integration of the attachment literature. Without such bridge building, however, the gap between theoretical and empirical advances in understanding adult attachment and the practice of individual psychotherapy will continue to widen.

This volume is a collective effort intended to be a comprehensive, friendly, and clinically minded starting place for therapists, clinical researchers, and graduate students new to attachment theory. We asked contributors to discuss not only the implications of attachment theory and research for

1

adult psychotherapy—that is, the consequences they have for how we think about clinical work—but to explore applications as well. Clinical researchers will also find this volume useful. Continuing the long empirical tradition within the attachment field (unique among psychoanalytic schools), contributors have supported their ideas with research findings and, when only theoretical speculations were possible, highlighted what areas needed more research.

Before orienting you, the reader, to the structure and content of this volume, we would like to draw attention to some common misunderstandings about attachment theory and research.

IS THERE SUCH A THING
AS "ATTACHMENT THERAPY" FOR ADULTS?

There is no school of therapy for adults called "attachment therapy." Moreover, attachment theory is not itself an independent therapeutic approach. Rather, it is a comprehensive theory of development, motivation, personality, and psychopathology. In an often-quoted passage, Slade (1999) reminds us that "an understanding of the nature and dynamics of attachment *informs* rather than *defines* intervention and clinical thinking" (p. 577; emphasis in original). This quotation is at once astute and unremarkable. Clinicians new to attachment theory may be sufficiently impressed by the theory's intuitive appeal and impressive array of empirical findings that they are inclined to believe that attachment theory is itself a clinical guide to practice. However—unlike, for example, Sigmund Freud or Aaron Beck—John Bowlby did not detail, beyond a rough outline, a therapeutic approach to complement his comprehensive theory. Though he sought to create a theory that was a better fit for his clinical experience than the dominant psychoanalytic theories of his day (Hunter, 1991), a task that occupied him for 30 years, he seemed generally satisfied with the techniques of psychodynamic psychotherapy. Whatever the reason, Bowlby hoped (indeed, expected) that clinicians would take over where he left off. To his disappointment, and for various historical reasons detailed by Karen (1994) and Holmes (1996), clinical applications of attachment theory did not quickly materialize.

On the other hand, no clinically oriented theory, no matter how brilliant, alone defines intervention; each is destined merely to inform clinical work if its technical aspects are left undeveloped. For example, psychoanalytic theory does not define intervention, but psychoanalytic psychotherapy does. It is our concern that some may understand Slade to mean that attachment theory cannot generate an independent adult psychotherapy, due to some inherent limitation of the theory. Our own view of attachment theory's clinical potential is, not surprisingly, more optimistic. To us, two types of therapies derived from attachment theory already exist. The first, which we call *attachment-informed* (or *attachment-oriented*) *psychotherapy*, is the subject of this volume. By *attachment-informed psychotherapy*, we mean a therapy that uses attachment theory and research as adjudicative sources of knowledge and that influences how presenting problems are conceptualized, assessed, and treated, but that relies on an established therapy for implementation in terms of approach and technique. Attachment-informed psychotherapy has assumed two forms. In one form, attachment concepts compose one of several theoretical pillars supporting the clinical approach, but are not necessarily evident in the approach's day-to-day practice. Exemplars include variations of interpersonal therapy, as outlined by Klerman, Weissman, Rounsaville, and Chevron (1984) and Teyber (2000); cognitive–analytic therapy (Ryle, 1990); and accelerated experiential–dynamic psychotherapy (Fosha, 2000). More informally, clinicians have used attachment concepts to shape case conceptualization, assessment, clinical listening, and interaction in a way that supplements the techniques of their preferred clinical orientation. Case examples of attachment-informed psychotherapy can be readily found in this volume and throughout the literature (e.g., Byng-Hall, 1998; Harris, 2003; Meyer & Pilkonis, 2002; Slade, 2004; Wallin, 2007).

The second type of therapy we call *attachment-based psychotherapy*. By this we mean a psychotherapy (1) that explicitly draws upon attachment theory to conceptualize development, psychopathology, personality, and intrapsychic and interpersonal dynamics; (2) that articulates attachment theory with a structure of psychotherapy; and (3) that attempts to demonstrate its effectiveness with outcome studies. Several approaches meet this definition, including the Circle of Security project for infant–parent dyads (Marvin, Cooper, Hoffman, & Powell, 2002; see Berlin, Ziv, Amaya-Jackson, & Greenberg, 2005, for more examples of attachment-based infant–parent psychotherapies), emotionally focused therapy (EFT) for couples (Johnson, 2004), and attachment-focused group therapy for relationship problems (Kilmann, Urbaniak, & Parnell, 2006). At least one family therapy is moving in this direction (attachment-based family therapy; Diamond, Siqueland, & Diamond, 2003). All of these therapies are related to attachment theory in the same way that cognitive-behavioral therapy (CBT), for example, is related to cognitive theory. As yet, there is no empirically supported attachment-based therapy for individual adult treatment, though at least four have been outlined by European clinicians: brief attachment-based therapy (Holmes, 2001), attachment-based psychoanalytic psychotherapy (White, 2004), attachment narrative therapy (Dallos, 2006), and an attachment-guided approach developed by Brisch (2002).

WHO'S ATTACHED TO WHOM?

The term *attachment*, as used in attachment theory, has a particular meaning quite different from the word *attachment* as it is casually used in the psychoanalytic and alliance literatures. *Attachment* refers to the enduring tie that one person has with another who fulfills needs for safety and comfort. Thus an infant is attached to a parent, but, strictly speaking, a parent is not attached to an infant; in all but the most disturbed parent–child relationships, a parent does not turn to a child for reassurance and comfort during times of distress. As development moves forward from infancy, children and adolescents gradually shift their attachments from their parents to their same-age peers. Courtship, dating, and commitment all consolidate an adult's attachment to another adult. Adults more often turn to their partners and friends when stressed.

At the broadest level, then, there are two relational domains of attachment: infant–parent and adult–adult. The first wave of attachment research focused on the quality of children's attachments to their parents and on the factors that appeared to influence the quality of such attachments. The second wave of attachment research attended to how attachment manifested itself in adult relationships.

CLASSIFICATION SCHEMES

Perhaps one of the more confusing aspects of attachment research is the proliferation of classification schemes (Table 1.1). Clinicians might ask several questions: Why are the terms slightly different? Which is the definitive scheme? How do these schemes relate to one another? Because each classification scheme was developed by independent researchers, is designed to tap different domains of attachment, and relies on different assessment methods, their respective labels for attachment security and insecurity tend to differ. Remarkably, and as a testament to attachment theory's validity, each set of schemes has similar correlates (for reviews, see Cassidy, 2000; Shaver & Mikulincer, 2004). Because attachment security is measured with respect to a particular person, and because attachment security is in part a consequence of relationship quality, there can be no definitive method of assessing attachment security; all are complementary. We encourage our readers to lay claim to all the assessment tools and their respective research traditions, regardless of the readers' own methodological preferences. As the contributions in this volume make clear, all tools have similar potential to inform clinical work.

A thornier, and as yet unresolved, issue is how attachment security should be measured. That is, do the data suggest that attachment security is fundamentally a categorical construct (i.e., secure or insecure) or a dimensional one (i.e., high or low in attachment-related avoidance or anxiety)? Though the natural inclination of clinicians is to think in terms of categories of people (e.g., seeing clients as secure, histrionic, or rationalizing), research findings at the moment suggest that describing people along a continuum of security is more accurate. In this book, contributors embrace both ways

TABLE 1.1. Commonly Used Classification Schemes of Attachment

Tool	Method	Attachment domain	Categories
Strange Situation	Observation	Infant–parent	Secure, anxious-ambivalent, anxious-avoidant
Adult Attachment Interview (AAI)	Interview	Infant–parent	Secure/autonomous, preoccupied, dismissing, unresolved/disorganized
Experiences in Close Relationships (ECR) questionnaire	Self-report	Adult–adult	Secure, preoccupied, dismissing, fearful

Note. Source for the Strange Situation: Ainsworth, Blehar, Waters, and Wall (1978). Sources for the AAI: George, Kaplan, and Main (1984, 1985, 1996). Source for the ECR: Brennan, Clark, and Shaver (1998).

of describing attachment security. Readers interested in measurement issues regarding attachment should consult the work of Fraley and colleagues (Fraley & Spieker, 2003; Fraley, & Waller, 1998; Roisman, Fraley, & Belsky, 2007; Roisman, Holland et al., 2007).

From a clinical perspective, assessing attachment is an important step in clinical formulation. However, several cautions, based on research and clinical experience, are warranted. First, a clinical assessment of attachment, especially an informal one, should be considered a working hypotheses, one that is used to organize clinical information but that is open to revision as new information is obtained and therapeutic change occurs (D. Wallin, personal communication, August 6, 2008). Second, the assessment cannot be treated as comprehensive and invariable. Research strongly suggests that people can have an insecure attachment with one attachment figure and, at the same time, a more secure one with another attachment figure (Bretherton, 1985). Similarly, research also suggests that while people appear to have one internal working model that is the most accessible and, therefore, the most used, they also have access to secure and insecure models (Baldwin, Keelan, Fehr, & Enns, 1996). Third, attachment style is not synonymous with the moment-to-moment or the session-to-session sense of felt-security. For example, a therapeutic climate that is accepting and encouraging can help even a dismissing client feel secure enough in the here and now to disclose a bit more or to explore a embarrassing issue for another minute or two (McCluskey, Hooper, & Miller, 1999). Finally, the assessment of attachment is merely a way to orient ourselves to attachment phenomena, as they are being played out in the consulting room and in the client's life, and to the functioning of the attachment system (Slade, 2004). Thus, the attachment-informed clinician considers the assessment of attachment not as an end unto itself but as a means to begin to understand the complexity of the client before them.

The answer to the question of how assessments of infant security relate to assessments of security made in adulthood is also still emerging. Based on available evidence, a reasonable conclusion is that attachment experiences in infancy and early childhood modestly influence attachment security in adult romantic relationships. To put this another way, early experience has an enduring, rather than a strong impact on the quality of latter attachments (Crowell & Treboux, 2001; Fraley & Brimbaugh, 2004; Roisman, Collins, Sroufe, & Egeland, 2005). This conclusion should be a relief to both clients and clinicians: The quality of early experiences does not determine the quality of later relationships. We are not doomed to repeat the drama of our early childhoods, nor does attachment security completely insulate us from the effects of later experience; later experience can have rehabilitative, aggravating, or undermining effects on attachment security and insecurity. Numerous studies and reviews point to this conclusion (for a review, see Mikulincer & Shaver, 2007).

ORGANIZATION OF THIS BOOK

All chapters in this book were designed to make attachment theory and research accessible to novice and experienced therapists unacquainted with the theory, to show how attachment research bears on the clinical enterprise, and to provide clear recommendations for incorporating attachment theory and research into clinical practice. The book includes five sections; the first four correspond roughly to major areas of clinical work. Part I, "Theoretical Foundations," gives an overview of the essentials of adult attachment theory and their clinical relevance. Part II presents three ways to assess adult attachment security, and Part III delves deeper into the clinical utility of attachment theory. In Part IV, contributors share their experience in supplementing a preferred clinical approach with attachment concepts to enhance therapeutic efforts. Part V reflects on the wisdom of preceding chapters, highlighting trends of thought and research needs.

In Chapter 2, Shaver and Mikulincer provide a clinician-friendly field guide to adult attachment theory and research. Although many are familiar with Mary Ainsworth's work on individual differences in attachment, Shaver and Mikulincer remind us that these differences emerge from the functioning of the attachment behavioral system—a biologically rooted system that promotes survival in humans. Their psychodynamic explication of this system and the adaptations it makes to experience (i.e., attachment strategies) are valuable heuristic tools for the attachment-informed clinician; much of a client's in-session behavior can be understood as the operation of the attachment behavioral system. Shaver and Mikulincer also highlight the clinical value of attachment theory—namely, its implications for understanding maladjustment and change, its reliance on empirical validation, its integration of intrapersonal and interpersonal aspects of experience, and its compatibility with existing clinical approaches.

Given that the quality of the therapeutic relationship is among the most robust predictors of psychotherapy outcome (Wampold, 2001), any approach to psychotherapy must address this reality. A strength of attachment theory is that it is at once a theory of relationships and of personality differences; these two characteristics make it well suited to conceptualize the complexity of the therapeutic relationship and broaden our understanding of it. Farber and Metzger (Chapter 3) examine the implications of viewing the therapeutic relationship in attachment terms. They make use of the secure-base concept to conceptualize client–therapist interactions, and they review empirical evidence demonstrating the impact of individual differences in attachment security on the behavior of clients and therapists alike.

Across clinical approaches, a common practice is to engage clients in reflecting on the mental states that drive their own and others' behavior. The crossroads of this activity, known as *mentalizing,* and attachment theory is the subject of Jurist and Meehan's chapter (Chapter 4). These authors explain the close relationship between attachment security and mentalizing; they then draw attention to one particular form of mentalizing, called *mentalized affectivity,* that focuses on emotional states.

Like most clinical theories, attachment theory has its own "take" on variations in personality. These variations are commonly referred to as attachment styles or individual differences in attachment security. In order to customize treatment, attachment-informed clinicians need to recognize the telltale signs of attachment styles. Rounding out Part I is Lopez's chapter (Chapter 5) on the clinical correlates of attachment style. Ordinarily, the authors of clinically oriented chapters on personality differences rely on blending clinical lore and experience. In contrast, Lopez culls the findings from the empirical literature and organizes them into areas that clinicians often attend to when formulating hypotheses about personality: developmental and family histories, patterns of cognitive–affective regulation, coping strategies, and types of interpersonal problems. He then weaves these findings into "profiles" of attachment security to help aspiring attachment-informed clinicians "know it when they see it." Lopez's chapter is a wonderful illustration of how the empirical tradition within the attachment field yields clinically meaningful data and moves us beyond sole reliance on theoretical speculation.

Part II highlights another strength of an attachment perspective: empirically grounded assessment of personality differences. Authors in this section advise us on how to use attachment assessment tools, tempered by 20 years of research, in clinical practice. Levy and Kelly (Chapter 6) give a thorough introduction to Mary Main's deservedly heralded Adult Attachment Interview (AAI), suggesting ways to incorporate aspects of the AAI into the clinical interview and pointing out challenges of using the interview with clinical populations. Fraley and Phillips (Chapter 7) review the lesser-known, but extremely well-researched, self-report measures of adult attachment. In addition to making practical suggestions about their use, they introduce an innovative online monitoring system, especially designed for working clinicians and their clients, that tracks changes in attachment security over time as well as other pertinent variables (e.g., depression and relationship satisfaction). This tool, called eSession, can be used in individual and couple therapy and has much potential for extending the study of attachment processes to the clinical arena. An important but rather new area of research in adult attachment assessment is leveraging the strengths of traditional personality measures to assess attachment security. Using empirical studies of attachment and projective measures, Berant (Chapter 8) convincingly shows that individual differences in attachment security are readily apparent on such measures as the Rorschach and the Thematic Apperception Test. In an extended clinical example, she demonstrates how projective measures can be used in tandem with a self-report measure of adult attachment to inform clinical work and monitor therapeutic change. Although the field of attachment assessment is still evolving, these chapters provide up-to-date guidance.

Leading off Part III is Cobb and Davila's review of internal working models (IWMs) and therapeutic change (Chapter 9). The IWM (attachment theory's equivalent of a schema, a mental representation, or the like) is the cognitive structure that is responsible for the attitudinal and behavioral manifestations of attachment. Cobb and Davila introduce the components of IWMs, highlight supporting research, and discuss the implications for therapeutic change. They arrive at the provocative conclusion that targeting any component of IWMs (e.g., beliefs, emotions, action tendencies) is likely to promote change. Mallinckrodt, Daly, and Wang (Chapter 10) discuss tailoring treatment to individual differences in attachment security. Drawing from the research literature and their own qualitative interviews of 12 expert therapists, they propose a model of therapeutic distance. After assessing attachment security, therapists can determine what degree of therapeutic distance or closeness the client "pulls" for and, depending on the stage of therapy, can accommodate or challenge maneuvers that maintain less optimal degrees of closeness (e.g., too much or too little).

In the next two chapters, the contributors delve into areas that are usually considered the domains of other schools of psychodynamic thought: transference and psychological defenses. Bowlby described transference as a client's tendency to rigidly apply his or her internal working model and, as a result, to misconstrue experiences. Marshaling findings from the social-cognitive literature as well as modern psychoanalytic thought, Tolmacz (Chapter 11) updates and extends Bowlby's ideas. Of particular interest is his exposition of two approaches to transference: one using traditional notions of IWMs, and another using mentalization. He presents several vignettes that clearly illustrate the role of attachment security in how transference manifests itself. In Chapter 12, Mikulincer, Shaver, Cassidy, and Berant address another neglected aspect of attachment theory: its ability to conceptualize defensive functioning. Building on recent developments in attachment theory and attachment-inspired research, Mikulincer and colleagues firmly establish that an attachment perspective can explain a wide variety of defensive maneuvers and can empirically connect sets of defenses with with differences in attachment security. Clinical examples vividly illustrate their arguments.

Not only can attachment theory give a fresh perspective on psycho-therapy process and psychological functioning, but its depth can support new theoretical extensions. A prime example is Nelson's (Chapter 13) work on crying. Crying, though commonplace in adult psychotherapy (no office is complete without a box of tissues), has rarely been given theoretical attention. Nelson persuasively argues that crying in adults is an attachment behavior that serves the same function as it does infancy: to rally the support of attachment figures. Using her taxonomy of crying, she encourages us to consider how crying bears on the assessment of attachment security and on therapeutic process.

An increasingly popular (and sensible) trend in psychotherapy is the integrative perspective (Holmes & Bateman, 2002)—the view that no one clinical theory monopolizes ideas about psychological health and interven-tion. Informed integration of clinical theories may better capture presenting problems and be better equipped to facilitate change. In this spirit, the chap-ters in Part IV explore how attachment theory can supplement some of the more dominant approaches to psychotherapy and help translate and back-translate parallel terms and concepts. Attachment theory and psychody-namic thinking share several assumptions (Shaver & Mikulincer, 2005)—no wonder, given that Bowlby was a psychoanalyst—so it is natural to consider how they complement each other in treatment. Eagle and Wolitzky take up this topic in Chapter 14. They highlight the importance of attachment ideas for psychoanalytic work, but also encourage us to appreciate that attach-ment styles "will always be idiosyncratic and embedded in a complex indi-vidual life in which conflicts, defenses, wishes, and fantasies are present" (p. 373). Eagle and Wolitzky point out that a psychoanalytic frame draws attention to clients' attitudes toward their own attachment-related desires (i.e., "wishes"); the conflict between these can cause considerable anguish, and its resolution is a valuable source of change.

Florsheim and McArthur (Chapter 15) discuss the advantages of inter-personal assessment and interventions in remediating insecurity. They pro-pose that an interpersonal analysis of attachment style can help identify the client's particular intrapsychic and interpersonal problems, as well as pre-scribe the therapeutic actions necessary to foster new, security-based attach-ment strategies. In Chapter 16, Johnson, the originator of EFT for couples, shows how attachment theory and the principles and techniques of EFT are ideal partners. She argues that EFT can be tuned by attachment theory's attention to the caregiving qualities that foster secure attachment, its under-standing of the emotional fallout of disconnection and abandonment, and its perspective on how attachment needs are commonly communicated (or camouflaged). Moving vignettes poignantly underscore her ideas. In Chapter 17, McBride and Atkinson address the much-overlooked complementarity of CBT and attachment theory and research. They outline the numerous points of contact between cognitive theory and attachment theory, and show how an assessment of attachment security can guide the choice of psychotherapy and aid in the design of CBT interventions.

Part V consists of two chapters that stake out emerging points of consensus regarding attachment-informed work, as well as future research needs. As attachment theory gains "mindshare" with clinicians working with adults, it becomes necessary to temper enthusiasm with careful attention to how Bowlby's hypotheses play out empirically. In Chapter 18, the two of us present a qualitative review of clinically oriented attachment research conducted to date and organize findings into four areas: treatment seeking, engagement, and alliance; therapeutic intervention; transference and countertransference; and therapeutic outcome. In the final chapter, Holmes—Bowlby's biographer and a long-time proponent of attachment theory's clinical utility—surveys the volume's contributions. Using his characteristic style of integrating theory, clinical experience, and research knowledge, he captures themes that stretch across chapters, outlines the essential contributions of attachment theory and research, and highlights aspects of theory and research in need of further attention in order for attachment-informed psychotherapy to move forward.

ACKNOWLEDGMENTS

This book began in Grand Teton National Park on a piece of paper riddled with notes. It would have stayed that way, were it not for a number of generous and talented people. Foremost among them are Phillip R. Shaver and Mario Mikulincer. Phil and Mario actively mentored us throughout the project. They connected us with each other, helped shape the volume's structure, led us to The Guilford Press, and generously shared their time and experience. Their support was unfailing. Their advocacy and widely respected reputations opened doors for us that we otherwise would have found difficult to pry open by ourselves.

Every edited volume exists only because of its contributors. Despite busy schedules, the authors greeted our idea for this book with enthusiasm; all were eager to share their interest and experience in applying attachment ideas and research to clinical work. Some participated despite expected or unexpected upheavals in their personal lives, and others worked under grueling deadlines. Though we purposely sought experts in each area for this book, we completed this project with an even greater admiration for the intellect, ingenuity, and clinical expertise of each contributor.

We feel very fortunate to have had the backing of The Guilford Press, a leader in bringing attachment theory and research to a wider audience. Seymour Weingarten, Editor in Chief, enthusiastically received our proposal. His warmth, unflinching support, and patience were indispensable. We also wish to thank Louise Farkas for keeping the volume's production on track in her firm but always friendly way; Marie Sprayberry, for her extraordinary copyediting; Paul Gordon, for the book's cover; and Gina Gerboth, for indexing.

Along the way, there were many folks who encouraged us and deepened our clinical understanding of attachment theory. I (Joseph H. Obegi) wish to thank Neil Ribner and Gary Lawson for making an edited volume sound doable; Donald Viglione for giving me my editing "sea legs" as a graduate student; and Jonathan Mohr for providing much-needed assistance and validation at a critical juncture. I feel lucky to have had three clinical supervisors with a strong foundation in attachment theory: Patricia Judd, Peter Wayson, and Ruth Newton. In different ways, each nourished my interest in applying attachment theory to clinical work. My deepest thanks goes to my wife, Amy. Although she at first believed that a book project was a grandiose, pie-in-the-sky idea, her love, support, and encouragement have been life-sustaining. Without her, I surely would have crumbled dozens of times under the strain of the project.

I (Ety Berant) wish to thank my two mentors, Mario Mikulincer and the late Victor Florian, both of whom encouraged me to become a researcher in addition to my existing work as a clinical psychologist. Their wisdom and "secure-base" presence accompanied me throughout this project. I also thank Rebecca Richer-Atir, Netta Horesh, and Hedva Segal for following me on this journey with interest and support, as well as Yael Yalovsky for her wise advice. I thank my coeditor, Joe, for inviting me to join him in this exciting project and for the trust he had in me throughout. Finally, I am grateful to my loving family—my parents; my husband, Michael; and my children, Roni, Orit, Jonathan, and Dafna—who, despite knowing that this project would lessen my free time with them, were constant in their love, support, patience, and pride. Their companionship made it all so much easier.

REFERENCES

Ainsworth, M. S., Blehar, M. C., Waters, E., & Wall, S. (1978). *Patterns of attachment: A psychological study of the Strange Situation.* Hillsdale, NJ: Erlbaum.

Baldwin, M. W., Keelan, J. P. R., Fehr, B., & Enns, V. (1996). Social-cognitive conceptualization of attachment working models: Availability and accessibility effects. *Journal of Personality and Social Psychology, 71,* 94–109.

Berlin, L. J., Ziv, Y., Amaya-Jackson, L., & Greenberg, M. T. (Eds.). (2005). *Enhancing early attachments: Theory, research, intervention, and policy.* New York: Guilford Press.

Bowlby, J. (1973). *Attachment and loss: Vol. 2. Separation: Anxiety and anger.* New York: Basic Books.

Bowlby, J. (1980). *Attachment and loss: Vol. 3. Loss: Sadness and depression.* New York: Basic Books.

Bowlby, J. (1982). *Attachment and loss: Vol. 1. Attachment* (2nd ed.). New York: Basic Books. (1st ed., 1969)

Brennan, K. A., Clark, C. L., & Shaver, P. R. (1998). Self-report measurement of adult attachment: An integrative overview. In J. A. Simpson & W. S. Rholes (Eds.), *Attachment theory and close relationships* (pp. 46–76). New York: Guilford Press.

Bretherton, I. (1985). Attachment theory: Retrospect and prospect. *Monographs of the Society for Research in Child Development, 50*, 3–35.

Brisch, K. H. (2002). *Treating attachment disorders: From theory to therapy* (K. Kronenberg, Trans.). New York: Guilford Press.

Byng-Hall, J. (1998). *Rewriting family scripts: Improvisation and systems change.* New York: Guilford Press.

Cassidy, J. (2000). Adult romantic attachments: A developmental perspective on individual differences. *Review of General Psychology, 4*, 111–131.

Cassidy, J., & Shaver, P. R. (Eds.). (1999). *Handbook of attachment: Theory, research, and clinical applications.* New York: Guilford Press.

Crowell, J., & Treboux, D. (2001). Attachment security in adult partnerships. In C. Clulow (Ed.), *Adult attachment and couple psychotherapy: The 'secure base' in practice and research* (pp. 28–42). New York: Brunner-Routledge.

Dallos, R. (2006). *Attachment narrative therapy: Integrating systemic, narrative, and attachment approaches.* Maidenhead, UK: Open University Press.

Diamond, G., Siqueland, L., & Diamond, G. M. (2003). Attachment-based family therapy for depressed adolescents: Programmatic treatment development. *Clinical Child and Family Psychology Review, 6*, 107–127.

Fosha, D. (2000). *The transforming power of affect: A model for accelerated change.* New York: Basic Books.

Fraley, R. C., & Brumbaugh, C. C. (2004). A dynamical systems approach to conceptualizing and studying stability and change in attachment security. In W. S. Rholes & J. A. Simpson (Eds.), *Adult attachment: Theory, research, and clinical implications* (pp. 86–132). New York: Guilford Press.

Fraley, R. C. & Spieker, S. J. (2003). Are infant attachment patterns continuously or categorically distributed? A taxometric analysis of Strange Situation behavior. *Developmental Psychology, 39*, 387–404.

Fraley, R. C., & Waller, N. G. (1998). Adult attachment patterns: A test of the typological model. In J. A. Simpson & W. S. Rholes (Eds.), *Attachment theory and close relationships* (pp. 77–114). New York: Guilford Press.

George, C., Kaplan, N., & Main, M. (1984). *Adult Attachment Interview protocol.* Unpublished manuscript, University of California, Berkeley.

George, C., Kaplan, N., & Main, M. (1985). *Adult Attachment Interview protocol* (2nd ed.). Unpublished manuscript, University of California, Berkeley.

George, C., Kaplan, N., & Main, M. (1996). *Adult Attachment Interview protocol* (3rd ed.). Unpublished manuscript, University of California, Berkeley.

Grossmann, K. E., Grossmann, K., & Waters, E. (Eds.). (2005). *Attachment from infancy to adulthood: The major longitudinal studies.* New York: Guilford Press.

Harris, T. (2003). Implications of attachment theory for developing a therapeutic alliance and insight in psychoanalytic psychotherapy. In M. Cortina & M. Marrone (Eds.), *Attachment theory and the psychoanalytic process* (pp. 62–91). London: Whurr.

Holmes, J. (1996). *Attachment, intimacy, autonomy: Using attachment theory in adult psychotherapy.* Northvale, NJ: Aronson.

Holmes, J. (2001). *The search for the secure base: Attachment theory and psychotherapy*. London: Brunner-Routledge.

Holmes, J., & Bateman, A. (Eds.). (2002). *Integration in psychotherapy: Models and methods*. New York: Oxford University Press.

Hunter, V. (1991). John Bowlby: An interview. *Psychoanalytic Review, 78*, 159–175.

Johnson, S. M. (2004). *The practice of emotionally focused couple therapy: Creating connection* (2nd ed.). New York: Brunner-Routledge.

Karen, R. (1994). *Becoming attached: First relationships and how they shape our capacity to love*. New York: Oxford University Press.

Kilmann, P. R., Urbaniak, G. C., & Parnell, M. M. (2006). Effects of attachment-focused versus relationship skills-focused group interventions for college students with insecure attachment patterns. *Attachment & Human Development, 8*, 47–62.

Klerman, G. L., Weissman, M. M., Rounsaville, B. J., & Chevron, E. S. (1984). *Interpersonal psychotherapy of depression*. New York: Basic Books.

Marvin, R., Cooper, G., Hoffman, K., & Powell, B. (2002). The Circle of Security project: Attachment-based intervention with caregiver–preschool child dyads. *Attachment & Human Development, 4*, 107–124.

McCluskey, U., Hooper, C.-A., & Miller, L. B. (1999). Goal-corrected empathic attunement: Developing and rating the concept within an attachment perspective. *Psychotherapy: Theory, Research, Practice, Training, 36*, 80–90.

Meyer, B., & Pilkonis, P. A. (2002). Attachment style. In J. C. Norcross (Ed.), *Psychotherapy relationships that work: Therapist contributions and responsiveness to patients* (pp. 367–382). London: Oxford University Press.

Mikulincer, M., & Shaver, P. R. (2007). *Attachment in adulthood: Structure, dynamics, and change*. New York: Guilford Press.

Roisman, G. I., Collins, W. A., Sroufe, L. A., & Egeland, B. (2005). Predictors of young adults' representations of and behavior in their current romantic relationship: Prospective tests of the prototype hypothesis. *Attachment & Human Development, 7*, 105–121.

Roisman, G. I., Fraley, R. C., & Belsky, J. (2007). A taxometric study of the Adult Attachment Interview. *Developmental Psychology, 43*, 675–686.

Roisman, G. I., Holland, A., Fortuna, K., Fraley, R. C., Clausell, E., & Clarke, A. (2007). The Adult Attachment Interview and self-reports of attachment style: An empirical rapprochement. *Journal of Personality and Social Psychology, 92*, 678–697.

Ryle, A., with Poynton, A. M., & Brockman, B. J. (1990). *Cognitive–analytic therapy: Active participation in change. A new integration in brief psychotherapy*. Chichester, UK: Wiley.

Shaver, P. R., & Mikulincer, M. (2004). What do self-report attachment measures assess? In W. S. Rholes & J. A. Simpson (Eds.), *Adult attachment: Theory, research, and clinical implications* (pp. 17–54). New York: Guilford Press.

Shaver, P. R., & Mikulincer, M. (2005). Attachment theory and research: Resurrection of the psychodynamic approach to personality. *Journal of Research in Personality, 39*, 22–45.

Slade, A. (1999). Attachment theory and research: Implications for the theory and practice of individual psychotherapy with adults. In J. Cassidy & P. R. Shaver (Eds.), *Handbook of attachment: Theory, research, and clinical applications* (pp. 575–594). New York: Guilford Press.

Slade, A. (2004). The move from categories to process: Attachment phenomena and clinical evaluation. *Infant Mental Health Journal, 25*, 269–283.

Sroufe, L. A., Egeland, B., Carlson, E., & Collins, W. A. (2005). *The development of the person: The Minnesota Study of Risk and Adaptation from Birth to Adulthood*. New York: Guilford Press.

Teyber, E. (1999). *Interpersonal process in psychotherapy: A relational approach*. Wadsworth.

Wallin, D. J. (2007). *Attachment in psychotherapy*. New York: Guilford Press.

Wampold, B. E. (2001). *The great psychotherapy debate: Models, methods, and findings*. Mahwah, NJ: Erlbaum.

White, K. (2004). Developing a secure-enough base: Teaching psychotherapists in training the relationship between attachment theory and clinical work. *Attachment & Human Development, 6*, 117–130.

Part I

THEORETICAL FOUNDATIONS

2

An Overview of Adult Attachment Theory

Phillip R. Shaver
Mario Mikulincer

Bowlby and Ainsworth's attachment theory (Ainsworth, Blehar, Waters, & Wall, 1978; Bowlby, 1969/1982) is one of the most successful psychological theories of the past half century. It has generated thousands of published studies and scores of books. It has appealed to all kinds of psychologists, including developmentalists, clinicians, personality and social psychologists, and even psychologists who study groups and organizations (see Mikulincer & Shaver, 2007, for a broad overview). There are several reasons for the theory's success.

First, attachment theory has roots in psychoanalysis, cognitive-developmental psychology, control systems theory, and primate ethology. No other theory is so deeply and broadly grounded in earlier conceptualizations of the social aspects of the human and nonhuman primate mind.

Second, the theory was expounded unusually clearly and systematically by Bowlby in his *Attachment and Loss* trilogy (Bowlby, 1969/1982, 1973, 1980). Most other psychoanalytic theorists had written (perhaps deliberately) in a convoluted and opaque manner, and their concepts (e.g., the id, cathexes, the death instinct) were difficult for researchers to operationalize. Bowlby reviewed diverse bodies of research and theory, somehow integrating them seamlessly and retaining both the depth and complexity of psychoanalytic ideas without losing track of the need for empirical grounding. Even Bowlby's boldest speculations were solidly rooted in established science.

Third, although Bowlby was primarily a clinician and a clinical theorist rather than a researcher, his close collaboration with Ainsworth resulted in measures and research paradigms that appealed to less clinical but empirically oriented researchers. No other object relations clinical theorist established a partnership with an astute observer and laboratory researcher like Ainsworth. Hence most of the other object relations theorists' ideas (whether good or bad—a distinction that is impossible to draw without evidence) have fallen by the wayside as empirical psychology has advanced. In contrast, attachment theory has continued to guide creative research—and, with Bowlby's blessings (see, e.g., Bowlby, 1988), the theory has continued to evolve in response to new research paradigms and findings.

The present chapter is an attempt to boil down the current version of the theory, especially as it applies to adults, to a workable set of ideas and constructs that will recur throughout the remaining chapters. A much more detailed examination of the same large territory, including a nearly exhaustive literature review, can be found in our recent book (Mikulincer & Shaver, 2007). At the end of the present chapter, we briefly consider the ways in which Bowlby and Ainsworth's theory is compatible with but different from other psychological frameworks that have guided clinical practice, including Freudian psychoanalysis, behaviorism, cognitivism, and structural approaches to the analysis of social relationships.

THE ATTACHMENT BEHAVIORAL SYSTEM

We begin by covering the normative (species-universal) aspects of what Bowlby (1969/1982, 1973, 1980) called the *attachment behavioral system*. Attachment theorists and researchers are all familiar with a set of standard names for the theory's basic constructs, and we define and discuss these constructs in this section.

According to Bowlby (1969/1982), human infants are born with a repertoire of behaviors (*attachment behaviors*) "designed" by evolution to assure proximity to supportive others (*attachment figures*), who are likely to provide protection from physical and psychological threats, promote safe and healthy exploration of the environment, and help the infant learn to regulate emotions effectively. The child's proximity-seeking behaviors are organized by an adaptive behavioral system (the *attachment behavioral system*), which emerged over the course of evolution because it increased the likelihood of survival and reproduction in a species whose offspring are born with very immature abilities to acquire food, move about their environment, or defend themselves (from predators, stressors, and other dangers). This system is assumed to govern the choice, activation, and termination of proximity-seeking behaviors aimed at attaining protection and support from significant others in times of need. Although the attachment system is most important early in life, Bowlby (1988) claimed that it is active across the lifespan and is manifest in thoughts and behaviors related to proximity seeking in times of need. This claim provided the impetus for subsequent theorists and researchers to conceptualize and study *adult attachment*.

During infancy, primary caregivers (usually one or both parents, but also grandparents, neighbors, older siblings, day care workers, etc.) are likely to occupy the role of attachment figure. Ainsworth (1973) reported that infants tend to seek proximity to their primary caregiver when tired or ill, and Heinicke and Westheimer (1966) found that infants tend to be soothed in the presence of their primary caregivers. During adolescence and adulthood, other relationship partners often become targets of proximity seeking and emotional support, including close friends and romantic partners. Teachers and supervisors in academic settings or therapists in clinical settings can also serve as real or potential sources of comfort and support. Moreover, groups, institutions, and symbolic personages (e.g., God, the Buddha, the Virgin Mary) can be recruited as attachment figures. As a group, these real people and symbolic personages form what Bowlby (1969/1982) called a person's *hierarchy of attachment figures.*

In addition, mental representations of attachment figures and subroutines of the self that develop through the internalization of caring and soothing qualities of attachment figures can successfully provide a symbolic sense of comfort, support, and protection (Mikulincer & Shaver, 2004). They can also serve as internalized models of effective, loving behavior that guide a person in helping him- or herself in the absence of physically present attachment figures.

From an attachment perspective, a specific relationship partner is an attachment figure and a specific relationship is an attachment relationship only to the extent that a relationship partner accomplishes three important functions (e.g., Ainsworth, 1991; Hazan & Shaver, 1994; Hazan & Zeifman, 1994). First, the attachment figure should be viewed as a target for proximity seeking in times of stress or need, and unwanted separation from this person should elicit distress, protest, and efforts to achieve reunion. Second, the person should be viewed as a real or potential *safe haven,* because he or she provides comfort, support, protection, and security in times of need. Third, the person should be viewed as a *secure base,* allowing a child or adult to pursue non-attachment-related goals in a safe environment and to sustain exploration, risk taking, and self-expansion. In other words, interactions with attachment figures are not the same as other forms of social interaction. Attachment-related interactions are organized around the expectation of receiving protection, comfort, encouragement, or support from an attachment figure in times of need, and this protection or support is valued because it allows a person to restore emotional balance and return to effective behavior in the wider social and physical environment.

What attachment theory calls *activation of the attachment system* can be seen in the behavior of human infants, who tend to drop whatever they are doing (e.g., playing with interesting toys in a laboratory situation) and seek comfort and support from an attachment figure if an odd noise is heard or a stranger enters the room (Ainsworth et al., 1978). The same kind of activation is notable in the minds of adults who are subjected to conscious or unconscious threats. For example, we (Mikulincer, Gillath, & Shaver, 2002) conducted several experiments in which we subliminally presented threatening words (e.g., *failure, separation*) to adults and then assessed indirectly (using reaction times in a word identification task or word-color-naming task) which names of relationship partners became more available for mental processing following the unconscious threat. It turned out that the names of attachment figures (identified with the WHOTO questionnaire, developed by Hazan & Zeifman, 1994, and adapted by Fraley & Davis, 1997, and Trinke & Bartholomew, 1997) became more available following unconscious exposure to a threatening word. The threatening words had no effect on the mental availability or accessibility of names of other people who were not viewed as attachment figures. That is, attachment figures are not just any relationship partners; they are special people to whom one turns, even unconsciously, when comfort or support is needed.

According to Bowlby (1969/1982), the natural goal of the attachment system is to increase a person's sense of security (which Sroufe & Waters, 1977, labeled *felt security*)—a sense that the world is a safe place, that one can rely on others for protection and support, and that one can confidently explore the environment and engage in social and nonsocial tasks and activities without fear of damage. This goal is made particularly salient by encountering actual or symbolic threats, or by appraising an attachment figure as not sufficiently available or responsive. In such cases, the attachment system is activated and the individual is driven to reestablish actual or symbolic proximity to an attachment figure (which attachment researchers call the *primary strategy* of the attachment system; Main, 1990). These bids for proximity persist until the sense of security is restored, at which time the attachment system is deactivated or turned down in "volume," and the individual calmly and skillfully returns to other activities. That is, the search for support, protection, and security is not only a goal in itself, but also an important foundation for attaining many non-attachment-related goals.

During infancy, the primary attachment strategy includes nonverbal expressions of neediness, such as crying and pleading, and movements (crawling, walking, extending arms) aimed at reestablishing and maintaining proximity to the caregiver (Ainsworth et al., 1978). In adulthood, this attachment strategy includes many other methods of establishing contact (e.g., talking, calling someone on the telephone, sending an e-mail or text message), as well as mentally activating soothing, comforting representations of attachment figures or even self-representations associated with these figures (Mikulincer & Shaver, 2004). Such cognitive–affective representations can infuse a person with a heightened sense of security and allow him or her to continue pursuing other goals without having to interrupt them to engage in actual bids for proximity and protection.

Indeed, several studies (e.g., Green & Campbell, 2000; Mikulincer, Hirschberger, Nachmias, & Gillath, 2001; Mikulincer & Shaver, 2001; Mikulincer, Shaver, Gillath, & Nitzberg, 2005) have shown that a variety of experimental techniques designed to activate mental representations of attachment figures (e.g., subliminal presentation of the names of people nominated as attachment figures in the WHOTO questionnaire; visualization of the faces of these figures) infuse a person with positive affect; reduce hostility to outgroup members; facilitate empathy, compassion, and altruistic helping; and sustain relaxed and creative forms of exploration. They also reduce the stridency of hurt feelings among anxious individuals and open more avoidant individuals to such feelings that have been suppressed (Shaver, Mikulincer, Lavy, & Cassidy, in press), both of which are likely to be very useful clinically.

Bowlby (1988) summarized many of the adaptive benefits of proximity seeking. First, he viewed successful bids for proximity and the attainment of felt security as necessary for forming and maintaining successful relationships. Every attachment-related interaction that restores a person's sense of security reaffirms the value of closeness and strengthens affectional bonds with the relationship partner responsible for augmenting the sense of security. Moreover, successful bids for proximity and support play an important part in teaching a person how to regulate and deescalate negative emotions, such as anger, anxiety, and sadness (Bowlby, 1973, 1980). They therefore help a person maintain emotional balance and resilience in the face of stress. Bowlby (1973) also viewed attachment security as an important foundation for developing skills and competence of all kinds. A child or adult who feels threatened and inadequately protected or supported has a difficult time directing attention to free play, curious investigation of objects and environments, and affiliative relationships with peers. Extended over long periods of time, this kind of interference disrupts the development of self-efficacy, self-esteem, and positive, trusting social attitudes. Because of Bowlby's (1969/1982) emphasis on the value of felt security, he strongly rejected any theoretical formulation that equated attachment per se with excessive dependence or childishness. In his view, secure attachment provides a foundation for personal growth and mature autonomy, which should never be equated with a reduction in the importance of close relationships. In his estimation, claims that well-treated children are likely to be "spoiled" or overly dependent confuse anxious attachment with attachment per se.

INDIVIDUAL DIFFERENCES
IN ATTACHMENT SYSTEM FUNCTIONING

Attachment theory is a general theory of social and emotional development, but it would probably not have captured the attention of developmental, personality, social, and clinical researchers if it had been only that. What captured research psychologists' attention were the patterns or styles of attachment emphasized in Bowlby's theory and operationalized in Ainsworth's research on mother–infant dyads. Most of the research and clinical applications inspired by the theory deal with these individual differences.

Attachment Figure Availability and Secondary Attachment Strategies

Besides possessing a species-universal set of operating characteristics, the attachment behavioral system includes various regulatory parameters that can be influenced by a person's history of interactions with key attachment figures. In early infancy, the effects of experience can be conceptualized in terms of simple learning principles. If a particular behavioral strategy (e.g., crying for help, protesting angrily, down-regulating distress signals) works with a particular caregiver, it will be reinforced. If a particular strategy results in punishment or caregiver withdrawal, it will become weaker and less visible (perhaps by being actively suppressed) in the infant's behavioral repertoire. The same is true for young mammals from many other species.

In the case of developing human children, however, what is learned includes not only automatic behavior patterns, but also a set of vivid memories, abstracted beliefs, and expectations about caregivers' reactions and the effectiveness or ineffectiveness of one's own possible behaviors. Because Bowlby and Ainsworth were writing at about the time of what has been called, in retrospect, the "cognitive revolution" in psychology, they were sensitive to the role played by memories, cognitive schemas, and other mental representations in regulating the attachment system. In attachment theory, these mental structures and processes are called *internal working models* of self and others (Bartholomew, 1990; Bowlby, 1969/1982). Over time, a person's working models, which contain both conscious and unconscious elements, become molded by the quality of interactions with attachment figures; that is, the system is "programmed" to fit these figures' characteristic behaviors, thereby increasing the likelihood of reliable expectations and effective reactions in those particular relational environments. Through this process, a person learns to adjust his or her attachment system to fit contextual demands and rely on expectations about possible access routes to protection and security. These working models are thought to be the basis of both current individual differences in attachment strategies, or styles, and within-person continuity in the operation of the attachment system over time.

According to Bowlby (1973, 1988), variations in working models, and hence in attachment system functioning, depend on the availability, sensitivity, and responsiveness of attachment figures in times of need. When one's key relationship partner is available, sensitive, and responsive to one's proximity- and support-seeking efforts, one is likely to experience felt security and to have greater confidence in proximity seeking as an effective distress regulation strategy. During such interactions one also acquires procedural knowledge about distress management, which we can imagine being organized around a relational script (Waters, Rodrigues, & Ridgeway, 1998). This *secure-base script* includes something like the following "if–then" propositions: "If I encounter an obstacle and/or become distressed, I can approach a significant other for help; he or she is likely to be available and supportive; I will experience relief and comfort as a result of proximity to this person; I can then return to other activities."

However, when a primary attachment figure proves not to be available, sensitive, or responsive, felt security is not attained, and the distress that initially activated proximity-seeking efforts is compounded by serious attachment-related doubts (e.g., "Can I trust others in times of need?"). These frightening, frustrating interactions also signal that the primary attachment strategy is failing to accomplish its goal and that alternative strategies must be adopted to deal with current insecurities and distress. Attachment theorists (e.g., Cassidy & Kobak, 1988; Main, 1990) have called these alternative tactics *secondary attachment strategies,* which (based on Ainsworth et al.'s [1978] research) are thought to take two major forms: *hyperactivation* and *deactivation.*

Hyperactivated strategies are what Bowlby (1969/1982) called *protest* reactions to the frustration of attachment needs. Protest often occurs in relationships in which the attachment figure is sometimes responsive but unreliably so, placing the needy individual on a partial reinforcement schedule that seems to reward persistence of energetic, strident, noisy proximity-seeking attempts, because such attempts sometimes seem to succeed. In such cases, the individual does not give up on frustrating proximity-seeking bids, but in fact intensifies them to demand or coerce the attachment figure's attention, love, and support. The main goal of these strategies is to make an unreliable or insufficiently available and responsive figure provide support and security. The way to pursue this goal seems, to the hyperactivating individual, to be to keep his or her attachment system in a chronically activated state until support and comfort is attained. This involves exaggerating appraisals of danger and signs of the attachment figure's unavailability, and intensifying one's demands for attention, care, and love. It can, paradoxically, lead to intensifying one's needs, and emotional reactions to frustrated needs, as a way of "regulating" them (even though the term *emotion regulation* in psychological writings usually refers to down-regulation of negative emotions).

Deactivating strategies, in contrast, are efforts to escape, avoid, or minimize the pain and frustration caused by unavailable, unsympathetic, or unresponsive attachment figures. This kind of response seems to occur in relationships with attachment figures who disapprove of and punish closeness and expressions of need, dependence, and vulnerability. In such relationships, a needy individual learns to expect better outcomes if proximity-seeking bids are suppressed, the attachment system is deactivated, and one attempts to deal with threats and dangers alone. Bowlby (1969/1982) called this strategy *compulsive self-reliance.* The primary goal of deactivating strategies is to keep the attachment system turned off or down-regulated to avoid recurring frustration and distress arising from interactions with cold, neglectful, or punishing attachment figures. Such deactivation requires that a person deny attachment needs; avoid intimacy and interdependence in relationships; and distance him- or herself from threats that might cause unwanted and potentially unmanageable activation of attachment needs, thoughts, feelings, or behaviors.

INTERNAL WORKING MODELS

As mentioned earlier, Bowlby (1969/1982) theorized that important social interactions with attachment figures are internalized and stored as schemas in an associative memory network. This stored knowledge allows a person to predict the course and outcomes of future interactions with an attachment figure and to adjust future proximity-seeking bids. Repeated augmentation and editing of these models result, in most cases, in increasingly stable mental representations of self, attachment figures, and relationships. Bowlby (1969/1982) wrote about two major forms of working models: representations of attachment figures' responses and inclinations (*working models of others*) and representations of the self's lovability and competence (*working models of self*). Once the attachment system has operated for several years in the context of close relationships with key attachment figures, it includes complex representations of the availability, responsiveness, and sensitivity of these figures, as well as representations of the self's ability to elicit a partner's attention and affection when desired. These cognitive–affective structures organize a person's memories of interactions with attachment figures; guide future bids for proximity and support; and account for much of a person's sense of self, including his or her sense of being lovable and socially valuable.

During infancy and childhood, working models are based on the internalization of specific interactions, or kinds of interactions, with particular attachment figures. As a result, a child can hold multiple episodic (situation- or person-specific) representations of self and others that differ with respect to an interaction's outcome (especially success or failure at gaining felt security) and with respect to the secondary strategy used to deal with insecurity during that interaction (hyperactivating, deactivating). With experience and cognitive development, these episodic representations form excitatory and inhibitory associations with each other (e.g., experiencing or thinking about an episode of security attainment activates memories of similar security-enhancing episodes and renders memories of attachment insecurities and worries less accessible), and these associations favor the formation of more abstract and generalized attachment representations with a specific partner. Then, through excitatory and inhibitory links with models representing interactions with other attachment figures, even more generic working models are formed to summarize relationships in general. This process of continual model building and integration results, over time, in a hierarchical associative network that includes episodic memories, relationship-specific models, and generic working models of self and others. Recently, Overall, Fletcher, and Friesen (2003) provided statistical evidence for the hierarchical nature of the cognitive network of attachment working models.

The attachment literature has sometimes made it seem that working models are simple and univocal with respect to important relationship issues. However, research evidence suggests—in line with Bowlby's (e.g., 1980) own ideas about multiple models, conflicting models, and conscious and unconscious models—that most people can remember and be affected by both security-enhancing interactions and security-eroding interactions with attachment figures (e.g., Baldwin, Keelan, Fehr, Enns, & Koh Rangarajoo, 1996; Mikulincer & Shaver, 2001). It therefore matters a great deal what a particular person is reminded of, or is thinking about, when attachment-related processes and outcomes are assessed by psychologists. The mental representation of one relationship may differ from the representation of another, and focusing on a particular issue (e.g., sexual infidelity) may make related previous experiences become more mentally accessible and psychologically influential than usual.

The notion that everyone has multiple attachment models organized within a hierarchical memory network raises questions about which model will be accessible (readily activated and used to guide attachment-related expectations, defenses, and behaviors) in a given situation. As with other mental representations, the accessibility of an attachment working model is determined by the amount of experience on which it is based, the number of times it has been applied in the past, the density of its neural connections with other working models, and the issues made salient in a particular situation (e.g., Baldwin, 1992; Collins & Read, 1994; Shaver, Collins, & Clark, 1996). At the relationship-specific level, the model representing the typical interaction with an attachment figure has the highest likelihood of being accessible and guiding subsequent interactions with that person. At the generic level, the model that represents interactions with major attachment figures (e.g., parents and romantic partners) typically becomes the most commonly available representation and has the strongest effect on attachment-related expectations, feelings, and behaviors across relationships and over time.

According to Bowlby (1973), consolidation of a regularly available working model is the most important psychological process accounting for the enduring, long-term effects of attachment interactions during infancy, childhood, and adolescence on attachment-related cognitions and behaviors in adulthood. Given a fairly consistent pattern of interactions with primary caregivers during infancy and childhood, the most representative working models of these interactions become part of a person's implicit procedural knowledge about close relationships, social interactions, and distress regulation. They tend to operate automatically and unconsciously and are resistant to change. Thus what began as representations of specific interactions with particular primary caregivers during childhood tend to be applied in new situations and relationships, and eventually they have an effect on attachment-related experiences, decisions, and actions even in adulthood.

Beyond the pervasive effects of attachment history on the accessibility of working models, attachment theory also emphasizes, as we have mentioned, the importance of contextual factors that influence the availability of particular models or components of models (e.g., Collins & Read, 1994; Shaver et al., 1996). Recent studies have shown that contextual cues related to the availability and responsiveness of attachment figures, as well as actual or imagined encounters with supportive or unsupportive figures, can affect which working models become active in memory, even if they are incongruent with a person's more general and more typically available working models (e.g., Mikulincer & Shaver, 2001; Mikulincer et al., 2005). In other words, the generally accessible and more generic models coexist with less typical working models in a person's associative memory network, and the less typical models can be influenced by contextual factors and become crucial to understanding a person's behavior in a particular situation. This suggests that in a clinical setting, a therapist would be wise to hold in mind both a client's general attachment orientation and the client's particular memories and reactions when specific issues become contextually salient.

AN INTEGRATIVE MODEL OF ATTACHMENT SYSTEM FUNCTIONING IN ADULTHOOD

We have proposed a three-component theoretical model of attachment system dynamics in adulthood (e.g., Mikulincer & Shaver, 2003, 2007; Shaver & Mikulincer, 2002) as a way to integrate the immense and still growing empirical research literature on the topic (see Figure 2.1). The first component concerns the monitoring and appraisal of threatening events and is responsible for activation of the attachment system (along with associated memories, feelings, expectations, and actions). The second component concerns the monitoring and appraisal of the availability, sensitivity, and responsiveness of attachment figures and is responsible for variations in the sense of attachment security. Once the attachment system is activated, an affirmative answer to the question "Is an attachment figure available and likely to be responsive to my needs?" results in a sense of security, fosters the application of the secure-base script mentioned earlier (Waters et al., 1998), and facilitates calm and confident engagement in other life activities. The third component concerns the appraisal of the viability of proximity seeking as a means of coping with attachment insecurity and is responsible for variations in the use of hyperactivating or deactivating secondary attachment and affect-regulation strategies.

The three components can be summarized in three "if–then" propositions. First, if threatened, seek proximity and protection from an attachment figure (or some temporarily equivalent stronger, wiser, and supportive

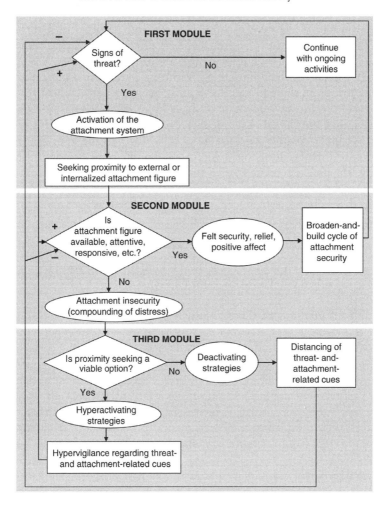

FIGURE 2.1. An integrative model of the activation and dynamics of the attachment system in adulthood. From Mikulincer and Shaver (2007). Copyright 2007 by The Guilford Press. Reprinted by permission.

actual person or symbolic personage). Second, if an attachment figure is available and supportive, relax, enjoy, and appreciate the feeling of being loved and comforted, and confidently return to other activities. Third, if an attachment figure is unavailable or unresponsive, either intensify efforts to achieve proximity and comfort (i.e., hyperactivate the attachment system) or deactivate the system, suppress thoughts of vulnerability or need, and rely steadfastly on oneself. As we explain in subsequent sections of this chapter, these propositions are crucial for understanding the relevance of attachment theory to counseling and psychotherapy.

The model is sensitive to both context and personality. On the one hand, each component of the model can be affected by specific contextual factors (e.g., actual threats, information about the availability of a specific attachment figure), which initiate a bottom-up process in a person's cognitive network of working models, activating congruent attachment representations and producing immediate changes in attachment-related cognitions and behaviors. On the other hand, each component of the model is affected by chronically accessible working models, which bias the appraisal of and reactions to threats, attachment figure availability, and proximity-seeking viability. In sum, we acknowledge the importance of both the context in which attachment cognitions, emotions, and behaviors are activated, and chronic dispositions (which can be conceptualized as personality traits) resulting from a person's attachment history.

CONCEPTUALIZATION AND MEASUREMENT OF ATTACHMENT PATTERNS OR STYLES

According to attachment theory (Bowlby, 1988; Fraley & Shaver, 2000; Shaver & Hazan, 1993), a particular history of attachment experiences and the resulting consolidation of chronically accessible working models lead to the formation of relatively stable individual differences in *attachment style*—the habitual pattern of expectations, needs, emotions, and behavior in interpersonal interactions and close relationships (Hazan & Shaver, 1987). Depending on how it is measured, attachment style characterizes a person's typical attachment-related mental processes and behaviors in a particular relationship (*relationship-specific* style) or across relationships (*global* style).

The concept of attachment patterns was first proposed by Ainsworth (1967) to describe infants' patterns of responses to separations from and reunions with their mothers in the Strange Situation, a laboratory procedure designed to activate the infants' attachment systems. Based on this procedure, infants were originally classified into one of three categories: *secure, anxious-ambivalent,* or *anxious-avoidant.* Main and Solomon (1990) later added a fourth category, *disorganized/disoriented,* characterized by odd, awkward behavior and unusual fluctuations between anxiety and avoidance.

Infants classified as secure in the Strange Situation typically react to separation from their mothers with observable signs of distress, but they recover quickly upon reunion with their mothers and return to exploring the many interesting toys provided in the Strange Situation room. They greet their mothers with joy and affection, initiate contact with them, and respond positively to being picked up and held (Ainsworth et al., 1978). Avoidant infants' reactions are quite different and seem to indicate attachment system deactivation. These infants express little distress when separated from their mothers and may actively turn away from or avoid them upon reunion. Anxious infants' reactions are hyperactivated. These infants cry and protest angrily during separation and show angry, resistant, hyperaroused reactions (i.e., protest) upon reunion, making it difficult for them to be soothed and return to creative play.

In the 1980s, researchers from different psychological subdisciplines (developmental, clinical, personality, and social) constructed new measures of attachment style to extend attachment research into adolescence and adulthood. Taking a developmental and clinical approach, Main and her colleagues (George, Kaplan, & Main, 1984, 1985, 1986; Main, Kaplan, & Cassidy, 1985; see Hesse, 1999, 2008 for a review) devised the Adult Attachment Interview (AAI) to study adolescents' and adults' mental representations of attachment to their parents during childhood. In the AAI, interviewees provide oral answers to open-ended questions about their childhood relationships with parents. The interview transcripts are then used to classify respondents into three categories paralleling Ainsworth's infant typology: *secure* or *autonomous* (with respect to attachment), *dismissing* (of attachment), or *preoccupied* (with attachment). Using the AAI coding system (Hesse, 1999; Main & Goldwyn, 1984; Main, Goldwyn, & Hesse, 2003), a person is classified as secure if he or she substantiates descriptors of parents as available and responsive, and/or if his or her memories of relationships with parents are presented in a clear and coherent manner even when the memories are negative. An adult is classified as dismissing of attachment if he or she downplays the importance of attachment relationships and tends to recall few concrete experiences with parents. Adults are classified as preoccupied with attachment if they are still angry with parents and can easily retrieve negative memories, but have trouble discussing them coherently without anger or anxiety.

In addition to the three main classification categories, there is also a way to note that a person seems *unresolved* with respect to trauma or abuse, which has proven to be especially important clinically (e.g., Lyons-Ruth, Yellin, Melnick, & Atwood, 2005), and there are categories for interviews that cannot be simply classified (see Hesse, 1999). An adult's AAI classification has been shown to predict his or her infant child's attachment pattern in the Strange Situation (see van IJzendoorn, 1995, for a review), even if the interview is completed well before the infant is born. In other words, there is good empirical evidence for the intergenerational transmission of attachment patterns, and this transmission seems not to be primarily attributable to heritable aspects of personality (e.g., O'Connor, 2005).

In an independent line of research, Hazan and Shaver (1987), who wished to apply Bowlby and Ainsworth's ideas to the study of adolescent and adult romantic relationships, developed a self-report measure of attachment style. In its original form, the measure consisted of three brief descriptions of constellations of feelings and behaviors in close relationships that were intended to parallel the three infant attachment patterns identified by

Ainsworth et al. (1978). College student and community adults were asked to read the three descriptions and then place themselves in one of the three attachment categories according to their predominant feelings and behavior in romantic relationships. (See also Table 7.1 of Fraley & Phillips, Chapter 7, this volume, for additional discussion.) The three descriptions were as follows:

> *Secure:* I find it relatively easy to get close to others and am comfortable depending on them and having them depend on me. I don't worry about being abandoned or about someone getting too close to me.
>
> *Avoidant:* I am somewhat uncomfortable being close to others; I find it difficult to trust them completely, difficult to allow myself to depend on them. I am nervous when anyone gets too close and often, others want me to be more intimate than I feel comfortable being.
>
> *Anxious:* I find that others are reluctant to get as close as I would like. I often worry that my partner doesn't really love me or won't want to stay with me. I want to get very close to my partner and this sometimes scares people away.

Hazan and Shaver's (1987) study was followed by hundreds of others that used the simple forced-choice self-report measure to examine the interpersonal and intrapersonal correlates of adult attachment style (see reviews by Shaver & Hazan, 1993; Shaver & Mikulincer, 2002). Over time, attachment researchers made methodological and conceptual improvements to the original self-report measure and reached the conclusion that attachment styles are best conceptualized as regions in a two-dimensional space (e.g., Bartholomew & Horowitz, 1991; Brennan, Clark, & Shaver, 1998; Simpson, 1990). The first dimension, which we call attachment-related *avoidance,* is concerned with discomfort with closeness and dependence on relationship partners and a preference for emotional distance and self-reliance. Avoidant individuals identified with self-report measures use deactivating attachment and affect-regulation strategies to deal with insecurity and distress. The second dimension, attachment-related *anxiety,* includes a strong desire for closeness and protection, intense worries about one's partner's availability and responsiveness and one's own value to the partner, and the use of hyperactivating strategies for dealing with insecurity and distress. People who score low on both dimensions are said to be secure or to have a secure attachment style.

The two attachment style dimensions can be measured with the 36-item Experiences in Close Relationships (ECR) scale (Brennan et al., 1998), which is reliable in both the internal-consistency and test–retest senses and has high construct, predictive, and discriminant validity (Crowell, Fraley, & Shaver, 1999). Eighteen items tap the avoidance dimension (e.g., "I try to avoid getting too close to my partner," "I prefer not to show a partner how I feel deep down"), and the remaining 18 items tap the anxiety dimension (e.g., "I need a lot of reassurance that I am loved by my partner," "I resent it when my partner spends time away from me"). The two scales were conceptualized as independent and have been found to be empirically uncorrelated, or only weakly correlated, in most studies. Studies based on self-report measures of adult attachment style—some based on three categories, some on four categories (including two kinds of avoidance, labeled *fearful* and *dismissive*), and some on two dimensions—have confirmed theoretically predictable attachment style variations in relationship quality, mental health, social adjustment, ways of coping, emotion regulation, self-esteem, interpersonal behavior, and social cognitions (see Mikulincer & Shaver, 2003, 2007, for reviews; see Fraley & Phillips, Chapter 7, this volume, for an overview of self-report measures of adult attachment).

There is relatively little research on the heritability of the forms of attachment insecurity measured with self-report scales or the AAI, but Crawford et al. (2007) reported preliminary evidence for the heritability of attachment anxiety and no evidence for the heritability of avoidant attachment. And Torgersen, Grova, and Sommerstad (2007) reported preliminary evidence for a genetic contribution to adult twins' concordance on the AAI. This is a topic that will receive heightened attention over the next few years, because it is now possible to measure particular genes (e.g., specific polymorphisms of particular genetic alleles that affect brain development and performance).

There is still no agreement on the degrees of association between the different measures of adult attachment (e.g., Shaver, Belsky, & Brennan, 2000; Shaver & Mikulincer, 2004). Nevertheless, in our review of the broad literature on adult attachment (Mikulincer & Shaver, 2007), we have noted many cases in which similar results were obtained with the AAI and with one of the major self-report measures. For the time being, the differences between measures and associated theoretical conceptions have to be kept in mind when one applies attachment theory and research clinically. The AAI has been validated mainly through its ability to predict the quality of attachment an adult's child has to that adult in the Strange Situation. The self-report measures have been validated mainly through their ability to predict processes and qualities related to adult relationships. The measures differ, in other words, in both their focus and their method, and some are more appropriate for particular clinical purposes than others. For clinicians interested in using the self-report measures, they can be found in the appendices of the Mikulincer and Shaver (2007) book.

ATTACHMENT FIGURE AVAILABILITY AND THE BROADEN-AND-BUILD CYCLE OF ATTACHMENT SECURITY

We have now outlined attachment theory's main constructs, the operating characteristics of the attachment system, major individual differences in system functioning, and methods of assessing these differences in adolescence and adulthood. We turn now to some of the personal, dyadic, and social-systemic consequences of variations in attachment system functioning. We are especially interested in this section in positive effects of attachment figure availability and the resulting sense of security on social judgments, self-image, personality development, mental health, and relationship quality. In the following section, we consider defensive biases produced by secondary attachment strategies, as well as emotional and adjustment problems resulting from these biases (see also Mikulincer, Shaver, Cassidy, & Berant, Chapter 12, this volume, for a detailed discussion of defenses).

According to our model of attachment system functioning in adulthood, discussed earlier and diagrammed in Figure 2.1, the physical and emotional availability of an actual security provider, or access to mental representations of supportive attachment figures, results in a sense of felt security and fosters what we (following Fredrickson, 2001) call a *broaden-and-build cycle* of attachment security. This cycle is a cascade of mental and behavioral events that augment a person's resources for maintaining emotional stability in times of stress, encourage intimate and deeply interdependent bonds with others, maximize personal adjustment, and expand the person's perspectives and capacities. In the long run, repeated experiences of attachment figure availability have an enduring effect on intrapsychic organization and interpersonal behavior. At the intrapsychic level, such experiences act as a resource for resilience, sustaining emotional well-being and personal adjustment, and they create positive working models of self and others that are highly accessible in memory. At the interpersonal level, repeated experiences of attachment figure availability create a secure attachment style, which facilitates the formation and maintenance of warm, satisfying, stable, and harmonious relationships. We suspect that this process is partly responsible for the well-documented association between a good therapeutic alliance and positive psychotherapy outcomes (e.g., Martin, Garske, & Davis, 2000).

The most immediate psychological effects of having reliable access to an available, sensitive, and responsive attachment figure in times of need are effective management of distress and restoration of emotional equanimity. As a result, secure people remain relatively unperturbed during times of stress and experience longer periods of positive affect, which contribute to mental health. Indeed, several studies have found that secure attachment is positively associated with measures of well-being (e.g., Berant, Mikulincer, & Florian, 2001; Birnbaum, Orr, Mikulincer, & Florian, 1997) and negatively associated with measures of negative affect, depression, and anxiety (e.g., Cooper, Shaver, & Collins, 1998; Mickelson, Kessler, & Shaver, 1997; Roberts, Gotlib, & Kassel, 1996).

Experiences of attachment figure availability also contribute to an extensive network of positive mental representations, which plays an important role in maintaining emotional stability and adjustment. The first set of beliefs concerns the appraisal of life problems as manageable, which helps a person maintain an optimistic and hopeful stance toward life's inevitable difficulties. Relatively secure people can appraise and reappraise stressful events in positive ways and thereby deal more effectively with them. Studies have consistently yielded positive associations between self-reports of attachment security and constructive, optimistic appraisals of stressful events (e.g., Berant et al., 2001; Birnbaum et al., 1997).

Another set of security-related mental representations concerns other people's intentions and traits. Numerous studies have shown that more securely attached people possess a more positive view of human nature (e.g., Collins & Read, 1990; Hazan & Shaver, 1987), use more positive trait terms to describe relationship partners (e.g., Feeney & Noller, 1991; Levy, Blatt, & Shaver, 1998), perceive relationship partners as more supportive (e.g., Davis, Morris, & Kraus, 1998; Ognibene & Collins, 1998), and are more likely to trust their partners (e.g., Collins & Read, 1990; Hazan & Shaver, 1987). In addition, securely attached people have more positive expectations concerning their partners' behavior (e.g., Baldwin et al., 1996) and tend to explain a partner's hurtful behavior in less negative ways (e.g., Collins, 1996).

Interactions with available and sensitive relationship partners reduce worries about being rejected, criticized, or abused. Such interactions indicate that a caring partner is unlikely to betray one's trust, react coldly or abusively to expressions of need, or respond unfavorably to bids for closeness and comfort. Numerous studies have shown that more secure individuals score higher on measures of self-disclosure, support seeking, intimacy, trust, open communication, pro-relational behavior, and relationship satisfaction (for reviews, see Feeney, 1999; Mikulincer, Florian, Cowan, & Cowan, 2002; Shaver & Mikulincer, 2006).

Interactions with security-enhancing attachment figures also strengthen a person's authentically positive sense of self-worth (Mikulincer & Shaver, 2003). That is, secure individuals generally feel safe and protected and perceive themselves as valuable, lovable, and special, thanks to being valued, loved, and regarded as special by caring relationship partners. Research consistently shows that more secure individuals have higher self-esteem (e.g., Bartholomew & Horowitz, 1991; Mickelson et al., 1997) and view themselves as more competent and efficacious (e.g., Cooper et al., 1998). Attachment security is also associated with possessing a coherent and well-organized model of self (Mikulincer, 1995). That is, attachment security not only encourages positive self-appraisals; it also seems to allow people to tolerate their own inevitable weaknesses and integrate them within a generally positive and coherent self-concept.

A relatively secure person's rich resources for dealing with stress make it less necessary to rely on psychological defenses that distort perception, limit coping flexibility, and generate interpersonal conflict. A secure person can devote mental resources that otherwise would be employed in preventive, defensive maneuvers to growth-oriented activities. Such people can attend to other people's needs and feelings rather than (or in addition to) their own. Moreover, being confident that support is available when needed, secure people can take calculated risks and accept important challenges; doing so contributes to the broadening of perspectives and skills and facilitates personal growth. Indeed, research has shown that attachment security is associated with enhanced curiosity and learning; encourages relaxed exploration of new, unusual information and phenomena; and favors the formation of open and flexible cognitive structures, despite the uncertainty and confusion that broadening experiences might entail (e.g., Elliot & Reis, 2003; Green & Campbell, 2000; Mikulincer, 1997).

Studies have documented the "broadening" effect of attachment security on a person's willingness to provide support and care to others who are chronically dependent or temporarily in need. Specifically, attachment security is associated with higher scores on self-report measures of responsiveness to a relationship partner's needs (e.g., Kunce & Shaver, 1994) and with more supportive reactions to a distressed partner (e.g., Fraley & Shaver, 1998; Simpson, Rholes, & Nelligan, 1992). In a series of studies, Mikulincer et al. (2005) found that both dispositional and situationally augmented attachment security were associated with heightened compassion for a suffering individual and willingness to relieve the person's distress.

Overall, studies have shown that both actual and symbolic (i.e., internalized) relationships with supportive attachment figures move a person toward the ideal advocated by "positive" psychologists (e.g., Maslow, 1968; Rogers, 1961; Seligman, 2002): a calm, confident person with a genuine, deep sense of personal value; a person who is willing and able to establish intimate, caring relationships and take risks to help others and broaden his or her skills and perspectives. In other words, attachment figure availability and responsiveness act as growth-enhancing catalysts—fostering prosocial motives and attitudes, and promoting personal development and improved relationships.

As explained in subsequent chapters, the broaden-and-build cycle of attachment security and its causes, especially attachment figure availability and responsiveness, are the building blocks of Bowlby's (1988) model of therapeutic change. He believed that a therapist should serve as an available, responsive, and hence security-enhancing attachment figure for his or her clients by providing a reliable safe haven and secure base. A good therapist effectively promotes the client's felt security within the therapeutic setting. The therapist's behaving as a good attachment figure allows the client to muster the courage for self-exploration: to delve deeply into partially occluded memories and distorted wishes and feelings, while developing greater self-understanding, revising working models of self and others, and getting back on the path to personal growth. Self-exploration in psychotherapy is bound to be difficult and painful, because clients must confront conflictual and distressing experiences, recall long-forgotten or heavily defended memories, encounter strong emotions, and explore perplexities that they have not been able to understand or cope with alone. Only with the support of an available attachment figure—in this case, taking the form of a skillful and caring therapist—can clients explore and understand deep-seated fears, well-practiced defenses, and distorted perceptions that interfere with revising working models and creating the conditions for more positive self-representations, more satisfying relationships, and a more creative and enjoyable life.

SECONDARY ATTACHMENT STRATEGIES, EMOTIONAL PROBLEMS, AND MALADJUSTMENT

According to attachment theory (Main, 1990; Mikulincer & Shaver, 2003, 2007; Shaver & Mikulincer, 2002), secondary attachment strategies (hyper-activation and deactivation) are defenses against the frustration and pain caused by attachment figures' unavailability in times of need (see Miku-lincer et al., Chapter 12, this volume, for a more complete analysis of these defenses). Although these secondary strategies are initially aimed at achiev-ing a workable relationship with an inconsistently available or consistently distant or unavailable attachment figure, they end up being maladaptive when used in later social situations where proximity, intimacy, and interde-pendence would be more productive and rewarding. Moreover, these strate-gies support distorted or constraining working models and affect-regulation techniques that are likely to interfere with psychological health, personal growth, and social adjustment.

According to Bowlby (1980, 1988), attachment insecurities are risk factors that reduce resilience in times of stress and contribute to emo-tional problems and poor adjustment. Anxious attachment encourages distress intensification and an uncontrollable stream of negative memories, thoughts, and emotions, which in turn interferes with cognitive organiza-tion and in some cases precipitates serious psychopathology (Mikulincer & Shaver, 2003). Although avoidant people can maintain a defensive façade of security and imperturbability, they ignore, misinterpret, or misunderstand their own emotions and have difficulty dealing with prolonged, demand-ing stressors that require active problem confrontation and mobilization of external sources of support (Mikulincer & Shaver, 2003). In addition, although avoidant people are able to suppress or ignore distress consciously, the distress can still be indirectly manifested in somatic symptoms, sleep problems, and other physical health problems. Moreover, avoidant individ-uals can transform unresolved distress into feelings of hostility, loneliness, and estrangement from others (Shaver & Hazan, 1993).

Many studies have shown that attachment-related anxiety is inversely related to well-being, and positively associated with global distress, depres-sion, anxiety, eating disorders, substance abuse, conduct disorder, and severe personality disorders (see Mikulincer & Shaver, 2007, for a review). With regard to avoidant attachment, many studies have found no significant associations between avoidant attachment and self-report measures of well-being and global distress (see Mikulincer & Shaver, 2007, for a review). However, several studies indicate that avoidant attachment is associated with particular patterns of emotional and behavioral problems, such as a pattern of depression characterized by perfectionism, self-punishment, and self-criticism (e.g., Zuroff & Fitzpatrick, 1995); somatic complaints (e.g., Kidd & Sheffield, 2005); substance abuse and conduct disorder (e.g., Brennan & Shaver, 1995; Cooper et al., 1998; Mickelson et al., 1997); and schizoid and avoidant personality disorders (e.g., Brennan & Shaver, 1998; Levy, Meehan, Weber, Reynoso, & Clarkin, 2005). In addition, whereas no consistent association has been found in community samples between avoidant attachment and global distress, studies that focus on highly demanding and stressful events (e.g., giving birth to a seriously disabled infant) reveal that avoidance is related to higher levels of distress and poorer long-term outcomes (e.g., Berant et al., 2001).

These effects of secondary attachment strategies are also important for understanding differences across clients in the client–therapist relationship and for understanding why this relationship sometimes produces therapeutic failures. As explained in more detail in subsequent chapters, attachment insecurities tend to color the client–therapist relationship—and, as in other relationships between adults, the attachment styles of both parties (client and therapist) can affect the quality of the therapeutic alliance, the client's transference reactions to the therapist, and the therapist's countertransference reactions to the client and his or her personal disclosures. Evidence is accumulating (see detailed reviews in subsequent chapters) that attachment insecurities of either the anxious or avoidant type interfere with the development of a strong and stable therapeutic alliance, intensify destructive and hostile forms of transference and countertransference, and reduce the likelihood of favorable therapeutic outcomes. Adult attachment studies also show, however, that skilled and caring therapists can work around these attachment insecurities, create a satisfactory alliance with insecure clients, increase the clients' sense of felt security, and help them achieve better adjustment and enhanced personal growth.

CONCLUSIONS

We hope this chapter provides a useful foundation for the chapters that follow. As already mentioned, the attachment literature is large and still mushrooming, so the best one can do, when wishing to clinically apply the theory and the studies it has generated, is to master the core ideas, terms, and constructs in the theory; read some of the overviews of attachment research (e.g., Cassidy & Shaver, 1999, 2008; Grossmann, Grossmann, &

Waters, 2005; Mikulincer & Goodman, 2006; Mikulincer & Shaver, 2007; Rholes & Simpson, 2004; Simpson & Rholes, 1998); and consider how the other chapter authors in this volume are using attachment theory and research in clinical practice.

One of the reasons for attachment theory's remarkable popularity and influence is that Bowlby and his successors acknowledged insights from other therapeutically useful theories, integrated them conceptually, and illustrated the value of empirical research for clinical theory and practice. In closing, we wish to say something about the compatibility of attachment theory and other classical theoretical frameworks that have influenced clinical work.

First of all, Bowlby was a psychoanalyst; although he eventually reworked much of psychoanalytic theory, he continued to emphasize the childhood origins of personality and psychopathology, the reality of unconscious defenses, and the importance and complexity of close relationships. In our own work (e.g., Banai, Mikulincer, & Shaver, 2005; Berant, Mikulincer, Shaver, & Segal, 2005; Mikulincer et al., 2004), we have found good empirical support for some of Bowlby's more psychodynamic hypotheses. Thus attachment theory and research continue to benefit from the insights of generations of psychoanalysts. It should be possible for psychoanalytically oriented clinicians to benefit from what has been learned so far by attachment researchers.

Second, Bowlby and Ainsworth's insights about how attachment patterns arise in infancy, as the infant adapts to its primary caregiver's (or caregivers') parenting behavior, are highly compatible with a behavioral approach to clinical work. The secure attachment pattern or style is rooted in experiences in which a caregiver responded favorably to a child or adult's primary attachment strategy—seeking protection, comfort, or encouragement in response to difficulties or threats. During infancy, this pattern clearly arises before a child has much in the way of cognitive or linguistic capacities, so it is likely to be due to a combination of natural (instinctual) behavioral tendencies and reinforcement contingencies.

The avoidant attachment pattern or style is rooted in experiences in which the natural, instinctual tendency to seek proximity and protection when distressed was met with punishment, distancing, or neglect. The avoidant infant is forced to learn, without complex thoughts or language, to suppress his or her attachment behavior in order to receive adequate or minimal care. With development, this suppressive, avoidant, self-reliant style takes on cognitive richness, but it would be a mistake to think of it as overly cognitive at, say, the age of 10 months.

The anxious attachment pattern or style is rooted in parental anxiety and inconsistency. The anxious infant feels rewarded for hyperactivating its attachment system—protesting loudly when a caregiver is self-preoccupied, distracted, or inattentive; crying loudly and persistently; being vigilant about possible separations and loss of support. Again, this pattern can be greatly elaborated during social and cognitive development, but the core behavioral tendencies were probably acquired before much in the way of thought or language was available. Thus therapeutic change may be partly a matter of extinction, relearning, and new reinforcement patterns that do not necessarily require thought or linguistic formulations.

To the extent that the adult forms of the major attachment patterns, or styles, involve cognitive "working models," ideas advanced by cognitive therapists beginning with Ellis (1962) and Beck (1976) are easy to integrate with attachment theory. Each major attachment pattern is characterized by a particular kind of self- and other-appraisal, and changing the pattern can be accomplished in part by changing key beliefs and schemas through identifying dysfunctional cognitions, teaching constructive alternatives, role-playing the alternatives, modeling them in one's own therapeutic comments, and so on (Mikulincer & Shaver, 2007).

One other approach to psychotherapy has evolved from basic researchers' analyses of the structure of dyadic interactions. Many different theorists and researchers (e.g., Benjamin, 1994; Kiesler, 1996; Leary, 1957) have noticed that dyadic interactions can be characterized in terms of two bipolar dimensions: warm–cold and dominant–submissive. Similarly, important personality traits can also be arrayed in a circular pattern (called a *circumplex*; Wiggins, 1979), such that people can be described as relatively dominant or submissive, warm or cold, dominant and cold versus warm and submissive, and so on. Moreover, interpersonal difficulties that cause people to enter psychotherapy can be arrayed around the same circumplex. Some people are too dominant or too submissive for their own good, and being too warm and expressive or too cool can damage relationships both at home and in the workplace.

Bartholomew and Horowitz (1991) used a circumplex model of interpersonal problems in conjunction with an early four-category measure of adult attachment style to see what kinds of interpersonal problems were associated with particular patterns of adult attachment. They found that secure individuals had relatively few interpersonal problems, and that the problems they did have were fairly evenly distributed around the circumplex. In contrast, avoidant people generally had problems with nurturance (being overly cold, introverted, or competitive), and anxious people had problems related to their insistent demands for love and support (being overly expressive). Fearfully avoidant participants (those who were high on both the anxious and avoidant attachment dimensions) had problems associated with lack of dominance (i.e., being overly submissive and exploitable). In other words, there was a systematic pattern of interpersonal problems associated with each attachment style.

To us, the scientific and therapeutic advantages of attachment theory are numerous. First, while clarifying psychoanalytic insights by translating them into testable propositions about cognition, emotion, and behavior, attachment theory continues to take childhood antecedents and psychodynamic defenses seriously. This recovers much of the viable psychodynamic "baby" thrown out with the cloudy theoretical "bathwater" by behavioral and cognitive theorists and researchers. Second, attachment theory is inherently social. Unlike behaviorally oriented clinical theories, which arose primarily from laboratory experiments involving rats and pigeons, attachment theory resulted from looking carefully at human and nonhuman primate infant–mother dyads. Its key concepts—attachment, emotion regulation aided by attachment figures, working models of self and relationship partners—are therefore easy to apply in dyadic psychotherapy and couple therapy. Unlike cognitive therapies (which arose during the "cognitive revolution," before cognitive insights were adopted by social psychologists), the cognitions emphasized in attachment theory are ones that arise and derive from dyadic interactions. They are therefore not just cool, "dry" beliefs or cognitions; they are emotionally hot, hormonally "wet" beliefs, worries, and expectations generated in the context of highly charged social relationships. These cognitions are likely to be of utmost importance in psychotherapy.

Third, unlike circumplex analyses of dyadic relationships, which (like attachment theory) are highly social in focus, attachment theory emphasizes relationships and interactions in which one person seeks proximity, protection, comfort, and support from another. These relationships and interactions are likely to have special features that make them somewhat distinct from other kinds of relationships and interactions. Moreover, circumplex models do not explain why the two dimensions of dyadic interactions are important. Attachment theory, rooted in primate ethology and infant cognitive-developmental psychology, emphasizes the human need for affection and support and the fundamental influence of one person on another—not because one person is submissive and the other is dominant, but because one is vulnerable, at least at the moment, and the other is a potential safe haven and secure base.

Finally—perhaps because of Bowlby's eclecticism, amazingly broad reading, and interest in a wide range of empirical studies (ranging from infant cognitive-developmental studies to community psychiatry studies of adult depression)—attachment research has been methodologically diverse and has benefited from the use of projective, observational, self-report, and physiological measures, as well as from cognitive and social-cognitive research paradigms. The research literature on attachment is exceptionally rich and conducive to diverse clinical applications. We hope that this book encourages such applications, which can then be rigorously assessed with appropriate research methods. Eventually we will have theoretically sound and truly evidence-based clinical practices, working in harmony with a research literature that is sensitive to clinical discoveries and applications.

RECOMMENDATIONS FOR FURTHER READING

Cassidy, J., & Shaver, P. R. (Eds.). (2008). *Handbook of attachment: Theory, research, and clinical applications* (2nd ed.). New York: Guilford Press.—The second edition of this handbook summarizes classic and recent contributions to attachment theory, and provides up-to-date reviews of many basic and applied research areas influenced by the theory.

Grossmann, K. E., Grossmann, K., & Waters, E. (Eds.). (2005). *Attachment from infancy to adulthood: The major longitudinal studies.* New York: Guilford Press.—A major accomplishment of attachment researchers has been tracking the correlates and sequelae of attachment orientations from infancy through childhood and into adulthood; this volume summarizes the major longitudinal studies, some spanning 20 years.

Mikulincer, M., & Shaver, P. R. (2007). *Attachment in adulthood: Structure, dynamics, and change.* New York: Guilford Press.—This book summarizes research on adult attachment and contains an in-depth discussion of ideas and findings mentioned in this chapter.

REFERENCES

Ainsworth, M. D. S. (1967). *Infancy in Uganda: Infant care and the growth of love.* Baltimore: Johns Hopkins University Press.

Ainsworth, M. D. S. (1973). The development of infant–mother attachment. In B. M. Caldwell & H. N. Ricciuti (Eds.), *Review of child development research* (Vol. 3, pp. 1–94). Chicago: University of Chicago Press.

Ainsworth, M. D. S. (1991). Attachment and other affectional bonds across the life cycle. In C. M. Parkes, J. Stevenson-Hinde, & P. Marris (Eds.), *Attachment across the life cycle* (pp. 33–51). New York: Routledge.

Ainsworth, M. D. S., Blehar, M. C., Waters, E., & Wall, S. (1978). *Patterns of attachment: A psychological study of the Strange Situation.* Hillsdale, NJ: Erlbaum.

Baldwin, M. W. (1992). Relational schemas and the processing of social information. *Psychological Bulletin, 112,* 461–484.

Baldwin, M. W., Keelan, J. P. R., Fehr, B., Enns, V., & Koh Rangarajoo, E. (1996). Social-cognitive conceptualization of attachment working models: Availability and accessibility effects. *Journal of Personality and Social Psychology, 71,* 94–109.

Banai, E., Mikulincer, M., & Shaver, P. R. (2005). "Selfobject" needs in Kohut's self psychology: Links with attachment, self-cohesion, affect regulation, and adjustment. *Psychoanalytic Psychology, 22,* 224–260.

Bartholomew, K. (1990). Avoidance of intimacy: An attachment perspective. *Journal of Social and Personal Relationships, 7,* 147–178.

Bartholomew, K., & Horowitz, L. M. (1991). Attachment styles among young adults: A test of a four-category model. *Journal of Personality and Social Psychology, 61,* 226–244.

Beck, A. (1976). *Cognitive therapy and the emotional disorders.* New York: International Universities Press.

Benjamin, L. S. (1994). SASB: A bridge between personality theory and clinical psychology. *Psychological Inquiry, 5,* 273–316.

Berant, E., Mikulincer, M., & Florian, V. (2001). Attachment style and mental health: A one-year follow-up study of mothers of infants with congenital heart disease. *Personality and Social Psychology Bulletin, 8,* 956–968.

Berant, E., Mikulincer, M., Shaver, P. R., & Segal, Y. (2005). Rorschach correlates of self-reported attachment dimensions: Dynamic manifestations of hyperactivating and deactivating strategies. *Journal of Personality Assessment, 84,* 70–81.

Birnbaum, G. E., Orr, I., Mikulincer, M., & Florian, V. (1997). When marriage breaks up: Does attachment style contribute to coping and mental health? *Journal of Social and Personal Relationships, 14,* 643–654.

Bowlby, J. (1973). *Attachment and loss: Vol. 2. Separation: Anxiety and anger.* New York: Basic Books.

Bowlby, J. (1980). *Attachment and loss: Vol. 3. Loss: Sadness and depression.* New York: Basic Books.

Bowlby, J. (1982). *Attachment and loss: Vol. 1. Attachment* (2nd ed.). New York: Basic Books. (1st ed., 1969)

Bowlby, J. (1988). *A secure base: Clinical applications of attachment theory.* London: Routledge.

Brennan, K. A., Clark, C. L., & Shaver, P. R. (1998). Self-report measurement of adult attachment: An integrative overview. In J. A. Simpson & W. S. Rholes (Eds.), *Attachment theory and close relationships* (pp. 46–76). New York: Guilford Press.

Brennan, K. A., & Shaver, P. R. (1995). Dimensions of adult attachment, affect regulation, and romantic relationship functioning. *Personality and Social Psychology Bulletin, 21,* 267–283.

Brennan, K. A., & Shaver, P. R. (1998). Attachment styles and personality disorders: Their connections to each other and to parental divorce, parental death, and perceptions of parental caregiving. *Journal of Personality, 66,* 835–878.

Cassidy, J., & Kobak, R. R. (1988). Avoidance and its relationship with other defensive processes. In J. Belsky & T. Nezworski (Eds.), *Clinical implications of attachment* (pp. 300–323). Hillsdale, NJ: Erlbaum.

Cassidy, J., & Shaver, P. R. (Eds.). (1999). *Handbook of attachment: Theory, research, and clinical applications.* New York: Guilford Press.

Cassidy, J., & Shaver, P. R. (Eds.). (2008). *Handbook of attachment: Theory, research, and clinical applications* (2nd ed.). New York: Guilford Press.

Collins, N. L. (1996). Working models of attachment: Implications for explanation, emotion, and behavior. *Journal of Personality and Social Psychology, 71,* 810–832.

Collins, N. L., & Read, S. J. (1990). Adult attachment, working models, and relationship quality in dating couples. *Journal of Personality and Social Psychology, 58,* 644–663.

Collins, N. L., & Read, S. J. (1994). Cognitive representations of attachment: The structure and function of working models. In K. Bartholomew & D. Perlman (Eds.), *Advances in personal relationships: Vol. 5. Attachment processes in adulthood* (pp. 53–92). London: Jessica Kingsley.

Cooper, M. L., Shaver, P. R., & Collins, N. L. (1998). Attachment styles, emotion regulation, and adjustment in adolescence. *Journal of Personality and Social Psychology, 74,* 1380–1397.

Crawford, T. N., Livesley, W. J., Jang, K. L., Shaver, P. R., Cohen, P., & Ganiban, J. (2007). Insecure attachment and personality disorder: A twin study of adults. *Journal of Personality Disorders, 21,* 191–208.

Crowell, J. A., Fraley, R. C., & Shaver, P. R. (1999). Measurement of individual differences in adolescent and adult attachment. In J. Cassidy & P. R. Shaver

(Eds.), *Handbook of attachment: Theory, research, and clinical applications* (pp. 434–465). New York: Guilford Press.

Davis, M. H., Morris, M. M., & Kraus, L. A. (1998). Relationship-specific and global perceptions of social support: Associations with well-being and attachment. *Journal of Personality and Social Psychology, 74,* 468–481.

Elliot, A. J., & Reis, H. T. (2003). Attachment and exploration in adulthood. *Journal of Personality and Social Psychology, 85,* 317–331.

Ellis, A. (1962). *Reason and emotion in psychotherapy.* New York: Lyle Stuart.

Feeney, J. A. (1999). Adult romantic attachment and couple relationships. In J. Cassidy & P. R. Shaver (Eds.), *Handbook of attachment: Theory, research, and clinical applications* (pp. 355–377). New York: Guilford Press.

Feeney, J. A., & Noller, P. (1991). Attachment style and verbal descriptions of romantic partners. *Journal of Social and Personal Relationships, 8,* 187–215.

Fraley, R. C., & Davis, K. E. (1997). Attachment formation and transfer in young adults' close friendships and romantic relationships. *Personal Relationships, 4,* 131–144.

Fraley, R. C., & Shaver, P. R. (1998). Airport separations: A naturalistic study of adult attachment dynamics in separating couples. *Journal of Personality and Social Psychology, 75,* 1198–1212.

Fraley, R. C., & Shaver, P. R. (2000). Adult romantic attachment: Theoretical developments, emerging controversies, and unanswered questions. *Review of General Psychology, 4,* 132–154.

Fredrickson, B. L. (2001). The role of positive emotions in positive psychology: The broaden-and-build theory of positive emotions. *American Psychologist, 56,* 218–226.

George, C., Kaplan, N., & Main, M. (1984). *Adult Attachment Interview protocol.* Unpublished manuscript, University of California, Berkeley.

George, C., Kaplan, N., & Main, M. (1985). *Adult Attachment Interview protocol* (2nd ed.). Unpublished manuscript, University of California, Berkeley.

George, C., Kaplan, N., & Main, M. (1985). *Adult Attachment Interview protocol* (3rd ed.). Unpublished manuscript, University of California, Berkeley.

Green, J. D., & Campbell, W. K. (2000). Attachment and exploration in adults: Chronic and contextual accessibility. *Personality and Social Psychology Bulletin, 26,* 452–461.

Grossmann, K. E., Grossmann, K., & Waters, E. (Eds.). (2005). *Attachment from infancy to adulthood: The major longitudinal studies.* New York: Guilford Press.

Hazan, C., & Shaver, P. R. (1987). Romantic love conceptualized as an attachment process. *Journal of Personality and Social Psychology, 52,* 511–524.

Hazan, C., & Shaver, P. R. (1994). Attachment theory as an organizational framework for research on close relationships. *Psychological Inquiry, 5,* 1–22.

Hazan, C., & Zeifman, D. (1994). Sex and the psychological tether. In K. Bartholomew & D. Perlman (Eds.), *Advances in personal relationships: Vol. 5. Attachment processes in adulthood* (pp. 151–177). London: Jessica Kingsley.

Heinicke, C., & Westheimer, I. (1966). *Brief separations.* New York: International Universities Press.

Hesse, E. (1999). The Adult Attachment Interview: Historical and current perspectives. In J. Cassidy & P. R. Shaver (Eds.), *Handbook of attachment: Theory, research, and clinical applications* (pp. 395–433). New York: Guilford Press.

Hesse, E. (2008). The Adult Attachment Interview: Protocol, method of analysis, and empirical studies. In J. Cassidy & P. R. Shaver (Eds.), *Handbook of attachment: Theory, research, and clinical applications* (2nd ed., pp. 552–598). New York: Guilford Press.

Kidd, T., & Sheffield, D. (2005). Attachment style and symptom reporting: Examining the mediating effects of anger and social support. *British Journal of Health Psychology, 10,* 531–541.

Kiesler, D. J. (1996). *Contemporary interpersonal theory and research: Personality, psychopathology, and psychotherapy.* New York: Wiley.

Kunce, L. J., & Shaver, P. R. (1994). An attachment-theoretical approach to caregiving in romantic relationships. In K. Bartholomew & D. Perlman (Eds.), *Advances in personal relationships: Vol. 5. Attachment processes in adulthood* (pp. 205–237). London: Jessica Kingsley.

Leary, T. (1957). *Interpersonal diagnosis of personality.* New York: Ronald Press.

Levy, K. N., Blatt, S. J., & Shaver, P. R. (1998). Attachment styles and parental representations. *Journal of Personality and Social Psychology, 74,* 407–419.

Levy, K. N., Meehan, K. B., Weber, M., Reynoso, J., & Clarkin, J. F. (2005). Attachment and borderline personality disorder: Implications for psychotherapy. *Psychopathology, 38,* 64–74.

Lyons-Ruth, K., Yellin, C., Melnick, S., & Atwood, G. (2005). Expanding the concept of unresolved mental states: Hostile/helpless states of mind on the Adult Attachment Interview are associated with disrupted mother–infant communication and infant disorganization. *Development and Psychopathology, 17,* 1–23.

Main, M. (1990). Cross-cultural studies of attachment organization: Recent studies, changing methodologies, and the concept of conditional strategies. *Human Development, 33,* 48–61.

Main, M., & Goldwyn, R. (1984). *Adult attachment scoring and classification system.* Unpublished manuscript, University of California, Berkeley.

Main, M., Goldwyn, R., & Hesse, E. (2003). *Adult attachment scoring and classification system.* Unpublished manuscript, University of California, Berkeley.

Main, M., Kaplan, N., & Cassidy, J. (1985). Security in infancy, childhood, and adulthood: A move to the level of representation. In I. Bertherton & E. Waters (Eds.), Growing points of attachment theory and research. *Monographs of the Society for Research in Child Development, 50,*(1–2, Serial No. 209), 66–104.

Main, M., & Solomon, J. (1990). Procedures for identifying infants as disorganized/disoriented during the Ainsworth Strange Situation. In M. T. Greenberg, D. Cicchetti, & M. Cummings (Eds.), *Attachment in the preschool years: Theory, research, and intervention* (pp. 121–160). Chicago: University of Chicago Press.

Martin, D. J., Garske, J. P., & Davis, M. K. (2000). Relation of the therapeutic alliance with outcome and other variables: A meta-analytic review. *Journal of Consulting and Clinical Psychology, 68,* 438–450.

Maslow, A. H. (1968). *Toward a psychology of being.* New York: Van Nostrand.

Mickelson, K. D., Kessler, R. C., & Shaver, P. R. (1997). Adult attachment in a nationally representative sample. *Journal of Personality and Social Psychology, 73,* 1092–1106.

Mikulincer, M. (1995). Attachment style and the mental representation of the self. *Journal of Personality and Social Psychology, 69,* 1203–1215.

Mikulincer, M. (1997). Adult attachment style and information processing: Individual differences in curiosity and cognitive closure. *Journal of Personality and Social Psychology, 72,* 1217–1230.

Mikulincer, M., Florian, V., Cowan, P. A., & Cowan, C. P. (2002). Attachment security in couple relationships: A systemic model and its implications for family dynamics. *Family Process, 41,* 405–434.

Mikulincer, M., Gillath, O., & Shaver, P. R. (2002). Activation of the attachment system in adulthood: Threat-related primes increase the accessibility of mental representations of attachment figures. *Journal of Personality and Social Psychology, 83,* 881–895.

Mikulincer, M., & Goodman, G. S. (Eds.). (2006). *Dynamics of romantic love: Attachment, caregiving, and sex.* New York: Guilford Press.

Mikulincer, M., Hirschberger, G., Nachmias, O., & Gillath, O. (2001). The affective component of the secure base schema: Affective priming with representations of attachment security. *Journal of Personality and Social Psychology, 81,* 305–321.

Mikulincer, M., & Shaver, P. R. (2001). Attachment theory and intergroup bias: Evidence that priming the secure base schema attenuates negative reactions to out-groups. *Journal of Personality and Social Psychology, 81,* 97–115.

Mikulincer, M., & Shaver, P. R. (2003). The attachment behavioral system in adulthood: Activation, psychodynamics, and interpersonal processes. In M. P. Zanna (Ed.), *Advances in experimental social psychology* (Vol. 35, pp. 53–152). San Diego, CA: Academic Press.

Mikulincer, M., & Shaver, P. R. (2004). Security-based self-representations in adulthood: Contents and processes. In W. S. Rholes & J. A. Simpson (Eds.), *Adult attachment: Theory, research, and clinical implications* (pp. 159–195). New York: Guilford Press.

Mikulincer, M., & Shaver, P. R. (2007). *Attachment in adulthood: Structure, dynamics, and change.* New York: Guilford Press.

Mikulincer, M., Shaver, P. R., Gillath, O., & Nitzberg, R. A. (2005). Attachment, caregiving, and altruism: Boosting attachment security increases compassion and helping. *Journal of Personality and Social Psychology, 89,* 817–839.

O'Connor, T. G. (2005). Attachment disturbances associated with early severe deprivation. In C. S. Carter, L. Ahnert, K. E. Grossmann, S. B. Hrdy, M. E. Lamb, S. W. Porges, et al. (Eds.), *Attachment and bonding: A new synthesis* (pp. 257–268). Cambridge, MA: MIT Press.

Ognibene, T. C., & Collins, N. L. (1998). Adult attachment styles, perceived social support, and coping strategies. *Journal of Social and Personal Relationships, 15,* 323–345.

Overall, N. C., Fletcher, G. J. O., & Friesen, M. (2003). Mapping the intimate relationship mind: Comparisons between three models of attachment representations. *Personality and Social Psychology Bulletin 29,* 1479–1493.

Rholes, W. S., & Simpson, J. A. (Eds.). (2004). *Adult attachment: Theory, research, and clinical implications.* New York: Guilford Press.

Roberts, J. E., Gotlib, I. H., & Kassel, J. D. (1996). Adult attachment security and symptoms of depression: The mediating roles of dysfunctional attitudes and low self-esteem. *Journal of Personality and Social Psychology, 70,* 310–320.

Rogers, C. R. (1961). *On becoming a person.* Boston: Houghton Mifflin.

Seligman, M. E. P. (2002). *Authentic happiness: Using the new positive psychology to realize your potential for lasting fulfillment.* New York: Free Press.

Shaver, P. R., Belsky, J., & Brennan, K. A. (2000). The Adult Attachment Interview and self-reports of romantic attachment: Associations across domains and methods. *Personal Relationships, 7,* 25–43.

Shaver, P. R., Collins, N., & Clark, C. L. (1996). Attachment styles and internal working models of self and relationship partners. In G. J. O. Fletcher & J. Fitness (Eds.), *Knowledge structures in close relationships: A social psychological approach* (pp. 25–61). Hillsdale, NJ: Erlbaum.

Shaver, P. R., & Hazan, C. (1993). Adult romantic attachment: Theory and evidence. In D. Perlman & W. Jones (Eds.), *Advances in personal relationships* (Vol. 4, pp. 29–70). London: Jessica Kingsley.

Shaver, P. R., & Mikulincer, M. (2002). Attachment-related psychodynamics. *Attachment & Human Development, 4,* 133–161.

Shaver, P. R., & Mikulincer, M. (2004). What do self-report attachment measures assess? In W. S. Rholes & J. A. Simpson (Eds.), *Adult attachment: Theory, research, and clinical implications* (pp. 17–54). New York: Guilford Press.

Shaver, P. R., & Mikulincer, M. (2006). Attachment theory, individual psychodynamics, and relationship functioning. In D. Perlman & A. Vangelisti (Eds.), *Handbook of personal relationships* (pp. 251–272). New York: Cambridge University Press.

Shaver, P. R., Mikulincer, M., Lavy, S., & Cassidy, J. (in press). Understanding and altering hurt feelings: An attachment-theoretical perspective on the generation and regulation of emotions. In A. L. Vangelisti (Ed.), *Feeling hurt in close relationships.* New York: Cambridge University Press.

Simpson, J. A. (1990). Influence of attachment styles on romantic relationships. *Journal of Personality and Social Psychology, 59,* 871–980.

Simpson, J. A., & Rholes, W. S. (Eds.). (1998). *Attachment theory and close relationships.* New York: Guilford Press.

Simpson, J. A., Rholes, W. S., & Nelligan, J. S. (1992). Support seeking and support giving within couples in an anxiety-provoking situation: The role of attachment styles. *Journal of Personality and Social Psychology, 62,* 434–446.

Sroufe, L. A., & Waters, E. (1977). Attachment as an organizational construct. *Child Development, 48,* 1184–1199.

Torgersen, A. M., Gorva, B. K., & Sommerstad, R. (2007). A pilot study of attachment patterns in adult twins. *Attachment & Human Development, 9,* 127–138.

Trinke, S. J., & Bartholomew, K. (1997). Hierarchies of attachment relationships in young adulthood. *Journal of Social and Personal Relationships, 14,* 603–625.

van IJzendoorn, M. (1995). Adult attachment representations, parental responsiveness, and infant attachment: A meta-analysis on the predictive validity of the Adult Attachment Interview. *Psychological Bulletin, 117,* 387–403.

Waters, H. S., Rodrigues, L. M., & Ridgeway, D. (1998). Cognitive underpinnings of narrative attachment assessment. *Journal of Experimental Child Psychology, 71,* 211–234.

Wiggins, J. S. (1979). A psychological taxonomy of trait descriptive terms: The interpersonal domain. *Journal of Personality and Social Psychology, 37,* 395–412.

Zuroff, D. C., & Fitzpatrick, D. K. (1995). Depressive personality styles: Implications for adult attachment. *Personality and Individual Differences, 18,* 253–365.

3

The Therapist as Secure Base

Barry A. Farber
Jesse A. Metzger

Real therapy is about creating a brand-new experience of safety,
a kind of safety never before experienced in the patient's life. This
kind of safety provides the atmosphere for inspired guidance and,
for the patient, the courage to attempt new behavior.
—FIRESTONE (2000, p. 4)

The idea that a psychotherapist functions as a secure base for his or her
clients has gradually taken hold within the psychotherapeutic community,
especially among clinicians and researchers influenced by contemporary
psychodynamic concepts. This metaphor has been adopted within the context of similar widespread acceptance over the past two decades of the primacy of the therapeutic relationship as a mutative ingredient in psychotherapy (e.g., Norcross, 2002), and the value of conceptualizing the process of
therapy within an object-relational or schema-influenced framework (e.g.,
Scarvalone, Fox, & Safran, 2005).

Nevertheless, although the idea of a therapist as a secure base has been
heuristically valuable and makes intuitive clinical sense, the parallels between
therapists' provision of a secure base for clients and parents' provision of
a secure base for children are at best inexact. Therapists are not equivalent
to parents, and clients are not the same as offspring. Moreover, like many
other evocative clinical metaphors (e.g., the Oedipus complex, mirroring,
the transitional object), the therapist as secure base is one that has been
stretched in ways that go far beyond its original meaning. The primary aims
of this chapter are to (1) discuss the ways in which the therapist serves as
a secure base for clients, explicating the differences between this process
and similar concepts (e.g., the therapeutic alliance); (2) review the empirical
evidence of secure-base and other attachment-related therapeutic phenom-

ena; (3) note possible markers in the process by which clients achieve and maintain a secure attachment to their therapist; and (4) examine the ways in which clients' use of a secure base may be influenced by their attachment status as well as that of their therapist.

One of Ainsworth's (1967) important contributions to attachment theory was the secure-base concept: When a mother provides an atmosphere of safety, she raises a "child's threshold for fear of the unfamiliar," thereby subduing the activation of attachment behavior and increasing the child's confidence to use her as a base of exploration (Ainsworth, 1972, p. 117). Along these lines, Bowlby (1977) suggested that it is important for a therapist to become a reliable and trustworthy figure—a secure base. The therapist, thought Bowlby (1988), should be a companion in the client's explorations rather than an interpreter of these experiences.

Farber, Lippert, and Nevas (1995) elaborated on these ideas, delineating specific ways in which the therapist functions as a secure base. Clients, they noted, use the safety of the therapist's office to discuss and attempt new ways of being in the world. Their anxiety and distress—emotions that ordinarily inhibit exploring new thoughts, feelings, or behaviors—are likely to be contained (managed) in the relative safety of the therapeutic setting. When their typical ways of interacting with others, based on their childhood attachment patterns, are responded to with the therapist's acceptance and care, mutual inquiry into alternative ways of seeing themselves and others become possible. Thus feelings or experiences that have been disavowed, repressed, or otherwise fraught with negative associations (e.g., assertiveness, trust, expressions of positive self-regard, healthy sexuality, emotional intimacy) may gradually reemerge, or in fact may emerge for the first time. Clients may derive particular benefit from using the secure therapeutic base to further their understanding of earlier and current attachment relationships, and to try out new, more adaptive relational patterns—initially with the therapist him- or herself, and then, assuming a good-enough result in the safety of the therapeutic environment, with others in the "real world."

Furthermore, Farber et al. (1995) have argued, therapists generally function as attachment figures for their clients. Not only do therapists provide a secure base for exploration, but their roles are consistent with the criteria posited by Bowlby in his writings (1969/1982, 1973, 1977) on the nature of attachment figures: They are typically considered by clients to be "wiser and stronger"; they serve as "insurers of survival" (at least in a psychological sense); they are the specific foci of attachment behavior (i.e., they are sought out preferentially in times of need); and they are the objects of intense affect during the formation, maintenance, disruption, renewal, and loss of the therapeutic relationship.

However, Farber et al. (1995) have also noted that "because its function is so distinctive and because it is defined by unique temporal, financial, logistic, and ethical boundaries, the patient–therapist dyad is significantly different from childhood attachment relationships" (p. 205). As an example, they note that the therapist is usually a more objective and less emotionally involved figure in a client's life than is a parent with his or her child.

Dozier and Tyrrell (1998) have maintained that a therapist's work with a client is more difficult than a parent's work with an infant. Their contention rests on the fact that the therapist must compensate for the failures in sensitive responsiveness of prior attachment figures, most notably parents. Thus clients tend to react to sensitive, responsive therapists as if they were uncaring, unavailable, or rejecting—a phenomenon that Freud would surely have included under the rubric of transference. Furthermore, according to these authors, a therapist's task is complicated by a client's need to begin work on exploring aspects of him- or herself (including the possibility of representing and interacting with others in alternative ways) before a secure base has been firmly established. "Thus, exploration of prior working models cannot wait until after a secure base is established; rather, the processes occur in tandem" (Dozier & Tyrrell, 1998, p. 222).

In this regard, it strikes us that contemporary clinical interpretations of Bowlby's work (e.g., Dozier & Tyrrell, 1998; Farber et al., 1995) imply that the notion of "secure" base should be reconceptualized along the lines of Winnicott's (1960/1965) "good-enough" base. The therapist does not have to be a firmly established attachment figure in order to be helpful—a virtual impossibility in the early stages of work with clients who have insecure attachment histories—but rather someone whose presentation is consistent with the characteristics of a security-enhancing attachment figure. Such a context enables the client to gradually, even nonlinearly, use the therapist as a secure-enough base to do the necessary exploratory work of therapy.

If we assume that the therapist generally functions as an attachment figure—in particular, by providing a secure-enough base for client exploration—two questions need to be more fully considered: What characteristics of the therapist facilitate the establishment of this secure base? And how does the provision of a secure base lead to therapeutic change?

CHARACTERISTICS AND FUNCTIONS OF A SECURE BASE

The therapist's "constancy, availability, sensitivity, and responsiveness" (Farber et al., 1995, p. 207) are what allow for the establishment of a secure base. To a certain extent, therapists recapitulate the conditions in childhood that facilitate secure attachments. They strive to be consistently and predictably responsive to the needs of their clients. They are attuned to their clients' affective worlds, attending to both verbal and nonverbal material (McCluskey, Hooper, & Miller, 1999). Within the prototypical structure of regularly scheduled appointments (and their availability at other times for emergencies), therapists attempt to help clients assuage distressful feelings and develop "positive new experiences" (Shane & Shane, 2001, p. 683). Working toward these goals may mean at times providing comfort, empathy, and understanding; at other times working to generate new solutions to problems; and at still other times offering explicit encouragement, mentoring, or advice (Bowlby, 1988).

Even therapists whose style is seemingly insensitive (e.g., like that of Albert Ellis or Fritz Perls) may serve as a secure base. In part, this is because therapists are imbued with enough socially sanctioned credibility (Frank, 1974) to offset personal characteristics that would otherwise be experienced as inimical to personal safety or a secure therapeutic relationship. But, more important, therapists of widely divergent theoretical orientations and styles have in common an attentiveness to and respect for the needs of their clients. Across the silence of classical analysts, the two-person approach of contemporary psychodynamically oriented clinicians, the confrontations of Gestalt and short-term dynamic therapists, the technology of biofeedback providers, the brusqueness of (some) rational–emotive practitioners, the manualized efficiency of cognitive-behavioral therapists, and the "get-real" tactics of some current media therapists, there is a common striving to hear and help. Thus sensitivity to a client's distress may take many forms.

Still, in most therapeutic systems, the characteristics of a therapist endeavoring to be a secure base are barely distinguishable from Rogers's (1957) delineation of the necessary and sufficient ingredients of therapeutic change. In fact, Leiper and Casares (2000), adopting some of the ideas of Mackie (1981), have suggested that "to provide a secure base for the client, the therapist must be perceived to be real, genuine, concerned and in touch with the patient's feelings" (p. 452). From a person-centered perspective, the therapist who is positively regarding, empathic, and genuine is able to provide fertile soil for the client (not patient!) to grow in new directions. Similarly, the therapist who provides a secure-enough base has inevitably established a positive working alliance—one in which the client feels a strong enough bond with the therapist to do the necessary work, including exploratory work, of therapy. Furthermore, as Bowlby (1988) himself noted, the concept of a secure base overlaps considerably with Winnicott's (1960/1965) notion of a psychologically protective holding environment. Is there anything truly distinctive, then, in the idea of the therapist as secure base?

Bowlby's (1988) work, as well as that of Dozier and colleagues (Bernier & Dozier, 2002; Dozier, Cue, & Barnett, 1994; Dozier & Tyrrell, 1998; Tyrrell, Dozier, Teague, & Fallot, 1999), suggests that there is something unique about the behavior of a therapist serving as a secure base. Their contention is that within an attachment-based model, therapists must go beyond Rogerian-like conditions of empathy and sensitivity; they must have sufficient ego strength—emanating perhaps from their own attachment security—to respectfully challenge clients' internal working models. The therapist, thought Bowlby (1988), must react to the demands of the client in ways that challenge the client's relational beliefs. This idea provides another means of understanding why confrontational therapists may be helpful. In their own fashion, these therapists not only offer a good-enough secure base for exploration, but also an often-needed persistent challenge to their clients to take advantage of these exploratory opportunities. Thus Perls, in the famous "Gloria" tape (Shostrom, 1965), justifies his seemingly rude comments by explaining to his client that he respects her too much to allow her to continue with her little-girlish, self-indulgent ways.

According to this perspective, therapists err when their customarily respectful stance inhibits them from confronting clients' maladaptive assumptions (working models). "The therapist's task," contend Dozier and Tyrrell (1998), "is to resist the pull to respond in ways that are consistent with expectations and complementary to behavioral strategies" (p. 237). They believe, for example, that therapists working with clients who rely on deactivating strategies must work with those clients to explore why the therapeutic environment feels unsafe. Conversely, therapists working with individuals who rely on hyperactivating strategies must avoid the pull to be overly protective and must make this dynamic a focus of the therapeutic dialogue. (See Shaver & Mikulincer, Chapter 2, this volume, for a discussion of attachment strategies.)

Although these recommendations make both clinical and theoretical sense, they overlook the fact that a therapeutic stance featuring respect and sensitivity is in itself antithetical to the negative self-representations held by many clients. Furthermore, these authors' emphasis on challenging internal working models, including the client's model of the therapist, is quite reminiscent of classical analysts' focus on the transference and the essential value of transference-related interpretations. In addition, their call for mutual exploration of therapeutic reenactments of clients' recurrent behavioral patterns is entirely congruous with the goals of contemporary relational psychotherapy (e.g., Aron, 1996).

An additional uniqueness about the secure-base concept is that it is grounded in a larger theory of individual differences in development, personality, and affect regulation. As we will discuss later, a client's response to the provision of a secure base is like a window into the organization of his or her attachment system, revealing the extent to which the client relies on security-based, hyperactivating, or deactivating attachment strategies to cope with distress. In turn, this allows therapists to develop hypotheses (based on the attachment research literature) about presenting problems, and to make adaptive changes in their therapeutic approach.

Given these considerations, we can return to the question of the distinctiveness of the secure-base concept. We would argue that although features of this concept overlap with those of the therapeutic alliance, and its provision leads to clinical material that is coextensive with traditional transference phenomena as well as more contemporary relational dynamics, there is still something in the concept that, if not sui generis, is nevertheless of considerable value. At its best, the secure-base aspect of an overall attachment model provides a template for understanding specific kinds of client internal working models, in turn allowing for consistent, focal efforts to change a particular form of insecure attachment to that of secure attachment behavior (or to enhance the solidity of a secure attachment). It offers a point of reference to which therapists can always return. Moreover, the secure-base concept provides the ground for therapist–client discussions of what is and "should be" happening between them. "Why, and in what ways," a therapist might well ask, "do I still feel unsafe to you?" "What is it that you keep expecting me to do that keeps us at a distance?" And "What is it you need from me to feel more connected/more disclosing/more hopeful?" Trust versus mistrust—that most elemental of Eriksonian stages—is exactly what we are talking about when we talk about a secure base.

The uniqueness of the secure-base concept, then, lies not in its essential features (inasmuch as these have been valued by one or another therapeutic system for many decades), but rather in what its use can lead to: in-depth exploration of the self in relationship to others, and, relatedly, the reworking of old, maladaptive mental models of self and others to form more secure and positively valenced representations, as well as more adaptive behavioral patterns. Regarding this last point, the therapist's task is to "prove wrong" the insecurely attached client's attributions of unresponsiveness and unavailability by being responsive, available, and even at times "noncomplementary," creating the possibility of a new, more secure kind of attachment to another person. To state the obvious, secure attachment (or, in some cases, a more secure attachment) is the overarching goal of an attachment-informed therapy.

Shane and Shane (2001) have also suggested that a secure therapeutic base should lead toward decreases in painful affect, as well as increases in clients' self-reflective capacities and self-esteem, awareness of others' mental states, and ease and mutuality in relating to others (including their therapists). Whereas these goals are not unique to an attachment-informed treatment model, again they do represent directions that are more consistent with a contemporary object-relational, rather than a Rogerian or cognitive-behavioral approach to therapy. They are reminders, then, that Bowlby understood his model as a variant of object relations theory.

EMPIRICAL STUDIES OF SECURE-BASE PHENOMENA

One means of determining whether a therapist serves as a secure base is to gauge the extent of client disclosure in therapy. Do clients tend to find psychotherapy a generally safe environment within which to explore their thoughts, feelings, and relationships with others? Although there is an inevitable tension in psychotherapy between the press to disclose and the often shameful and/or painful nature of what is discussed, empirical studies have indicated that clients do find therapy a generally safe place to disclose intimate issues. Although clients keep secrets from their therapists (especially those of a sexual nature), they tend to perceive themselves as highly disclosing (Farber, 2003, 2006; Hill, Gelso, & Mohr, 2000; Quintana & Meara, 1990).

In one study (Hill, Thompson, Cogar, & Denman, 1993), clients reported, on average, only one thing they failed to say to their therapist in a given session. In response to the question "Overall, how self-disclosing have you been to your therapist?", clients' mean scores in a series of studies (Berano & Farber, 2006; Farber & Sohn, 1997; Pattee & Farber, 2004) have ranged from 5.5 to 5.9 on a 7-point scale. Similarly, in response to the question "What percentage of 'who you truly are' have you revealed to your therapist?", clients' average scores in these studies have been between 79 and 82 on a 100-point scale. In addition, studies indicate that over time, individuals become more disclosing to their therapists (Farber, 2003).

It is also notable that clients perceive their disclosures as safe. When clients were asked to evaluate a variety of emotions experienced following disclosure on a 1–7 Likert-type scale, the mean score for "safe" was 5.0 (Farber, Berano, & Capobianco, 2004). Other highly ranked items in this study were "relieved" ($M = 5.6$), "vulnerable" ($M = 5.4$), and "authentic" ($M = 5.1$). Despite their considerable degree of vulnerability, clients do tend to feel safe (and helped) when disclosing to their therapists—a strong indication of the presence of a secure base. Furthermore, when clients evoke representations of their therapist between sessions, the most predominant theme is that of continuing the therapeutic dialogue (Rosenzweig, Farber, & Geller, 1996). Thus, even in his or her physical absence, the therapist continues to be utilized as a secure base for therapeutic work.

Using variables other than disclosure per se, two recent studies have also linked attachment security to clients' exploratory behavior. In one study, clients' perceived level of security with the therapist was positively related to the degree to which negative transference emerged—a finding supporting the idea that a secure therapeutic base can be used to explore difficult issues (Woodhouse, Schlosser, Crook, Ligiero, & Gelso, 2003). In a second study, researchers found a significant association between secure attachment to one's therapist and greater session "depth" (i.e., client exploration; Mallinckrodt, Porter, & Kivlighan, 2005).

In a series of articles, Geller and colleagues have found evidence for attachment-related processes in the therapist–client relationship that are conceptually linked, though not identical, to secure-base phenomena. For example, Geller and Farber (1993) have shown that both current and former therapy clients are most likely to evoke representations of their therapists when painful affects (e.g., sadness, anxiety, depression, guilt, fear, stress, self-hate) are being experienced—an indirect indication that they seek the emotional proximity of their therapists, and that the therapy relationship provides a safe haven to turn to for comfort in times of need (Bowlby,

1969/1982). Corroborating the notion of therapist as safe haven, Rosenzweig et al. (1996) found that when clients evoke therapist representations, they are most likely to experience feelings of being comforted, safe, and accepted. According to Geller and Farber (1993), "In contrast to merely 'remembering' information about their therapists, patients bring forth representations of themselves in relation to their therapists to, among other things, regular painful affects, assuage feelings of loneliness, and facilitate problem-solving and conflict resolution" (p. 176). That is, patients' use of internal representations of their therapists reflects multiple aspects of a therapist as attachment figure: someone who provides a secure base and safe haven, is considered stronger and wiser, and is sought out for emotional connection.

Yet another means of assessing the extent to which the therapist serves as an attachment figure is to examine the effects of the therapist's absence—that is, the extent of separation protest. Bowlby's (1969/1982) work on separation anxiety suggests that clients may experience both anxiety and anger in the face of this perceived loss. He believed that individuals tend to feel anxious as long as they retain hope for the return of the object; their anger, he thought, should be seen as an adaptive mechanism, catalyzing intense efforts to retrieve the lost object. Consistent with Bowlby's formulations, Kohut (1971) hypothesized that clients view therapist separations as de facto lapses in empathy that are likely to provoke "rage, despondency, and regressive retreat" (p. 91).

Barchat's (1989) research investigated clients' feelings during a therapist's absence. Adopting an object-relational perspective, she studied the "August phenomenon"—clients' reactions to the traditional month-long summer vacation that many therapists take. She found that clients' thoughts of their therapist during this vacation period were marked by feelings of longing for and missing him or her. She also found a significant positive relationship between the number of therapy sessions attended and the extent of clients' fear: Those who had presumably established the strongest secure base experienced the most fear of losing this relationship or felt more secure in acknowledging this reaction. In addition, Barchat's results indicated that the greater the combined intensity of clients' anger, sadness, and fear, the more difficult their transition from separation to resuming meaningful contact (reunion). In short, the results of this study strongly corroborate the idea of the therapist as an attachment figure whose absence provokes strong separation protest.

The most direct empirical assessment of the extent to which a therapist serves as an attachment figure was carried out by Parish and Eagle (2003). Using a sample of 105 adults currently in therapy for at least 6 months, these researchers attempted to determine the overall nature of attachment behavior toward a therapist. More specifically, they focused on differences between this attachment and that to a primary attachment figure (i.e., spouse, friend, or relative). Not surprisingly, they found that the relationship with a primary attachment figure had more components of an attachment relationship than the relationship with the therapist had. (Although Parish and Eagle use terms like *strength* and *intensity* of attachment, we prefer to stay away from these descriptors because of early controversies, described by Cassidy [1999], about *quality* vs. *quantity* of attachment. Many researchers mistook anxious attachment for intense attachment.) They also found, however, that, of nine discrete attachment components assessed (including Proximity Seeking, Separation Protest, Safe Haven, Wiser/Stronger, and Availability), Secure Base was the only factor on their measure (the Components of Attachment Questionnaire, or CAQ; Parish, 2000) for which there was no significant difference between participants' perceptions of their therapist and their primary attachment figure. In other words, therapists were perceived as offering as effective a secure base (i.e., a place from which to explore the world) as other identified attachment figures.

Consistent with the data of Woodhouse et al. (2002), Parish and Eagle also found that the number of attachment components in the therapeutic relationship, as perceived by clients, was positively and significantly correlated with duration of treatment and frequency of sessions. Noteworthy, too, was the finding that female clients with male therapists tended to report more components of attachment in the therapeutic relationship than clients in other kinds of gender pairs—a result consistent with earlier findings (Farber & Geller, 1994). Of all therapist–client gender configurations, female clients working with male therapists are most likely to daydream about therapy and acknowledge missing their therapists between sessions.

In addition, Parish and Eagle found that the CAQ Secure Base component of attachment to the therapist was positively correlated ($r = .31$, $p < .01$) with duration of therapy. Consistent with our arguments above, these authors also found that the CAQ Secure Base component was highly correlated ($r = .65$, $p < .001$) with the Working Alliance Inventory (WAI; Horvath & Greenberg, 1989). In a multiple-regression analysis, only Secure Base and Availability (of the nine CAQ attachment components studied) emerged as significant predictors of the WAI.

Finally, confirming some basic tenets of attachment theory, Parish and Eagle demonstrated that clients who scored high on attachment security reported that their therapeutic relationships had more components of attachment. Of particular relevance to this chapter, scores on the Secure dimension of the Relationship Questionnaire (Bartholomew & Horowitz, 1991) were significantly correlated with scores on the Secure Base component ($r = .22$, $p < .05$), the Safe Haven component ($r = .38$, $p < .01$), and the (perceived) Availability component ($r = .25$, $p < .01$) of the CAQ. Those with a secure attachment style were better able to use the therapist as a secure base for exploration, and were also better able to experience the therapist as a safe, available figure.

MARKERS OF THE DEVELOPMENT OF A SECURE BASE
(AND OTHER ATTACHMENT PHENOMENA) IN THERAPY

The research evidence points strongly to the fact that the therapist generally functions as a secure base. This section, based on Hazan, Gur-Yaish, and Campa's (2004) work on the formation of adult attachments and on Obegi's (in press) application of this model to the client–therapist relationship, attempts to identify markers for the gradual unfolding of attachment phenomena in therapy. Questions addressed here are these: What is the typical developmental sequence of the process of client–therapist attachment? And what are the manifestations of each stage in the process?

In a review of the research on normative patterns of attachment (i.e., what it means to be attached, regardless of individual differences in attachment), Hazan et al. (2004) have outlined specific behavioral, cognitive, physiological, and emotional markers of adult attachment, and speculated about how these markers unfold within the context of Bowlby's (1969/1982) four phases of attachment (preattachment, attachment in the making, clear-cut attachment, and goal-corrected partnership). According to Hazan et al. (2004), the adult counterpart of the infant preattachment phase is characterized by flirtation and playful, sexually charged exchanges; the quality of the interaction is not yet suggestive of a true attachment. As the couple moves into the throes of romantic infatuation, however, such behaviors as prolonged mutual gazing, cuddling, and nuzzling (which also characterize infant–caregiver behavior) begin to emerge and are indicative of attachment in the making. Clear-cut attachment, according to Hazan et al., is indicated by new attachment behaviors whose defining feature is their "organization around a single caregiver" (p. 59). Finally, the goal-corrected partnership phase in adult attachment is characterized by a decline in overt displays of attachment behavior.

Applying this framework to the client–therapist relationship, Obegi (in press) has offered a list of markers indicating the formation of an attachment at each of the four phases (see Table 3.1). As can be seen, the markers of attachment in the client–therapist relationship are different from those of adult (romantic) attachment in some ways, but also similar in other important ways. For example, in the preattachment phase, there is (ideally) not much sexually charged flirtation, but the behavioral, cognitive, physiological, and emotional markers—like those in adult attachment—are not yet indicative of a full-fledged attachment; the therapist does not yet serve any of the functions of an attachment figure. As the therapy progresses into the attachment-in-the-making phase, however, some of these functions begin to take hold. The therapist can begin to serve, for example, as a secure base (as the client feels more comfortable disclosing) and as a safe haven (as the client's emotional and physiological arousal declines in the presence of the therapist). In the clear-cut attachment phase, although the therapist may not be the only or primary attachment figure in the client's life, the client may

**TABLE 3.1. Hypothetical Markers in the Development
of Client–Therapist Attachment**

Behavioral	Cognitive	Physiological	Emotional
	Preattachment		
• Initial contact • Informed consent • Initial problem disclosure • Queries about therapist's competence	• Construction of IWM of therapist begins • Covert assessment of interpersonal safety	• High arousal • Presence of therapist has modest effect on physiological arousal	• High level of distress • Presence of therapist has modest effect on emotional regulation
	Attachment in the making		
• Regular session attendance (proximity seeking) • Fuller, more detailed problem disclosure (secure base) • Transference tests of interpersonal safety • More responsive to therapist's actions • Requests for reassurance • Appeals to therapist's expertise (requests for clarification, information, advice) • Sharing accomplishments	• Active construction of IWM of therapist (beliefs, expectations re: responsiveness and availability) • Thinking of therapist outside of sessions • Historical IWMs more chronically accessible, but IWM of therapist begins to compete • Increased likelihood that ruptures in alliance will be perceived as attachment injuries	• Pattern of arousal in presence of therapist begins to form • Moderate reductions in arousal with contact (safe haven)	• Pattern of emotional co-regulation begins to form • More displays of feeling • Contact is pleasurable and leads to soothing
	Clear-cut attachment		
• Reaction to separations from therapist • Reports desire to consult between sessions • Comes to session with questions/agenda • Interest in personal life/well-being of therapist • Gift giving • Reluctance to rely on the "on-call therapist"	• IWM of therapist complete • IWM available and influences information processing and behavior • IWM evoked during times of distress • Severe ruptures may be perceived as attachment injuries	• Moderate reductions in arousal with contact	• Modest/moderate positive impact on emotional regulation • Depthful displays of feeling • Evoking IWM of therapist leads to soothing • Uninhibited, genuine displays of feeling
	Goal-corrected partnership		
• Fewer transference tests of interpersonal safety • Focused attention on presenting problems • Decline in overt proximity-seeking behavior • Genuine consultation	• Further elaboration of IWM of therapist • Increased influence of IWM of therapist on information processing and behavior	• Moderate reductions in arousal with contact	• Modest/moderate positive impact on emotional regulation • Depthful displays of feeling

Note. IWM, internal working model. Based on Obegi (in press). Reprinted by permission.

begin to rely on the therapist for support or assistance that only he or she can provide. For example, the cognitive shift whereby internalized representations of the therapist become more fully accessible to conscious recall and influence thoughts and behaviors suggests that the therapist may in fact be a primary figure in terms of modifying the client's way of looking at the world. Finally, similar to the goal-corrected partnership in adult attachment, in the client–therapist relationship there is a decline in overt displays of attachment behaviors (e.g., assessments of interpersonal safety become less frequent and the relationship becomes more genuinely collaborative).

Work with one of our clients provides a good clinical example of the kinds of attachment phenomena that occur over time in a therapeutic relationship. (The therapist in this case, Barry A. Farber, is the "I" in what follows.)The client (disguised here for purposes of confidentiality), "J," is a married woman in her 40s who, because of early sexual and physical trauma, has been dealing for many years—and with a great deal of tenacity and courage—with issues of trust. Many of the behaviors described by Obegi's (in press) model did in fact transpire in our relationship.

For example, early in therapy we struggled together, sometimes painfully, to get through what Obegi (in press) terms, after Weiss (1993), "transference tests of interpersonal safety": J would vigilantly monitor my words, my body language, and my tone of voice, often finding "evidence" that I was unsafe and that trusting me would inevitably lead to my betraying her trust by rejecting or hurting her. We did eventually get through this stage—by going over, again and again, what I said (and did not say), what I did (and did not do), and who I was (and was not—i.e., her abusing father). I was, in her words, "authentic" and "consistent," and provided "a sense of stability" to her life. She began to believe that I did indeed value and accept her—and she became better able to accept her own imperfections. Thus I began to serve as a secure base for far more explicit (and difficult) disclosures surrounding her abuse.

In the clear-cut attachment stage, J professed a desire to increase the frequency of our sessions and often communicated in between sessions via phone calls and/or e-mail messages. Also, during this stage—one that lasted for several years—she would ask personal questions (e.g., regarding my musical taste) or find out through the Internet about my research interests. We are now, I believe, in what Obegi (in press) calls the "goal-corrected partnership" phase, one in which there is "genuine consultation" and collaboration and far fewer "transference tests." I am, for the most part, a safe haven and secure base: Misunderstandings are discussed in an atmosphere of mutual respect; disclosures are considerably less guarded; and intense emotions are revealed with far less apprehension that I will abuse the privilege of this intimacy. Recently, J had the following to say about this current phase of our work:

> "I find it so paradoxical that I used to think that being safe was to not be in pain. I have come to realize that being safe is being able to express

when I am in pain, and trusting that the intimacy communicated during those times will embrace me and help me to feel protected."

This model, then, is of considerable heuristic value, offering normative, clinically relevant guidelines for the client–therapist attachment process. Nevertheless, it is somewhat limited by its generic approach to these attachment phenomena. Whereas it describes a normative sequence of events, it does not take into consideration variations due to such factors as client age, attachment status, relationship status, and diagnosis (especially the presence or absence of personality disorders [PDs]); nor does it allow for differences in therapist attachment status, years of experience, or theoretical orientation. We believe that diagnosis, especially the presence of a PD, significantly affects the process of forming and maintaining an attachment with one's therapist. Fonagy et al. (1996), in fact, documented significant distortion in attachment representations in clients with PDs, noting, for example, the link between borderline pathology and preoccupied attachment. Similarly, Bender, Farber, and Geller (2001) found borderline tendencies (in an outpatient sample) to be significantly correlated with several attachment dimensions, including proximity seeking, separation protest, perceived unavailability of objects, and fear of object loss. Thus, clients with borderline PD are likely to experience earlier, more intense emotional reactions to the presence of therapists than those experienced by other clients (especially those without PDs). They are also likely to suffer from reactions to separations before the clear-cut attachment stage, and struggle more than most clients to reduce their overt proximity-seeking behavior toward their therapist. Variations in the attachment process due to other diagnoses and clinical factors are also to be expected. Empirical investigations of the validity of this model will, of course, be needed; still, the model holds much promise as an investigative and clinical tool.

CLIENT ATTACHMENT STYLES
AND SECURE-BASE DYNAMICS

In this section, we discuss the ways in which client attachment styles influence secure-base dynamics in therapy; we focus primarily on the insecure styles of preoccupied, fearful, and dismissing clients (see Shaver & Mikulincer, Chapter 2, and Lopez, Chapter 5, this volume, for full descriptions of these styles). The ideas outlined in this section are primarily based on our clinical judgment; however, in some cases, research on both clinical and nonclinical populations lends support to these formulations.[1]

Preoccupied Clients

To the extent that an attachment figure provides both safety and a firm ground for exploration, we suggest that clients high in attachment anxiety (i.e., those who manifest a preoccupied style of attachment) are able to take partial advantage of the first function of the therapist (provision of felt security), but have greater difficulty utilizing the second (provision of a secure base for exploration). Research has identified some characteristics of preoccupied individuals that may bear directly on the ways in which they are able to use the therapist as a secure base. For example, Bartholomew and Horowitz (1991) found that preoccupied individuals (as compared to those who displayed different attachment styles) scored high on measures of self-disclosure, emotional expressiveness, frequency of crying, crying in the presence of others, reliance on others, and use of others as a secure base. They also scored low on measures of coherence (in discussing relationships) and self-confidence.

A similar portrait emerges from the work of Mikulincer (e.g., Mikulincer & Nachshon, 1991; Mikulincer & Shaver, 2003), who found that although preoccupied individuals are prone to self-disclosure, they tend to disclose indiscriminately to those who are not prepared for intimate interactions and also tend to be unresponsive to their partners' disclosures. Taken together, these findings support the notion that whereas preoccupied individuals may be "well suited" to some of the primary activities of therapy (relying on the therapist, expressing emotions, self-disclosing), the ways in which they use or exhibit these behaviors may serve as obstacles in the therapeutic endeavor and prevent them from using the therapist for the "extended" purpose of exploration. In other words, although they may find the therapeutic relationship safe enough to self-disclose—to let their therapist know their deepest feelings—they may be unable to accept the reassurance, support, or invitations to explore new ways of being and relating that the therapist offers. Similarly, these clients may be unresponsive to the connections and associations the therapist makes among aspects of their experience. A preoccupied client's extensive focus on the therapist and the therapist's other clients (Mallinckrodt, Gantt, & Coble, 1995) interferes with the ability to do effective exploratory work.

It is as if, for preoccupied clients, the base is only semisecure: "I trust you enough to dump my stuff on you, but not enough to take in whatever wisdom you have to offer." It does help that the therapist hears these clients' disclosures, and we might hypothesize that this can have a cathartic effect— one of the primary benefits of self-disclosure (Farber, 2006). Still, it may take a long time before this client can trust the therapist enough to use him or her as a secure-enough base to explore not only extant thoughts, but also possibilities for new ways of framing experience that can ultimately lead to change. Moreover, there may be a halting quality to disclosures among preoccupied clients; they seem to convey to the therapist that "you were there [empathically] for me the last time we met, but I still cannot be entirely sure that you'll be here for me that way this time." In other words, disclosures tend not to move linearly toward greater depth, with trust building upon trust; rather, these clients respond to the therapist in a manner more reflective of their expectation that he or she will be only inconsistently responsive.

Fearful Clients

Unlike preoccupied individuals, those who display a fearful attachment style tend to avoid close involvement with others for fear of rejection; they have been found to score significantly lower than preoccupied individuals on measures of self-disclosure, intimacy, reliance on others, and the use of others as a secure base (Bartholomew & Horowitz, 1991). As a result of their sense that others are untrustworthy and rejecting, fearful individuals may not feel safe enough in the therapeutic relationship to self-disclose with depth or express themselves fully, let alone use the therapist as a secure base for exploring new ways of being or relating.

Consistent with these hypotheses, Mallinckrodt et al. (2005) found that an attachment to one's therapist characterized by fears of rejection and withdrawal was negatively correlated with session exploration, and Reis and Grenyer (2004) have hypothesized that the early difficulties in therapy typically experienced by clients with a fearful attachment style are attributable to the requirements of "a degree of disclosure that they may not initially be comfortable with" (p. 420). Furthermore, research examining the effects of an interpersonally oriented treatment on a sample of depressed women found that among those who benefited from the treatment, those with a highly fearful style took longer to stabilize (Cyranowski et al., 2002). The authors speculated that these clients, "who view the self as unlovable and others as unreliable, and thus experience heightened discomfort with social interaction, took longer to develop a trusting therapeutic alliance" (p. 211). This research, as well as our clinical sense, suggests that fearful clients struggle both to accept the therapeutic situation as a safe place and to use it as a context for exploration and self-disclosure.

Dismissing Clients

Although dismissing clients are similar to fearful clients in their avoidance of close relationships and reliance on others, they differ significantly in that they do not share the fearful clients' conscious sense of personal unworthiness and social insecurity (Bartholomew & Horowitz, 1991). This distinction has important implications for dismissing clients' use of the therapist as a secure base. Dismissing individuals are often reluctant to come to therapy in the first place, because of their characteristic disinclination to reach out to others for emotional support. However, if they do get to therapy (usually in response to others' requests), they are more likely than either preoccupied or fearful clients to use the secure base to discuss and explore others' problems rather than their own. They may use therapy as a way to prove to themselves that they are okay—to confirm their belief that "it's the world that's screwed up, not me." A dismissing client, convinced of the "consistent unresponsiveness" of attachment figures, repeatedly sends this message to the therapist: "I don't really need you; you aren't important in my life; you could be anyone. I won't use you to work on myself, but I can use you to criticize others in my life, which is far less dangerous."

When dismissing clients do speak about themselves, their disclosures tend to be intellectualized rather than affectively charged. Their disclosures may sound complaining or superficial, owing to their characteristic avoidance of real feelings and connection. They may disclose more in breadth than in depth, filling up the time with descriptions of their own accomplishments, day-to-day activities, or (as noted above) others' flaws; rarely is there an exploration of their own dynamics, or of the possibility that they themselves have flaws or have contributed significantly to a problematic interaction. The therapist feels prevented from getting to know who such a client really is, and often feels emotionally distant within the relationship. Lending support to these impressions, Bartholomew and Horowitz (1991) found that these individuals tend to score low on measures of emotional expressiveness and warmth, and low on all measures reflecting closeness in personal relationships (self-disclosure, intimacy, capacity to rely on others, and use of others as a secure base). Based on Mikulincer and Nachshon's (1991) findings with young adults, we might also expect that dismissing individuals will be less likely than those with other attachment styles to be responsive to therapist disclosures.

Although preoccupied, fearful, and dismissing clients clearly differ in their use of the secure base and the ways in which they resist taking in what the therapist has to offer, none believe in the reliable responsiveness of attachment figures. Ultimately, therefore, the therapist's work with these individuals involves moving the therapy to the point where the therapist's (alternative, paradigm-challenging) point of view can be better heard. To return to an earlier point, it is perhaps useful to think of the "base" in the relationship as neither "secure" nor "not secure," but rather as existing on a continuum, with degrees of felt security as markers in the therapeutic process. It may be that, especially for insecurely attached clients in therapy, the secure base is something that is tenuously held—experienced as a good-enough base at times and then resisted, or gradually built up toward ever greater security.

A client's process may be one of testing the therapist—persistently, and often without conscious intent—to determine the degree to which he or she can function as a secure base. Insecurely attached clients repeatedly enact their attachment paradigms with their therapist, trying to prove that the therapist isn't really available; the therapist's process therefore becomes one of "hanging in there," gently pointing out the clients' resistances to newly perceiving the therapist in a trusting way, as well as maintaining that perception. For example, to a fearful person, the therapist might convey this thought: "Although I try to convey to you that I respect and care for you, it feels to me as if you hear my words as primarily critical and rejecting." Or the therapist might say this to a dismissing person: "I feel like I could be anyone in here; there is something affectively missing between us. I wonder whether in between sessions you think about what we've discussed, or about the nature of our relationship."

Secure Clients

Work with securely attached clients is likely to differ from therapy with insecurely attached individuals. Secure individuals are predisposed to use the therapist as a secure base and to use him or her in the service of "tuning up" an attachment paradigm that is already operative and valuable. Satterfield and Lyddon (1998) confirmed this hypothesis with respect to the working alliance; they found that securely attached clients—who viewed themselves as worthy of love and support, and believed that others were generally trustworthy, accessible, and responsive—were more likely to form emotional bonds and negotiate meaningful goals with their mental health counselors. Similarly, Mallinckrodt et al. (1995) found that securely attached clients tended to report positive working alliances and to perceive their therapists as emotionally responsive and accepting.

Indeed, work with a client whose basic orientation is toward trusting and using the therapist to explore the self is very different from work toward transforming a deep-seated and insecure attachment paradigm. Clearly, it would be a mistake to assume that secure individuals don't present problems or dilemmas. Nevertheless, with respect to the ways in which attachment-related phenomena influence their use of the therapist as a secure base, these individuals are generally able to disclose intimate thoughts and feelings (including those that bear on the therapist him- or herself), acknowledge that their relational patterns affect their experiences and others in their life, and use that knowledge relatively nondefensively in the service of growth.

Several studies (Grabill & Kerns, 2000; Keelan, Dion, & Dion, 1998; Mikulincer & Nachshon, 1991) have found that securely attached individuals report higher levels of self-disclosure than individuals in other attachment categories (ambivalent and avoidant) do. These studies have also shown that secure individuals are better able to appropriately regulate the amount of their disclosure in accord with the demands and features of various situations and disclosure targets. We believe that these dynamics extend to the therapeutic situation: Secure clients are generally comfortable with disclosure to their therapists and are able to perceive more accurately than clients with other attachment styles when, what, and to what extent self-disclosures are most appropriate. In fact, as noted earlier, Mallinckrodt et al. (1995) found a significant association between secure attachment to one's therapist and greater in-session exploration.

THE EFFECTS OF THERAPIST ATTACHMENT
STYLE ON SECURE-BASE DYNAMICS

How does a therapist's attachment style affect secure-base dynamics in therapy? Although little research has been devoted to this topic, there is evidence that insecure therapists, relative to secure therapists, have greater difficulty maintaining a strong working alliance (Sauer, Lopez, & Gormley, 2003) and tend to respond to clients less empathically (Rubino, Barker, Roth, & Fearon, 2000). To the extent that a strong, enduring working alliance and a client's experience of therapist empathy can be considered preconditions for the establishment of a secure base, insecure therapists may face greater challenges in this area than their more secure counterparts.

Sauer et al. (2003) measured the attachment styles of clients and therapists, as well as the working alliance at the first, fourth, and seventh sessions of therapy. They found that therapists high in attachment anxiety had a significant positive effect on client working alliance ratings after the first session, but significant negative effects over time. (No other therapist or client attachment variables had a significant effect on client working alliance ratings.) Clients initially reported having a stronger connection and sense of collaboration with therapists high in attachment anxiety, but as the therapy progressed, these ratings were not maintained. Specifically, the more therapists reported attachment anxiety, the more client ratings of the working alliance decreased over the course of therapy.

In providing an explanation for the unexpected finding that anxious therapists had a positive effect on the alliance, if only initially, the authors suggest that these therapists "are better at perceiving variation in others and responding differently depending on the needs of the other person because they are highly invested in establishing connections" (Sauer et al., 2003, p. 379). Our sense is that, much like an anxious client—who self-discloses to feel close to the therapist, but who is uncomfortable with unexplored variations on this theme—an anxious therapist may be able initially to create a close connection, but is less able to respond flexibly as the relationship deepens. Anxious therapists are eager to please and establish a good relationship, but they ultimately struggle to provide firm enough boundaries for their clients; in particular, they may resist doing the kind of confrontive, discomfirmatory work (in regard to the attachment expectations of their clients) that is often required. In addition, therapists high in attachment anxiety, with their tendency to fear rejection, may have a harder time handling inevitable ruptures in the therapeutic alliance. Insecure therapists may interpret ruptures as an indication of their clients' desire to terminate therapy—a situation that would then trigger their own sensitivity to abandonment and diminish their capacity to respond therapeutically (Rubino et al., 2000). It is not difficult to imagine that such reactions would have a detrimental effect upon a therapist's ability to provide a good-enough secure base for a client's disclosures and attempts to change.

In one of the few empirical studies in this area, Rubino et al. (2000) examined the relationship between therapists' ways of resolving therapeutic alliance ruptures and therapist attachment styles. Although all therapists in this analogue study demonstrated "adequate levels of empathy" (p. 416), the more anxious therapists tended to respond less empathically than their less anxious counterparts to taped client vignettes. The authors suggest that therapists' attachment styles influence their ability to empathize with clients' concerns in a manner similar to the ways in which parents' ability to be attuned to their children's needs may be influenced by their own attachment histories (Fonagy, Steele, Steele, Moran, & Higgitt, 1991, as cited in Rubino et al., 2000). It should also be noted, however, that client attachment styles also affect the nature and resolution of alliance ruptures; Eames and Roth (2000), for example, found a significant positive correlation between preoccupied attachment style and client reports of ruptures.

Despite methodological weaknesses (e.g., the ratings of therapist empathy were based on single responses to videotaped clients), the Rubino et al. (2000) study offers further evidence that a therapist's attachment style affects important elements of the therapeutic relationship. An interesting secondary finding was that therapists higher in attachment anxiety were particularly less empathic in response to fearful and secure clients. The authors suggest that this finding could indicate that "similarities between the attachment patterns of therapists and those of their patients [may] affect the former's ability to be empathic" (p. 416)—specifically, in the direction of being less empathic.

Although Rubino et al. (2000) found no other evidence to support this notion (i.e., no other therapist–client match effects were observed), at least one other study has shown that there may be such dynamics at work with respect to the interaction of clinician and client attachment styles. Tyrrell et al. (1999), who studied the relationship between client and case manager attachment classifications in the Adult Attachment Interview (AAI; George, Kaplan, & Main, 1984, 1985, 1996), found that a mismatch of attachment styles resulted in better outcomes. Specifically, positive outcomes were predicted by differences in deactivating versus hyperactivating strategies. Clients who were more deactivating with respect to attachment had better alliances and functioned better with less deactivating case managers, whereas clients who were less deactivating worked better with more deactivating case managers. (According to Mikulincer & Shaver, 2003, deactivating strategies tend to be used by avoidant individuals in the service of diverting their attention away from attachment-related cues.) Tyrrell et al. (1999) concluded that client interaction with a case manager who utilizes different emotional and interpersonal strategies may result in disconfirmation of the client's working models, and that it is therefore important for clinicians and clients to be matched in ways that balance their interpersonal and emotional strategies.

Other work on the therapeutic impact of therapist attachment patterns has yielded some clinically provocative findings. Dozier et al. (1994), for example, found that clinical case managers' state of mind regarding early attachment (as assessed with the AAI) were related to their clinical intervention strategies, such that secure case managers were more likely to respond to clients' underlying needs, whereas insecure case managers attended to only the most obvious need. The results also indicated that case managers who relied on hyperactivating strategies intervened more intensely than did their counterparts who relied on deactivating strategies. The authors concluded that secure case managers may be better able than insecure case managers to resist clients' pull to behave in a way that is confirmatory of their internal working models: "Clinicians who are insecure appear to feel the pull of the client's attachment strategies and react accordingly" (p. 798). Why might this be? Rubino et al. (2000) suggest, and we concur, that secure individuals' working models serve as more effective guides in tailoring individualized, flexible responses to others. It should be noted however, that while these studies (Dozier et al., 1994, Dozier & Tyrrell, 1998; Tyrrell et al., 1999) provide interesting and relevant data with respect to the interaction of client–helper attachment styles, a case manager–client relationship may differ significantly from a therapist–client relationship with respect to secure-base dynamics.

CONCLUSIONS

Although it is well established that the therapeutic relationship is a significant contributor to treatment outcome (Horvath & Bedi, 2002), researchers have long sought to understand the specific ingredients underlying the potency of this relationship. Attachment theory provides a new and powerful perspective from which to examine this question. The therapist's provision of a secure base, in ways similar to the development of an effective alliance, allows clients to feel psychologically "held" enough to explore new aspects of themselves—most importantly, their intimate relationships with others.

Empirical work indicates that therapy provides sufficient safety for most clients to disclose to at least a moderate extent, and that the attachment status (or style) of clients and therapists significantly affects the ways in which a secure therapeutic base is established and used. Nevertheless, much work remains to be done in this area. Studies focused on client disclosure have not examined the effects of client attachment styles. In comparison to studies on client attachment styles, there is a paucity of research on the therapeutic effects (including the extent of client disclosure and exploration) of therapist attachment style. Moreover, more studies are needed on the issue of client–therapist matching—that is, on the ways in which complementary and non-complementary attachment tendencies affect the process of establishing and using a secure therapeutic base. Work to date (e.g., Dozier et al., 1994;

Dozier & Tyrrell, 1998; Tyrrell et al., 1999) has suggested that noncomplementarity is beneficial to treatment outcome, but this research has been conducted with clients who have severe psychopathology and are working with case managers, not psychotherapists. It may also be of great clinical significance to determine whether effective resolution of ruptured alliances in therapy is affected by client and therapist attachment styles. These inevitable ruptures can be seen as temporary disruptions in the secure-base system, and their effective resolution has been shown to contribute significantly to therapeutic success (Safran, Muran, Samstag, & Stevens, 2002).

In short, Bowlby's concept of a secure base for therapeutic work, based partly on Ainsworth's (1967) fertile theoretical reasoning and research, has led to new and important ways of understanding clinical phenomena; these include the development of therapeutic relationships, the process of client disclosure, the impact of therapist separations, and the importance of noncomplementarity in challenging old, maladaptive attachment paradigms. Further empirical work on these and related issues will continue to improve clinicians' ability to utilize attachment concepts to help clients improve their lives.

NOTE

1. The focus of this section is on how individual differences in attachment affect secure-base behavior, rather than on adaptations therapists might make to these variations. For discussion of this latter topic, see Mallinckrodt, Daily, and Wang (Chapter 10, this volume).

RECOMMENDATIONS FOR FURTHER READING

Dozier, M., & Tyrrell, C. (1998). The role of attachment in therapeutic relationships. In J. A. Simpson & W. S. Rholes (Eds.), *Attachment theory and close relationships* (pp. 221–248). New York: Guilford Press.—A comprehensive overview of attachment dynamics within psychotherapy.

Farber, B. A., Lippert, R. A., & Nevas, D. B. (1995). The therapist as an attachment figure. *Psychotherapy, 32,* 204–212.—One of the first attempts to examine the correspondence between Bowlby's ideas about attachment figures and the roles played by psychotherapists.

Mallinckrodt, B., Porter, M. J., & Kivlighan, D. M., Jr. (2005). Client attachment to therapist, depth of in-session exploration, and object relations in brief psychotherapy. *Psychotherapy: Theory, Research, Practice, Training, 42,* 85–100.—Well-done empirical investigation of the effects of attachment dynamics on therapy process and outcome.

Parish, M., & Eagle, M. N. (2003). Attachment to the therapist. *Psychoanalytic Psychology, 20,* 271–286.—Examines empirically the ways in which therapists serve multiple attachment functions.

REFERENCES

Ainsworth, M. D. S. (1967). *Infancy in Uganda: Infant care and the growth of love.* Baltimore: Johns Hopkins University Press.

Ainsworth, M. D. S. (1972). Attachment and dependency: A comparison. In J. L. Gewirtz (Ed.), *Attachment and dependency* (pp. 97–137). Washington, DC: V. H. Winston.

Aron, L. (1996). *A meeting of minds: Mutuality in psychoanalysis.* Hillsdale, NJ: Analytic Press.

Barchat, D. (1989, June). *Representations and separations in therapy: The August phenomenon.* Paper presented at the meeting of the Society for Psychotherapy Research, Toronto.

Bartholomew, K., & Horowitz, L. M. (1991). Attachment styles among young adults: A test of four-category model. *Journal of Personality and Social Psychology, 61,* 226–244.

Bender, D., Farber, B. A., & Geller, J. D. (2001). Cluster B personality traits and attachment. *Journal of the American Academy of Psychoanalysis, 29,* 551–563.

Bernier, A., & Dozier, M. (2002). The client–counselor match and the corrective emotional experience: Evidence from interpersonal and attachment research. *Psychotherapy: Theory, Research, Practice, Training, 39,* 32–43.

Berano, K., & Farber, B. A. (2006, June). *A comparison of Asian-American and Caucasian-American patterns of disclosure in psychotherapy.* Paper presented at the meeting of the Society for Psychotherapy Research, Edinburgh, Scotland, UK.

Bowlby, J. (1973). *Attachment and loss: Vol. 2. Separation: Anxiety and anger.* New York: Basic Books.

Bowlby, J. (1977). The making and breaking of affectional bonds: II. Some principles of psychotherapy. *British Journal of Psychiatry, 130,* 421–431.

Bowlby, J. (1982). *Attachment and Loss: Vol. 1. Attachment* (2nd ed.). New York: Basic Books. (1st ed., 1969)

Bowlby, J. (1988). *A secure base: Parent–child attachment and healthy human development.* New York: Basic Books.

Cassidy, J. (1999). The nature of the child's ties. In J. Cassidy & P. R. Shaver (Eds.), *Handbook of attachment: Theory, research, and clinical applications* (pp. 3–20). New York: Guilford Press.

Cyranowski, J. M., Bookwala, J., Feske, U., Houck, P., Pilkonis, P., Kostelnik, B., et al. (2002). Adult attachment profiles, interpersonal difficulties, and response to interpersonal psychotherapy in women with recurrent major depression. *Journal of Social and Clinical Psychology, 21,* 191–217.

Dozier, M., Cue, K. L., & Barnett, L. (1994). Clinicians as caregivers: Role of attachment organization in treatment. *Journal of Consulting and Clinical Psychology, 62,* 793–800.

Dozier, M., & Tyrrell, C. (1998). The role of attachment in therapeutic relationships. In J. A. Simpson & W. S. Rholes (Eds.), *Attachment theory and close relationships* (pp. 221–248). New York: Guilford Press.

Eames, V., & Roth, A. (2000). Patient attachment orientation and the early working alliance: A study of patient and therapist reports of alliance quality and ruptures. *Psychotherapy Research, 10,* 421–434.

Farber, B. A. (2003). Patient self-disclosure: A review of the research. *Journal of Clinical Psychology, 59,* 589–600.

Farber, B. A. (2006). *Self-disclosure in psychotherapy.* New York: Guilford Press.

Farber, B. A., Berano, K. C., & Capobianco, J. A. (2004). Clients' perceptions of the process and consequences of self-disclosure in psychotherapy. *Journal of Counseling Psychology, 51,* 340–346.

Farber, B. A., & Geller, J. D. (1994). Gender and representation in psychotherapy. *Psychotherapy, 31,* 318–326.

Farber, B. A., Lippert, R. A., & Nevas, D. B. (1995). The therapist as an attachment figure. *Psychotherapy, 32,* 204–212.

Farber, B. A., & Sohn, A. (1997, August). *Patient disclosure and denial: A delicate balance.* Paper presented at the annual convention of the American Psychological Association, Chicago.

Firestone, R. (2000, July 23). Mockingbird years. *The New York Times Book Review* (Letters), p. 4.

Fonagy, P., Leigh, T., Steele, M., Steele, H., Kennedy, R., Mattoon, G., et al. (1996). The relation of attachment status, psychiatric classification, and response to psychotherapy. *Journal of Consulting and Clinical Psychology, 64,* 22–31.

Frank, J. D. (1974). *Persuasion and healing, A comparative study of psychotherapy* (rev. ed.). New York: Schocken Books.

Geller, J. D., & Farber, B. A. (1993). Factors influencing the process of internalization in psychotherapy. *Psychotherapy Research, 3,* 166–180.

George, C., Kaplan, N., & Main, M. (1984). *Adult Attachment Interview protocol.* Unpublished manuscript, University of California, Berkeley.

George, C., Kaplan, N., & Main, M. (1985). *Adult Attachment Interview protocol* (2nd ed.). Unpublished manuscript, University of California, Berkeley.

George, C., Kaplan, N., & Main, M. (1996). *Adult Attachment Interview protocol* (3rd ed.). Unpublished manuscript, University of California, Berkeley.

Grabill, C. M., & Kerns, K. A. (2000). Attachment style and intimacy in friendship. *Personal Relationships, 7,* 363–378.

Hazan, C., Gur-Yaish, N., & Campa, M. (2004). What does it mean to be attached? In W. S. Rholes & J. A. Simpson (Eds.), *Adult attachment: Theory, research, and clinical implications* (pp. 55–85). New York: Guilford Press.

Hill, C. E., Gelso, C. J., & Mohr, J. J. (2000). Client concealment and self-presentation in therapy: Comment on Kelly (2000). *Psychological Bulletin, 126,* 495–500.

Hill, C. E., Thompson, B. J., Cogar, M., & Denman, D. W. (1993). Beneath the surface of long-term therapy: Therapist and client reports of their own and each other's covert processes. *Journal of Counseling Psychology, 40,* 278–287.

Horvath, A. O., & Bedi, R. P. (2002). The alliance. In J. C. Norcross (Ed.), *Psychotherapy relationships that work: Therapist contributions and responsiveness to patients* (pp. 37–69). New York: Oxford University Press.

Horvath, A., & Greenberg, L. (1991). Development and validation of the Working Alliance Inventory. *Journal of Counseling Psychology, 36,* 223–233.

Keelan, J. P. R., Dion, K. K., & Dion K. L. (1998). Attachment style and relationship satisfaction: Test of a self-disclosure explanation. *Canadian Journal of Behavioural Science, 30,* 24–35.

Kohut, H. (1971). *The analysis of the self: A systematic approach to the psychoana-*

lytic treatment of narcissistic personality disorders. New York: International Universities Press.

Leiper, R., & Casares, P. (2000). An investigation of the attachment organization of clinical psychologists and its relationship to clinical practice. *British Journal of Medical Psychology, 73,* 449–464.

Mackie, A. J. (1981). Attachment theory: Its relevance to the therapeutic alliance. *British Journal of Medical Psychology, 54,* 203–212.

Mallinckrodt, B., Gantt, D. L., & Coble, H. M. (1995). Attachment patterns in the psychotherapy relationship: Development of the Client Attachment to Therapist Scale. *Journal of Counseling Psychology, 42,* 307–317.

Mallinckrodt, B., Porter, M. J., & Kivlighan, D. M., Jr. (2005). Client attachment to therapist, depth of in-session exploration, and object relations in brief psychotherapy. *Psychotherapy: Theory, Research, Practice, Training, 42,* 85–100.

McCluskey, U., Hooper, C. A., & Miller, L. B. (1999). Goal-corrected empathic attunement: Developing and rating the concept within an attachment perspective. *Psychotherapy, 36,* 80–90.

Mikulincer, M., & Nachshon, O. (1991). Attachment styles and patterns of self-disclosure. *Journal of Personality and Social Psychology, 61,* 321–331.

Mikulincer, M., & Shaver, P. R. (2003). The attachment behavioral system in adulthood: Activation, psychodynamics, and interpersonal processes. In M. P. Zanna (Ed.), *Advances in experimental social psychology* (Vol. 36, pp. 53–152). San Diego, CA: Academic Press.

Norcross, J. C. (Ed.). (2002). *Psychotherapy relationships that work: Therapist contributions and responsiveness to patients.* New York: Oxford University Press.

Obegi, J. H. (in press). The development of the client–therapist bond through the lens of attachment theory. *Psychotherapy Theory, Research, Practice, Training.*

Parish, M. (2000). The nature of the patient's ties to the therapist. *Dissertation Abstracts International, 60,* 6378-B.

Parish, M., & Eagle, M. N. (2003). Attachment to the therapist. *Psychoanalytic Psychology, 20,* 271–286.

Pattee, D., & Farber, B. A. (2004, November). *Gender and client self-disclosure in psychotherapy.* Paper presented at the meeting of the Society for Psychotherapy Research (North American Chapter), Springdale, UT.

Quintana, S. M., & Meara, N. M. (1990). Internationalization of therapeutic relationships in short-term therapy. *Journal of Counseling Psychology, 37,* 123–130.

Reis, S., & Grenyer, B. (2004). Fearful attachment, working alliance and treatment response for individuals with major depression. *Clinical Psychology and Psychotherapy, 11,* 414–424.

Rogers, C. (1957). The necessary and sufficient conditions of therapeutic personality change. *Journal of Consulting Psychology, 21,* 95–103.

Rosenzweig, D. L., Farber, B. A., & Geller, J. D. (1996). Clients' representations of their therapists over the course of psychotherapy. *Journal of Clinical Psychology, 52,* 197–207.

Rubino, G., Barker, C., Roth, T., & Fearon, P. (2000). Therapist empathy and depth of interpretation in response to potential alliance ruptures: The role of therapist and patient attachment styles. *Psychotherapy Research, 10,* 408–420.

Safran, J. D., Muran, J. C., Samstag, L. W., & Stevens, C. (2002). Repairing alliance ruptures. In J. C. Norcross (Ed.), *Psychotherapy relationships that work: Therapist contributions and responsiveness to patients* (pp. 235–244). New York: Oxford University Press.

Satterfield, W. A., & Lyddon, W. J. (1998). Client attachment and the working alliance. *Counseling Psychology Quarterly, 11*, 407–415.

Sauer, E. M., Lopez, F. G., & Gormley, B. (2003). Respective contributions of therapist and client adult attachment orientations to the development of the early working alliance: A preliminary growth modeling study. *Psychotherapy Research, 13*, 371–382.

Scarvalone, P., Fox, M., & Safran, J. D. (2005). Interpersonal schemas: Clinical theory, research, and implications. In M. W. Baldwin (Ed.), *Interpersonal cognition* (pp. 359–387). New York: Guilford Press.

Shane, M. G., & Shane, M. (2001). The attachment motivational system as a guide to an effective therapeutic process. *Psychoanalytic Inquiry, 21*, 675–687.

Shostrom, E. L. (Producer). (1965). *Three approaches to psychotherapy (Part 2)* [Film]. Orange, CA: Psychological Films.

Tyrrell, C. L., Dozier, M., Teague, G. B., & Fallot, R. D. (1999). Effective treatment relationships for persons with serious psychiatric disorders: The importance of attachment states of mind. *Journal of Consulting and Clinical Psychology, 67*, 725–733.

Weiss, J. (1993). *How psychotherapy works: Process and technique.* New York: Guilford Press.

Winnicott, D. W. (1965). Ego distortion in terms of true and false self. In D. W. Winnicott (Ed.), *The maturational processes and the facilitating environment* (pp. 140–152). New York: International Universities Press. (Original work published 1960)

Woodhouse, S., Schlosser, L. Z., Crook, R. E., Ligiero, D. P., & Gelso, C. J. (2003). Client attachment to therapist: Relations to transference and client recollections of parental caregiving. *Journal of Counseling Psychology, 50*, 395–408.

4

Attachment, Mentalization, and Reflective Functioning

Elliot L. Jurist
Kevin B. Meehan

Mentalization theory represents an important new contribution to the field of clinical psychology. It offers a developmental perspective on psychopathology and provides guidance in terms of technique and treatment, integrating ideas and research from psychoanalytic theory and attachment theory—two theories that originally were not regarded as compatible. Moreover, mentalization theory is grounded in ideas and debates from neuroscience, cognitive psychology, and philosophy, and thus ought to be recognized as a theory that is truly interdisciplinary in scope (Jurist, 2008). Although mentalization theory has primarily been applied to the treatment of borderline personality disorder (BPD), it has broader ramifications for treating other kinds of psychopathology and carrying out therapeutic interventions. The notion of *mentalized affectivity* is used here to support the case for the wide-ranging significance of mentalization theory. Mentalized affectivity is the capacity to reflect on the meaning of affective states—a capacity that is closely related to affect regulation, since it is fair to presume that trying to understand affects will help people to be able to modify how these are experienced. Although mentalized affectivity is a new concept, all forms of psychotherapy aim to expand it, whether implicitly or explicitly.

In the first part of this chapter, we elaborate the issues described above by placing mentalization theory in the context of its roots in developmental research, neuroscience, and philosophy. In the second part of this chapter, we discuss recent research findings on reflective function (RF), the operationalization of mentalization, and the implications of both of these for our developing understanding of the concept. In the third part of this chapter, we discuss recent clinical applications of mentalization theory, using clinical examples and vignettes. In the conclusions, we consider some unresolved issues regarding mentalization that future study will need to address.

MENTALIZATION THEORY

The term *mentalization* is used by Peter Fonagy (2006) to capture the process of how the brain becomes a mind. More specifically, mentalization delineates the transformation in the child's emerging capacity to acknowledge and interpret the mind of another person, and to recognize the realm of the mental as representational. Fonagy's understanding of mentalization is grounded in early development, although it is a sensitive way of describing a crucial aspect of subjective experience for humans at any stage of life. According to Fonagy, the sociobiological origin of mentalization can be traced to competition, which originally spurred humans to be invested in reading the intentions of others, and later evolved further to help them negotiate complex social interactions.

Mentalization unfolds in the context of early relationships. The attachment bond between infant and caregiver provides a sense of security, but the quality of parent–child interactions can promote or impede the development of mentalization (Fonagy, 2001). More specifically, the minds of caregivers themselves offer opportunities for infants to understand and begin to explore what it means that others have mental states, and to have a dawning sense that they too possess mental states. A *theory of mind* unfolds from attachment, beginning with *psychic equivalence,* wherein the child holds the belief that what exists in the mind must exist in the world. This is transformed through play, resulting in the appreciation that the mind shapes and interprets what is real and external to the self (Fonagy, 2001; Fonagy, Gergely, Jurist, & Target, 2002; Fonagy & Target, 1996).

So mentalization is a skill that allows one to interpret others' minds, which in turn fosters the ability to read and understand one's own mental states, especially those mental states that are based on emotions. Secure attachment facilitates the capacity to regulate affects; it presides over the movement from co-regulation to self-regulation. Initially, infants are dependent upon caregivers to help them contain strong negative affects and to promote tolerance for positive affects. As their capacity for affect regulation develops in the second half of the first year of life, the sense of self emerges, which in turn results in a better capacity for regulation. Affect regulation relies on discerning the intentions of others and learning to see oneself as a being with its own (affective) intentions. Thus it prepares the way for mentalization, which unfolds at about the age of 4 years, coinciding with the ability to identify false-belief tasks correctly.[1] According to Fonagy et al. (2002), affect regulation is the basis for mentalization; however, mentalization then fosters a new, more differentiated kind of affect and self-regulation, such as mentalized affectivity.

As a theory, mentalization offers a powerful tool for integrating ideas from attachment and psychoanalysis. Attachment theory has evolved beyond Bowlby's (1969/1982, 1980) original formulation that the goal of attachment is to provide proximity to the caregiver with the amendation of the goal of *felt security* (Sroufe, 1996; Sroufe & Waters, 1977). It has transcended a tendency toward *naïve realism,* the philosophical term for the belief that our minds reflect the world in a direct and unmediated way, in the way that *internal working models* have typically been construed. Main has spearheaded a movement to grapple with the realm of mental representation more seriously—for example, recognizing how the reworking of memory alters internal working models (Main, Kaplan & Cassidy, 1985).

Fonagy's proposal that the goal of attachment is to produce a representational system seems to reflect idealism, the opposite philosophical pole from realism, in affirming the belief that the way our minds work alters our perception and conception of reality (Fonagy, 2001; Fonagy et al., 2002). It is most perspicuous, in fact, to see Fonagy's proposal as incorporating elements of both realism and idealism, rather than siding with one over the other. For Fonagy, the realm of mental representation reflects Sandler and Rosenblatt's (1962/1987) affectively tinged notion of the *representational world,* incorporating both *fantasy* from psychoanalytic theory and *internal working models* from attachment theory. Fonagy views the representational system as deriving from cognitive–affective schemas, but it must also be understood in connection with theory-of-mind activities, such as social reality testing and imaginary play. His perspective mitigates differences that previously divided attachment theory and psychoanalysis.

Fonagy's understanding of the relation between attachment and mentalization has been evolving (Fonagy, 2006; Fonagy & Bateman, 2006). Originally, it was hypothesized that mentalization comes into being through secure attachment—that the very capacity for mentalization is rooted in the attachment relationship (Fonagy, 2001; Fonagy et al., 2002). Bateman and Fonagy (2004) viewed attachment as propelling cognitive development (p. 58), and affirmed that mentalization is "greatly facilitated by secure attachment" (p. 72). A key part of this argument included the claim that borderline pathology is characterized by a lack of mentalization—with the capacity to mentalize at times failing, while at other times manifesting itself as a *pseudomentalization* (i.e., mentalization characterized by hypervigilant monitoring of others, but no realistic understanding of their mental states).

More recently, Fonagy and Bateman (2006) have shifted their thinking toward the notion that there is a "loose coupling" between attachment and mentalization. They acknowledge that the neural systems underlying mentalization and attachment not only are separate, but also may also have a mutually inhibiting impact on one another. Following Bartels and Zeki (2004), Fonagy and Bateman (2006) posit that *neural system A*—which includes the middle prefrontal, inferior parietal, and middle temporal cortices mainly in the right hemisphere, as well as the posterior cingulate cortex—functions to integrate cognition and emotions, and may contribute to the typology of attachment. The second system, *neural system B,* includes the temporal poles, parietotemporal junction, amygdala, and mesial prefrontal cortex; it is activated by negative emotion, judgments of social trustworthiness, moral judgments, theory-of-mind tasks, and attention to one's own emotions. Fonagy and Bateman note that neural systems A and B have a reciprocal relationship in which the activation of system A leads to the inhibition of system B. In other words, the neural system that underlies the ability to recognize and interpret one's own mental states as well as the mental states of others is deactivated by the activation of the attachment system.

Fonagy and Bateman (2006) squarely face the potential conflict between findings of a "positive correlation" between attachment and mentalization, and the fact that they exist in a reciprocal relationship. However, there is nothing contradictory, according to these authors, in recognizing that secure attachment promotes the development of mentalization in such a way that the attachment system can be put aside in favor of mentalization. Secure attachment affords a child the opportunity to experiment with mentalization in a setting where the stakes are lower than in the real world (i.e., the child can count on the regard of the attachment figure). As Fonagy (2006) suggests, evolution has selected attachment as the "principal training ground" for the acquisition of mentalization. Indeed, persons with BPD get into trouble because their attachment systems become hyperactivated precisely when being able to mentalize would help them avoid acting out. A significant revision of borderline pathology follows here: It is not so much that patients with BPD lack the capacity to mentalize, but that for these patients the capacity to mentalize becomes inhibited by the heightened activation of the attachment system.

This qualification in Fonagy's thinking betokens the emergence of a more complex model of mentalization. Fonagy (2006) speculates about underlying neurocognitive aspects of mentalization—including the capacity to withhold impulsive responses, as well as *selective attention,* first proposed by Leslie (2000)—from which he traces a detailed outline of the evolution of the concept developmentally. Fonagy suggests, but does not develop, a two-level system that defines mentalization: a *frontocortical system* that involves declarative representation, and a *mirror neuron system,* which provides a more immediate and direct understanding of others (p. 58).

It is important to appreciate that Fonagy imports the idea of mentalization from the theory-of-mind literature in neuroscience, cognitive psychology, and philosophy (Frith & Happé, 1994; Harris, 1989), where the emphasis is more on cognition—that is, on awareness of thoughts and beliefs. Two alternative points of view can be differentiated in the theory-of-mind literature: *theory-theory* and *simulation theory* (Baron-Cohen, Tager-Flusberg, & Cohen, 2000; Carruthers & Smith, 1996).

According to the proponents of theory-theory, the capacity to interpret the mind of another is based upon formulating a theory of how minds work, which corresponds to our shared beliefs or "folk psychology." Some theory-theory proponents liken the child to a scientist who formulates a theory and then tests it in the real world (Gopnik, 1993; Gopnik, Capps, & Meltzoff, 2000). According to simulationists, the capacity to interpret the mind of another is predicated upon placing oneself in the other person's situation. Simulationists argue that we extrapolate from ourselves in reading others and that no theory is necessary. Mentalization, in this account, relies on our imaginative ability to put ourselves in the "mental shoes" of others (Goldman, 2006). Gordon (1996) emphasizes that the virtue of the simulationist view is that it is based on so-called "hot cognition," which includes emotions, rather than on "cold cognition," which the theory-theory presumes.

The debate between these two positions continues to the present, and we do not review the arguments in any detail here. One key new development is the challenge to the linchpin of the theory-theory position: that caution needs to be exercised in interpreting "false beliefs" experiments based upon switched-location tasks (see endnote 1), given research that supports an appreciation of mentalizing abilities in children under 4 years old (Gergely & Unoka, 2008, Onishi & Baillargeon, 2005). It should be noted that evidence in support of early mentalization does not mean that there is not an important shift taking place at 4–5 years of age. What it seems to suggest, however, is that mentalization is not ideally conceived of as an either–or capacity, but as a continuum from immature to mature forms of mentalizing.

It is important to clarify the differences between the psychoanalytic and the theory-of-mind approaches to mentalization. The psychoanalytic approach to mentalization highlights the interaction between parent and child; that is, the child learns to mentalize because the parent has mentalized about the child. Mentalization is understood to be as much about reading oneself as it is about reading others. The psychoanalytic approach also places a greater emphasis on emotions, which are constitutive of relationships. Simulationists pay attention to emotions, but they do not go far enough in recognizing their centrality in terms of the self. The psychoanalytic approach is based upon attachment style—that is, on characteristic and consistent patterns of responses that govern specific emotional behaviors and expressions. We return to this point in connection with mentalized affectivity.

RESEARCH ON MENTALIZATION

Mentalization has been operationalized by Fonagy and colleagues (Fonagy et al., 1995; Fonagy, Steele, Steele, & Target, 1998). The Reflective Function (RF) Scale was developed to empirically measure the capacity to mentalize the thoughts, intentions, feelings and beliefs of oneself and of others in the context of attachment relationships. This scale has been applied to transcripts of the Adult Attachment Interview (AAI), a semistructured clinical interview assessing early attachment relationships (George, Kaplan, & Main, 1984, 1985, 1996).

The RF Scale identifies four dimensions of RF: explicit efforts to make connections between mental states underlying behavior ("Well, I think he felt obligated to do that because he felt guilty ..."); awareness of the characteristics and limitations of recognizing mental states ("... or at least that's how it appeared; sometimes you feel different inside from how things appear"); acknowledgment of the impact of development on mental states ("It's only as an adult that I understand this; as a child I was confused why he did that"); and recognition of mental states in relation to the interviewer ("I'm not sure if that makes sense to you; should I explain further?"). Passages are rated on a scale of −1 (negative RF—concrete, totally barren of mentalization, or grossly distorting of the mental states of others) to 9 (exceptional RF—complex, elaborate, or original reasoning about mental states), and these scores are then aggregated to provide an overall score for the transcript.

The role of RF has been examined in relation to adult attachment security and its implications for infant attachment patterns in the Strange Situation (Ainsworth, Blehar, Waters, & Wall, 1978). Fonagy and colleagues (Fonagy, Steele, & Steele, 1991; Fonagy, Steele, Steele, Moran, & Higgitt, 1991) found that mothers who were classified as secure on the AAI and who had high RF when discussing their own attachment history were more likely to have infants who showed more secure-base behaviors in the Strange Situation. Furthermore, mothers classified as insecure on the AAI were more likely to have securely attached babies when their RF was high (Fonagy, Steele, Steele, Moran, et al., 1991).

Consistent with this finding, Slade and colleagues (Slade, Grienenberger, Bernbach, Levy, & Locker, 2005; Grienenberger, Kelly, & Slade, 2005) found that mothers who exhibited high RF in discussing their relationships with their infants on the Parent Development Interview (Aber, Slade, Berger, Bresgi, & Kaplan, 1985) were more likely to have infants categorized as secure in the Strange Situation. They also found that mothers' RF mediated the relationship between atypical maternal behaviors (i.e., fearful/disorganized behaviors, role or boundary confusion, intrusiveness, withdrawal) and attachment security in their infants. Taken together, these findings indicate that a mother's capacity to mentalize the experience of her child may function as a buffer against intense, overwhelming, or disorganizing experiences that have the potential to interfere with the development of a secure internal working model of attachment.

Additional research on the potential buffering effect of RF comes from studies of clinical populations of adults. In a sample of psychiatric inpatients, Fonagy et al. (1996) found that RF mediated the relationship between early experiences of abuse and the later development of BPD; abused patients with lower RF were more likely to be diagnosed with BPD than patients who were abused but evidenced higher RF. In a study of a forensic population, Levinson and Fonagy (2004) found that prisoners evidenced lower RF than that of patient populations, and that violent offenders evidenced the greatest deficits in RF. The authors note that in response to experiences of severe childhood trauma, the capacity to mentalize in an attachment context may be inhibited, and this impairment in reflective capacity may lead to acting in an impulsive or violent manner.

However, the relationship between RF and trauma remains unclear. In a study of maternal representations of children in a sample of traumatized women, Schechter et al. (2005) found that while RF and severity of violence-related PTSD symptoms were each found to independently predict the level of integration of mothers' representations of their children, RF and the severity of PTSD symptoms were not correlated with each other. Furthermore, in a sample of patients with BPD, Levy et al. (2006) found that RF was unrelated to lack of resolution of loss and trauma on the AAI. These findings are surprising, given the fact that many links have been theorized among mentalization, trauma, and the coherence and integration of object representations (Fonagy et al., 2002). Further research will be necessary to delineate whether these constructs interact with one another (and, if so, how) or whether they function independently.

Bateman and Fonagy (2004) hypothesize a relationship between RF and the capacity to inhibit an urge to respond to stimuli impulsively. Preliminary data from Levy et al. (2005) on a series of computer-based neurocognitive tasks—the Wisconsin Card Sorting Test (WCST; Heaton, 1981) and the Conners' Continuous Performance Test II (CPTII; Conners & Multi-Health Systems Staff, 2002)—lend support to this notion. On the CPTII, in a sample of clients with BPD and comparison groups, it was found that a low RF score correlated with impulsivity but not with sustained attention. On the WCST, a low RF score was correlated with more perseverative errors and failures in maintaining the set, both of which indicate problems using feedback to either maintain or shift to more accurate behavioral patterns. Taken together, these findings indicate that while low RF is not associated with a general impairment of attention, there may be a relationship between RF and the capacity to inhibit one's immediate response in order to assess and respond to feedback, including both internal appraisals and data from the environment.

Recent research indicates that the capacity to mentalize may improve during the course of psychotherapy. Levy et al. (2006), in a study comparing Kernberg's transference-focused psychotherapy (TFP) to supportive psychotherapy and dialectical behavior therapy, found that only clients in TFP evidenced significant increases in RF after 1 year of treatment. The change in RF noted exclusively in TFP is hypothesized to be related to this treatment's explicit focus on integrating disparate object representations, which should lead to a greater capacity to reflect on one's own and others' thoughts, intentions, feelings, and beliefs.

Furthermore, Meehan (2007) found that in TFP there was a sufficient but not overwhelming degree of emotional engagement in the relationship between client and therapist within which this change in RF occurred. Positive change in RF was predicted by therapists' ratings of optimal emotional engagement (i.e., there was connectedness but not overinvolvement) and an optimal level of affect in treatment (i.e., sessions were neither emotionally barren nor laden with negative affect). Based on these findings, Meehan speculated that the improvement in RF that was unique to TFP could be attributed to TFP's explicit effort to promote RF (via clarifications, confrontations, and interpretations) in the context of heightened but modulated affective moments in the attachment relationship with the therapist.

Reflective capacity has been found to change as a function not only of treatment type, but also of client characteristics. Vermote (2005), who analyzed RF in the transcripts of therapy sessions, identified a differential pattern of change in *anaclitic* clients, who struggle with issues of relatedness, and *introjective* clients, who struggle with issues of self-definition (Blatt & Ford, 1994). Whereas introjective clients progressively increased their reflective capacity over the course of treatment, anaclitic clients showed a decrease in their reflective capacity in the early stage of treatment, but this gradually improved as treatment went on. Vermote notes that this decreased RF corresponds with anaclitic clients' displaying a regression to a more primitive level of functioning within the treatment.

CLINICAL APPLICATIONS OF MENTALIZATION THEORY

The theory of mentalization has been applied most extensively to borderline pathology. Bateman and Fonagy (2004) have manualized what they call *mentalization-based treatment* (MBT), and initial research has demonstrated positive outcomes for the treatment of BPD. In an 18-month treatment, partially hospitalized patients with BPD who received MBT demonstrated significant improvement compared to a control group across a range of outcome measures: fewer suicide attempts and acts of self-harm; fewer and shorter inpatient admissions; decreased use of psychotropic medication; decreased self-reports of depression; anxiety, and general symptom distress; improved interpersonal functioning; and improved social adjustment (Bateman & Fonagy, 1999). Even more impressive, however, is that in a follow-up study evaluating whether the gains were sustained, the clients actually had a statistically significant continued improvement on most measures compared to the control group (Bateman & Fonagy, 2001).

Bateman and Fonagy (2004) deliver MBT to clients with BPD in the context of an integrated hospital-based day treatment program that combines individual therapy, analytic group therapy, and medication management. Although each client has a primary therapist, it is more accurate to say that the client is working with a treatment team whose members impart a mentalizing stance to every aspect of the client's care. However, Bateman and Fonagy suggest that most of the principles behind this treatment are transferable to working privately with patients with BPD.

The goal of MBT is to help clients adopt a mentalizing stance in the service of developing a more stable sense of self and more secure relationships. This involves inviting patients to become curious about their thoughts, intentions, and beliefs, and especially their awareness of manifest affects about themselves and others. Clients are often asked to reflect on disparities between their internal affective experience and the external expression of affect outside their awareness. The focus of treatment is thus on the here and now, and while the past may be discussed, it is in the service of better elucidating the clients' present experience.

As in other contemporary dynamic therapies, MBT focuses on the transference in the here and now; however, in contrast to other treatments, MBT emphasizes that for clients with BPD the transference is experienced as "real" and "accurate," and therefore should be responded to as such. Rather than challenging the aspects of the transference that involve distortion or displacement from past experiences, MBT focuses on the self-protective function of the transference and works with it to help a client stay in and progress in treatment. It should be noted that MBT emphasizes a consistent and reliable treatment structure, as this stability assists clients (and therapists) in adopting a mentalizing stance and protects the treatment from boundary transgressions.

Mentalization theory has also been applied clinically to parenting programs, with the goal of helping mothers increase their capacity to reflect on the internal experience of their children. Slade (2006) notes that while most effective interventions with parents implicitly encourage increased RF, recent programs based on mentalization theory explicitly engage parents in taking a reflective stance toward their children. Treatment for low-risk mothers typically occurs in group settings (Goyette-Ewing et al., 2003; Grienenberger et al., 2004). Mothers are encouraged to be curious about their children's internal states and thoughts, rather than to focus solely on the children's manifest behaviors. In a treatment for high-risk mothers called Minding the Baby (Slade, Sadler, & Mayes, 2005), weekly home visits that promote the emotional and physical health of mother and child foster an increased level of stability in the home, which has been found to support a secure, reflective environment in which the child can internalize a sense of security. In other words, being mindful of the mother's own needs allows that mother to attend more closely to the needs of her child.

Though the treatments described by Slade (2006) involve organized treatments for mothers, the principles of reflective parenting can be applied to individual therapy with children and their families as well.

Clinical Vignette on Promoting Reflective Parenting

Chris was a 9-year-old boy being raised by a single mother with his two siblings. He presented for individual treatment with one of us (Kevin B. Meehan, the "I" in what follows) with a then-undiagnosed attention disorder that led to significant behavioral problems and intense frustration on the part of his mother, who could not understand why her son acted in the ways that he did. During the initial stages of treatment (which included neuropsychological testing to determine his attention problems), the therapy focused on helping Chris through words and play to develop a language for his experience of feeling "confused" and his attempts to ground himself at such times with repetitive behaviors (e.g., doodling, singing, digging holes with a pen) that got him in trouble at school.

Chris came into a session one day playing his Game Boy. When I asked him about it, he said, "Why is everybody always talking about my game? No way! No! Nope!" and then began to mumble about how he got in trouble with a teacher for playing his game at school, angering his mother. I said, "I think that sometimes when you feel 'confused,' you play your Game Boy or sing to help distract you from what you're worried about, and if you focus on the game or singing, you don't have to think about what's worrying you." His face lit up as he responded, "Can you tell my mother that? Don't say no!" He then pulled out the pad and wrote, "When Chris sings or play his game he calms down. Mr. Kevin will explain it to Chris's mother." He gave the paper to me and told me to practice, and then took the paper back and added the line "Practice saying it."

In the following session, Chris and I decided that we would invite his mother to a session for the first 5 minutes. I prepared her for the meeting by telling her that Chris and I had been recently talking about things that he wanted to share with her. I let her know that Chris was a little nervous about the meeting, and that therefore he might drift off as if he was not paying attention, but that this was fine.

A week later, his mother joined us at the beginning of the session. As we were walking to the room, his mother reported that Chris had been in trouble at school that day for knocking his papers all over the floor. When we entered the room, Chris immediately began anxiously to play basketball and did not make eye contact with either me or his mother. I said to his mother:

> "We wanted to talk to you about when Chris has difficulty, like he had at school today. When he gets stressed and overwhelmed, he doesn't look like what other kids who are stressed look like. He glazes over, looks clumsy, and that's when he has trouble controlling himself. Like now, he was worried about this meeting, and I think we're seeing some of that right now. [He looked extremely clumsy while playing his basketball game.] When he gets overwhelmed, it's hard for him to control

himself. Me and Chris were talking about one way he tries to calm himself down is by singing or playing his Game Boy. He's really trying to behave and control himself, and with the Game Boy he seems to try to calm himself down by focusing on that and tuning out everything else that's worrying him. The Game Boy and singing aren't the best ways to do that; sometimes they get him in trouble. But right now it's the best he can do, and that is him trying really hard to control himself. But he's worried that other people see what he's doing and think he's trying to be bad, when really this is him trying to calm himself down."

She was quite moved by this, and she called Chris over and gave him a hug with misty eyes. We talked for a few more minutes about a discussion that his mother had with his teacher. As his mother stood to leave, she hugged Chris again. After she left, Chris said that the meeting was "the coolest," but seemed not to want to talk about what had happened. However, he seemed happy as we played the basketball game for the rest of the session.

As illustrated by this vignette, the clinical aim of intervention is to help the mother (or other caregiver) increase her capacity to reflect on her child's internal experience rather than focus solely on manifest behaviors. When Chris's mother was helped to shift her focus from Chris's playing his Game Boy to the anxiety underlying this behavior, she was able to respond more empathically. Furthermore, this intervention helped Chris internalize a sense that his thoughts and feelings could be identified, put into words, and communicated to others.

A focus on helping the caretakers of children shift away from responding to manifest behaviors and toward reflecting on the children's internal experience has also been applied to school settings. Twemlow, Fonagy, and Sacco (2005) have developed the Peaceful Schools project, which is designed to address school bullying and aggressive behavior among peers by helping teachers create a mentalizing environment that encourages reflective rather than reactive responses from both children and teachers.

It is reasonable to expect that in the near future, we will see theorists apply mentalization theory's explanatory power to other forms of psychopathology. Mentalization is surely germane to any personality-based pathology in which reading and interpreting others accurately are at the source of the problem. For example, Fonagy (2006) has been focusing more attention on trauma and recently has turned his attention to eating disorders. There is also some emerging work on applying mentalization theory to substance abuse and dependence (Jurist, 2007; Allen, 2006).

Clinical Vignette on Substance Dependence

Barbara was a woman in her early 40s who was seen in psychotherapy by one of us (Elliot L. Jurist, the "I" in what follows). She had grown up in

Scotland and came to the United States along with her husband because he was offered an ideal job opportunity. She had had a stellar career in business before they left London, but she never worked in this country, and her drinking escalated over the course of a decade while she was home alone with their treasured dog (they had no children). Barbara drank only white wine—but up to three or four bottles a day—prior to entering a detoxification unit. Her alcohol intoxication initially served to make her feel less depressed and lonely, but the results of it, not surprisingly, exacerbated both. After completing detox Barbara was referred to me as a substance abuse specialist. She was dubious about psychotherapy, but a bit less dubious than she was about a Twelve-Step program (which she had previously tried and loathed). When I inquired about her substance use and asked whether she had used any other drugs besides alcohol, she looked at me as if I were nuts.

Barbara was a shy, proper woman who rarely revealed her internal suffering to anyone, including her husband. She was the daughter of strict parents. Her mother in particular abhorred alcohol, though she was the daughter of a pub owner. Her father was more kindly, but remote. Barbara showed signs of avoidance in the transference, and this was confirmed by stories she told about growing up in a cool atmosphere in which there was no room for expressed feelings. From an early stage, Barbara had sought gratification through success at school, and she was proud of having been an excellent student. Since she had had a serious and challenging job before moving to the United States, it perplexed me that she never worked here. Over time, it emerged that Barbara had already developed a fairly serious problem with alcohol even before her move, which she had taken precautions to hide. Barbara sustained a pseudoindependence through adolescence and young adulthood, masking her problems by overmodulating and barely expressing affects.

My treatment with Barbara went well at first. She maintained 7 months of sobriety, but then traveled back to London on a business trip with her husband and suffered a lapse that verged on a relapse. She returned to the States and was able to become sober again for a brief period of a month or so. Subsequently, she had another relapse and underwent detox again. We resumed work together until she suffered another relapse about 5 months later. When her husband threatened to divorce Barbara over her drinking problems, she finally consented to inpatient treatment. She has not resumed outpatient psychotherapy since then, as far as I am aware.

The vicissitudes of Barbara's experience in psychotherapy were not so unusual for a person with serious substance dependence. In one sense, her addiction overpowered her readiness and willingness to receive help, confirming the standard wisdom that psychotherapy is more effective once substance use problems have been brought under control. In another, very important sense, however, psychotherapy had an impact on Barbara's life, and we made significant progress in understanding what was underlying her need to use alcohol during the last 5 months of the treatment. This makes me hopeful for Barbara in the future.

Through psychotherapy, Barbara greatly improved her awareness of the cost of her style of attachment and affect regulation. She was able to see how her avoidant attachment style made it difficult to connect with her family and husband—and how it both precipitated and was reinforced by her drinking. Barbara used alcohol as a way to alleviate painful feelings, but she came to appreciate how obscuring feelings was not a successful strategy for making them disappear. Barbara struggled to identify affects as they occurred; she also had trouble expressing them, and my work involved helping her to stay with and make sense of her feelings and not to be afraid of revealing them.

Barbara and I had a crucial interaction that occurred after she had lapsed in London and then returned to New York and suffered another relapse. Barbara's description of her relapse in New York was as follows: She was coming from the gym and instructed her taxi driver to take a detour, during which, it just so happened, they passed her favorite liquor store. What ensued was predictable: She stopped, bought several bottles of wine, and immediately went home and drank them. At first, Barbara insisted that she had acted impulsively, without premeditation. As a matter of fact, she brusquely dismissed the idea that something might have precipitated her choice. I was persistent, and this led her to see the self-deception that she had perpetrated on herself. Barbara became tearful as she reported that during her workout she became distracted after seeing a man who reminded her of an ex-boyfriend—a man whom she had loved but had become aloof with over time. This set off a chain of thoughts that left her feeling vulnerable and unnerved, which she tried to push aside; she then found herself in a desperate state of mind and in need of some way to comfort herself.

This was a key moment in psychotherapy. We had discussed what prompted previous relapses, but this time was different—partly because the incident was raw, but mainly, I think, because Barbara glimpsed the complexity of her internal life and was becoming more vulnerable and able to acknowledge her feelings. More specifically, Barbara came face to face with how her attempts to banish her emotions—both at the gym and in her relationship with the old boyfriend—had backfired and hurt her. We were able to explore how she had suffered in her family because her parents had been so unresponsive to her needs, discouraging her from seeking their help. Barbara was inching toward mentalized affectivity in opening herself to how her family culture had left her ill equipped to deal with painful emotions, and how alcohol was a way to perpetuate this way of being in the world (albeit at great cost).

Barbara had serious alcohol dependence, and psychotherapy twice a week was not sufficient to help her overcome her addiction. Yet this certainly does not mean that Barbara did not benefit from psychotherapy. She became attached to me and began to show a warmth in her transference, noting that she appreciated the fact that I never dealt with her alcoholism in a moralistic way. At the time of her second detox, I took pleasure in hearing from her psychiatrist that he was impressed with the change he saw in Barbara—in particular, her investment in conveying her emotions. Barbara needed to have the immersion of an inpatient stay; however, her experience in psychotherapy facilitated her choice to make that decision for herself, which she had heretofore resisted. In recalling Barbara, my emotions pull toward great sadness—because the treatment was interrupted; because we never had the opportunity to resume it; and because such strong unmodulated feelings, I would surmise, might be displacements from her own overly regulated affective world.

During our work together, Barbara moved from skepticism to some openness about psychotherapy, which perhaps means that she might consider psychotherapy again in the future. In conclusion, my work with Barbara helped her to evolve away from reflexive avoidance of emotions to the realization that emotions are complex, rich, and worth understanding. We were still in an early stage of developing mentalized affectivity, but she clearly took a few steps in this direction.

In terms of the broader implications of mentalization theory, the concept seems to be clinically relevant not just to specific kinds of psychopathology, but to psychotherapy in general. One argument in support of this notion is the fact that all treatment involves the enhancement of affect regulation (given the extent to which virtually all forms of suffering can be construed in terms of affect dysregulation). Emotions are more exposed in the clinical realm than in everyday life; they are both lived and recalled, and it is a crucial part of all psychotherapy to help clients to recognize, manage, and modulate them. Mentalization theory, under the influence of psychoanalysis, emphasizes that such regulation is not simply about emotions. Ultimately, it is about exploring the self and the mind (Fonagy et al., 2002).

The exploration of the self and the mind is precisely where the concept of mentalized affectivity comes to the foreground (Fonagy et al., 2002; Jurist, 2005, 2008). Mentalized affectivity captures what is most challenging in adult affect regulation: that new meaning can be created and specified by reflecting upon affective experience. In engaging in such reflection, it is desirable to remain within or recapture the feeling of that state. The term suggests that this process is not simply a matter of exercising cognition over affective states. Mentalized affectivity is also not just a matter of modulating affects; it entails the struggle to revalue affects, which includes various elements such as naming, distinguishing, and expressing them inwardly and outwardly. The inward expression of emotions is particularly important, as it is crucial to know and experience what one feels, regardless of whether one acts on it or not. Let us illustrate this with an example.

One of our clients became aware of how angry he was at his wife for blaming him for her pregnancy; yet, just as he came to realize this, he also became aware that his wife was feeling too vulnerable to hear his reaction.

It was helpful for this client to recognize and experience his anger more fully than he had done, but it was equally important for him to confirm the choice not to convey his affect directly to his wife. In this instance, mentalized affectivity served to help the client know what he felt, and to appreciate that it was counterproductive to suppress his own reaction. This actually alleviated his impulse to have a confrontation with his wife.

Mentalized affectivity allows people to appreciate new meanings in old affects, but may lead to new or different affects. For example, a client who found herself engaging in conflicts with coworkers, and especially bosses, realized that this sort of thing happened particularly when she was anxious. She had never thought of herself as anxious, but this shift in self-understanding allowed her to monitor herself in situations where previously she would have asserted herself insensitively. It is fair to infer that an aim of mentalized affectivity is to promote positive affect, but it is also fair to presume that it should help individuals to be able to tolerate and cope with negative affect. One of the most striking aspects of mentalized affectivity is that it underscores the value of reinterpreting, not just labeling, altering, and acting on one's affects.

Underlying the concept of mentalized affectivity is the notion that affective experience is mediated by attachment style—in other words, that current (and future) affects are experienced through the lens of past experiences, both real and imagined. Some affects may well occur in a pure, universal form without such mediation, but this should not obscure the fact that affects are connected to relationships with others—sometimes in obvious ways, sometimes in ways that are hidden. Mentalized affectivity enables people to conceptualize an aspect of emotional experience that is not obvious: that such experience is often confusing, complex, and fluid.

Clinical Vignette on Mentalized Affectivity

Rob was a bright and sensitive young man in his mid-20s who came from a close family, which included a younger sister. Rob was particularly close to his mother; he remembered coming home from school and sitting down with her as she attentively listened to him describe his day while he enjoyed milk and cookies.

Rob began therapy with one of us (Elliot L. Jurist, again the "I" here) because he became depressed after splitting up with his girlfriend of 5 years. Their relationship had started during his freshman year in college—the same year, it turned out, that his parents announced their divorce. His parents informed him of their decision by flying out together to visit him and discussing their intention. Rob had had no idea that his parents' relationship was in trouble. The family dynamic mixed sensitive parenting with a strong undercurrent of needing conflict to be suppressed.

At first, Rob was somewhat resistant to my suggestion that he might be reexperiencing the pain of his parents' divorce through the current breakup with his girlfriend. But as he gained more distance from the end of the relationship and formed a connection to me, he began to realize that he had avoided dealing with his reactions to his parents' divorce. More specifically, Rob recalled how in college he threw himself into activity—his work, politics, and sports—right after the divorce. He had not had much experience with women up to that point, but soon commenced his first serious relationship (with the woman he broke up with just before entering treatment). A couple of years into the treatment, Rob became interested in how his depression at the end of this relationship had reactivated older feelings about his parents' divorce. Not only could he see that he had much stronger feelings about the divorce than he realized at the time, but he came to be in touch with his anger at his father, whom he saw as responsible for breaking up the family.

As his involvement in therapy deepened, Rob and I explored new and different angles of his past. His understanding of what had happened in his romantic relationship shifted. He began to reinterpret the breakup in terms of diverging interests between them and the inherent difficulty of sustaining a relationship that began in college, rather than as being "left" by his girlfriend. Rob eventually became able to acknowledge aspects of his own dissatisfaction in the relationship. He also became aware of some differences between his parents' divorce, which had occurred without warning and without his input, and the breakup of the relationship, which at least to some degree reflected his choice. Rob and I developed a complex interpretation of his flight into a relationship in the face of his parents' divorce. The relationship helped him to avoid feeling hopeless about relationships and to be a little less involved with his family in the aftermath of his parents' divorce, but it also served to distance himself from the full range of his feelings about the divorce. Finally, Rob developed insights about how the divorce, while looming largely in his late adolescent experience, itself reenacted much earlier developmental issues. The divorce had an aspect of being an Oedipal victory for him: His mother turned to him more during and after the divorce, and this heightened conflict between himself and his father. Yet the divorce also evoked intense anxiety, because Rob felt that it had forced him prematurely to fend for himself, and to do so with less support than he imagined he would have received if his parents had remained married.

Rob was and remained deeply sad about the breakup of his family. He wept in a session as he realized that leaving home for him coincided with there being no more home left. Over the next year, Rob moved from feeling despair about relationships and isolating himself to being sad on occasion but ready to move ahead in his life. He became involved in a new relationship. Our work began to focus more on his tendency to drift into thinking about how he should feel rather than staying with his genuine experience.

Since the divorce, Rob's mother had not gotten involved in a new relationship, and she remained very much involved in her children's lives. Rob's father did get remarried a few years ago, to a younger woman; his father made an effort to maintain a relationship with him, but Rob felt that it was perfunctory. Rob did not like his stepmother and resented that she controlled his father, although he was also critical of his father for allowing her to do so.

During a family gathering that concluded a long weekend together, Rob's father made an announcement in front of Rob and his younger sister (as well as their grandmother and some cousins) that startled Rob: His wife and he planned to adopt a baby. Rob was aware that they were contemplating having a child, but figured the matter had been resolved when his stepmother did not get pregnant. Rob had a negative reaction to how the issue of adopting a child was raised—just at the conclusion of the gathering, as if to ensure that there would be no discussion, causing him to feel doubly left out. In therapy, we considered whether Rob ought to disclose his feelings to his father. He wrote his father a letter; his father answered promptly with an e-mail—not responding to what Rob said, but affirming the value in talking and openly exchanging their opinions.

No heart-to-heart talk ensued. Rob felt that his father was obliged to be the one to follow up. On the next occasion they were together, neither Rob nor his father initiated a serious conversation. Rob began to think that perhaps his father and stepmother had cooled to the idea of adoption. Several months later, Rob received a phone call from his father, explaining that on short notice, they were leaving to pick up a baby girl to adopt. Rob felt angry and betrayed. He understood that part of his reaction was irrational—that on some level he knew this might happen, that his father was perfectly entitled to choose to have a new family, and that this need not exclude him. The inception of this new family, however, meant that Rob was facing anew the demise of his old family. Rob acknowledged his anxiety over both being rejected by his father and being stuck with his mother.

This experience repeated elements of his parents' divorce: The announcement was precipitous, and his father voiced the right sentiments but failed to follow through. Rob's negative reaction to his father was exacerbated when his father called after the baby was at home. He did not have time to talk and mentioned offhandedly that he had thought Rob would not be at home and had planned to leave a message. Unfortunately, Rob's mother did not refrain from being critical of her ex-husband.

Although Rob exhibited a wide range of affects, the influence of his family's style, which minimized affects and interfered with their regulation, was apparent. Rob could be vulnerable to both depression and anxiety. In spite of his tendency to intellectualize how he felt, Rob's problems with affect regulation should not be overly pathologized; he was successful in his work and well adjusted socially. It was evident that Rob brought to therapy a capacity for mentalized affectivity and was able to put it to good effect in the treatment. Rob's affectivity was apparent in his reassessment(s) of what he felt about his parents' divorce, allowing him to experience his own feelings in a more open and complex way. He came to see that he had opted not to fully experience negative affects connected with an important event from the past, and that this avoidance continued to influence his relationships in the present; he thus came to value reexamining and reinterpreting his emotional experiences.

Rob's recognition that he had warded off feelings of depression about the divorce spurred new affective experiences. He was able to move from feeling morose to feeling sad in a way that was accompanied by an affirmative sense of self-understanding. His sadness pertained to the demise of both his parents' and his own (first) relationship, but he also now appreciated that while he had no control over what happened with his parents, the end of his own relationship was neither out of his control nor opposed to his real wishes. As he came to accept what he felt, his sense of agency was enhanced, and his overall sense of gloom lessened.

Rob's capacity for mentalized affectivity still had room for growth. He had a tendency to suppress his feelings; a good example of this was revealed in his reaction to his father's new family. Rob knew that he was displeased with this development, and, to a certain extent, he was able to communicate this. However, there was something restrained about his reaction, reflecting his wish to sound reasonable and to edit his real feelings. Rob's tendency to restrain free expression of his feelings produced countertransference responses on my part; I was aware of putting more affect into my voice, as if to provide examples of immediate affective reactions and to compensate for his low-keyed responses.

Rob was someone who struggled to allow himself to express his affects, but this should not be construed to mean that the solution was for him to express them outwardly. The inward expression of affects was equally important. For example, Rob was starting to become progressively more aware of his anger toward his father. Apart from whether and how he chose to communicate this to his father, it was crucial for Rob to allow himself to feel his resentment and to begin to separate himself from his family style of downplaying affective responses. In his new realization that his father might not be willing to respond to his attempts to communicate with him, Rob's expression of his affects inwardly and the exploration of the meaning of his feelings served as valuable affirmations of his own experience of the new family situation.

The mentalized affectivity that Rob did exhibit in coming to terms with his parents' divorce and the impact it had on his life came under stress with the fresh reminder (the adoption) that his own nuclear family had dissolved. This did not contradict the suggestion that he possessed mentalized affectivity; rather, it highlighted that circumstances could temporarily undermine his mentalized affectivity, or at least make it difficult to sustain. Indeed, mentalized affectivity can break down at the moment when the impact of a strong affect is felt. Normally, mentalized affectivity requires gaining some perspective, which in the heat of the moment can be beyond a person's capacity. It is certainly possible to acquire mentalized affectivity in situations where one previously lacked it, but it would be imprudent to ignore how much of a struggle it is to maintain it consistently. Rob brought a high level of mentalized affectivity with him into therapy; the treatment served to help him to deepen it significantly.

CONCLUSIONS

As mentalization theory receives greater interest in the field, both as a research construct and in terms of its clinical utility, the meaning and boundaries of the concept continue to be defined. Our increasingly complex understanding of mentalization has raised many questions that will need to be elucidated in the future.

Jurist (2008) has noted differences in the degree of complexity that various authors have attributed to mentalizing processes: a low-level form involving an implicit detection of emotions (primarily through facial expressions), and a high-level form involving complex evaluations and decision making about relationships. Fonagy and Bateman (2006) allude to a distinction between subcortical and frontocortical aspects of mentalization; the former is based on the mirror neuron system that produces an immediate and unconscious kind of mind reading, and the latter (whose neurocircuitry is not well understood) allows us to make the differentiated and complex social judgments about ourselves and others that are manifested in mentalized affectivity. However, it remains unclear whether there are in fact these different levels of mentalization, and, if so, how they relate to one another. The close connection between mentalization and other constructs, such as empathy and mindfulness, is a topic that also deserves further attention (for a discussion of constructs related to mentalization, see Allen, 2006).

As we continue to refine our understanding of mentalization, questions also arise as to how mentalization may interact with other constructs, such as personality, attachment style, and character style. Furthermore, as discussed in the "Research on Mentalization" section, the relationship between mentalization and trauma remains unclear. We also do not know how culture might influence the nature and quality of mentalization. Although there is clearly much to resolve in mentalization theory, this should not prevent us from recognizing it as a promising tool for explicating how the mind works and how psychotherapy helps clients.

NOTE

1. According to Carruthers and Smith (1996), "The original false-belief task involved a character, Maxi, who places some chocolate in a particular location and then leaves the room; in his absence the chocolate is then moved to another

location. The child is then asked where Maxi will look for the chocolate on his return. In order to succeed in this task, the child must understand that Maxi still *thinks* that the chocolate is where he left it—the child must understand that Maxi has a false belief, in fact" (p. 2).

RECOMMENDATIONS FOR FURTHER READING

Bateman, A. W., & Fonagy, P. (2004). *Psychotherapy for borderline personality disorder: Mentalization-based treatment.* Oxford: Oxford University Press.—This book elaborates the principles of working from a mentalization-based perspective.

Fonagy, P., & Bateman, A. W. (2006). Mechanisms of change in mentalization-based treatment of BPD. *Journal of Clinical Psychology, 62,* 411–430.—This article reflects Fonagy and Bateman's latest thinking on the relationship among mentalization, attachment, and BPD.

Fonagy, P., Gergely, G., Jurist, E., & Target, M. (2002). *Affect regulation, mentalization, and the development of the self.* New York: Other Press.—This book is the most thorough accounting of the development of mentalization.

Jurist, E. L. (2005). Mentalized affectivity. *Psychoanalytic Psychology, 22,* 426–444.—This article further elaborates the role of affect in mentalizing.

Jurist, E. L., Slade, A., & Bergner, S. (Eds.). (2008). *Mind to mind: Infant research, neuroscience and psychoanalysis.* New York: Other Press.—An edited volume based on a conference with the most recent views of mentalization.

Levy, K. N., Meehan, K. B., Kelly, K. M., Reynoso, J. S., Weber, M., Clarkin, J. F., et al. (2006). Change in attachment patterns and reflective function in a randomized control trial of transference-focused psychotherapy for borderline personality disorder. *Journal of Consulting and Clinical Psychology, 74,* 1027–1040.—This study is the first to document the efficacy of TFP in improving reflective functioning among clients with BPD.

REFERENCES

Aber, J., Slade, A., Berger, B., Bresgi, I., & Kaplan, M. (1985). *The Parent Development Interview.* Unpublished manuscript, City University of New York.

Ainsworth, M. S., Blehar, M. C., Waters, E., & Wall, S. (1978). *Patterns of attachment: A psychological study of the Strange Situation.* Hillsdale, NJ: Erlbaum.

Allen, J. (2006). Mentalizing in practice. In J. Allen & P. Fonagy (Eds.), *Handbook of mentalization-based treatment* (pp. 3–30). Hoboken, NJ: Wiley.

Baron-Cohen, S., Tager-Flusberg, H., & Cohen, D. (Eds.). (2000). *Understanding other minds.* Oxford: Oxford University Press.

Bartels, A., & Zeki, S. (2004). The neural correlates of maternal and romantic love. *NeuroImage, 21,* 1155–1166.

Bateman, A. W., & Fonagy, P. (1999). Effectiveness of partial hospitalization in the treatment of borderline personality disorder: A randomized controlled trial. *American Journal of Psychiatry, 156,* 1563–1569.

Bateman, A. W., & Fonagy, P. (2001). Treatment of borderline personality disorder with psychoanalytically oriented partial hospitalization: An 18-month follow-up. *American Journal of Psychiatry, 158,* 36–42.

Bateman, A. W., & Fonagy, P. (2004). *Psychotherapy for borderline personality disorder: Mentalization-based treatment.* Oxford: Oxford University Press.

Blatt, S. J., & Ford, R. Q. (1994). *Therapeutic change: An object relations perspective.* New York: Plenum Press.

Bowlby, J. (1980). *Attachment and loss: Vol. 3. Loss: Sadness and depression.* London: Hogarth Press and the Institute of Psycho-Analysis.

Bowlby, J. (1982). *Attachment and loss: Vol. 1. Attachment* (2nd ed.). London: Hogarth Press and the Institute of Psycho-Analysis. (1st ed., 1969)

Carruthers, P., & Smith, P. K. (1996). Introduction. In P. Carruthers & P. K. Smith (Eds.), *Theories of theories of mind* (pp. 1–10). Cambridge: Cambridge University Press.

Conners, C. K., & Multi-Health Systems Staff. (2002). *Manual for the Conners' Continuous Performance Test II.* Toronto: Multi-Health Systems.

Fonagy, P. (2001). *Attachment theory and psychoanalysis.* New York: Other Press.

Fonagy, P. (2006). The mentalization-focused approach to social development. In G. Allen & P. Fonagy (Eds.), *Handbook of mentalization-based treatment* (pp. 53–101). Hoboken, NJ: Wiley.

Fonagy, P., & Bateman, A. W. (2006). Mechanisms of change in mentalization-based treatment of BPD. *Journal of Clinical Psychology, 62,* 411–430.

Fonagy, P., Gergely, G., Jurist, E., & Target, M. (2002). *Affect regulation, mentalization, and the development of the self.* New York: Other Press.

Fonagy, P., Leigh, T., Steele, M., Steele, H., Kennedy, R., Mattoon, G., et al. (1996). The relation of attachment status, psychiatric classification, and response to psychotherapy. *Journal of Consulting and Clinical Psychology, 64,* 22–31.

Fonagy, P., Steele, H., & Steele, M. (1991). Maternal representations of attachment during pregnancy predict the organization of infant–mother attachment at one year of age. *Child Development, 62,* 891–905.

Fonagy, P., Steele, M., Steele, H., Leigh, T., Kennedy, R., Mattoon, G., et al. (1995). Attachment, the reflective self, and borderline states. In S. Goldberg & J. Kerr (Eds.), *Attachment theory: Social, developmental, and clinical perspectives* (pp. 233–278). Hillsdale, NJ: Analytic Press.

Fonagy, P., Steele, M., Steele, H., Moran, G. S., & Higgitt, A. C. (1991). The capacity for understanding mental states: The reflective self in parent and child and its significance for security of attachment. *Infant Mental Health Journal, 12,* 201–218.

Fonagy, P., Steele, M., Steele, H., & Target, M. (1998). *Reflective-functioning manual: Version 5.0 for application to the Adult Attachment Interview.* Unpublished manuscript, University College London.

Fonagy, P., & Target, M. (1996). Playing with reality: I. Theory of mind and the normal development of psychic reality. *International Journal of Psycho-Analysis, 77,* 217–233.

Frith, U., & Happé, F. (1994). Autism: Beyond 'theory of mind'. *Cognition, 50,* 115–132.

George, C., Kaplan, N., & Main, M. (1984). *Adult Attachment Interview protocol.* Unpublished manuscript, University of California, Berkeley.

George, C., Kaplan, N., & Main, M. (1985). *Adult Attachment Interview protocol* (2nd ed.). Unpublished manuscript, University of California, Berkeley.

George, C., Kaplan, N., & Main, M. (1996). *Adult Attachment Interview protocol* (3rd ed.). Unpublished manuscript, University of California, Berkeley.

Gergely, G., & Unoka, Z. (2008). Attachment, affect regulation and mentalization: The developmental origins of the representational affective self. In C. Sharp, P. Fonagy, & I. Goodyer (Eds.), *Social cognition and developmental psychopathology* (pp. 303–340). Oxford: Oxford University Press.

Goldman, A. (2006). *Simulating minds: The philosophy, psychology and neuroscience of mindreading.* Oxford: Oxford University Press.

Gopnik, A. (1993). How we know our minds. *Behavioral and Brain Sciences, 16,* 1–14.

Gopnik, A., Capps, L., & Meltzoff, A. (2000). Early theories of mind: What the theory can tell us about autism. In S. Baron-Cohen, H. Tager-Flusberg, & D. Cohen (Eds.), *Understanding other minds: Perspectives from autism and cognitive neuroscience.* Oxford: Oxford University Press.

Gordon, R. M. (1996). 'Radical' simulationism. In P. Carruthers & P. K. Smith (Eds.), *Theories of theories of mind* (pp. 11–21). Cambridge, UK: Cambridge University Press.

Goyette-Ewing, M., Slade, A., Knoebber, K., Gilliam, W., Truman, S., & Mayes, L. (2003). *Parents first: A developmental parenting program.* Unpublished manuscript, Yale Child Study Center.

Grienenberger, J., Kelly, K., & Slade, A. (2005). Maternal reflective functioning, mother–infant affective communication, and infant attachment: Exploring the link between mental states and observed caregiving behavior in the intergenerational transmission of attachment. *Attachment & Human Development, 7,* 299–311.

Grienenberger, J., Popek, P., Stein, S., Solow, J., Morrow, M., Levine, N., et al. (2004). *The Wright Institute reflective parenting program workshop training manual.* Unpublished manuscript.

Harris, P. (1989). *Children and emotion: The development of psychological understanding.* Oxford: Blackwell.

Heaton, R. K. (1981). *A manual for the Wisconsin Card Sorting Test.* Odessa, FL: Psychological Assessment Resources.

Jurist, E. L. (2005). Mentalized affectivity. *Psychoanalytic Psychology, 22*(3), 426–444.

Jurist, E. L. (2007). *Mentalization and substance abuse.* Unpublished manuscript (revision of a paper presented at the meeting of Division 39 of the American Psychological Association, New York, April 2005, and at the Mentalization Conference, Budapest, Hungary, June 2006).

Jurist, E. L. (2008). Minds and yours: New directions for mentalization theory. In E. L. Jurist, A. Slade, & S. Bergner (Eds.), *Mind to mind: Infant research, neuroscience and psychoanalysis* (pp. 88–114). New York: Other Press.

Leslie, A. M. (2000). "Theory of mind" as a mechanism of selective attention. In M. S. Gazzaniga (Ed.), *The new cognitive neurosciences* (2nd ed., pp. 1235–1247). Cambridge, MA: MIT Press.

Levinson, A., & Fonagy, P. (2004). Offending and attachment: The relationship between interpersonal awareness and offending in a prison population with psychiatric disorder. *Canadian Journal of Psychoanalysis, 12,* 225–251.

Levy, K. N., Meehan, K. B., Kelly, K. M., Reynoso, J. S., Weber, M., Clarkin, J. F., et al. (2006). Change in attachment patterns and reflective function in a randomized control trial of transference focused psychotherapy for borderline personality disorder. *Journal of Consulting and Clinical Psychology, 74,* 1027–1040.

Levy, K. N., Meehan, K. B., Reynoso, J. S., Lenzenweger, M. F., Clarkin, J. F., & Kernberg, O. F. (2005, January). *The relation of reflective function to neurocognitive functioning in patients with borderline personality disorder.* Poster presented at the 2005 Annual Winter Meeting of the American Psychoanalytic Association, New York.

Main, M., Kaplan, N., & Cassidy, J. (1985). Security in infancy, childhood and adulthood: A move to the level of representation. In I. Bretherton & E. Waters (Eds.), Growing points of attachment theory and research. *Monographs of the Society for Research in Child Development, 50*(1–2, Serial No. 209), 66–104.

Meehan, K. B. (2007). *Affective communication as a mechanism of change in the treatment of borderline personality disorder.* Unpublished doctoral dissertation, City University of New York.

Onishi, K., & Baillargeon, R. (2005). Do 15-month-old infants understand false beliefs? *Science, 308,* 255–258.

Sandler, J., & Rosenblatt, B. (1987). The representational world. In J. Sandler, *From safety to superego: Selected papers of Joseph Sandler* (pp. 58–72). New York: Guilford Press. (Original work published 1962)

Schechter, D. S., Coots, T., Zeanah, C. H., Davies, M., Coates, S. W., Trabka, K. A., et al. (2005). Maternal mental representations of the child in an inner-city clinical sample: Violence-related posttraumatic stress and reflective functioning. *Attachment & Human Development, 7,* 313–331.

Slade, A. (2006). Reflective parenting programs: Theory and development. *Psychoanalytic Inquiry, 26,* 640–657.

Slade, A., Grienenberger, J., Bernbach, E., Levy, D., & Locker, A. (2005). Maternal reflective functioning, attachment, and the transmission gap: A preliminary study. *Attachment & Human Development, 7,* 283–298.

Slade, A., Sadler, L. S., & Mayes, L. C. (2005). Minding the Baby: Enhancing parental reflective functioning in a nursing/mental health home visiting program. In L. J. Berlin, Y. Ziv, L. Amaya-Jackson, & M. T. Greenberg (Eds.), *Enhancing early attachments: Theory, research, intervention, and policy* (pp. 152–177). New York: Guilford Press.

Sroufe, L. A. (1996). *Emotional development: The organization of emotional life in the early years.* New York: Cambridge University Press.

Sroufe, L. A., & Waters, E. (1977). Attachment as an organizational construct. *Child Development, 48,* 1184–1199.

Twemlow, S. W., Fonagy, P., & Sacco, F. C. (2005). A developmental approach to mentalizing communities: II. The Peaceful Schools experiment. *Bulletin of the Menninger Clinic, 69,* 282–304.

Vermote, R. (2005). *Psychoanalytically informed hospitalization-based treatment of personality disorders: A process–outcome study.* Unpublished doctoral dissertation, Katholieke Universiteit Leuven, Leuven, Belgium.

5

Clinical Correlates of Adult Attachment Organization

Frederick G. Lopez

> A great deal of work needs doing before we can be confident which
> disorders of attachment and care-giving behaviour are treatable
> by psychotherapy and which are not and, if treatable, which of
> the various methods is to be preferred. Much turns on a clinician's
> experiences, capabilities, and facilities.
>
> —BOWLBY (1977, p. 422)

John Bowlby recognized that attachment theory would need to rest on a solid, integrated platform of academic and clinical inquiry before it could be established as a bona fide framework for clinical practice. His expressed caution was well considered. At the time he wrote these words, nearly another decade would pass before two lines of research on adult attachment emerged—one emanating from developmental psychology (Main, Kaplan, & Cassidy, 1985) and the other from social psychology (Hazan & Shaver, 1987). For most of the subsequent years, these streams formed largely independent lines of inquiry, each developing and preferring different assessment tools and methodologies, and each progressively creating a steady cascade of insightful findings on adult psychological functioning and adjustment.

Indeed, Bowlby would no doubt be pleased with the "great deal of work" that has already been done. Yet, despite the remarkable growth of this scholarly literature, the theory has had little impact on clinical theory and practice until recently (Slade, 1999). Currently, few practitioners of adult psychotherapy use attachment theory as a primary means of conceptualizing client problems and therapeutic processes and of guiding their therapeutic interventions. Why? Perhaps researchers have not often tried to bridge the gap between the burgeoning research literature and its clinical application because the available knowledge on adult attachment has been

94

illuminated by two distinct academic traditions, creating an understandable degree of confusion about the different ways in which adult attachment has been conceptualized and assessed. Moreover, findings generated by these two assessment traditions have rarely been organized into a more comprehensive understanding of the larger construct, thereby hampering clinicians' abilities to discern how consistent empirical findings across studies may have their parallels (which I term *correlates*) in particular observations that can emerge within therapy-relevant domains of inquiry and activity. As a result, many clinicians may not appreciate how the available theory-grounded research on adult attachment can now offer practical case conceptualization guidance for interrelating various aspects of clients' histories, disclosures, behaviors, and problems.

Fortunately, the winds of change are blowing. Recent calls for a greater integration of inquiry in the developmental and social psychology traditions (Kobak, 2002; Shaver & Mikulincer, 2002) are heralding a time when the confluence of these two research streams is forming a deep pool of knowledge that is increasingly relevant to both clinicians and scholars. Still, if Bowlby's expressed hope that more clinicians would contribute to this effort by using their own "experiences, capabilities, and facilities," then there is more work to be done. In short, clinicians must be persuaded that the available research can inform their practice.

This chapter is an effort in this direction. I begin with a brief overview of the two major assessment traditions in the adult attachment literature, with emphasis on clarifying the language of their respective classification systems. Next, I summarize key findings in three broad domains of inquiry that are also common venues of clinical observation and assessment.[1] Lastly, I attempt to organize these clinically relevant correlates into more integrated, holistic patterns (*profiles*) that may aid clinicians in discerning individual differences in adult attachment, and thereby in using attachment theory as a guide for case conceptualization.

ADULT ATTACHMENT STYLES, DIMENSIONS, AND STATES OF MIND: LEARNING THE LANGUAGE OF RESEARCH ON ADULT ATTACHMENT

Elsewhere (Lopez, 2003), I have reviewed several prominent measures of adult attachment security and provided a brief historical perspective on the two major assessment traditions—interview and self-report. I have also delved into some of the controversies and lingering questions regarding the appropriate conceptualization and measurement of adult attachment. The reader is referred to that chapter, as well as to the next three chapters in this volume, for more detailed information on these matters. My purpose here is not to revisit this territory; rather, it is to orient the reader to subtle yet important differences in the language of adult attachment, which are linked to differences in the inquiry domains and goals of these two assessment traditions.

Interview-Based Assessment of Adult Attachment

Interview-based measures, such as the Adult Attachment Interview (AAI; George, Kaplan, & Main, 1984, 1985, 1996), were initially developed and have been preferentially used by attachment scholars in the developmental psychology tradition. (For an in-depth review, see Levy & Kelly, Chapter 6, this volume.) Developmental psychologists are largely concerned with understanding processes and patterns of typical and atypical behavioral organization across the lifespan. The AAI is an approximately hour-long semistructured and audiotaped interview that probes participants' early memories and relationship experiences centered around incidents or themes of distress, loss, and separation. The domain of attachment emphasized in the AAI is the *early parent–child attachment relationship*; experiences with adults other than primary attachment figures is omitted. Moreover, the AAI was validated in terms of its ability to predict the attachment classification of an adult interviewee's *infant*. So its purpose is to find indications in an adult's discussion of attachment-related memories from childhood of residues of childhood experiences that might affect a person's parenting style.

Hesse (1999), in a comprehensive published description of the AAI, cautioned that because the AAI explores early experiences with multiple caregivers, it is not meant to assess whether one is securely or insecurely attached to any particular person. Rather, the AAI attempts to determine whether one is in a secure or insecure *state of mind* regarding attachment. Toward this end, interview transcripts are reviewed and coded by independent raters with extensive training in the use of a standardized system of discourse analysis and attachment classification (Main & Goldwyn, 1984; Main, Goldwyn, & Hesse, 2003). The goal of these analyses is to discern important differences in implicit cognitive–affective representations (*internal working models*; Bretherton & Munholland, 1999) of experiences in early attachment relationships, by attending to whether or not respondents follow typical rules of social discourse when responding to interview questions about these experiences.

Following this analysis, interviewees are typically classified into one of five groups (*secure-autonomous, dismissing, enmeshed-preoccupied, unresolved-disorganized, cannot classify*) on the basis of their ability to provide a coherent narrative account of their early attachment experiences. Interviewees identified as secure-autonomous demonstrate the capacity to provide thoughtful, reflective answers and appropriate elaborations (i.e., they are "free to evaluate" their state of mind regarding attachment). By contrast, interviewees assigned to one of the three main insecure adult attachment categories demonstrate distinctive difficulties in responding to AAI questions without lapsing into defensive, dysfluent, or dissociative speech patterns. The final category, cannot classify, is used when an interview shows conflicting indicators of state of mind with respect to attachment. (This sometimes happens because relationships with key figures have been very different, or because salient experiences have not been well integrated.)

AAI transcripts can also be rated to yield an overall, continuously scaled *coherence-of-narrative* score, or subjected to an alternative scoring system (Kobak, 1989) that provides continuous scores on two independent dimensions: *security–anxiety* and *hyperactivation–deactivation*. The former dimension reflects the degree to which a person exhibits an autonomous state of mind versus one compromised by anxiety or insecurity; the latter dimension codes variability in tendencies to overfocus on attachment-related concerns versus divert attention away from such concerns.

Self-Report Assessment of Adult Attachment

Self-report measures of adult attachment were initially developed and have been preferentially used by scholars in the social-psychological research tradition, who are, among other things, interested in understanding social-cognitive processes in human relationships. Accordingly, most self-report measures of adult attachment direct respondents' attention to the domain of *intimate peer relationships* prior to having them use either standard checklists or rating scales to describe their typical cognitive, affective, and behavioral responses to the intimacy-related demands of these relationships. The goal of this assessment is to reliably measure distinctive and explicit *patterns of relating* to romantic partners that are representative of different *adult attachment styles*. These measures do not ask about childhood relationships with parents or other attachment figures, and they rely on self-reports of feelings and behavioral tendencies rather than on observations of discourse patterns.

The steady evolution of scale development in this method of assessment has now produced an array of psychometrically sound self-report instruments (Lopez, 2003; for an in-depth review, see Fraley & Phillips, Chapter 7, this volume). The most recent and sophisticated instruments contain up to several dozen continuously scored items designed to yield categorical and dimensional scores. For example, Brennan, Clark, and Shaver's (1998) 36-item Experiences in Close Relationships (ECR) inventory yields two factor-analytically derived scale scores. Items representing the first dimension, Avoidance, tap expressed discomfort with closeness and interdependence whereas items loading on the second dimension, Anxiety, assess strong fears of rejection and abandonment by romantic partners and intense desires to maintain intimate contact. In the self-report tradition, high scores on Avoidance indicate *deactivation* of the attachment system (i.e., inhibition or suppression of proximity-seeking tendencies; see Shaver & Mikulincer, Chapter

2, this volume, for a discussion of the attachment system). High scores on Anxiety indicate a pattern of relating characterized by *hyperactivation* of the attachment system (i.e., frequent and intense efforts to maintain proximity to a relationship partner and intense expression of emotions related to attachment and separation, such as hurt feelings, needs for support, and anger or jealousy in response to perceived inadequacy of support). These two dimensions are remarkably similar in focus to the two dimensions found in the AAI when it is scored on a continuous scale (Shaver, Belsky, & Brennan, 2000; Shaver & Mikulincer, 2004; Mikulincer & Shaver, 2007).

Because the two dimensions are fairly independent, the four quadrants of the two-dimensional conceptual space they form can be viewed as different attachment styles (Bartholomew & Horowitz, 1991; Bartholomew & Shaver, 1998). Secure persons are those who report low levels of both Avoidance and Anxiety, whereas fearful (or fearfully avoidant) persons are those who receive high scores on both dimensions. Persons with a preoccupied style report low levels of Avoidance but high levels of Anxiety, and dismissing (or dismissingly avoidant) persons exhibit the opposite pattern (high scores on Avoidance, low scores on Anxiety).

Toward an Integration of Research Findings

Although early findings of (at best) only modest correspondence between interview and self-report classifications of adult attachment raised preliminary doubts about the overall integrity and coherence of the literature on adult attachment (Crowell & Treboux, 1995), others (Bartholomew & Shaver, 1998) argued that such differences are probably due to differences in the targets of inquiry (i.e., parent–child vs. intimate peer relationships) and methodological focus (discourse coherence vs. self-reported feelings and behavioral tendencies in close relationships). Evidence of some convergence between measures, especially those that yield dimensional scores, has been presented (Bartholomew & Shaver, 1998; Shaver et al., 2000; Shaver & Mikulincer, 2004). Shaver et al. (2000) found, for example, that continuous coherence-of-narrative ratings on the AAI were moderately correlated with dimensions of self-reported adult attachment. And many studies done with one kind of measure or the other produce similar results when attachment-related phenomena are studied (see Mikulincer & Shaver, 2007, for a comprehensive review). Still, as Fraley and Phillips discuss in Chapter 7 of the present volume, a meta-analysis of all studies using both methods still suggests little overall measurement congruence. In general, it seems best to keep in mind the different foci of the different measures and accept that each measurement tradition offers distinctive yet potentially complementary perspectives on the still somewhat malleable construct of adult attachment (Collins, Guichard, Ford, & Feeney, 2004).

Interview methods are meant to uncover (through discourse analysis) some of the less conscious and more implicit features of adult attachment organization that may be rooted in childhood experiences with parental figures, whereas self-report methods more directly assess what a person has noticed about his or her feelings and behaviors in close relationships in adulthood. This is not to say that self-report measures cannot function as valid indicators of covert or less conscious processes; indeed, a number of recent experimental studies have linked self-reported adult attachment styles with various nonconscious forms of information processing (Shaver & Mikulincer, 2004). Across many studies, the self-report measures have been linked with dreams, Thematic Apperception Test stories, scores on the Rorschach, and implicit cognitive and emotional responses assessed in laboratory tasks and magnetic resonance imaging scans. With both kinds of measures, inferences about underlying unconscious processes require interpretation; neither kind of measure provides a transparent window onto the unconscious mind. Therefore, there is considerable value in integrating research findings from both assessment traditions.

In line with this perspective, I now consider key findings from both assessment traditions that are relevant to clinical practice. More specifically, I will summarize selected findings in three broad domains of inquiry—developmental and family histories; cognitive–affective patterns and coping processes; and types of interpersonal problems and relationship difficulties—because these domains parallel likely arenas of therapeutic exploration, and as such may hold particular promise as guideposts for the differential assessment of clients' adult attachment organization.

CLINICAL CORRELATES OF ADULT ATTACHMENT ORGANIZATION

Developmental and Family History Correlates

A core assumption of attachment theory (now supported by several longitudinal studies; see Grossmann, Grossmann, & Waters, 2005) is that attachment security in adulthood is the likely outcome of a favorable childhood characterized by stable, loving, noninvasive, and responsive relationships with parents and other caregiving figures, whereas insecurity has its origins in less stable and more disrupted child-rearing environments and in more neglectful, controlling, or traumatic experiences with primary caregivers. Furthermore, because variations in these critical formative experiences are presumed to differentially shape the internal working models of self and other that guide expectations and behavior in subsequent relationships, differences in adult attachment security and insecurity are likely to dispose individuals toward different trajectories of life course adjustment. This broad lifespan perspective raises several important questions about adult attachment that are especially relevant to clinicians. For example, are differences in adult attachment organization distinguishable from basic temperament and personality differences? Are they related to different accounts of early family experiences? Do they predict the quality of life course adjustment?

Evidence

There is evidence that AAI classifications are largely independent of general personality measures (van IJzendoorn, 1995), although Pianta, Egeland, and Adam (1996) found that preoccupied adults tended to overreport symptoms, whereas those classified as dismissing were likely to underreport distress. More consistent associations between self-report measures of adult attachment and personality have been observed. Self-report measures of insecure adult attachment styles and orientations have been moderately associated in expected directions with measures of negative affect (Simpson, 1990), self-esteem (Collins & Read, 1990; Feeney & Noller, 1990), and neuroticism (Noftle & Shaver, 2006; Shaver & Brennan, 1992). Diehl, Elnick, Bourbeau, and Labouvie-Vief (1998) also reported findings differentiating secure and insecure adult attachment (and especially fearful and preoccupied types) across such personality dimensions as sociability, dominance, social presence, empathy, communality, and capacity for status. Despite these associations, self-reported adult attachment styles are not reducible to basic personality dimensions, because they can predict both laboratory reactions in social cognition tasks and romantic relationship outcomes after basic personality variables are controlled for (Mikulincer & Shaver, 2007; Noftle & Shaver, 2006; Shaver & Brennan, 1992).

Although the AAI specifically explores early attachment-related memories, research correlating AAI classifications with independent measures of family history or parental representations has thus far been sparse and has yielded inconsistent findings (Bernier & Dozier, 2002). Manassis, Owens, Adam, West, and Sheldon-Keller (1999) found that people classified as secure-autonomous on the AAI reported higher levels of maternal (but not paternal) care and lower levels of maternal (but not paternal) overprotection on a retrospective measure of experienced parenting [the Parental Bonding Instrument; Parker, Tupling, & Brown, 1979]. However, Crowell, Treboux, and Waters (1999) found that secure and insecure AAI groups did not differ in their reports of mothers and peers on a self-report measure (Mother–Father–Peer Scale; Epstein, 1983), whereas secure and insecure attachment style groups based on self-report measures did differ from one another on these comparisons. More recently, Lyons-Ruth, Yellin, Melnick, and Atwood (2003) observed within a sample of 45 mothers that references to fearful affect on the AAI were specifically related to their reports of having witnessed or experienced physical violence. Within the coding scales of the AAI, there is a fairly high correlation between an interviewee's discourse coherence and description of his or her mother as "loving" (e.g., Fonagy, Steele, & Steele, 1991).

There is more consistent evidence linking self-report measures of adult attachment to retrospective reports of early family environments and parental representations. Relative to their less secure peers, adults with secure attachment styles report more positive early bonds with parents (Collins & Read, 1990; Feeney & Noller, 1990; Hazan & Shaver, 1987), fewer experiences of childhood adversity (Mickelson, Kessler, & Shaver, 1997), generally well-differentiated and benevolent representations of parental figures (Levy, Blatt, & Shaver, 1998), and more positive interactions within their families of origin (Diehl et al., 1998). Persons reporting a fearful attachment style, by contrast, are more likely to acknowledge that one or both parents had a serious drinking problem (Brennan, Shaver, & Tobey, 1991) and to report childhood experiences with physical and sexual abuse (Shaver & Clark, 1994). More recently, Gallo, Smith, and Ruiz (2003) observed that when compared to their secure counterparts, preoccupied people described their fathers' behavior as more hostile, whereas fearful persons described early experiences with both parents as hostile.

Thus far there is little direct evidence (i.e., long-term prospective studies) that adult attachment security (whether assessed via interview or self-report) should forecast more favorable life trajectories, whereas insecurity should prefigure more problematic life outcomes.[2] However, some preliminary data support this assumption. Scharf, Mayseless, and Kivenson-Baron (2004) found that Israeli high school students classified as secure-autonomous on the AAI demonstrated better coping with basic military training 1 year later, and exhibited a higher capacity for mature intimacy 3 years later than their less secure peers did. In another short-term prospective study, young women who maintained a secure attachment style over a 2-year period were somewhat more likely to report fewer stressful life events and less symptomatology than were either peers with stable insecure styles or peers who changed from a secure to an insecure style (Davila, Burge, & Hammen, 1997). In 1-year longitudinal studies of mothers of children with congenital heart disease, Berant and her colleagues found that attachment anxiety and avoidance were related to poor mental health and lower marital satisfaction, and that avoidance scores uniquely predicted deterioration in mental health and perceived coping abilities over as long as 7 years (Berant, Mikulincer, & Florian, 2001, 2003; Berant, Mikulincer, Shaver, & Segal, 2008).

Klohnen and Bera (1998) found, within a sample of women studied over 31 years, that self-reported adult attachment styles assessed at age 52 were significantly related to adjustment and relationship history variables first assessed when these women were age 21 and again at regular periods thereafter. Unlike their peers with avoidant styles, the lives of securely attached women were marked by less distressing affect and by warmer, more durable, and satisfying relationships. In a more recent and well-designed prospective study covering a 6-year interval, adolescents with avoidant styles later evidenced less satisfying and more poorly functioning romantic relationships—patterns that in part were associated with their selections of less well-adjusted partners (Collins, Cooper, Albino, & Allard, 2002).

Cognitive–Affective Correlates

The more favorably organized internal working models of people with a secure attachment style or state of mind are also presumed to optimize their capacities for open, flexible cognitive processing and memory retrieval of attachment information, thereby facilitating more competent affect regulation. As noted earlier, being classified as secure-autonomous in the AAI hinges heavily on a person's ability to access, retrieve, and appropriately describe both positive and painful attachment-related memories without emotionally dissembling or lapsing into irrelevant or dysfluent discourse. Such competencies suggest the presence of a more stable, integrated, and resilient self-structure capable of engaging in both self-reflective and self-soothing operations when stressed, and, when necessary, orienting the person toward appropriately enlisting social support. These assumptions raise questions of potential relevance to clinicians. For instance, are differences in adult attachment security related to different patterns of cognition and information processing when it comes to attachment-related information? Are differences in adult attachment security related to differential access to painful memories? Are adult attachment differences related to distinct patterns of affect regulation and stress-related coping?

Evidence

Much of the research pertaining to whether adult attachment differences influence cognition and information processing has used self-report measures. The resulting evidence indicates that, when compared to secure persons, preoccupied individuals explain relationship events in more negative ways and report greater distress, whereas avoidant persons, while similarly characterizing events more negatively, report less distress (e.g., Collins, 1996). Relatedly, although both secure and preoccupied persons describe themselves as more curious than their avoidant peers, only secure persons demonstrate the lowest levels of premature *cognitive closure*; that is, they are more likely to rely on and to better assimilate new information when making both generic social judgments (Mikulincer, 1997) and relationship-specific appraisals (Mikulincer & Arad, 1999). By contrast, anxiously attached adults are more likely to perceive conflict and to anticipate conflict escalation, and less likely to adjust relationship schemas in response to their partners' actions (Campbell, Simpson, Boldry, & Kashy, 2005).

These variations may in part reflect important differences in people's access to and management of attachment-related memories, which in turn contribute to the formation of adaptive or maladaptive cognitive appraisals and expectations. In this regard, and in line with AAI-related observations, studies have found that secure persons demonstrate easier access to negative memories than do their insecure peers; preoccupied persons, while capable of accessing these memories, are overwhelmed by so-called "emotional spreading," and avoidant persons demonstrate low accessibility to negative affects (Mikulincer & Orbach, 1995) and poor immediate recall of information regarding attachment-related threats and losses (Fraley, Garner, & Shaver, 2000). There is also evidence that whereas dismissing individuals are generally successful in suppressing attachment-related affects and behaviors (Fraley & Shaver, 1997), the diminished emotional expressiveness of people with the fearful style belies an acute awareness and deep experience of emotions (Searle & Meara, 1999). Mikulincer, Dolev, and Shaver (2004) found that even dismissing persons' ability to suppress painful thoughts can break down under a cognitive load, suggesting that their defenses have limitations.

In experimental studies using a lexical decision-making task for examining interpersonal expectancies, subjects with a secure attachment style were quicker to identify words associated with positive interpersonal outcomes, whereas insecure subjects were quicker in identifying negative outcome words (Baldwin, Fehr, Keedian, Seidel, & Thompson, 1993). Elsewhere, Mikulincer (1998) showed that secure adults exhibited higher accessibility to trust-related memories and used more constructive strategies for coping with the violation of trust-related memories than did insecure adults. When compared with their anxious and avoidant counterparts, adults with a secure adult attachment style exhibit more balanced, complex, and coherent self-structures, which enable them to examine both strong and weak points of the self (Mikulincer, 1995) and to engage in the exploratory pursuit of achievement- and mastery-related goals (Elliott & Reis, 2003).

These findings mesh well with generally consistent observations across other studies that have related differences in adult attachment security to distinctive styles of affect regulation and stress-related coping (Fuendeling, 1998). In one early landmark study using the AAI, Kobak and Sceery (1988) found that secure college students were rated by their peers as more ego-resilient and less anxious than their preoccupied and dismissing peers. Similarly, in their review of studies examining links between self-reported adult attachment styles and various coping outcomes, Mikulincer and Florian (1998) concluded that secure attachment functions as an "inner resource" that helps a person to positively appraise an array of threatening and stressful experiences (e.g., dealing with interpersonal losses, war- and parenting-related stresses, or physical pain) and to engage in constructive coping strategies, whereas either avoidant or anxious attachment styles appear to function as risk factors that contribute to poorer coping and less optimal adjustment.

In general, when stressed, secure adults demonstrate adaptive forms of coping and, when necessary, appropriately enlist the emotional support of others (Davis, Shaver, & Vernon, 2003). By contrast, preoccupied adults are more likely to engage in ruminative, emotion-focused coping that exacerbates their distress, while avoidant adults tend to engage in distancing coping behaviors such as denying the experience of negative affect, directing attention away from attachment-related stimuli, inhibiting emotional displays, and engaging in social withdrawal. Drawing upon these and other research findings, Mikulincer and Shaver (2004, 2007) have proposed a model for explaining how repeated security-enhancing interactions with attachment figures promote autonomous self-regulation. In their model, the coupling of favorable representations of attachment figures and favorable representations of the self with an attachment figure results in complementary and mutually nested cognitive structures, which can be more readily accessed to serve self-soothing functions.

Social Competencies and Relationship Problems

Most clients' presenting problems are interpersonal in nature (Horowitz, 1979), and attachment theory offers useful insights and predictions regarding the likely emergence of different types of interpersonal problems and relationship distress. Because people with a strongly avoidant attachment orientation (i.e., a dismissing or fearful attachment style) are presumed to share a common discomfort with closeness, both should exhibit greater difficulties with intimacy-related tasks (e.g., self-disclosure, soliciting feedback and social support, and engaging in caregiving and collaborative problem solving). By the same token, critical differences in their respective levels of attachment anxiety should result in observably different expressions of these difficulties, with dismissing individuals evidencing more consistent patterns of interpersonal distancing and detachment, and fearful individuals demonstrating more anxious, conflicted, and prematurely aborted efforts to establish intimacy. On the other hand, because of their powerful need to maintain relationships and to avoid rejection, people with a predominantly anxious orientation (i.e., a preoccupied attachment style) are likely to be persistently hypervigilant regarding their partners' availability and may thus overtax them with excessive demands for reassurance and support. Once again, these assumptions raise clinically relevant questions. Are differences in adult attachment security related to particular social competencies and to different patterns of interpersonal behavior? Are they related to different ways of managing relationship conflict and to different types of relationship problems?

Evidence

There are convergent findings from both interview and self-report studies that people classified as securely attached typically display more competent and adaptive interpersonal behaviors and are more satisfied with their intimate relationships. For example, although both secure and preoccupied adults similarly acknowledge engaging in high levels of self-disclosure with their partners, secure adults prefer to disclose to partners rather than strangers, are better able to elicit disclosures, and to stay on topic when responding to another's disclosure (Keelan, Dion, & Dion, 1998; Mikulincer & Nachshon, 1991). Relative to their less secure peers, secure individuals are also more open to receiving and valuing feedback from their partners (Brennan & Bosson, 1998), more likely to respect them (Frei & Shaver, 2002), and more frequently report engaging them in collaborative forms of problem solving (Corcoran & Mallinckrodt, 2000; Kobak & Hazan, 1991).

Theory-consistent differences in adult attachment security have been related to both self-reported and observed support-seeking and caregiving behaviors across several studies (Collins & Feeney, 2000; Kunce & Shaver, 1994; Larose & Bernier, 2001; Mikulincer, Shaver, Gillath, & Nitzberg, 2005; Simpson, Rholes, & Nelligan, 1992). For example, Larose and Bernier (2001) examined relations between AAI-derived dimensions of hyperactivation (i.e., a preoccupied state of mind) and deactivation (i.e., a dismissing state of mind) and college students' perceptions of social support and seeking help from teachers during the first-year college transition. They found that a dismissing tendency was related to difficulties in getting assistance from peers and teachers, and to peer-reported withdrawal, but not to self-reported distress. By contrast, a preoccupied tendency was related to reported transition-related distress and distrust in potential support providers, as well as to reported loneliness. In other research using self-report measures, persons with high levels of attachment anxiety predictably demonstrated excessive reassurance seeking in their close relationships (Shaver, Schachner, & Mikulincer, 2005). In a related vein, Bogaert and Sadava (2002) found that anxious attachment was modestly yet significantly related (especially among women) to several indices of sexual experiences and behavior, including perceived physical attractiveness, age of first intercourse, number of sexual partners, and episodes of infidelity.

In line with findings from independent studies using self-report measures of adult attachment, Creasey and Hesson-McInnis (2001) reported that adolescents with more insecure attachment orientations (i.e., those with either anxious or avoidant orientations) used more negative conflict management strategies than did their secure counterparts. Using the AAI, Creasey (2002) classified each member of a dating couple as secure or insecure, prior to observing how they attempted to resolve a conflict in their relationship. He observed that couples containing a secure female were more likely to engage in positive behaviors, whereas couples containing an insecure male were more likely to engage in negative behaviors. This finding suggests that gender and attachment security may interact in predicting the quality of a couple's efforts to resolve conflict. In this regard, there is evidence that fearful men are more prone to hostility and partner abuse than are their preoccupied and dismissing counterparts (Bartholomew & Allison, 2006; Dutton, Starzomski, & Ryan, 1996).

Finally, evidence exists that different patterns of adult attachment organization are related to different configurations of interpersonal problems derived from both self-reports and friends' reports. For instance, Bartholomew and Horowitz (1991) found that dismissing persons were likely to exhibit interpersonal problems characterized by coldness and aloofness, while preoccupied persons were more likely to be viewed by peers as overly expressive and domineering, and fearful persons more likely to demonstrate problems reflecting passivity, social inhibition and unassertiveness. Securely attached persons, by contrast, did not reveal particular elevations in any measured domain of interpersonal problems, suggesting a more balanced form of interpersonal relatedness.

THINKING INTEGRATIVELY ABOUT THE EVIDENCE: FOUR PROFILES OF ADULT ATTACHMENT ORGANIZATION

Using different methods and focusing on different facets of the larger construct of attachment security in adulthood, research studies in the interview-based and self-report assessment traditions, when viewed inclusively, form a deep pool of findings concerning the nature of adult attachment organization. In so doing, they affirm the capacity of attachment theory to interrelate diverse features of early experiences, cognitive organization, affect regulation strategies, and interpersonal behaviors in ways that differentiate healthy and unhealthy patterns of adult functioning (Lopez & Brennan, 2000). Nevertheless, if attachment theory is to fulfill its potential as a good *clinical* theory, clinicians need tools to apprehend this interrelatedness when forming a coherent conceptualization of a client and the client's problems. As Slade (1999) has noted, clinicians often rely on metaphors that efficiently capture such interrelatedness when applying theory to practice. In these closing sections, I borrow and extend Waters et al.'s metaphor of a *secure-base script* (Waters, Rodrigues, & Ridgeway, 1998) by proposing that convergent research findings describing differences in adult attachment organization may form the "subtext" of four distinct *scripts* or *profiles* that may be discernible in the therapy context (see Table 5.1). Because the term *script* is frequently used in social psychology for particular kinds of internal cognitive representations, I use the word *profile* here to indicate a set of characteristics or qualities that identify a certain kind of person.

TABLE 5.1. Summary of Adult Attachment Organization Correlates across Three Clinically Relevant Domains

Developmental/ family history	Cognitive–affective processes	Social competencies/ relationship problems
Secure attachment organization		
• Favorable early parental bonds; positive, differentiated parental representations • Stable, satisfying relationship histories • Less childhood adversity • Mature, integrated personality orientation	• Enhanced capacity for self-reflection; flexible cognitive processing of attachment information • Greater access to both positive and negative affect, memories; more adaptive coping • More resilient, coherent, positive self-structure	• Higher-quality self-disclosure • More collaborative problem-solving orientation • More stable, satisfying intimate relationships • Need-contingent support seeking, caregiving
Preoccupied attachment organization		
• Less warm, more enmeshed parental relationships • Parental representations as both punitive and benevolent • Dependent personality orientation	• Reflective capacities impaired by negative associations • Reactive, emotion-focused coping; low self-esteem • Less open to assimilating new information about others	• Excessive reassurance seeking; controlling • Seeks but devalues social feedback • Poor caregiving skills
Dismissing attachment organization		
• Early parental bonds as less warm and caring • Less differentiated, more punitive parental representations • Counterdependent personality orientation	• Poor recall, integration of attachment memories • Distancing, denial, and distraction as coping strategies • Suppresses attachment-related affect; defensive self-esteem	• Low self-disclosure; viewed as aloof, detached • Unlikely to seek social support when stressed • Neither seeks nor values social feedback
Fearful attachment organization		
• More disrupted, traumatic early bonds • Well-differentiated, malevolent parental representations • More likely exposure to physical/sexual abuse • Socially avoidant personality orientation	• Chronic vulnerability to stress • Tendency to dissemble, dissociate when faced with attachment-related threats • Self-critical depression; low self-esteem	• Passive, unassertive, exploitable • Poor social and support-seeking skills • Less satisfying and stable intimate relationships

The Secure Profile

The available findings suggest that clients with a secure profile are likely to engage readily and collaboratively in the therapeutic process. Although their pursuit of therapeutic help indicates the experience of current distress, they should disclose openly and reflectively when asked about their past and current relationships, and (with minimal encouragement) exhibit a willingness to critically examine their thought processes and behavioral involvements regarding these difficulties. These inquires are likely to confirm the presence of generally stable and satisfying relationships with others, as well as the relative absence of significant personal traumas. And in cases where prior relationship experiences with significant others have been painful and upsetting, the accounts of secure persons should evince a capacity to acknowledge this distress, to consider larger contextual influences that may have contributed to these undesired outcomes, and to express an authentic sense of loss and regret. Their descriptions of these disappointments should be appropriately detailed and focused, and should include indications that although they have retained an appreciation of the meaningfulness of these experiences, they have also "moved on" with their lives.

In short, these clients evidence a capacity to weave the threads of loss and learning into a coherent tapestry of life experience. They are also likely to use a flexible array of coping responses in dealing with stressors, and to be able to modify or change a coping strategy when it proves ineffective in managing their distress. The distress and interpersonal problems they present in therapy are more likely to be linked to acute, situational crises and adjustment difficulties (e.g., change in health status, loss of loved one) than to recurrent problem themes in their lives.

The Preoccupied Profile

By contrast, the available research clearly suggests that clients with a preoccupied profile present a more significant therapeutic challenge. To begin with, they are likely to report considerable distress and yet to evince corresponding difficulty in reflecting on their emotional experience, thus attesting to the powerfully dominant influence of attachment anxiety and chronic attachment system hyperactivation in their lives. General inquiries into their relationship histories are likely to reveal multiple experiences of intense, entangled, and disappointing relationships with family and intimate partners. Although these clients should be able to access attachment-related memories and self-disclose freely (if not excessively) to their therapists, their stories may have a rambling and "automatic" quality, often introducing contents that go well beyond the specific focus of therapeutic inquiry. Their accounts of their prior relationship difficulties are likely to distort their personal contributions and to fixate on themes of rejection and abandonment by others. In a parallel fashion, their coping strategies will be less flexible and considerably more ruminative and reactive than those of clients operating in accordance with the secure profile. The preoccupied profile's coupling of excessive reassurance seeking with limited capacities for self-soothing and persistent doubts about a caregiver's dependability is likely to tax the empathic capabilities of most therapists. Indeed, as the therapeutic relationship proceeds, clients operating within a preoccupied script should be frustrated by a therapist's efforts to maintain appropriate interpersonal boundaries, and may repeatedly "test" the therapist's expressed concerns and assurances.

The Dismissing Profile

The dominance of avoidance and attachment system deactivation in the dismissing person will orient him or her toward defensively maintaining self-esteem, denying personal vulnerability, and diverting attention away from attachment-related stresses and threats. As a result, these individuals are unlikely to seek therapeutic help volitionally and should be proportionally underrepresented within clinical samples. For those who nonetheless enter therapy, the same motivations and orientations should similarly present significant early obstacles to their effective engagement in the therapeutic process. The research findings suggest that many direct and implicit demands of therapy conversations (self-disclosure, affective exploration, self-reflection) may themselves represent attachment-related threats that could exacerbate the deactivating tendencies of dismissing persons. As a result, therapists are likely to experience these early conversations as superficial, vapid, and affectively flat.

   In a similar vein, explorations of these clients' early family experiences are likely to exhibit a superficial quality. However, as suggested by AAI research, careful listening and observing may reveal clues—such as inappropriate laughter or other incongruent behaviors when describing childhood experiences typically associated with pain, disappointment, or frustration—that are consistent with a dismissing profile. Research findings further suggest that dismissing clients' narratives of close relationships will be poorly differentiated and thinly elaborated, and that denial, intellectualization, and preemptive social withdrawal will be their preferred coping strategies for dealing with problems in these relationships.

The Fearful Profile

Available evidence indicates that the fearful pattern includes chronic approach–avoidance conflicts with regard to the intimacy demands of close relationships and the absence of a coherent strategy for managing threats to attachment security. Unlike the more clearly counterdependent and vulnerability-denying features of the dismissing profile, and unlike the more desperate intimacy-related approach themes evident in the preoccupied profile, the experience of fearfully avoidant persons is likely to include a confusing vacillation among detached, dependent, and controlling postures with others. Inquiries into their relationship histories are likely to uncover significant and unresolved experiences of traumatic psychological loss and injury, and generally distressful and frightening experiences with family members and other intimates. Persistent themes of interpersonal distrust, vulnerability, and passive withdrawal should also be apparent in their personal narratives, and their efforts to recall and recount these painful experiences may exhibit fragmented and dissociative qualities. Explorations of their current relationships are similarly likely to reveal recurring examples of passive, unassertive involvements with others, coupled with acknowledged hypersensitivity to cues of social rejection and noteworthy deficits in collaborative problem-solving skills.

Although there is scholarly disagreement as to whether fearful avoidance represents a special ("collapsed defenses") version of dismissing avoidance (Shaver & Mikulincer, 2002) or an etiologically unique form of adult attachment organization (Simpson & Rholes, 2002), there is evidence that, given their combined impairments in affective self-regulation and social competencies, fearful individuals appear to be the most troubled in terms of personality disorders (Brennan & Shaver, 1998) and may present the greatest challenges to successful therapeutic outcomes (Reis & Grenyer, 2004).

CONCLUSIONS

Over 30 years ago, Bowlby recognized that if attachment theory was to serve as a viable framework for clinical practice, both academics and clinicians would need to establish its predictive power and practical utility. Although sustained scholarly inquiry over the past two decades has created a deep fund of knowledge concerning the nature of adult attachment, clinicians have been slow to embrace attachment theory as a means of conceptualizing client problems. This chapter is intended to accelerate this movement by briefly reviewing the two major assessment traditions in the adult attachment literature and clarifying important terminological distinctions and correspondences in their respective systems. Selected empirical findings from both traditions, organized within three clinically relevant domains of inquiry, have been summarized to highlight noteworthy features of different adult attachment organizations. Lastly, four profiles of adult attachment organization have been proposed as potentially serviceable metaphors for interrelating diverse features of clients' developmental experiences, cognitive and coping processes, and interpersonal difficulties that may be revealed through the therapy process.

I hope that clinicians consider these profiles as complementary to more traditional modes of assessment, and as useful in customizing their treatment approaches to clients demonstrating different patterns of adult attachment organization. In this regard, it is important to keep in mind that a client's attachment-related presentation is not fixed, but may change in response to treatment processes and conditions. Indeed, it was John Bowlby's fervent hope that an attachment-theory-informed approach to clinical work would not only facilitate the therapeutic revision of problematic working models, but also illuminate our understanding of the change process itself.

NOTES

1. The focus of this chapter is on the adult attachment literature, rather than on the similarities in findings between it and the literature on infant attachment. That said, there is a remarkable degree of overlap among individual differences in adult attachment and infant attachment patterns. For an excellent review of this topic, see Cassidy (2000).
2. It is important to clarify here that whereas a number of longitudinal studies tracking the developmental sequelae of infant attachment security (as measured by the Strange Situation) into childhood, adolescence, and early adulthood have been conducted (see Grossmann et al., 2005, for an overview), longitudinal studies of adult attachment security (as measured by self-report and interview methods) are considerably rarer.

RECOMMENDATIONS FOR FURTHER READING

Collins, N. L., Guichard, A. C., Ford, M., & Feeney, B. C. (2004). Working models of attachment: New developments and emerging themes. In W. S. Rholes & J. A. Simpson (Eds.), *Adult attachment: Theory, research, and clinical implications* (pp. 196–239). New York: Guilford Press.—This chapter provides a comprehensive review and discussion of theory and research relevant to the development, contents, functions, and structural organization of attachment models.

Hesse, E. (2008). The Adult Attachment Interview: Protocol, method of analysis, and empirical studies. In J. Cassidy & P. R. Shaver (Eds.), *Handbook of attachment: Theory, research, and clinical applications* (2nd ed., pp. 395–433). New York: Guilford Press.—This chapter offers an excellent and thorough introduction to the development and refinement of the AAI, including its classification and coding systems.

Lopez, F. G., & Brennan, K. A. (2000). Dynamic processes underlying adult attachment organization: Toward an attachment theoretical perspective on the healthy and effective self. *Journal of Counseling Psychology, 47,* 283–300.—This integrative review of the adult attachment literature underscores important associations between adult attachment security and indicators of positive self-development and optimal functioning.

Shaver, P. R., & Mikulincer, M. (2002). Attachment-related psychodynamics. *Attachment & Human Development, 4,* 133–161.—This impressive paper

integratively reviews attachment-theory-informed investigations of psychodynamic processes, and underscores convergent findings from studies using inter-
view- and self-report-based measures of adult attachment.
Slade, A. (2008). The implications of attachment theory and research for adult psychotherapy: Research and clinical perspectives. In J. Cassidy & P. R. Shaver
(Eds.), *Handbook of attachment: Theory, research, and clinical applications*
(2nd ed., pp. 762–782). New York: Guilford Press.—This chapter thoughtfully
explores associations between interview-based classifications of adult attachment and several prominent clinical processes, including transference and
countertransference dynamics.

REFERENCES

Baldwin, M. W., Fehr, B., Keedian, E., Seidel, M., & Thompson, D. W. (1993). An
exploration of the relational schemata underlying attachment styles: Self-report
and lexical decision approaches. *Personality and Social Psychology Bulletin,
19,* 746–754.

Bartholomew, K., & Allison, C. J. (2006). An attachment perspective on abusive
dynamics in intimate relationships. In M. Mikulincer & G. S. Goodman (Eds.),
Dynamics of romantic love: Attachment, caregiving, and sex (pp. 102–127).
New York: Guilford Press.

Bartholomew, K., & Horowitz, L. (1991). Attachment styles among young adults:
A test of a four category model. *Journal of Personality and Social Psychology,
61,* 226–244.

Bartholomew, K., & Shaver, P. R. (1998). Methods of assessing adult attachment:
Do they converge? In J. A. Simpson & W. S. Rholes (Eds.), *Attachment theory
and close relationships* (pp. 25–45). New York: Guilford Press.

Berant, E., Mikulincer, M., & Florian, V. (2001). Attachment style and mental
health: A 1-year follow-up study of mothers of infants with congenital heart
disease. *Personality and Social Psychology Bulletin, 27,* 956–968.

Berant, E., Mikulincer, M., & Florian, V. (2003). Marital satisfaction among mothers of infants with congenital heart disease: The contributions of illness severity, attachment style, and the coping process. *Anxiety, Stress, and Coping, 16,*
399–415.

Berant, E., Mikulincer, M., Shaver, P. R., & Segal, Y. (2008). Mothers' attachment
styles, their mental health, and their children's emotional vulnerabilities: A
7-year study of children with congenital heart disease. *Journal of Personality,
76,* 31–65.

Bernier, A., & Dozier, M. (2002). Assessing adult attachment: Empirical sophistication and conceptual biases. *Attachment & Human Development, 4,* 171–179.

Bogaert, A. F., & Sadava, S. (2002). Adult attachment and sexual behavior. *Personal
Relationships, 9,* 191–204.

Bowlby, J. (1977). The making and breaking of affectional bonds: II. Some principles of psychotherapy. *British Journal of Psychiatry, 130,* 421–431.

Brennan, K. A., Shaver, P. R., & Tobey, A. E. (1991). Attachment styles, gender and
parental problem drinking. *Journal of Social and Personal Relationships, 8,*
451–466.

Brennan, K. A., & Bosson, J. K. (1998). Attachment style differences in attitudes toward and reactions to feedback from romantic partners: An exploration of the relational basis of self-esteem. *Personality and Social Psychology Bulletin, 24,* 699–714.

Brennan, K. A., Clark, C. L., & Shaver, P. R. (1998). Self-report measurement of adult attachment: An integrative overview. In J. A. Simpson & W. S. Rholes (Eds.), *Attachment theory and close relationships* (pp. 46–76). New York: Guilford Press.

Brennan, K. A., & Shaver, P. R. (1998). Attachment styles and personality disorders: Their connections to each other and to parental divorce, parental death, and perceptions of parental caregiving. *Journal of Personality, 66,* 835–878.

Bretherton, I., & Munholland, K. A. (1999). Internal working models in attachment relationships: A construct revisited. In J. Cassidy & P. R. Shaver (Eds.), *Handbook of attachment: Theory, research, and clinical applications* (pp. 89–111). New York: Guilford Press.

Campbell, L., Simpson, J. A., Boldry, J., & Kashy, D. A. (2005). Perceptions of conflict and support in romantic relationships: The role of attachment anxiety. *Journal of Personality and Social Psychology, 88,* 510–531.

Cassidy, J. (2000). Adult romantic attachments: A developmental perspective on individual differences. *Review of General Psychology, 4,* 111–131.

Collins, N. L. (1996). Working models of attachment: Implications for explanation, emotion, and behavior. *Journal of Personality and Social Psychology, 71,* 810–832.

Collins, N. L., Cooper, M. L., Albino, A. & Allard, L. (2002). Psychosocial vulnerability from adolescence to adulthood: A prospective study of attachment style differences in relationship functioning and partner choice. *Journal of Personality, 70,* 965–1008.

Collins, N. L., & Feeney, B. C. (2000). A safe haven: An attachment theory perspective on support seeking and caregiving in intimate relationships. *Journal of Personality and Social Psychology, 78,* 1053–1073.

Collins, N. L., Guichard, A. C., Ford, M., & Feeney, B. C. (2004). Working models of attachment: New developments and emerging themes. In W. S. Rholes & J. A. Simpson (Eds.), *Adult attachment: Theory, research, and clinical implications* (pp. 196–239). New York: Guilford Press.

Collins, N. L., & Read, S. J. (1990). Adult attachment, working models, and relationship quality in dating couples. *Journal of Personality and Social Psychology, 58,* 644–663.

Corcoran, K. O., & Mallinckrodt, B. (2000). Adult attachment, self-efficacy, perspective taking and conflict resolution. *Journal of Counseling and Development, 78,* 478–489.

Creasey, G. (2002). Associations between working models of attachment and conflict management behavior in romantic couples. *Journal of Counseling Psychology, 49,* 365–375.

Creasey, G., & Hesson-McInnis, M. (2001). Affective responses, cognitive appraisals, and conflict tactics in late adolescent romantic relationships: Associations with attachment orientations. *Journal of Counseling Psychology, 48,* 85–96.

Crowell, J. A., & Treboux, D. (1995). A review of adult attachment measures: Implications for theory and research. *Social Development, 4,* 294–327.

Crowell, J. A., Treboux, D., & Waters, E. (1999). The Adult Attachment Interview and the Relationship Questionnaire: Relations to reports of mothers and partners. *Personal Relationships, 6,* 1–18.

Davila, J., Burge, D., & Hammen, C. (1997). Why does attachment style change? *Journal of Personality and Social Psychology, 73,* 826–838.

Davis, D., Shaver, P. R., & Vernon, M. L. (2003). Physical, emotional, and behavioral reactions to breaking up: The roles of gender, age, emotional involvement, and attachment style. *Personality and Social Psychology Bulletin, 29,* 871–884.

Diehl, M., Elnick, A. B., Bourbeau, L. S., & Labouvie-Vief, G. (1998). Adult attachment styles: Their relations to family context and personality. *Journal of Personality and Social Psychology, 74,* 1656–1669.

Dutton, D. G., Starzomski, A. J., & Ryan, L. (1996). Antecedents of abusive personality and abusive behavior in wife assaulters. *Journal of Family Violence, 11,* 113–132.

Elliott, A. J., & Reis, H. T. (2003). Attachment and exploration. *Journal of Personality and Social Psychology, 85,* 317–331.

Epstein, S. (1983). *The Mother–Father–Peer Scale.* Unpublished manuscript, University of Massachusetts at Amherst.

Feeney, J. A., & Noller, P. (1990). Attachment style as a predictor of adult romantic relationships. *Journal of Personality and Social Psychology, 58,* 281–291.

Fonagy, P., Steele, H., & Steele, M. (1991). Maternal representations of attachment during pregnancy predict the organization of infant–mother attachment at one year of age. *Child Development, 62,* 891–905.

Fraley, R. C., Garner, J. P., & Shaver, P. R. (2000). Adult attachment and the defensive regulation of attention and memory: Examining the role of preemptive and postemptive defensive processes. *Journal of Personality and Social Psychology, 79,* 816–826.

Fraley, R. C., & Shaver, P. R. (1997). Adult attachment and the suppression of unwanted thoughts. *Journal of Personality and Social Psychology, 73,* 1080–1091.

Frei, J. R., & Shaver, P. R. (2002). Respect in close relationships: Prototype definition, self-report assessment, and initial correlates. *Personal Relationships, 9,* 121–139.

Fuendeling, J. M. (1998). Affect regulation as a stylistic process within adult attachment. *Journal of Social and Personal Relationships, 15,* 291–322.

Gallo, L. C., Smith, T. W., & Ruiz, J. M. (2003). An interpersonal analysis of adult attachment style: Circumplex descriptions, recalled developmental experiences, self-representations, and interpersonal functioning in adulthood. *Journal of Personality, 71,* 141–181.

George, C., Kaplan, N., & Main, M. (1984). *Adult Attachment Interview protocol.* Unpublished manuscript, University of California, Berkeley.

George, C., Kaplan, N., & Main, M. (1985). *Adult Attachment Interview protocol* (2nd ed.). Unpublished manuscript, University of California, Berkeley.

George, C., Kaplan, N., & Main, M. (1996). *Adult Attachment Interview protocol* (3rd ed.). Unpublished manuscript, University of California, Berkeley.

Grossmann, K. E., Grossmann, K., & Waters, E. (Eds.). (2005). *Attachment from infancy to adulthood: The major longitudinal studies.* New York: Guilford Press.

Hazan, C., & Shaver, P. R. (1987). Romantic love conceptualized as an attachment process. *Journal of Personality and Social Psychology, 52,* 511–524.

Hesse, E. (1999). The Adult Attachment Interview: Historical and current perspectives. In J. Cassidy & P. R. Shaver (Eds.), *Handbook of attachment: Theory, research, and clinical applications* (pp. 395–433). New York: Guilford Press.

Horowitz, L. (1979). On the cognitive structure of interpersonal problems treated in psychotherapy. *Journal of Consulting and Clinical Psychology, 47,* 5–15.

Keelan, J., Dion, K., & Dion, K. L. (1998). Attachment style and relationship satisfaction: Test of a self-disclosure explanation. *Canadian Journal of Behavioural Science, 30,* 24–35.

Klohnen, E. C., & Bera, S. (1998). Behavioral and experiential patterns of avoidantly and securely attached women across adulthood: A 31-year longitudinal perspective. *Journal of Personality and Social Psychology, 74,* 211–223.

Kobak, R. R. (1989). *The Attachment Interview Q-Set.* Unpublished manuscript, University of Delaware.

Kobak, R. R. (2002). Building bridges between social, developmental and clinical psychology. *Attachment & Human Development, 4,* 216–222.

Kobak, R. R., & Hazan, C. (1991). Attachment in marriage: Effects of security and accuracy of working models. *Journal of Personality and Social Psychology, 60,* 861–869.

Kobak, R. R., & Sceery, A. (1988). Attachment in late adolescence: Working models, affect regulation, and representations of self and other. *Child Development, 59,* 135–146.

Kunce, L. J., & Shaver, P. R. (1994). An attachment-theoretical approach to caregiving in romantic relationships. In K. Bartholomew & D. Perlman (Eds.), *Advances in personal relationships: Vol. 5. Attachment processes in adulthood* (pp. 205–237). London: Jessica Kingsley.

Larose, S., & Bernier, A. (2001). Social support processes: Mediators of attachment state of mind and adjustment in late adolescence. *Attachment & Human Development, 3,* 96–120.

Levy, K. N., Blatt, S. J., & Shaver, P. R. (1998). Attachment styles and parental representations. *Journal of Personality and Social Psychology, 74,* 407–419.

Lopez, F. G. (2003). The assessment of adult attachment security. In S. J. Lopez & C. R. Snyder (Eds.), *Handbook of positive psychological assessment* (pp. 285–299). Washington, DC: American Psychological Association.

Lopez, F. G., & Brennan, K. A. (2000). Dynamic processes underlying adult attachment organization: Toward an attachment theoretical perspective on the healthy and effective self. *Journal of Counseling Psychology, 47,* 283–300.

Lyons-Ruth, K., Yellin, C., Melnick, S., & Atwood, G. (2003). Childhood experiences of trauma and loss have different relations to maternal unresolved and hostile-helpless states of mind on the AAI. *Attachment & Human Development, 5,* 330–352.

Main, M., & Goldwyn, R. (1984). *Adult attachment scoring and classification system.* Unpublished manuscript, University of California, Berkeley.

Main, M., Goldwyn, R., & Hesse, E. (2003) *Adult attachment scoring and classification system.* Unpublished manuscript, University of California, Berkeley.

Main, M., Kaplan, N., & Cassidy, J. (1985). Security in infancy, childhood, and adulthood: A move to the level of representation. *Monographs for the Society for Research in Child Development, 50*(1–2, Serial No. 2019), 66–104.

Manassis, K., Owens, M., Adam, K. S., West, M., & Sheldon-Keller, A. E. (1999). Assessing attachment: Convergent validity of the Adult Attachment Interview and the Parental Bonding Instrument. *Australian and New Zealand Journal of Psychiatry, 33,* 559–567.

Mickelson, K. D., Kessler, R. C., & Shaver, P. R. (1997). Adult attachment in a nationally representative sample. *Journal of Personality and Social Psychology, 73,* 1092–1106.

Mikulincer, M. (1995). Attachment style and the mental representation of the self. *Journal of Personality and Social Psychology, 69,* 1203–1215.

Mikulincer, M. (1997). Adult attachment style and information processing: Individual differences in curiosity and cognitive closure. *Journal of Personality and Social Psychology, 72,* 1217–1230.

Mikulincer, M. (1998). Attachment working models and the sense of trust: An exploration of interaction goals and affect regulation. *Journal of Personality and Social Psychology, 74,* 1209–1224.

Mikulincer, M., & Arad, D. (1999). Attachment working models and cognitive openness in close relationships: A test of chronic and temporary accessibility effects. *Journal of Personality and Social Psychology, 77,* 710–725.

Mikulincer, M., Dolev, T., & Shaver, P. R. (2004). Attachment-related strategies during thought suppression: Ironic rebounds and vulnerable self-representations. *Journal of Personality and Social Psychology, 87,* 940–956.

Mikulincer, M., & Florian, V. (1998). The relationship between adult attachment styles and emotional and cognitive reactions to stressful events. In J. A. Simpson & W. S. Rholes (Eds.), *Attachment theory and close relationships* (pp. 143–165). New York: Guilford Press.

Mikulincer, M., & Nachshon, O. (1991). Attachment styles and patterns of self-disclosure. *Journal of Personality and Social Psychology, 61,* 321–331.

Mikulincer, M., & Orbach, I. (1995). Attachment styles and repressive defensiveness: The accessibility and architecture of affective memories. *Journal of Personality and Social Psychology, 68,* 917–925.

Mikulincer, M., & Shaver, P. R. (2004). Security-based self-representations in adulthood: Contents and processes. In W. S. Rholes & J. A. Simpson (Eds.), *Adult attachment: Theory, research, and clinical implications* (pp. 159–195). New York: Guilford Press.

Mikulincer, M., & Shaver, P. R. (2007). *Attachment in adulthood: Structure, dynamics, and change.* New York: Guilford Press.

Mikulincer, M., Shaver, P. R., Gillath, O., & Nitzberg, R. A. (2005). Attachment, caregiving, and altruism: Boosting attachment security increases compassion and helping. *Journal of Personality and Social Psychology, 85,* 817–839.

Noftle, E. E., & Shaver, P. R. (2006). Attachment dimensions and the Big Five personality traits: Associations and comparative ability to predict relationship quality. *Journal of Research in Personality, 40,* 179–208.

Parker, G., Tupling, H., & Brown, L. B. (1979). A parental bonding instrument. *British Journal of Medical Psychology, 52,* 1–10.

Pianta, R. C., Egeland, B., & Adam, E. K. (1996). Adult attachment classification and self-reported psychiatric symptomatology as assessed by the Minnesota Multiphasic Personality Inventory–2. *Journal of Consulting and Clinical Psychology, 64,* 273–281.

Reis, S., & Grenyer, B. F. S. (2004). Fearful attachment, working alliance, and treatment response for individuals with major depression. *Clinical Psychology and Psychotherapy, 11,* 414–424.

Scharf, M., Mayseless, O., & Kivenson-Baron, I. (2004). Adolescents' attachment representations and developmental tasks in emerging adulthood. *Developmental Psychology, 40,* 430–444.

Searle, B., & Meara, N. M. (1999). Affective dimensions of attachment styles: Exploring self-reported attachment style, gender, and emotional experience among college students. *Journal of Counseling Psychology, 46,* 147–158.

Shaver, P. R., Belsky, J., & Brennan, K. A. (2000). The Adult Attachment Interview and self-reports of romantic attachment: Associations across domains and methods. *Personal Relationships, 7,* 25–43.

Shaver, P. R., & Brennan, K. A. (1992). Attachment styles and the "Big Five" personality traits: Their connections with each other and with romantic relationship outcomes. *Personality and Social Psychology Bulletin, 18,* 536–545.

Shaver, P. R., & Clark, C. L. (1994). The psychodynamics of adult romantic attachment. In J. M. Masling and R. F. Bornstein (Eds.), *Empirical perspectives on object relations theories* (pp. 105–156). Washington, DC: American Psychological Association.

Shaver, P. R., & Mikulincer, M. (2002). Attachment-related psychodynamics. *Attachment & Human Development, 4,* 133–161.

Shaver, P. R., & Mikulincer, M. (2004). What do self-report attachment measures assess? In W. S. Rholes & J. A. Simpson (Eds.), *Adult attachment: Theory, research, and clinical implications* (pp. 17–54). New York: Guilford Press.

Shaver, P. R., Schachner, D. A., & Mikulincer, M. (2005). Attachment style, excessive reassurance seeking, relationship processes, and depression. *Personality and Social Psychology Bulletin, 31,* 343–359.

Simpson, J. A. (1990). Influence of attachment styles on romantic relationships. *Journal of Personality and Social Psychology, 59,* 971–980.

Simpson, J. A., & Rholes, W. A. (2002). Fearful-avoidance, disorganization, and multiple working models: Some directions for future theory and research. *Attachment & Human Development, 4,* 223–229.

Simpson, J. A., Rholes, W. S., & Nelligan, J. S. (1992). Support seeking and support giving within couples in an anxiety-provoking situation: The role of attachment styles. *Journal of Personality and Social Psychology, 62,* 434–446.

Slade, A. (1999). Attachment theory and research: Implications for the theory and practice of individual psychotherapy with adults. In J. Cassidy & P. R. Shaver (Eds.), *Handbook of attachment: Theory, research, and clinical applications* (pp. 575–594). New York: Guilford Press.

van IJzendoorn, M. H. (1995). Adult attachment representations, parental responsiveness, and infant attachment: A meta-analysis on the predictive validity of the Adult Attachment Interview. *Psychological Bulletin, 117,* 387–403.

Waters, H. S., Rodrigues, L. M., & Ridgeway, D. (1998). Cognitive underpinnings of narrative attachment assessment. *Journal of Experimental Child Psychology, 71,* 211–234.

Part II

ASSESSING ATTACHMENT

6

Using Interviews
to Assess Adult Attachment

Kenneth N. Levy
Kristen M. Kelly

John Bowlby (1969/1982, 1973) provided psychology with a rich and cogent theory of personality development and interpersonal relating. From the beginning, he conceptualized attachment theory in terms of both typical and psychopathological development. Bowlby (1979) believed that attachment difficulties increase vulnerability to psychopathology and can help clinicians to identify and understand the specific kinds of psychological difficulties that arise. Bowlby (1977) contended that *internal working models* of attachment help to explain "the many forms of emotional distress and personality disturbances, including anxiety, anger, depression, and emotional detachment, to which unwilling separations and loss give rise" (p. 201). He held that childhood attachment underlies the "later capacity to make affectional bonds as well as a whole range of adult dysfunctions," including "marital problems and trouble with children, as well as ... neurotic symptoms and personality disorders" (p. 206). Thus Bowlby postulated that the effects of early attachment experiences tend to persist across the lifespan, are among the major determinants of personality organization, and have specific clinical relevance.

On the basis of Bowlby's attachment theory, Ainsworth, Blehar, Waters, and Wall (1978) identified three major styles of attachment in infancy—secure, anxious-avoidant, and anxious-ambivalent—and traced them to caregivers' parenting behavior. In Ainsworth's Strange Situation paradigm, attachment security was determined behaviorally. Babies who approached their mothers for comfort, soothing, and emotional refueling after a 3-minute separation from the mothers were deemed securely attached. Infants who avoided their mothers, ignored them, or were difficult to console after such a separation were coded as insecurely attached. Subsequent investigators replicated and extended Ainsworth et al.'s (1978) initial findings, both in the United States and in other countries (for a review, see van IJzendoorn, 1995). Longitudinal studies investigating the predictability of later functioning and adaptation from infant attachment styles have found considerable stability of attachment classification from infancy to adulthood, although the degree of stability is dependent on intervening experiences in relationships (for reviews, see Fraley, 2002, and Grossmann, Grossmann, & Waters, 2005).

On the basis of Bowlby's contention that the attachment system is active throughout the lifespan, Mary Main began focusing on adults' *state of mind with respect to attachment* as a predictor of the adults' infants' attachment classification in the Strange Situation. In so doing, she moved the assessment of attachment from the behavioral level to what she and her colleagues (e.g., Main, Kaplan, & Cassidy, 1985) called the *level of representation,* as reflected in the Adult Attachment Interview (AAI). In this chapter, we discuss the essential elements of AAI administration and coding. We also discus the AAI's clinical utility and the challenges involved in using the AAI with a clinical population. Since the AAI was created, a number of other interviews have been developed to assess attachment security in adults. These include the Current Relationship Interview (Crowell & Owens, 1996), a modified AAI (Crittenden, 1995), and the Patient–Therapist AAI (Diamond et al., 1999). Although we briefly describe these other interviews, we focus mainly on the AAI because (1) the design and scoring of all the variants are based on the AAI, and (2) the AAI has generated the most reliability and validity data.

THE ADULT ATTACHMENT INTERVIEW

Main and her colleagues (George, Kaplan, & Main, 1984, 1985, 1996; Main et al., 1985) developed the AAI, a 1-hour attachment history interview, as a way of beginning to determine what residues of attachment-related experiences exist in parents' minds and affect the ways in which they behave with their young children. The interview asks about early attachment relationships, as well as an interviewee's sense of how these experiences affected his or her adult personality, by probing for specific memories that corroborate and/or contradict the nature of the attachment history presented by the interviewee. Noting the discourse features in the interviews, Main and colleagues identified three major patterns of adult attachment: *secure-autonomous* (F), *dismissing* (Ds), and *enmeshed/preoccupied* (E). More recently, they have added two further categories: *unresolved/disorganized* (U/d) and *cannot classify* (CC). The first three categories parallel the attachment classifications originally identified in childhood by Ainsworth et al.

(1978), and the unresolved/disorganized classification parallels a pattern that Main earlier noticed in infants (Main & Weston, 1981; see also Main & Solomon, 1990). As hoped, Main found that the adult attachment patterns identified in adults reliably predict the Strange Situation behavior of their children (Main et al., 1985; for a review, see van IJzendoorn, 1995).

The AAI is a semistructured clinical-like interview designed to elicit thoughts, feelings, and memories related to early attachment experiences, and to assess an adult's state of mind with respect to attachment, or internal working model of attachment relationships. The interview consists of 18–20 questions asked in a set order with standardized probes. Interviewees are asked to describe their childhood relationships with their parents, choosing five adjectives or short phrases to describe each relationship and (later in the interview) supporting these descriptors with specific memories. To elicit attachment-related information, they are asked how their parents responded to them when they were in physical or emotional distress (e.g., during times when they were upset, injured, or ill as children). They are also asked about memories of separations, losses, experiences of rejection, and times when they might have felt threatened (including, but not limited to, times involving physical and sexual abuse). The interview requires that they reflect on their parents' styles of parenting and consider how their childhood experiences with their parents have influenced their lives. The interview technique has been described as "surprising the unconscious" (George et al., 1985), and it provides numerous opportunities for an interviewee to elaborate upon, contradict, or fail to support previous statements. Although the AAI is a semistructured interview, it yields information similar to what is obtained in a less structured clinical interview.

Coding

The AAI is transcribed verbatim and very carefully, and trained coders score the typed transcripts by using several scale ratings (Main & Goldwyn, 1984; Main, Goldwyn, & Hesse, 2003), which are then used to assign the person interviewed to one of five primary attachment classifications (secure-autonomous, dismissing, preoccupied, unresolved/disorganized, and cannot classify). The unresolved classification can be a primary or secondary designation, and a person given this designation is also assigned the one of three main organized styles that best fits the transcript (secure, dismissing, or preoccupied). Primary attachment classifications are derived from three classes of scale ratings:

1. The first class contains scales based on the rater's (i.e., coder's) *inferences* about the individual's experiences with parents during childhood (e.g., the extent to which each parent was or was not loving, rejecting, neglecting, involving, and role-reversing). It is important

to note that the AAI does not purport to assess an individual's actual experiences, but only the content and structure of the person's current representations of those experiences.

2. The second group of scales assesses the individual's style of discourse (including coherence of the transcript, idealization of parents, insistence on lack of recall, expression of anger or other strong feelings, lack of resolution of loss or trauma, and overall coherence of thought).

3. The third group contains scales that assess the individual's overall state of mind with respect to attachment (e.g., degree of derogation of attachment).

The scale ratings are usually made along a 9-point continuum, where 1 refers to absence or very low levels and 9 refers to high levels of the quality in question. Although all of the subscales are used to classify interviewees' overall state of mind with respect to attachment, research indicates that the coherence-of-the-narrative scale is the best single indicator of attachment security ($r = .96$, $p < .001$) (Waters, Treboux, Crowell, Fyffe, & Crowell, 2001).

Classification

Individuals classified as *secure-autonomous* describe the positive and negative aspects of their childhood experiences with parents in an open, coherent, and consistent manner. Their responses are typically spontaneous and fresh, and at times indicate that they are actively reflecting on their own thought processes. Security is also characterized by a well-organized, undefended discourse style in which emotions are freely expressed and by a high degree of coherence in discussing attachment relationships, regardless of how positively or negatively those relationships might have been described. (Because security, according to the scoring system, is mostly a matter of coherence, coherent discourse about negative relationship experiences is also counted toward security.) Secure individuals are collaborative during the interview process, maintain a balanced and realistic-seeming view of their early relationships, value attachment relationships, and view attachment-related experiences as highly influential in their development.

Individuals classified as *dismissing* devalue attachment relationships or portray them in an idealized fashion while being unable to provide corroborating concrete examples. As the interview proceeds, inconsistencies usually appear between vaguely positive generalizations and "leaked" concrete evidence to the contrary. In contrast with secure individuals, dismissing individuals typically exhibit discomfort with the interview, either implicitly or explicitly, often responding to the relationship questions as if they are foreign and unexpected. They also have difficulty recalling specific events, but gradually reveal an early history of rejection; they may attempt to normalize this and to deny or minimize any untoward effects. They are judged to have low *coherence of mind* because of the vagueness and sparseness of their descriptions, as well as the inconsistency between the vaguely positive generalizations and the "leaked" concrete evidence of negative experiences.

Individuals who are classified as *preoccupied* with respect to attachment are confused and entangled with previous attachment relationships or experiences. While typically speaking about their parents and past experiences in an open, unguarded manner, they produce narratives that are unfruitful and lack objectivity. Perhaps most importantly, preoccupied individuals have a tendency toward incoherence in their accounts. Their interviews are often excessively long and characterized by the use of lengthy, grammatically entangled sentences; jargon and nonsense words; reversions to childlike speech; or confusion regarding past and present relationships—all of which convey a lack of distance or an adult perspective. They often describe early relationships with parents as overinvolved or as guilt-inducing. Descriptions of their current relationships with parents are often characterized by pervasive anger, passivity, and/or attempts to please parents. Preoccupied answers often fail to address the interviewer's original questions, as if the person is so enmeshed in past negative feelings that he or she loses track of the interviewer's needs (or existence).

Individuals classified as *unresolved/disorganized* (concerning trauma or loss) may speak largely in a coherent manner, yet make fleeting, confused statements in relation to traumatic attachment-related events. Because their interviews may have prominent features of either the secure, dismissing, or preoccupied attachment style, these interviews are given a corresponding secondary classification. The unresolved classification is assigned when an individual displays lapses in the monitoring of reasoning or discourse when discussing experiences of loss or abuse. These lapses include highly implausible statements regarding the causes and consequences of traumatic attachment-related events, loss of memory for attachment-related traumas, and confusion and silence during discussions of trauma or loss.

The fifth category, *cannot classify,* was developed because Hesse (1996) found that approximately 18–20% of people in typical community samples and 40% of clinical samples could not be classified within the four-category system. The cannot classify designation is assigned when an individual displays a combination of contradictory or incompatible attachment patterns, or when no single state of mind with respect to attachment is predominant. The person may shift attachment patterns in midinterview, display different attachment patterns when discussing different attachment figures, or exhibit a mixture of different discourse styles within the same portion of the transcript.

As with the Strange Situation coding procedure for infants, there are subclassifications within each of the major adult attachment categories. We do not attempt to delve into those details here, although it is worth noting that they may eventually prove clinically important and useful.

The AAI is generally administered by interviewers who have completed a 2-week training workshop conducted by Mary Main and Erik Hesse or by one of the trainers they have certified. However, many research teams have found that a range of individuals, from graduate students in developmental and clinical psychology to clinicians in the community, can be trained to administer the AAI (but *not* code it) by an experienced AAI interviewer, preferably one who has completed the 2-week training workshop. The AAI is administered face to face in a single session, and because the time needed to complete it varies, the interviewer needs to schedule sufficient time. We have had interviews take as little as 20 minutes and as long as 3–4 hours. The median is somewhere between 1 and 3 hours. Because the interview is lengthy and emotional, we recommend a comfortable room, complete with tissues and bottled water. The interview is audiotaped; although it can be videotaped, this makes it more difficult and expensive to transcribe, because VCR/DVD transcription machines are expensive. We recommend using a digital recorder with separate clip-on microphones to ensure the best-quality recording.

Because the AAI is designed to parallel the infant Strange Situation procedure by surprising the unconscious and activating the attachment system, and because it flows differently than a therapy session does, we recommend that therapists not administer the AAI to their own patients. When using the AAI in a clinical setting, an interviewer needs to be able to assess the interviewee's emotional state and be prepared to end the interview if clinically indicated. We should mention, however, that in conducting over 200 interviews with patients who had borderline personality disorder (BPD), we had to end an interview prematurely on only one occasion.

How Is the AAI Coded?

The AAI is transcribed verbatim according to transcription rules developed by Mary Main. It usually takes a person using a foot-pedaled transcription machine 6–12 hours to transcribe an AAI, depending on such factors as the length of the interview, clearness of the speakers, and typing speed. Once transcribed and checked for accuracy, the AAI is scored for attachment classification by coders who have been properly trained and have achieved reliability on an extensive set of training transcripts. Raters must remain unaware of each participant's identifying characteristics, including clinical status, diagnosis, and (if the AAI is being administered as part of a research project) the nature and purpose of the study and the participant's placement in the design.

Distribution of Attachment Patterns

In a meta-analytic study with a combined sample of 584 nonclinical mothers, when the three-way classification system was used, 58% of participants were classified as secure-autonomous, 24% as dismissing, and 18% as preoccupied. When the four-way system was used with 487 nonclinical mothers, 55% were classified as secure-autonomous, 16% as dismissing, 9% as preoccupied, and 19% as unresolved. In two nonclinical samples, 6.6% and 10% of participants received the cannot classify designation (Allen, Hauser, & Borman-Spurrell, 1996; Holtzworth-Monroe, Stuart, & Hutchinson, 1997).

Interrater Reliability

Studies indicate a range of interrater reliabilities from 75% to 100% agreement in overall classification (Allen et al., 1996; de Haas, Bakermans-Kranenburg, & van IJzendoorn, 1994; Levy et al., 2006; Pianta, Egeland, & Adam, 1996; Sagi, van IJzendoorn, Scharf, & Koren-Karie, 1994), and a greater range of scores across rating scales. In our own study of patients with BPD (Levy et al., 2006), raters agreed on 86% of the categorical classifications ($\kappa = .80$, $t = 6.11$, $p < .001$). The intraclass correlation for dimensional ratings of narrative coherence was .88.

Test–Retest Reliability

Much research has shown that the secure, dismissing, and preoccupied classifications are stable over long periods of time (Bakermans-Kranenburg & van IJzendoorn, 1993; Benoit & Parker, 1994; de Haas et al., 1994; Sagi et al., 1994). Bakermans-Kranenburg and van IJzendoorn (1993) found 78% stability ($\kappa = .63$) across the three organized attachment categories. Sagi et al. (1994) reported a reliability of 90% ($\kappa = .79$) over a 3-month period. Benoit and Parker (1994) found 90% three-category stability between prebirth interviews and interviews conducted when the participants' infants were 11 months old. Crowell, Waters, Treboux, and O'Connor (1996) reported a stability of 86% (three-category; $\kappa = .73$). Ammaniti, van IJzendoorn, Speranza, and Tambelli (2000), over a 4-year period, found 95% secure–insecure correspondence and 70% three-category correspondence.

Validity

The validity of the AAI has been judged primarily in terms of its ability to predict the quality of an adult's attachment relationship with his or her infant, as observed in the Strange Situation, and to predict parents' responsiveness to their infants' attachment signals. Much of this work has been done with nonclinical samples, although there is some evidence that the AAI is predictive in clinical samples (Fonagy, Steele, Steele, Moran, & Higgitt, 1991).

Predictive Validity

van IJzendoorn (1995) conducted a meta-analytic review of studies assessing secure versus insecure parental attachment representations and the quality of infant attachment as observed in the Strange Situation, as well as observations of parents' sensitivity, warmth, structure, and supportiveness toward their infants or preschool-age children. In 18 samples (N = 854), the combined effect size for predicting infant secure versus insecure attachment was 1.06 in the expected direction. For a portion of the studies, the percentage of correspondence between parents' state of mind with respect to attachment and their infants' attachment security could be computed, and the resulting percentage was 75% (k = .49). There was a strong association between AAI and Strange Situation classifications (r = .49, biserial r = .59).

With regard to responsiveness to infants' attachment signals, a meta-analysis of 10 studies (N = 389) yielded a combined effect size of 0.72. Whereas the match between the AAI and the infants' Strange Situation classifications was somewhat lower in those studies (although still strong, d = 0.80) for fathers than for mothers, the predictability of caregiving responsiveness from the AAI was greater for fathers than for mothers. These effect sizes are considered large (Cohen, 1992). The effect size discriminating clinical from nonclinical populations (d = 1.03) was almost identical to that discriminating parents of secure infants from parents of insecure infants (d = 1.06; van IJzendoorn & Bakermans-Kranenburg, 1996).

Long-Term Continuity

Several studies have examined long-term continuity by following infants into young adulthood (Hamilton, 2000; Lewis, Feiring, & Rosenthal, 2000; Waters, Merrick, Treboux, Crowell, & Albersheim, 2000; Weinfield, Sroufe, & Egeland, 2000; Zimmerman, Fremmer-Bombik, Spangler, & Grossmann, 1997). The results of these studies have been somewhat inconsistent, but overall they are consistent with Sroufe's concept of *lawful discontinuity* (Stroufe, 1979; Weinfield et al., 2000). Two studies found high continuity (Hamilton, 2000; Waters et al., 2000). Hamilton (2000) found a 75% correspondence for secure–insecure attachment status between infancy and late adolescence, with the strongest stability in the preoccupied group. Waters et al. (2000) followed 50 individuals for 20 years, finding 64% stability in attachment classification. Three other studies found less continuity, but have found evidence of lawful discontinuity. Weinfield et al. (2000) were able to differentiate stable from unstable groups on the basis of child maltreatment, maternal depression, and family functioning in early adolescence. Lewis et al. (2000) found that parental divorce during childhood was related to later insecure attachment. Waters et al. (2000) also found evidence of lawful discontinuity. They found greater than 70% stability for individuals with no major negative life events, and less than 50% stability for those who had lost a parent, endured parental divorce, or the like. These findings provide evidence that the stability of attachment representations over time vary as a function of family environment and difficult and chaotic life experiences.

In a meta-analytic study, Fraley (2002) tested two mathematical models of stability and change: (1) a *revisionist* model, which holds that early attachment patterns are subject to continual change on the basis of new experience; and (2) a *prototype* model, which holds that despite some capacity for change, core attachment patterns are sustained over time and continue to influence attachment behavior later in adulthood. Results indicated that the moderate stability of attachment security over the first 19 years of life is better accounted for by the prototype model.

Discriminant Validity

van IJzendoorn (1995) found that in five out of six studies, secure versus insecure adult attachment status was unrelated to intelligence, and Bakermans-Kranenburg and van IJzendoorn (1993) found that AAI classifications were independent of non-attachment-related memory. Crowell et al. (1996) studied the discriminant validity of the AAI vis-à-vis measures of intelligence, social desirability, discourse style, and general social adjustment in a sample of 53 married women with preschool children. There was no relation between AAI classifications and discourse style or social desirability, but there were modest but significant correlations with IQ scores and social adjustment. With regard to dismissing attachment, Bakermans-Kranenburg and van IJzendoorn (1993) found the AAI to be unrelated to social desirability. In general, then, the AAI appears to be an attachment-related measure rather than a measure of some other, more general trait.

INCORPORATING THE AAI INTO CLINICAL PRACTICE

There are at least two ways that the AAI might be incorporated into clinical practice. First, it can be administered before beginning therapy or during the evaluation process to provide clinically relevant data; it can also be administered periodically to assess change in the coherence of a client's narrative and improvement on some of the attachment coding scales. This first kind of assessment would probably take place outside the therapy hour, and, as mentioned earlier, it would be best in this case for the AAI to be administered by someone other than the therapist. However, for most clinicians it may be difficult to use the AAI for formal assessments of attachment state of mind. Thus it is worthwhile to consider a second manner in which the AAI can be used in clinical practice—employing the central constructs and principles in the AAI to understand and guide clinical work.

Once the AAI coding system is learned, a clinician can listen to clinical process with attachment organization in mind (Slade, 1999). For example, when a patient is describing relationships with important attachment figures, a clinician can listen for cues that may suggest the individual's state of mind with respect to attachment.

Using the AAI in Clinical Diagnosis

The AAI was not designed as a clinical diagnostic tool and should not be used as a substitute for diagnosis, particularly a formal psychiatric diagnostic-and-statistical-manual-based diagnosis. However, it provides useful clinical information about the way in which an individual organizes his or her thought processes and copes with stress, and it may aid in distinguishing subtypes within particular diagnostic classifications (e.g., Levy & Blatt, 1999).

As mentioned earlier, the AAI was intended to "surprise the unconscious" and to serve as an adult version of the Strange Situation procedure by activating an individual's attachment system. The interview achieves these goals through presenting questions that catch the interviewee off guard by directing attention to images, memories, and representations of childhood attachment experiences, and it calls upon the person to evaluate these emotion-laden experiences while maintaining appropriate interview discourse and reasoning. The interviewee has to integrate challenging thoughts and feelings in a way that allows the interviewer to observe and evaluate the person's self-regulatory abilities. In this way, the AAI is similar to Kernberg's (1984) structural interview, which assesses the degree of differentiation and integration of representations of self and others to determine a person's personality organization, although the AAI is much more structured. It is interesting to note that object relations theorists like Kernberg and Blatt, and developmental psychologists like Main, independently developed assessment procedures to examine the organization of mental representations revealed in discourse; they also invented similar questions and coding schemes (although Kernberg's procedure was meant to be used clinically, whereas Blatt and Main developed their respective systems for research purposes).

There are few data regarding the potential diagnostic value of the AAI for relating a particular disorder or groups of disorders to specific attachment patterns. For example, unresolved attachment has been related to a host of different psychopathological outcomes, including substance abuse (Riggs & Jacobvitz, 2002), BPD (Barone, 2003; Fonagy et al., 1996; Levy et al., 2006; Patrick, Hobson, Castle, & Howard, 1994), psychiatric hospitalization (Adam, Sheldon-Keller, & West, 1996; Allen et al., 1996; van IJzendoorn & Bakermans-Kranenburg, 1996), suicidal ideation (Allen et al., 1996; Riggs & Jacobvitz, 2002), posttraumatic stress disorder (PTSD) (Stovall-McClough & Cloitre, 2006), and dissociation (Carlson, 1998).

AAI States of Mind as Predictors of Treatment Use and Response

The AAI may be useful for understanding important aspects of psychotherapy, particularly the therapeutic relationship, transference–countertransference dynamics, and psychotherapy dropout.

The AAI and Treatment Use

A number of studies have related AAI states of mind to treatment use (Dozier, 1990; Korfmacher, Adam, Ogawa, & Egeland, 1997; Riggs & Jacobvitz, 2002). Not surprisingly, those with secure states of mind have proven to be more collaborative, more receptive, and better able to utilize treatment. In contrast, those with dismissing states of mind have been found to be less engaged in treatment. Those with preoccupied states of mind have presented as more needy, but have not necessarily been compliant with treatment.

Dozier (1990) found that dismissing patients were often resistant to treatment, had difficulty asking for help, and retreated from help when it was offered. Riggs and Jacobvitz (2002) found that dismissing adults were less likely to report having ever been in therapy than those who were secure, preoccupied, or unresolved with respect to attachment. Interestingly, secure adults reported the highest rates of couple therapy. Korfmacher et al. (1997), in a study of treatment use among pregnant mothers receiving home visitation services, found that those with secure states of mind were rated as more collaborative in the treatment process than those who were less secure-autonomous. Clients who were more dismissing were rated as rejecting treatment. This can be understood by noticing that a person seems to act toward therapists as he or she acts toward AAI interviewers.

Using the AAI as a Guide to Therapeutic Interventions

Treating People Who Have Secure-Autonomous States of Mind

Given that secure individuals are more open to exploring their surroundings and relationships, it is not surprising that they tend to be open, engaged, collaborative, compliant, committed, and proactive in treatment (Dozier, 1990; Korfmacher et al., 1997; Riggs & Jacobvitz, 2002). Although they may enter treatment distressed, they tend to be trusting of therapists and, most importantly, able to integrate what their therapists say and suggest. In addition, anecdotal evidence suggests that they tend to be more able to show gratitude toward their therapists for providing treatment.

Treating People Who Have Preoccupied States of Mind

Because preoccupied individuals can be so interpersonally engaged, initially they may appear to be easier to treat. They are often so distressed and interpersonally oriented that they are eager to discuss their worries and both past and current relationship difficulties (Dozier, 1990). However, both clinical and empirical evidence suggests that they may nevertheless be extremely difficult to treat. Because their chaotic and contradictory representations of self and others are so rich, they may be fairly readily "mentalized" by therapists (Allen & Fonagy, 2006). However, they often leave their therapists feeling confused and overwhelmed. In a number of publications, Slade (1999, 2000, 2004) has written about the unique challenges faced by clinicians working with preoccupied clients. She warns that "Progress is ... hard-won" (Slade, 1999, p. 588), and that therapists must be prepared for the "slow creation of structures for the modulation of affect" (Slade, 1999, p. 586). She contends that change occurs because of a therapist's long-term "emotional availability and tolerance for fragmentation and chaos" (Slade, 1999, p. 588). Consistent with these ideas, Dozier (1990) found that inpatient clients with preoccupied attachment patterns tended to present themselves as needy, but were not more compliant with treatment plans than dismissing individuals. In addition, Fonagy et al. (1996) found that preoccupied clients, compared with those classified as dismissing, were less likely to show improvement. The preoccupied patients may have been more difficult to treat because their representational systems were intricately linked with emotions that were intense and well elaborated by entrenched rumination on the difficult events in their lives.

In our own work with preoccupied individuals, we have encountered a number of difficulties that could have been identified in their AAI narratives. These have included: (1) rigid mental states, (2) rapid vacillations or oscillations between contradictory mental states, (3) current anger and confusion, and (4) self-blame and self-derogation.

The following vignette illustrates these issues. The patient was an unmarried 35-year-old woman of Southeast Asian descent who, despite being very attractive, highly intelligent, and educated at an Ivy League college, found herself unemployable and unable to date—mainly because, despite being emotionally needy, she could not get along with others and frequently engaged in angry outbursts. At 35, she was highly dependent on her parents (particularly for financial support, but also for emotional support). Her parents were at their wits' end and perceived her as wasting her life away. Although they were very traditional and perceived psychotherapy as a corrupt endeavor practiced by charlatans, they were willing to pay for therapy. The patient's relationship with her parents was anchored at two equally uncomfortable extremes, so she vacillated between wanting to live at home and wanting to break away and become independent and self-reliant. At times, she would plead with the therapist in a loud, pressured voice, "Dr. X, Dr. X, please, please tell me what to do! Should I try to work it out with my parents, or should I just forget about them?" She rapidly flipped between desperately wanting to be close to her parents and wanting to have nothing to do with them. In each of these stances she was adamant and inflexible about her position, despite frequently flipping back and forth. When she was in one mental state, she did not appear to recall being in the other. However, when she asked the therapist to make a decision for her, both mental states were briefly represented at the same time.

Any hesitation on the therapist's part was interpreted as withholding valuable information and was met with anger. The therapist felt backed into a corner with no good solution, but he wanted to make use of these moments when both options were mentally available. He pointed out that if he told her to reconcile with her parents, he imagined that she might see that as a criticism of her: They were right, she was wrong, and she should submit to their will. On the other hand, if he told her to resist them and leave, she would feel as if the therapy was pointless, and she would feel abandoned by her parents and more dependent on the therapist. When both of the affective states were acknowledged and tolerated by the therapist, the patient was able to refrain from her rapid oscillations long enough to have a productive discussion and develop a more integrated perspective on her and her parents' situation.

In work with patients classified as preoccupied, it is important to set and maintain a structured frame. Doing so may help keep the therapist from becoming overly entangled with the patients, particularly the ones who can be diagnosed as having BPD. In addition, a high degree of structure and predictability may provide the containment necessary to hold preoccupied individuals in treatment.

Treating People Who Have Dismissing States of Mind

As noted earlier, Dozier (1990) found that dismissing patients were often resistant to treatment, had trouble asking for help, and retreated from help when it was offered. Consistent with Dozier's findings, Diamond and colleagues (Diamond, Clarkin, et al., 2003; Diamond, Stovall-McClough, Clarkin, & Levy, 2003) find that dismissing patients often evoke countertransference feelings of being excluded from the patients' lives. In our own study, a patient classified as dismissing came into a session one morning and announced, to her therapist's surprise, that she was getting married that afternoon. Although the therapist had known of her engagement, it had been many months since she had brought up any aspect of her upcoming marriage. In addition, dismissing individuals often become more distressed and confused when confronted with emotional issues in therapy (Dozier, Lomax, Tyrrell, & Lee, 2001). Another dismissing patient, when reflecting on her experience in therapy, stated:

"He [the therapist] would start digging into things and find out why I was angry, and then I would realize that something really made me mad, but I didn't want to be mad. With my parents, for example, I didn't want to be angry at them."

Finally, a therapist working with a dismissing patient may be pulled into an enactment analogous to the "chase and dodge" sequence with mothers and infants identified by Beebe and Lachmann (1988), which leaves the patient feeling intruded upon only to withdraw further. Conversely, a patient with a dismissing state of mind may curtail the therapist's ability to engage with, visualize, or evoke the individual's representational world, or identify with the patient.

Treating People Who Have Unresolved States of Mind

In our experience, unresolved individuals with BPD are also very difficult to treat. In two studies, we found that between 32% and 60% of patients with BPD were classified as unresolved (Diamond, Stovall-McClough, et al., 2003; Levy et al., 2006). In our randomized clinical trial (Levy et al., 2006), we found a nonsignificant decrease from pre- to posttreatment in the number of patients with BPD classified as unresolved (32% vs. 22%). We also have some unpublished data suggesting that those patients with BPD who were unresolved were more likely to drop out of treatment. However, in a small sample of women with PTSD related to childhood sexual and physical abuse, Stovall-McClough and Cloitre (2003) found that 62% of unresolved patients lost their unresolved status following treatment. This effect was more prominent in the group receiving exposure plus affect regulation skills than in the group receiving affect regulation skills only. Interestingly, in this sample, unresolved attachment was more robustly related to BPD symptoms (Stovall-McClough & Cloitre, 2003) and PTSD avoidant symptoms than to dissociative symptoms (Stovall-McClough & Cloitre, 2006). The difference in outcome was probably related to differences in the severity of the disorders characterizing the two samples of patients. Ours were all diagnosed with BPD, and only 5% were classified as securely attached. In the Stovall-McClough and Cloitre (2006) study, patients were suffering from PTSD (although some had BPD symptoms), and 50% were securely attached. Many of their unresolved patients were securely attached, whereas all of our unresolved patients were insecurely attached. Thus unresolved attachment in the context of secure attachment may be a positive predictor of favorable change.

Dropping Out of Therapy

Patients with different attachment patterns may be differentially at risk for dropping out of psychotherapy, may differentially drop out of specific treatments, or may be at risk of dropping out for different reasons. For example, individuals with a dismissing state of mind may be at risk for dropping out of treatment because they are not fully committed to, attached to, or engaged with the therapist and/or the treatment (Dozier, 1990). In addition, they may be at risk for leaving treatment because they find that psychotherapy emotionally unravels them. In contrast, preoccupied states of mind may leave patients at risk of dropping out after what they perceive to be an abandonment experience, such as an emergency cancellation, a scheduled vacation, or a long wait for a phone call to be returned. Patients who fit the *fearfully preoccupied* subclassification (called E3, but not explicitly discussed here), which has been related to high rates of dropout (Fonagy et al., 1995), may be prone to drop out in response to feeling overly connected, attached, or dependent on the therapist and treatment.

Although the dynamics we have discussed here are familiar to clinicians who treat patients with BPD, our hypotheses are speculative regarding the relationship of these dynamics to specific attachment patterns. Further research is needed to delineate the prognostic and prescriptive significance of attachment patterns for treating patients.

THE AAI AND THERAPEUTIC OUTCOME

The AAI has been useful for assessing clinical outcome in treatment (Fonagy et al., 1996; Diamond, Stovall-McClough, et al., 2003; Levy, Diamond, Yeomans, Clarkin, & Kernberg, 2007; Levy et al., 2006; Stovall-McClough & Cloitre, 2003). However, it is important to administer the AAI prior to treatment in order to have a baseline for comparison. Furthermore, the trained raters coding the interviews should be kept unaware of initial classifications and rating scores, as well as clinical status and diagnoses.

The first large-scale treatment study involving the AAI was conducted by Fonagy et al. (1996). They examined the relation between patterns of attachment and psychiatric status in 82 nonpsychotic inpatients (treated at Cassel Hospital in west London with psychoanalytically oriented therapy) and 85 case-matched controls. They found that individuals classified as dismissing on the AAI were more likely to display clinically significant improvements (93%) on the Global Assessment of Functioning scale. Forty-three percent of the preoccupied and 33% of the secure subjects, respectively, showed significant clinical improvement. This surprising result deserves replication and further explication.

In a book chapter, Fonagy et al. (1995) reported partial findings from a subset of 35 of the 82 inpatients in the Cassel Hospital inpatient study. All 35 inpatients were classified as insecure during their initial interview. However, 14 (40%) of the 35 inpatients were assigned a secure classification upon discharge. This increase in the proportion of secure classifications was highly significant ($p < .001$). On the individual scale ratings, bland or idealized pictures of parents and a pattern of pervasive memory blockages were more characteristic of the AAIs at intake than at discharge, and they appear to have been changed by treatment. These findings are important, because they show that attachment patterns can change as a function of treatment. However, neither the specific psychopathology nor the treatment was well specified. In addition, no more detailed description of the changes in AAI status observed in this study has been published, making reports of these findings difficult to interpret.

In our own work at the Personality Disorders Institute at Cornell University, changes in attachment organization and *reflective function* (RF; i.e., the ability to mentalize; for a review, see Jurist & Meehan, Chapter 4, this volume) were assessed as putative mechanisms of change in one of three year-long psychotherapy treatments for patients with BPD. In pilot work (Diamond, Stovall-McClough, et al., 2003; Levy et al., 2007), we used the AAI to examine changes in attachment and RF in 10 patients treated in a year-long modified psychodynamic treatment called transference-focused psychotherapy (TFP). We were able to show changes in both attachment and RF. Of the 9 (90%) insecure patients, 2 became secure (22%), which resulted in 33% of the patients with BPD being classified as secure. Of the 6 unresolved patients (60%), 4 (67%) lost their unresolved status, resulting in only 40% of the sample being classified as unresolved after a year of treatment. We were also able to show significant increases in coherence and RF at the end of treatment (Levy et al., 2007).

In a randomized controlled trial (Levy et al., 2006), 90 reliably diagnosed patients with BPD were randomly assigned to TFP, an integrative cognitive-behavioral therapy called dialectical behavior therapy, or a modified psychodynamic supportive psychotherapy. Attachment organization was assessed with the AAI and the RF Scale (see "Mentalization and RF," below). After 12 months of treatment, there was a significant increase in the number of patients classified as secure in the group receiving TFP, but not in the other two treatment groups. Significant changes in narrative coherence and RF were found as a function of treatment, with the patients receiving TFP showing increases in both constructs during the course of treatment.

As mentioned previously, Stovall-McClough and Cloitre (2003) found that 8 of 13 (62%) patients with PTSD lost their unresolved classification during the course of treatment. They also found that the posttreatment unresolved scores were significantly lower for those who received prolonged exposure than for those who received skills training in affect and interpersonal regulation (2.8 vs. 5.4).

PROBLEMS WITH USING THE AAI IN CLINICAL SAMPLES

The AAI is a complicated measure whose reliable administration and coding require extensive and rigorous training. Its complexity is amplified for the interviewer and coder when clinical populations are examined, particularly with clients who have serious personality problems or violent and traumatic backgrounds. Having administered and coded AAIs in both normative and clinical samples, we have encountered a number of problems that tend to differentiate clinical from nonclinical interviews.

Eliciting a Clear Attachment Biography

Eliciting a clear attachment biography at the start of the interview can be difficult with clinical interviewees for two reasons. Many clinical intervie-wees have had multiple transient caregivers, making it difficult to identify key attachment figures. Patients may have resided in multiple institutions or foster homes. Many patients may have had strong attachments to a grand-parent, an older sibling, or an aunt or uncle who allowed a less malevo-lent relationship to develop. We have also found that some patients insist that a friend's parent was an attachment figure to them. Some interviewers will deal with these problems by erring on the side of inclusiveness, but it is important not to inquire about too many attachment figures, because it dilutes the intensity of the interview and tires both the interviewer and the interviewee. Conversely, it is important to avoid omitting an important attachment figure (which happens more often than one would think, despite the interviewer's best intentions).

We have found it useful to inquire about the time frame in which the care was provided, as well as the kind of care provided and whether the per-son is still in contact with the care provider. Often grandparents, aunts, and uncles were not seen very frequently or for extended periods of time. Like-wise, grandparents, aunts/uncles, siblings, and friends' parents were usually not involved in an interviewee's direct and intimate care. Finally, clients often have not been in contact for years with individuals when they present as important attachment figures. Any one or two of these heuristics used in isolation may not be sufficient in making a determination, but they can be valuable in narrowing the scope of an interview with a person who has had a chaotic life with multiple caregivers.

The second issue that interferes with producing a clear attachment biography is the presence of unintegrated and/or rigid representations and mental states. Such mental states can prevent clinical interviewees from adhering to the structure of the AAI, and as a result can make coding dif-ficult. Compounding the problem is the fact that many clinical interviewees have had multiple therapies, and to the extent that the AAI feels like a typi-cal therapy session, many clinical interviewees have a hard time responding to the somewhat different structure of the AAI. For example, we have found that many patients, particularly those with trauma histories, have difficulty answering the opening question. After a brief introduction, the AAI begins by asking the interviewee to give an overview of his or her *early* family situ-ation. The goal is to get a sense of the family's structure, but many patients launch directly into their relationship with their parents, including details about abuses, mistreatment, and grievances they have against one or both parents. Although this is useful information about lack of coherence and/ or lack of resolution, it is extremely important to redirect the interviewee. Otherwise, the interviewer is licensing the interviewee to violate the structure of the interview, which may seriously dilute the information needed for coding.

Similar difficulties arise in answers to the second question of the AAI ("I'd like you to try and describe your relationship with your parents as a young child. If you could start from as far back as you can remember ... "), which is meant as a lead-in or warm-up for asking about the five adjectives. Answers should be brief, but a less coherent interviewee may spend 20 minutes chronicling, for example, an extensive abuse history that pulls the interviewer into deviating from the interview's structure. In such a situation, it is useful to politely acknowledge the importance of the material, inform the interviewee that there will be an opportunity to discuss these events in more detail later in the interview, and then guide him or her to the next question.

Identifying Attachment Figures for Whom Resolution of Loss Should Be Probed

Another difficulty with clinical samples is deciding which losses should be probed for level of resolution. The coding of unresolved/disorganized attachment is of particular importance with clinical interviewees (who are likely to have suffered separations, losses, and abuse), so determining which losses to probe is critical. The AAI protocol dictates that interviewees be questioned about any significant figure who has died. However, just as it can be difficult to determine who is actually an attachment figure, it can be difficult to determine what counts as a significant loss, in part because some clients have experienced so many losses and appear to have the same intensity of affect attached to each one. Moreover, questioning about loss or trauma may have to be interrupted if the interviewee becomes too distressed. Finally, some interviewees have experienced traumatic loss of a parent through abandonment rather than death. Adam et al. (1996) suggest that severe or traumatic separation experiences may result in unresolved attachment.

Managing Extreme Violations of Discourse and Monitoring

We have found that some patients with BPD vacillate so quickly between contradictory and conflicting mental states that making sense of the narrative feels impossible. It is important to make sure that the interviewee understands the question and to clarify what the interviewee is saying, rather than making assumptions about inconsistent responses. On the other hand, the interviewer needs to guard against filling in content that a patient may acquiesce to, or providing structure and elaboration that may interfere with accurate assessment of coherence. In contrast, some patients are so terse or vague that it is difficult to elicit usable information. The interviewer needs to be skillful in finding the optimal level of probing.

Problems Related to Medication, Nonprescription Drug Use, and Neuropsychological or Cognitive Impairment

Certain clinical problems or somatic treatments for these problems may affect thinking and thought content. Most notably, disorders such as schizophrenia, particularly if a patient is floridly psychotic, may seriously interfere with the ability to carry out and code the AAI. Likewise, some patients may show up for the interview "high," intoxicated, or overmedicated. We have found that occasionally a nonpsychotic patient will arrive and appear over-medicated or "out of it," but during the course of the interview, the person perks up. Likewise, we have seen patients who arrive appearing fine but then become "out of it" after being asked certain questions or getting angry at the interviewer. In both cases, it is important to employ clinical skill in order to continue the interview.

Other Difficulties

We hope that this discussion of problems conveys some of the difficulties of using the AAI with clinical populations. Rather than go into the remaining problems in detail, we will count on clinician-readers' own experiences to flesh out these problems, which we simply list here:

   1. Some clients or patients may have been in therapy so long or so many times that they have developed a rehearsed telling of their life stories. In these cases, the AAI may not "surprise the unconscious," and the narrative may appear coherent.
   2. During the interview, some patients may behave in an erratic/chaotic manner (e.g., running out of the interview without warning), an aggressive fashion (e.g., screaming at or threatening the interviewer), or a controlling manner (e.g., trying to control the discourse, not answering questions, asking irrelevant questions, or asking that the recording be stopped). The trained clinical interviewer needs to be ready to deal with such developments.
   3. Some interviews exhibit what we call *pseudosecurity* (Levy, 2005); that is, the patient's narrative appears coherent (e.g., has clear supporting examples, is free of derogations, and lacks preoccupied anger), but is marked by descriptions of insecure behavior in response to attachment figures (e.g., self-injury following a recent interaction with a parent) and/or by a lack of the forgiveness, collaboration, and valuing of attachment shown by those

with secure states of mind. Coders need to be especially attentive because these indications can be subtle.

4. Because the AAI coding system was developed for typical community samples of adults living in the United States, difficulties may arise when it is used with clinical samples and/or samples in other cultures. The AAI has been successfully used in Canada (e.g., Atkinson et al., 2005), England (e.g., Fonagy et al., 1996), Mexico (Gojman de Millán & Millán, 2004), Israel (e.g., Sagi et al., 1994), Italy (e.g., Barone, 2003), Germany (e.g., Scheidt et al., 2000), the Netherlands (Bakermans-Kranenburg & van IJzendoorn, 1993), Spain (e.g., Fava, Simonelli, & Petena, 2000), and Japan (e.g., Onishi & Gjerde, 2002).

Although the prevalence of particular attachment patterns has differed somewhat across cultures, the general consensus regarding the cross-cultural validity of attachment is that it is universal but context-dependent (van IJzendoorn & Sagi, 1999). That is, although the premises of attachment theory appear universally valid, the AAI or aspects of its coding system may not be valid in every culture or may require modifications. For example, one indicator of preoccupied attachment is a high score on the *current anger* scale. Current anger is scored when a speaker fails to maintain past tense when discussing past grievances with parents. However, in some languages, such as Chinese, there is no conjugation of verbs or specific grammar that differentiates between past and present tense. Instead, past and present are distinguished by contextual indicators; therefore, someone coding Chinese transcripts will have to be sensitive to this issue. To take another example, Onishi and Gjerde (2002) noted that modified, translated Japanese AAIs used in pilot studies showed that many Japanese phrases, when directly translated from the English-language AAI, did not accurately convey the intended meaning of the original questions. In addition, they noted that evidence of collaboration with the interviewer may be manifested differently in Japanese culture. Truthfulness is sometimes indicated in Japanese by prolonged silence, which in the United States is often interpreted as defensive (editing of thought processes) or as indicating a lapse in discourse monitoring.

OTHER ATTACHMENT INTERVIEWS AND CODING SCHEMES

Since the AAI was developed in the 1980s, several adaptations, additional coding schemes, and interviews have been developed from it or modeled on it. Here, we cannot go into all of these modifications and adaptations in detail, but we list them in case they are of special interest to some clinician-readers. For example, two common modifications of the AAI involve either asking about the interviewee's relationship or imagined relationship with his or her own children, or asking about the interviewee's current romantic relationship (Gjerde, Miyoko, & Carlson, 2004).

The Adult Attachment Q-Sort

The Adult Attachment Q-Sort (Kobak,1993), a 100-item Q-sort scoring system for the AAI, identifies the three organized attachment categories: secure, preoccupied, and dismissing. Raters score transcripts along two dimensions: security versus anxiety and deactivation versus hyperactivation. Hyperactivating emotional strategies are typical of preoccupied individuals, whereas deactivitating strategies are typical of dismissing individuals. Scores are compared to a criterion or "ideal" prototype sort created by attachment experts to represent each of the three organized attachment categories. Two raters (one of whom should be trained in the AAI scoring system) independently read and sort the interview data. A third rater is used if adequate agreement is not achieved. Research has found overlap between the Q-sort system and the standard AAI scoring system ranging from 71% to 79% (Borman-Spurrell, Allen, Hauser, Carter, & Cole-Detke, 1998; Kobak, Cole, Ferenz-Gillies, & Fleming, 1993). A number of important studies have employed the Q-sort system, producing interesting and replicable findings.

Mentalization and RF

Peter Fonagy, drawing on the work of philosophers like Dennett and Brentano, has articulated a theory of mind based on what he calls *mentalization:* a person's ability to reflect on what is going on in his or her own mind and accurately understand wishes, intentions, and motivations underlying the person's own behavior and that of others. Fonagy proposed that good RF should relate to a range of positive outcomes, from successful parenting to satisfying relationship functioning and resilience in the face of stressors. In order to test his theory, he developed a scale to assess various aspects of RF (e.g., understanding a developmental perspective, understanding the opaqueness of mental states, and the possible defensive nature of mental states). Consistent with his theory, Fonagy et al. (1991) found that caregiver RF predicted a baby's functioning in a laboratory testing procedure. In a later study, Fonagy et al. (1996) found that high RF acted as a buffer against the negative effects of traumatic experiences.

To evaluate the quality of mentalization, Fonagy, Target, Steele, & Steele (1998) created the RF Scale, which ranges from −1 (negative RF, in which interviews are totally barren of mentalization or grossly distorting of the mental states of others) to 9 (exceptional RF, in which interviews show unusually complex, elaborate, or original reasoning about mental states). The midpoint of the scale is 5, ordinary RF, which indicates that an individual possesses a model of others' minds that is fairly coherent, if somewhat one-dimensional, naïve, or simplistic. Initial research utilizing the RF Scale has been promising. In a study examining the role of the parents' mentalizing skills and the relation of these skills to their infant's attachment pattern, Fonagy et al. (1995) found that RF mediated the relationship between parental attachment security and infant attachment security in the Strange Situation (Ainsworth et al., 1978) at 12 and 18 months. That is, insecurely attached parents with high RF were more likely to have securely attached babies than were insecurely attached parents with low RF. Consistent with this finding, Slade and colleagues (Grienenberger, Kelly, & Slade, 2005) have recently found that a mother's RF mediates the relationship between atypical maternal behaviors (e.g., affective communication errors, role/boundary confusion, intrusiveness) and an infant's attachment security. Levy et al. (2005) found that RF was related to a number of neurocognitive mechanisms, including attentional capacities, executive functioning, and impulsivity. These capacities are central to the difficulties experienced by people with personality disorders. Subsequent clinical research has found that RF can improve during the course of psychotherapy, even for severely disturbed outpatients with personality disorders (Levy et al., 2006).

Hostile-Helpless Coding of the AAI

Lyons-Ruth, Yellin, Melnick, and Atwood (2003) developed a coding system to assess *hostile-helpless* states of mind. This coding system builds on the existing AAI coding system with additional codes to capture punitive, compulsive caregiving, or other highly defended states of mind associated with BPD psychopathology and with exposure to trauma, abuse, or hostile or violent family relationships. Recent research has shown that the additional codes do not overlap substantially with the unresolved/disorganized, cannot classify, or fearfully preoccupied by traumatic events (E3) categories and are associated with infant disorganization and maternal disrupted communication with the infant at 18 months of age. In a second study (Lyons-Ruth, Melnick, Patrick, & Hobson, 2007), patients with BPD were compared to dysthymic patients in regard to hostile-helpless states of mind. All of the women with BPD, compared with half of the group with dysthymia, displayed such states of mind. In addition, the women with BPD showed a higher frequency of globally devaluing representations, and there was a strong trend for more of this group to show identification with devalued hostile caregivers (58% with BPD vs. 18% with dysthymia). An additional significant finding was that 75% of the women with BPD, but only 27% of those with dysthymia, made reference to controlling behavior toward attachment figures in childhood—a pattern of behavior that had previously been linked with disorganized attachment (Main et al., 1985).

Other AAI-Based Interviews

Several other interviews are mentioned only very briefly, along with key references, so that readers can find these instruments on their own. The Family and Peer Attachment Interview (FPAI; Bartholomew & Horowitz, 1991) is

a semistructured interview designed to assess adult attachment styles on the
basis of information about parents and peers. The FPAI rates people on four
attachment styles (secure, fearful, preoccupied, and dismissing) described
by Bartholomew (1990), rather than categorizing them into one of the five
AAI categories. The FPAI provides a bridge between the literatures based on
interview and self-report measures of attachment patterns in close relationships (see Fraley & Phillips, Chapter 7, this volume).

Crittenden (1995) modified the AAI to permit analysis of a wide range
of distortions in information processing. This modification was based on
her "dynamic-maturation perspective" on attachment, which stresses that
maturation and experience enable children to construct increasingly sophisticated attachment strategies. Crittenden (1997) compared 62 (40 normative and 22 clinical) individuals coded with the original AAI system and
with her dynamic-maturation system. The two systems provided somewhat
different results, motivating Crittenden to develop her own coding scheme.
It is too early to tell from published sources how valuable this scoring system will be, but Crittenden and her colleagues, many of whom are Europe-
ans, have raised a number of important issues and have begun to publish
their research (e.g., Crittenden & Claussen, 2000).

The Current Relationship Interview (CRI; Crowell & Owens, 1996)
was developed to assess representations of attachment in a current romantic
or marital relationship. As in the AAI, the interviewee is asked for adjectives describing his or her relationship and for examples that support those
choices of descriptors; about such experiences as being upset, ill, or hurt;
and about separations. In addition, the interviewee is asked about influences
on the relationship and the effects of the relationship on his or her development. Preliminary research using the CRI was discussed by Crowell, Fraley,
and Shaver (1999) in their chapter on attachment measures, and subsequent publications by Crowell and her colleagues have provided additional
information (e.g., Crowell et al., 2002). A related instrument is the Marital
Attachment Interview (Dickstein, Seifer, St. Andre, & Schiller, 2001).

The Patient–Therapist AAI (PT-AAI; Diamond et al., 1999) was
designed by Diana Diamond and her colleagues to investigate patients' and
therapists' states of mind with respect to attachment in the therapeutic relationship. The PT-AAI follows the same format and order of questions as
does the AAI, with minor changes in the wording of questions to fit the
context of the patient–therapist relationship. It includes some additional
questions designed to explore patients' and therapists' experiences and
representations of the therapeutic relationship. As is done for the primary
attachment relationship(s) in the AAI, the interviewee is asked in the PT-
AAI to describe the therapeutic relationship generally, to give five words to
describe the therapist or patient (i.e., the partner in the relationship), and to
support these descriptors with specific examples or incidents. The interview
also includes questions about the individual's response to separations from
the therapeutic partner; about what he or she does when upset, hurt, or ill

in the course of therapy; and about times when the individual felt rejected or threatened by the patient or therapist in the course of treatment. In addition, speakers are asked why they think the therapeutic partner acted the way he or she did in the course of treatment, and how they would describe and evaluate the effects of psychotherapy. The PT-AAI can be scored not only for attachment classification, but also for RF with the RF Scale (Fonagy et al., 1998).

The PT-AAI has proven difficult to use in research, because it is difficult to administer to patients and therapists prior to treatment, and therefore difficult to compare baseline scores with later scores. Diamond et al. (1999) reported results for two clients with BPD treated with Kernberg's TFP procedure (Clarkin, Yeomans, & Kernberg, 1999) by the same therapist. Both clients progressed from insecure to secure states of mind within 1 year of treatment; however, consistent with previous research (Eames & Roth, 2000; Dolan, Arnkoff, & Glass, 1993; Dozier, Cue, & Barnett, 1994; Mallinckrodt, Gantt, & Coble, 1995; Tyrrell, Dozier, Teague, & Fallot, 1999), each patient interacted with and affected the therapist in very different ways, and the therapist responded to each patient very differently. The therapist was engaged and active in the treatment of the client initially classified as preoccupied, whereas the same therapist was much less engaged, often felt dismissed, and developed a much weaker therapeutic bond with the dismissing client. The therapist's RF was higher with the patient he was more engaged with, and much lower with the patient he was less engaged with. Both patients entered treatment with equally low RF, and the patient with whom the therapist was more engaged was actually more mentally disturbed by objective standards.

Later, Diamond, Stovall-McClough, et al. (2003) reported findings on a sample of 10 patients. Patients were assessed at 4 months into treatment with the AAI, and after 1 year of treatment with the AAI and the PT-AAI, administered to both the patients and the therapists. Each of these interviews was coded for RF. The PT-AAI ratings of the 10 patients at 1 year varied considerably. In all but one case, the patient's attachment state of mind with respect to the therapist on the PT-AAI was concordant with one or more aspects of the attachment state of mind on the AAI at time 1 and/ or time 2. For example, if the patient displayed a secure, dismissing, or preoccupied attachment state of mind (or some admixture of these) with respect to childhood relationships in the AAI, she was likely to receive the parallel attachment classification(s) with respect to the therapist on the PT-AAI. These findings suggest that the PT-AAI in combination with the AAI, administered over the course of therapy, may be useful in tracking aspects of the transference as it unfolds over time, and particularly in identifying which aspects of the early relationship with the parents are recapitulated with the therapist after 1 year of therapy.

Diamond, Stovall-McClough, et al. (2003) also found that over the course of psychotherapy, a number of patients were classified as secure with respect to attachment to their therapists, but they continued to report (albeit coherently) engaging in self-destructive behaviors, keeping secrets from their therapists, and experiencing intense fears of abandonment by their therapists. These patients were able to describe coherently their apprehension in telling their therapists about their thoughts and feelings, or withholding information from their therapists. Clearly, they were not behaving or feeling like securely attached individuals. Nevertheless, they were clearly more coherent with respect to attachment representations, which might result eventually in better integration of experience, increased flexibility of thought processes, and better self-regulation. It might put them on the road to more secure behavior.

CONCLUSIONS

The ability to integrate the assessment of attachment processes into the clinical situation requires a thorough understanding of attachment theory and research. This can be accomplished by becoming familiar with the procedures and scoring approaches used in the AAI. (There are also several useful volumes that outline the development of attachment theory and research in a broad and comprehensive way, as well as a number of review articles that outline basic findings and methods of attachment research.) The AAI is an extremely rich and clinically relevant measure that generates narratives very similar to the narratives commonly told in psychotherapy. Despite the benefits of the AAI, it requires rigorous and time-consuming training, and its use requires energy and time. It may be possible, over time, to reduce the complexity of attachment interviews and the systems used to score them. In the meantime, the insights already obtained from attachment interview studies can prove extremely useful to therapists.

RECOMMENDATIONS FOR FURTHER READING

Fonagy, P., Gergely, G., Jurist, E., & Target, M. (2002). *Affect regulation, mentalization, and the development of the self.* New York: Other Press.—This book provides the most recent and thorough description of the development of mentalization.

Hesse, E. (2008). The Adult Attachment Interview: Protocol, method of analysis, and empirical studies. In J. Cassidy & P. R. Shaver (Eds.), *Handbook of attachment: Theory, research, and clinical applications* (pp. 575–594). New York: Guilford Press.—This chapter provides a comprehensive review of the AAI and its related research findings.

Levy, K. N. (2005). The implications of attachment theory and research for understanding borderline personality disorder. *Development and Psychopathology, 17*, 959–986.—This article reviews a number of important issues regarding attachment theory and research in clinical populations.

Levy, K. N., Kelly, K. M., Meehan, K. B., Reynoso, J. S., Clarkin, J. F., Lenzenweger, M. F., et al. (2006). Change in attachment patterns and reflective function in the treatment of borderline personality disorder with transference focused psychotherapy. *Journal of Consulting and Clinical Psychology, 74,* 1027–1040.—This article discusses our research findings regarding attachment security and RF.

Main, M., Kaplan, N., & Cassidy, J. (1985). Security in infancy, childhood, and adulthood: A move to the level of representation. In I. Bretherton & E. Waters (Eds.), Growing points of attachment theory and research. *Monographs of the Society for Research in Child Development, 50*(1–2, Serial No. 209) 66–104.—This is the original article detailing the AAI and provides the conceptual rationale for the measure.

Slade, A. (2008). The implications of attachment theory and research for adult psychotherapy: Research and clinical perspectives. In J. Cassidy & P. R. Shaver (Eds.), *Handbook of attachment: Theory, research, and clinical applications* (2nd ed., pp. 762–782). New York: Guilford Press.—Using case examples, Slade beautifully describes how central constructs and principles in the AAI can be used in clinical practice to understand and guide clinical work.

REFERENCES

Adam, K. S., Sheldon-Keller, A. E., & West, M. (1996). Attachment organization and history of suicidal behavior in clinical adolescents. *Journal of Consulting and Clinical Psychology, 64,* 264–272.

Ainsworth, M. S., Blehar, M. C., Waters, E., & Wall, S. (1978). *Patterns of attachment: A psychological study of the Strange Situation.* Hillsdale, NJ: Erlbaum.

Allen, J. G., & Fonagy, P. (Eds.). (2006). *Handbook of mentalization-based treatment.* Chichester, UK: Wiley.

Allen, J. P., Hauser, S., & Borman-Spurrell, E. (1996). Attachment theory as a framework for understanding sequelae of severe adolescent psychopathology: An 11-year follow-up study. *Journal of Consulting and Clinical Psychology, 6,* 254–263.

Ammaniti, M., van IJzendoorn, M. H., Speranza, A. M., & Tambelli, R. (2000). Internal working models of attachment during late childhood and early adolescence: An exploration of stability and change. *Attachment & Human Development, 2,* 328–346.

Atkinson, L., Goldberg, S., Raval, V., Pederson, D., Benoit, D., Moran, G., et al. (2005). On the relation between maternal state of mind and sensitivity in the prediction of infant attachment security. *Developmental Psychology, 41,* 42–53.

Bakermans-Kranenburg, M. J., & van IJzendoorn, M. H. (1993). A psychometric study of the Adult Attachment Interview: Reliability and discriminant validity. *Developmental Psychology, 29,* 870–879.

Barone, L. (2003). Developmental protective and risk factors in borderline personality disorder: A study using the Adult Attachment Interview. *Attachment & Human Development, 5,* 64–77.

Bartholomew, K. (1990). Avoidance of intimacy: An attachment perspective. *Journal of Social and Personal Relationships, 7,* 147–178.

Bartholomew, K., & Horowitz, L. M. (1991). Attachment styles among young adults: A test of a four-category model. *Journal of Personality and Social Psychology, 61,* 226–244.

Beebe, B., & Lachmann, F. M. (1988). The contribution of mother–infant mutual influence to the origins of self- and object representations. *Psychoanalytic Psychology, 5,* 305–337.

Benoit, D., & Parker, K.C.H. (1994). Stability and transmission of attachment across three generations. *Child Development, 65,* 1444–1456.

Borman-Spurrell, E., Allen, J., Hauser, S., Carter, A., & Cole-Detke, H. (1998). *Assessing adult attachment: A comparison of interview-based and self-report models.* Unpublished manuscript.

Bowlby, J. (1973). *Attachment and loss: Vol. 2, Separation: Anxiety and anger.* New York: Basic Books.

Bowlby, J. (1977). The making and breaking of affectional bonds: I. Aetiology and psychopathology in light of attachment theory. *British Journal of Psychiatry, 130,* 201–210.

Bowlby, J. (1979). *The making and breaking of affectional bonds.* London: Tavistock.

Bowlby, J. (1982). *Attachment and loss: Vol. 1. Attachment* (2nd ed.). New York: Basic Books. (1st ed., 1969)

Carlson, E. A. (1998). A prospective longitudinal study of attachment disorganization/disorientation. *Child Development, 69,* 1107–1128.

Cohen, J. (1992). A power primer. *Psychological Bulletin, 112,* 155–159.

Clarkin, J. F., Yeomans, F. E., & Kernberg, O. F. (1999). *Psychotherapy for borderline personality.* New York: Wiley.

Crittenden, P. M. (1995). Attachment and psychopathology. In S. Goldberg, R. Muir, & J. Kerr (Eds.), *Attachment theory: Social, developmental, and clinical perspectives* (pp. 367–406). Hillsdale, NJ: Analytic Press.

Crittenden, P. M. (1997). The effect of early relationship experiences on relationships in adulthood. In S. Duck (Ed.), *Handbook of personal relationships* (2nd ed., pp. 99–119). Chichester, UK: Wiley.

Crittenden, P. M., & Claussen, A. H. (Eds.). (2000). *The organization of attachment relationships: Maturation, culture, and context.* New York: Cambridge University Press.

Crowell, J. A., Fraley, R. C., & Shaver, P. R. (1999). Measurement of individual differences in adolescent and adult attachment. In J. Cassidy & P. R. Shaver (Eds.), *Handbook of attachment: Theory, research, and clinical applications* (pp. 434–465). New York: Guilford Press.

Crowell, J.A., & Owens, G. (1996). *Current Relationship Interview and scoring system.* Unpublished manuscript, State University of New York at Stony Brook.

Crowell, J. A., Waters, E., Treboux, D., & O'Connor, E. (1996). Discriminant validity of the Adult Attachment Interview. *Child Development, 67,* 2584–2599.

Crowell, J.A., Treboux, D., & Waters, E. (2002). Stability of attachment representations: The transition to marriage. *Developmental Psychology, 38,* 467–479.

de Haas, M. A., Bakermans-Kranenburg, M. J., & van IJzendoorn, M. H. (1994). The Adult Attachment Interview and questionnaires for attachment style, temperament, and memories of parental behavior. *Journal of Genetic Psychology, 155,* 471–486.

Diamond, D., Clarkin, J. F., LeVine, H., Levy, K. N., Foelsch, P., & Yeomans, F.

(1999). Borderline conditions and attachment: A preliminary report. *Psychoanalytic Inquiry, 19,* 831–884.

Diamond, D., Clarkin, J. F., Stovall-McClough, K. C., Levy, K. N., Foelsch, P. A., Levine, H., et al. (2003). Patient–therapist attachment: Impact on the therapeutic process and outcome. In M. Cortina & M. Marrone (Eds.), *Attachment theory and the psychoanalytic process* (pp. 127–178). London: Whurr.

Diamond, D., Stovall-McClough, C., Clarkin, J. F., & Levy, K. N. (2003). Patient–therapist attachment in the treatment of borderline personality disorder. *Bulletin of the Menninger Clinic, 67,* 227–259.

Dickstein, S., Seifer, R., St. Andre, M., & Schiller, M. (2001). Marital Attachment Interview: Adult attachment assessment of marriage. *Journal of Social and Personal Relationships, 18,* 651–672.

Dolan, R. T., Arnkoff, D. B., & Glass, C. R. (1993). Client attachment style and the psychotherapist's interpersonal stance. *Psychotherapy, 30,* 408–411.

Dozier, M. (1990). Attachment organization and treatment use for adults with serious psychopathological disorders. *Development and Psychopathology, 2,* 47–60.

Dozier, M., Cue, K. L., & Barnett, L. (1994). Clinicians as caregivers: Role of attachment organization in treatment. *Journal of Consulting and Clinical Psychology, 62*(4), 793–800.

Dozier, M., Lomax, L., Tyrrell, C. L., & Lee, S. (2001). The challenge of treatment for clients with dismissing states of mind. *Attachment & Human Development, 3,* 62–76.

Eames, V., & Roth, A. (2000). Patient attachment orientation and the early working alliance: A study of patient and therapist reports of alliance quality and ruptures. *Psychotherapy Research, 10,* 421–434.

Fava, G., Simonelli, A., & Petena, L. (2000). Representaciones maternas y transmisión de los factores de riesgo y protección en hijos de madres drogodependientes [Maternal representations and intergenerational transmission of risk and protective factors in children of drug-addicted mothers] *Adicciones (Palma de Mallorca), 12,* 413–424.

Fonagy, P., Leigh, T., Steele, M., Steele, H., Kennedy, R., Mattoon, G., et al. (1996). The relation of attachment status, psychiatric classification, and response to psychotherapy. *Journal of Consulting and Clinical Psychology, 64,* 22–31.

Fonagy, P., Steele, M., Steele, H., Leigh, T., Kennedy, R., Mattoon, G., et al. (1995). Attachment, the reflective self, and borderline states: The predictive specificity of the Adult Attachment Interview and pathological emotional development. In S. Goldberg, R. Muir, & J. Kerr (Eds.), *Attachment theory: Social, developmental, and clinical perspectives* (pp. 233–278). Hillsdale, NJ: Analytic Press.

Fonagy, P., Steele, M., Steele, H., Moran, G.S., & Higgitt, A.C. (1991). The capacity for understanding mental states: The reflective self in parent and child and its significance for security of attachment. *Infant Mental Health Journal, 12,* 201–218.

Fonagy, P., Target, M., Steele, H., & Steele, M. (1998). *Reflective-functioning manual: Version 5.0 for application to the Adult Attachment Interview.* Unpublished manuscript, University College London.

Fraley, R. C. (2002). Attachment stability from infancy to adulthood: Meta-analysis and dynamic modeling of developmental mechanisms. *Personality and Social Psychology Review, 6,* 123–151.

George, C., Kaplan, N., & Main, M. (1984). *Adult Attachment Interview protocol.* Unpublished manuscript, University of California, Berkeley.

George, C., Kaplan, N., & Main, M. (1985). *Adult Attachment Interview protocol* (2nd ed.). Unpublished manuscript, University of California, Berkeley.

George, C., Kaplan, N., & Main, M. (1996). *Adult Attachment Interview protocol* (3rd ed.). Unpublished manuscript, University of California, Berkeley.

Gjerde, P. F., Onishi, M., & Carlson, K. S. (2004). Personality characteristics associated with romantic attachment: A comparison of interview and self-report methodologies. *Personality and Social Psychology Bulletin, 30,* 1402–1415.

Gojman de Millán, S., & Millán, S. (2004). *An attachment research project in rural and urban Mexican dyads.* Paper presented at the XVth Biennial International Conference on Infant Studies, Kyoto, Japan.

Grienenberger, J., Kelly, K., & Slade, A. (2005). Maternal reflective functioning, mother–infant affective communication and infant attachment: Exploring the link between mental states and observed caregiving. *Attachment & Human Development, 7,* 299–311.

Grossmann, K. E., Grossmann, K., & Waters, E. (Eds.). (2005). *Attachment from infancy to adulthood: The major longitudinal studies.* New York: Guilford Press.

Hamilton, C. E. (2000). Continuity and discontinuity of attachment from infancy through adolescence. *Child Development, 71,* 690–694.

Hesse, E. (1996). Discourse, memory, and the Adult Attachment Interview: A note with emphasis on the emerging cannot classify category. *Infant Mental Health Journal, 17,* 4–11.

Holtzworth-Munroe, A., Stuart, G. L., & Hutchinson, G. (1997). Violent vs. nonviolent husbands: Differences in attachment patterns, dependency, and jealousy. *Journal of Family Psychology, 11,* 314–331.

Kernberg, O. F. (1984). *Severe personality disorders: Psychotherapeutic strategies.* New Haven, CT: Yale University Press.

Kobak, R. R. (1993). *The Adult Attachment Q-Sort.* Unpublished manuscript, University of Delaware.

Kobak, R. R., Cole, H. E., Ferenz-Gillies, R., & Fleming, W. S. (1993). Attachment and emotion regulation during mother–teen problem solving: A control theory analysis. *Child Development, 64,* 231–245.

Korfmacher, J., Adam, E., Ogawa, J., & Egeland, B. (1997). Adult attachment: Implications for the therapeutic process in a home visitation intervention. *Applied Developmental Science, 1,* 43–52.

Levy, K. N. (2005). The implications of attachment theory and research for understanding borderline personality disorder. *Development and Psychopathology, 17,* 959–986.

Levy, K. N., & Blatt, S. J. (1999). Attachment theory and psychoanalysis: Further differentiation within insecure attachment patterns. *Psychoanalytic Inquiry, 19,* 541–575.

Levy, K. N., Diamond, D., Yeomans, F. E., Clarkin, J. F., & Kernberg, O. F. (2007). *Changes in attachment, reflective function, and object representation in the psychodynamic treatment of borderline personality disorder.* Unpublished manuscript.

Levy, K. N., Meehan, K. B., Kelly, K. M., Reynoso, J. S., Clarkin, J. F., Lenzenweger, M. F., et al. (2006). Change in attachment patterns and reflective function in the treatment of borderline personality disorder with transference focused psychotherapy. *Journal of Consulting and Clinical Psychology, 74,* 1027–1040.

Levy, K. N., Meehan, K. B., Reynoso, J. S., Lenzenweger, M. F., Clarkin, J. F., & Kernberg, O. F. (2005). The relation of reflective function to neurocognitive functioning in patients with borderline personality disorder. *Journal of the American Psychoanalytic Association, 53,* 1305–1309.

Lewis, M., Feiring, C., & Rosenthal, S. (2000). Attachment over time. *Child Development, 71,* 707–720.

Lyons-Ruth, K., Melnick, S., Patrick, M., & Hobson, R. P. (2007). A controlled study of hostile-helpless states of mind among borderline and dysthymic women. *Attachment & Human Development, 9,* 1–16.

Lyons-Ruth, K., Yellin, C., Melnick, S., & Atwood, G. (2003). Childhood experiences of trauma and loss have different relations to maternal unresolved and hostile-helpless states of mind on the AAI. *Attachment & Human Development, 5,* 330–352.

Main, M., & Goldwyn, R. (1984). *Adult attachment scoring and classification system.* Unpublished manuscript, University of California, Berkeley.

Main, M., Goldwyn, R., & Hesse, E. (2003) *Adult attachment scoring and classification system.* Unpublished manuscript, University of California, Berkeley.

Main, M., Kaplan, N., & Cassidy, J. (1985). Security in infancy, childhood, and adulthood: A move to the level of representation. In I. Bretherton & E. Waters (Eds.), Growing points of attachment theory and research. *Monographs of the Society for Research in Child Development (1–2, Serial No. 209), 50,* 66–104.

Main, M., & Solomon, J. (1990). Procedures for identifying infants as disorganized/disoriented during the Ainsworth Strange Situation. In M. T. Greenberg, D. Cicchetti, & E. M. Cummings (Eds.), *Attachment in the preschool years: Theory, research, and intervention* (pp. 121–160). Chicago: University of Chicago Press.

Main, M., & Weston, D. R. (1981). The quality of the toddler's relationship to mother and to father: Related to conflict behavior and the readiness to establish new relationships. *Child Development, 52,* 932–940.

Mallinckrodt, B., Gantt, D. L., & Coble, H. M. (1995). Attachment patterns in the psychotherapy relationship: Development of the Client Attachment to Therapist Scale. *Journal of Counseling Psychology, 42,* 307–317.

Onishi, M., & Gjerde, P. F. (2002). Attachment strategies in Japanese urban middle-class couples: A cultural theme analysis of asymmetry in marital relationships. *Personal Relationships, 9,* 435–455.

Patrick, M., Hobson, R. P., Castle, D., & Howard, R. (1994). Personality disorder and the mental representation of early social experience. *Development and Psychopathology, 6,* 375–388.

Pianta, R., Egeland, B., & Adam, E. (1996). Adult attachment classification and self-reported psychiatric symptomatology as assessed by the Minnesota Multiphasic Personality Inventory–2. *Journal of Consulting and Clinical Psychology, 64,* 273–281.

Riggs, S. A., & Jacobvitz, D. (2002). Expectant parents' representations of early attachment relationships: Associations with mental health and family history. *Journal of Consulting and Clinical Psychology, 70,* 195–204.

Sagi, A., van IJzendoorn, M. H., Scharf, M., & Koren-Karie, N. (1994). Stability

---

and discrimination validity of the Adult Attachment Interview: A psychometric study in young Israeli adults. *Developmental Psychology, 30,* 771–777.

Scheidt, C. E., Waller, E., Malchow, H., Ehlert, U., Becker-Stoll, F., Schulte-Monting, J., et al. (2000). Attachment representation and cortisol response to the Adult Attachment Interview in idiopathic spasmodic torticollis. *Psychotherapy and Psychosomatics, 69,* 155–162.

Slade, A. (1999). Attachment theory and research: Implications for the theory and practice of individual psychotherapy with adults. In J. Cassidy & P. R. Shaver (Eds.), *Handbook of attachment: Theory, research, and clinical applications* (pp. 575–594). New York: Guilford Press.

Slade, A. (2000). The development and organization of attachment: Implications for psychoanalysis. *Journal of the American Psychoanalytic Association, 48,* 1147–1174.

Slade, A. (2004). The move from categories to process: Attachment phenomena and clinical evaluation. *Infant Mental Health Journal, 25,* 269–283.

Stovall-McClough, K., & Cloitre, M. (2003). Reorganization of unresolved childhood traumatic memories following exposure therapy. *Annals of the New York Academy of Sciences, 1008,* 297–299.

Stovall-McClough, K., & Cloitre, M. (2006). Unresolved attachment, PTSD, and dissociation in women with childhood abuse histories. *Journal of Consulting and Clinical Psychology, 74,* 219–228.

Stroufe, L. A. (1979). The coherence of individual development: Early care, attachment, and subsequent developmental issues. *American Psychologist, 34,* 834–841.

Tyrrell, C. L., Dozier, M., Teague, G. B., & Fallot, R. D. (1999). Effective treatment relationships for persons with serious psychiatric disorders: The importance of attachment states of mind. *Journal of Consulting and Clinical Psychology, 67*(5), 725–733.

van IJzendoorn, M. H. (1995). Adult attachment representations, parental responsiveness, and infant attachment: A meta-analysis of the predictive validity of the Adult Attachment Interview. *Psychological Bulletin, 117,* 387–403.

van IJzendoorn, M. H., & Bakermans-Kranenburg, M. J. (1996). Attachment representations in mothers, fathers, adolescents, and clinical groups: A meta-analytic search for normative data. *Journal of Consulting and Clinical Psychology, 64,* 8–21.

van IJzendoorn, M. H., & Sagi, A. (1999). Cross-cultural patterns of attachment: Universal and contextual dimensions. In J. Cassidy & P. R. Shaver (Eds.), *Handbook of attachment: Theory, research, and clinical applications* (pp. 713–734). New York: Guilford Press.

Waters, E., Merrick, S., Treboux, D., Crowell, J., & Albersheim, L. (2000). Attachment security in infancy and early adulthood: A twenty-year longitudinal study. *Child Development, 71,* 684–689.

Waters, E., Treboux, D., Fyffe, C., & Crowell, J. (2001). *Secure versus insecure and dismissing versus preoccupied attachment representation scored as continuous variables from AAI state of mind scales.* Manuscript submitted for publication.

Weinfield, N.S., Sroufe, L.A., & Egeland, B. (2000). Attachment from infancy to young adulthood in a high-risk sample: Continuity, discontinuity and their correlates. *Child Development, 71,* 695–702.

Zimmerman, P., Fremmer-Bombik, E., Spangler, G., & Grossmann, K. E. (1997). Attachment in adolescence: A longitudinal perspective. In W. Koops, J. B. Hoeksema, & D. C. van den Boom (Eds.), *Development of interaction and attachment: Traditional and non-traditional approaches* (pp. 281–291). Amsterdam: North-Holland.

7

Self-Report Measures of Adult Attachment in Clinical Practice

R. Chris Fraley
Robert L. Phillips

According to Bowlby's (1969/1982) attachment theory, the affective bonds that develop between a person and his or her attachment figures play a central role in shaping the person's life. Secure bonds facilitate trust, autonomy, exploration, and growth; insecure ones contribute to distrust, inhibition, and withdrawal. Given the centrality of attachment dynamics in psychological functioning across the life course, a priority for both basic research and applied clinical work is to understand the ways in which people relate to their attachment figures.

As mentioned in other chapters in this volume, there are many methods available for assessing the nature of a person's attachment organization and attachment relationships. Some of them are based on semistructured interviews (e.g., the Adult Attachment Interview [AAI]; see Levy & Kelly, Chapter 6, this volume), others on projective techniques (e.g., the Adult Attachment Projective; George, West, & Pettem, 1999; see Berant, Chapter 8, this volume), and still others on self-report questionnaires. In this chapter, we review the literature concerning the self-report approach to assessing attachment organization, as it has evolved within social and personality psychology. However, our goal is not simply to summarize the ways in which self-reports have been employed; we also want to focus on ways to use self-report measures of attachment in the context of psychotherapy. To date, self-report instruments have been used largely for research purposes. Researchers administer self-report questionnaires to large samples of people and then study the statistical associations among variables (e.g., between attachment style and depressive symptoms). This approach is useful for learning how different variables are related to one another and why. The clinical context, however, often requires methods tailored to the study of individual lives rather than of variations within large populations.

Here, we propose a new method for using self-report attachment measures clinically—a method that is interactive, dynamic, and tailored to the clinical context. Specifically, we introduce a Web-based system called eSession that provides for the longitudinal assessment and monitoring of a client's attachment patterns and dynamics. Between therapy sessions, clients can log in to eSession to complete therapeutic "homework" and a 10- to 15-minute questionnaire. The questionnaire is designed to assess a client's attachment patterns in four distinct relationships, as well as other aspects of the client's interpersonal functioning (i.e., satisfaction with relationships, basic personality traits, and depressive symptoms). The therapist can monitor these reports and, alone or in consultation with the client, can use them to identify problem areas in the client's life and determine whether treatment plans are working as expected. In short, the method allows self-reports of attachment patterns to be assessed in a longitudinal, idiographic fashion, providing information that can be used clinically.

We begin by discussing social-psychological models of attachment patterns, highlighting both the history of self-report methods and some recent theoretical and empirical developments in the assessment of individual differences. We also provide an overview of the most popular ways of measuring attachment with self-report instruments. We then describe eSession and illustrate its potential by using the extended case study of "Bridget," a woman who sought counseling because heated arguments with her spouse had pushed her marriage almost to a breaking point. Finally, we offer recommendations for future developments in the use of self-report methods of assessing attachment organization and dynamics.

BACKGROUND: EARLY SELF-REPORT MEASURES OF ADULT ATTACHMENT

Hazan and Shaver's Three-Category Model

When Hazan and Shaver (1987) began their seminal work on adult attachment, they adopted Ainsworth's threefold typology of attachment patterns in infancy (Ainsworth, Blehar, Waters, & Wall, 1978) as a framework for organizing individual differences in the ways adults think, feel, and behave in romantic relationships (see Shaver & Mikulincer, Chapter 2, this volume). In their initial studies, Hazan and Shaver (1987, 1990) developed brief multisentence descriptions of the three proposed adult attachment types—*avoidant, secure,* and *anxious-ambivalent.* These descriptions are presented in Table 7.1. In this measure, respondents are asked to think back across their history of romantic relationships and indicate which of the three

TABLE 7.1. Hazan and Shaver's Attachment Style Descriptions

- I am somewhat uncomfortable being close to others; I find it difficult to trust them completely, difficult to allow myself to depend on them. I am nervous when anyone gets too close, and often, others want me to be more intimate than I feel comfortable being. (*Avoidant*)

- I find that others are reluctant to get as close as I would like. I often worry that my partner doesn't really love me or won't want to stay with me. I want to get very close to my partner, and this sometimes scares people away. (*Anxious-ambivalent*)

- I find it relatively easy to get close to others and am comfortable depending on them and having them depend on me. I don't worry about being abandoned or about someone getting too close to me. (*Secure*)

Note. From Hazan and Shaver (1987, p. 515). Copyright 1987 by the American Psychological Association. Reprinted by permission.

descriptions best captures the way they *generally* think, behave, and feel in romantic relationships.

These descriptions were based on a speculative extrapolation of the three infant patterns summarized in the final chapter of Ainsworth et al.'s (1978) book on infant–caregiver attachment. For example, the first paragraph captures the kinds of thoughts and feelings that Hazan and Shaver believed to characterize the adult analogue of anxious-avoidant attachment in infancy. This description targets feelings of insecurity, distancing strategies, and reluctance to open up to and depend on others. The second paragraph describes secure attachment. Embedded in this description is the secure person's belief that other people are likely to be warm, sensitive, and responsive. The final paragraph captures the adult analogue of the anxious-ambivalent infant. It describes a person who is insecure regarding whether or not close others will be available, accessible, and responsive. Moreover, it captures the inherent conflict of anxious-ambivalent children—the desire to be loved and comforted, coupled with the inability to feel adequately loved.

In their initial studies, Hazan and Shaver (1987) found that people's self-reported romantic attachment pattern was related to a number of theoretically relevant variables, including beliefs about love and relationships (working models of romantic relationships) and recollections of early experiences with parents. For example, people endorsing the secure description were more likely to report warm relationships with their parents, as well as harmonious relationships between their parents. With respect to their romantic relationships, they reported higher levels of happiness and trust. People endorsing the avoidant description perceived their mothers as cool and rejecting; in their romantic relationships, they reported a fear of intimacy, difficulty in accepting their partners, and a general belief that romantic love does not last. Anxious-ambivalent adults also reported conflicted relationships with parents and were more likely to report feelings of obsession and jealousy in romantic relationships.

The Hazan and Shaver three-category measure was adopted by many researchers in social, clinical, and personality psychology, partly because of its brevity, face validity, and ease of administration. In addition, this measure, coupled with the ideas articulated by Hazan and Shaver (1987), offered a promising means for building a psychodynamically informed empirical science.

Bartholomew's Four-Category Model

In 1990, Bartholomew published an important paper that challenged researchers to reconsider the three-category model of individual differences in adult attachment (see also Bartholomew & Horowitz, 1991; Griffin & Bartholomew, 1994a). Integrating ideas from Bowlby (1973), developmental research (e.g., Main, Kaplan, & Cassidy, 1985), psychodynamic concepts (Weinberger, 1995), and interpersonal theory (e.g., Leary, 1957), Bartholomew (1990) argued that people hold separate representational models of themselves (*model of self*) and their social world (*model of others*)—models that have distinct consequences for the way attachment behavior is organized. The model of others reflects the expectations, beliefs, and strategies that people have concerning close others in general and attachment figures in particular. Individuals with a positive model of others view attachment figures as trustworthy, reliable, and dependable. Individuals with negatively valenced models of others lack confidence in people's trustworthiness and dependability. The model of self reflects the valence of people's views of themselves. People with a positive model of self see themselves as competent, autonomous, and worthy of love. People with a negative model of self lack confidence, harbor self-doubts, and are vulnerable to psychological distress.

Bartholomew argued that when these two kinds of representational models are crossed with valence (i.e., the models' positivity or negativity), it is possible to derive four, rather than three, major attachment patterns (see Figure 7.1). She borrowed names for the four patterns from a mixture of the Ainsworth et al. (1978), Hazan and Shaver (1987, 1990), and Main et al. (1985) typologies, calling the positive–positive group *secure,* the negative–positive group *preoccupied,* the positive–negative group *dismissing,* and the negative–negative group *fearful.* Following Hazan and Shaver's lead, Bartholomew and Horowitz (1991) developed the Relationship Questionnaire (RQ), a short instrument containing descriptions of each of the four theoretical types. As with Hazan and Shaver's measure, respondents are asked to read each description and select the one that best captures the way they approach close relationships (see Table 7.2).

Notice that the wording of three of the four type descriptions (secure, preoccupied, and fearful-avoidant) is very similar to the wording of the three Hazan and Shaver descriptions (secure, anxious-ambivalent, and

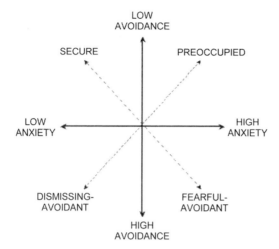

FIGURE 7.1. The two-dimensional model of individual differences in attachment organization.

avoidant). In fact, Bartholomew (1990) essentially equated the secure categories between the two systems, as well as the anxious-ambivalent and preoccupied patterns. In Bartholomew's model, however, the avoidant type is split into two distinct types. The first kind of avoidance, *fearful avoidance,* captures the vulnerable, insecure form of avoidance reflected in the Hazan and Shaver avoidant category. Fearful individuals, theoretically, are avoidant of intimacy because they fear being hurt by someone they love. The second kind of avoidance, *dismissing avoidance,* is not represented in

TABLE 7.2. Bartholomew's Four Attachment Types

- It is easy for me to become emotionally close to others. I am comfortable depending on them and having them depend on me. I don't worry about being alone or having others not accept me. (*Secure*)

- I am uncomfortable getting close to others. I want emotionally close relationships, but I find it difficult to trust others completely, or to depend on them. I worry that I will be hurt if I allow myself to become too close to others. (*Fearful,* or *fearful-avoidant*)

- I want to be completely emotionally intimate with others, but I often find that others are reluctant to get as close as I would like. I am uncomfortable being without close relationships, but I sometimes worry that others don't value me as much as I value them. (*Preoccupied*)

- I am comfortable without close emotional relationships. It is very important to me to feel independent and self-sufficient, and I prefer not to depend on others or have others depend on me. (*Dismissing,* or *dismissing-avoidant*)

Note. From Bartholomew and Horowitz (1991, p. 244). Copyright 1991 by the American Psychological Association. Reprinted by permission.

the Hazan and Shaver system. These kinds of individuals avoid intimacy, not because they consciously fear being hurt, but because they consciously value independence and autonomy. Bowlby (1980) referred to these kinds of people as compulsively self-reliant.

The Evolution of the Categorical Measurement System

Although both Hazan and Shaver's and Bartholomew's categorical, forced-choice measures became widely used, a few investigators quickly recognized the limitations of these instruments (e.g., Collins & Read, 1990; Levy & Davis, 1988; Simpson, 1990). For example, both measures force people to choose one category that best describes them, even if more than one category seems appropriate (Simpson, 1990). In addition, as Baldwin and Fehr (1995) pointed out, the test–retest stability of the Hazan and Shaver measure was only 70% (equivalent to a Pearson r of approximately .40)—a value that Baldwin and Fehr argued was extraordinarily low, given the theoretical emphasis placed on the stability of attachment patterns.

To address some of these issues, some attachment researchers began to use continuous rating scales (see Fraley & Waller, 1998). In the earliest such published report, Levy and Davis (1988) asked participants to rate how well each of the three Hazan and Shaver attachment patterns described their general approach to relationships. Subsequently, Collins and Read (1990) and Simpson (1990) decomposed the three Hazan and Shaver multisentence descriptions to form separate items that could be individually rated on Likert-type response scales. On average, these relatively brief multi-item scales have alpha and test–retest reliability estimates of .70 over periods ranging from 1 week to 2 years (Carpenter & Kirkpatrick, 1996; Collins & Read, 1990; Fuller & Fincham, 1995; Scharfe & Bartholomew, 1994; Simpson, Rholes, & Nelligan, 1992; Simpson, Rholes, & Phillips, 1996), suggesting that breaking the paragraphs into their component parts was a useful way to improve estimates of attachment stability.

As Bartholomew's four-category system became more popular, researchers began assessing the four types with continuous ratings. In fact, in Bartholomew's original empirical report, she recommended obtaining continuous ratings of each of the four attachment patterns in addition to the self-classification (Bartholomew & Horowitz, 1991). A few years after the RQ was published, Griffin and Bartholomew (1994b) developed a multi-item attachment inventory, the Relationship Scales Questionnaire (RSQ). This 30-item inventory contained content from both the Hazan and Shaver descriptions and Bartholomew's RQ descriptions. The RSQ can be scaled to create a continuous score for each person on each of Bartholomew's four attachment patterns (see *www.sfu.ca/psyc/faculty/bartholomew/rsq.htm* for a complete list of the RSQ items; these and other measures are also reproduced in the appendices of the book by Mikulincer & Shaver, 2007). That is, each individual can be assigned a score on security, a score on fearful avoidance, a score on preoccupation, and a score on dismissing avoidance. Due to its multi-item nature, the RSQ exhibits somewhat higher reliability estimates (r's about .65 for the brief scales assessing each of the four attachment patterns; Fraley & Shaver, 1997) than the single-item ratings of each RQ paragraph (about .50; see Scharfe & Bartholomew, 1994).

Types versus Dimensions

Although the gradual move from classifications to ratings was an important step toward improving the measurement of adult attachment, these shifts raised a larger theoretical question: Do people vary continuously or categorically with respect to these theoretical attachment patterns? This question, sometimes referred to as the "types versus dimensions" question, is a critical one for the study of adult attachment. If people actually vary continuously in attachment organization, but researchers assign people to categories, then potentially important information about the way people differ from one another is lost. This loss can have deleterious effects on the study of continuity and change; on mapping the developmental antecedents and consequences of attachment experiences; on understanding whether certain experiences affect attachment organization; and on bridging the gaps among attachment research in social, personality, clinical, and developmental psychology.

How can one determine whether variation in an unobservable construct, such as attachment organization, is continuous or categorical? Historically, researchers have relied on clustering techniques to identify groupings in data (e.g., Collins & Read, 1990; Feeney, Noller, & Hanrahan, 1994). One of the limitations of cluster analysis, however, is that it reveals groupings in data regardless of whether natural groupings actually exist. Fortunately, Meehl and his colleagues (e.g., Meehl & Yonce, 1996; Waller & Meehl, 1998) developed a suite of techniques that allow one to uncover the latent structure of a domain and rigorously test *taxonic* (i.e., typological) conjectures. Fraley and Waller (1998) adopted two of Meehl's techniques, MAXCOV and MAMBAC, to address the types-versus-dimensions question in the study of adult attachment. They administered Griffin and Bartholomew's (1994b) 30-item RSQ to a sample of over 600 undergraduates. Their taxometric analyses of the data provided no evidence for a categorical model of attachment. Instead, their results were more consistent with what would be expected if individual differences in attachment were continuously distributed. To complement this research, Fraley and Spieker (2003) conducted a MAXCOV analysis on a sample of over 1,000 infants observed in Ainsworth's Strange Situation test procedure at age 15 months. They also found no evidence for attachment categories. These findings suggest that individual differences in attachment organization, in both children and adults, are better conceptualized as continuous than as categorical.

The taxometric results reported by Fraley and his colleagues suggest that a dimensional system might be more appropriate than a categorical one for conceptualizing and assessing individual differences in attachment. The move from categorical to continuous measurement systems, however, raises a number of questions: What is the best dimensional system for conceptualizing variation in adult attachment? What measures should be used to assess this variation? And how can we think about dimensions, as opposed to types, in a clinical context?

What Are the Fundamental Dimensions Underlying Adult Attachment?

In the 1990s, a number of investigators began creating multi-item inventories of adult attachment—inventories that could be used to produce continuous attachment scores. Although each of these instruments was rooted in Bowlby and Ainsworth's attachment theory, the designers of these instruments emphasized different constructs and used different methods of test development. As noted previously, some researchers simply decomposed the items contained in the original Hazan and Shaver paragraphs. For example, Collins's (Collins & Read, 1990; Collins, 1996) Adult Attachment Scale was developed by taking the individual sentence fragments in the original Hazan and Shaver descriptions and creating 18 distinct items, each of which was rated on a continuous scale. From psychometric analyses of the items, Collins and Read (1990) derived three composites. The first, *close*, captured variation in the extent to which people felt comfortable being close to others. The second, *depend*, reflected variation in the degree to which people were comfortable depending on others and having others depend on them. The third composite, *anxiety*, captured variability in the extent to which people were worried that relationship partners might abandon or reject them.

Feeney et al. (1994) took a different approach to generating continuous measures of attachment. Rather than extracting fragments and phrases from the Hazan and Shaver or Bartholomew prototypes, they developed new items designed to capture some of the common themes in attachment theory, such as trust, dependence, and self-reliance. A factor analysis of responses to their items uncovered five factors: self-confidence, discomfort with closeness, need for approval, preoccupation with relationships, and the belief that relationships are of secondary importance. Brennan and Shaver (1995) followed a similar approach, generating a large pool of items and then factor-analyzing them. Brennan and Shaver (1995) reported seven factors: ambivalence, anxious clinging to partners, jealous and fear of abandonment, frustration with partners, proximity seeking, self-reliance, and trust.

By the mid- to late 1990s, researchers and clinicians new to the field were drowning in a sea of self-report measures of attachment. To address this problem, Brennan et al. (1998) gathered all the self-report measures of adult attachment known at the time and administered the nonredundant items to 1,086 undergraduates. Factor analyses of the responses revealed two major factors; the content of the items loading on these factors led Brennan and her colleagues to label them attachment-related *anxiety* and attachment-related *avoidance*. The anxiety factor was defined by such items as "I worry that my partner won't want to stay with me" and "I don't think my partner loves me." The avoidance factor was defined by such items as "I am uncomfortable depending on others" and, at the opposite end, "I turn to my partner for assurance."

The Brennan et al. (1998) paper was a breakthrough for three reasons. First, their analyses revealed that the diverse pool of self-report measures of adult attachment was essentially tapping two fundamental dimensions. Second, the Brennan et al. report showed how measures originally developed with different objectives could be mapped onto a common dimensional framework. This has allowed subsequent scholars to interpret the findings of studies based on different measures within the same two-dimensional system. Finally, Brennan and her colleagues used their data to produce a new questionnaire, the Experiences in Close Relationships (ECR) inventory—a 36-item questionnaire based on the items that best tapped the dimensions of anxiety and avoidance. In their original report, Brennan et al. (1998) showed that the 18 items for each subscale hung together well (<F"Symbol">a<F255>'s > .90), and the scales predicted a number of theoretically relevant outcomes, such as the enjoyment of touch, sexual preferences, and emotions experienced in an intimate context. The ECR and its derivatives (e.g., the ECR-R; Fraley, Waller, & Brennan, 2000) are currently the most commonly used self-report measures of adult attachment, and are commonly recommended for use as the primary self-report instruments for assessing adult attachment patterns.

What Is the Meaning of the Two Dimensions?

Although Brennan et al.'s (1998) analyses indicated that two major factors underlie individual differences in adult romantic attachment, they did not offer an interpretation of the factors that was rooted in a specific model of how the attachment system operates. In fact, there have been several distinct ways of conceptualizing these two factors over the years. Some researchers have favored a *model of self* and *model of others* interpretation, as put forward by Griffin and Bartholomew (1994a) (e.g., Klohnen & John, 1998; Carnelley, Pietromonaco, & Jaffe, 1994). Within this framework, individual differences are conceptualized as differences in the valence (i.e., the positivity vs. negativity) of the models people hold of themselves and others.

Accordingly, many researchers have attempted to specify the actual beliefs that people with different attachment orientations hold (e.g., Baldwin, Keelan, Fehr, Enns, & Koh-Rangarajoo, 1996; Collins, 1996; Klohnen & John, 1998).

Fraley and Shaver (2000) outlined several limitations of conceptualizing the dimensions within the model of self and model of others. First, the manifest content of the items typically used to assess variation in attachment, both in the ECR and in Bartholomew's original prototype descriptions, is more consistent with a conceptualization that focuses on sensitivity to rejection and strategies for regulating affect. Second, the interpretation based on the models of self and others requires that preoccupied individuals hold positive views of others (views of others as available, responsive, attentive, etc.). This characterization is at odds with the empirical literature, which suggests that highly preoccupied individuals are often angry, jealous, combative, and prone to feel that partners are insensitive to their needs (e.g., Collins, 1996; Simpson et al., 1996).

As an alterative to the models of self and others framework, Fraley and Shaver (2000) put forward an *affective–motivational framework* (see also Fraley & Shaver, 1998; Fraley & Spieker, 2003). From this perspective, the two dimensions can be conceptualized as reflecting variability in the functioning of two fundamental subsystems or components of the attachment behavioral system. Shaver and Mikulincer (Chapter 2, this volume) provide a control systems representation of the dynamics of these two subsystems (see Figure 2.1 in Chapter 2), based on theoretical discussions by Fraley and Shaver (1998), Kobak, Cole, Ferenz-Gillies, Fleming, & Gamble (1993), Lazarus and Folkman (1984), and Shaver, Hazan, and Bradshaw (1988). One component of the system involves monitoring and appraising events for their relevance to attachment-related goals, such as the attachment figure's physical or psychological proximity, availability, and responsiveness. When the system detects a discrepancy between the current set goal for sensitivity and proximity and the perceived behavior of the attachment figure, the individual feels anxious and becomes increasingly vigilant to attachment-related cues. Variation in people's threshold for detecting threats to security or cues of rejection corresponds to individual differences in what Brennan et al. (1998) call attachment-related *anxiety*. The second component is responsible for regulation of attachment behavior with respect to attachment-related goals. For example, to regulate attachment-related anxiety, people can orient their behavior toward their attachment figures (i.e., seeking contact or support) or withdraw and attempt to handle the threat alone. Variation in this behavioral/motivational component is responsible for individual differences in what Brennan et al. (1998) call attachment-related *avoidance*, and in many respects reflects whether a person is willing or unwilling to rely on another individual as a safe haven and secure base.

One of the advantages of this framework is that it allows Bartholomew's four theoretical types to be conceptualized as linear combinations of the two dimensions of anxiety and avoidance. For example, security and dismissing avoidance are characteristic of people who have high thresholds for detecting cues of rejection. Preoccupation and fearful avoidance are characteristic of individuals with low thresholds for detecting such cues, making concerns about love-worthiness and rejection particularly salient. Security and preoccupation characterize people who wish to be close to and intimate with their partners. Dismissing avoidance and fearful avoidance characterize people who try to deny the importance of close relationships or force themselves not to become vulnerable to them (see Figure 7.1).

Another advantage of this framework is that it has the potential to be clinically useful. Although it is typically easier to classify a client into one of several distinct categories (e.g., secure, dismissing, preoccupied, fearful) than to scale him or her with respect to two or more dimensions (especially given that clinicians are often trained to make categorical diagnoses by using the Diagnostic and Statistical Manual of Mental Disorders), it can be much easier to study change in personality organization when the fine-grained distinctions that are available in a dimensional system are made. It is possible, for example, for a client to exhibit gradual gains in security across therapy that would be evident in the use of dimensional measures. However, if clinicians were using classification systems across sessions, those changes might go undetected.

Finally, the fact that the two-dimensional system distinguishes between attachment-related insecurities and the motivational strategies people use to regulate their thoughts and feelings (i.e., as reflected in attachment-related avoidance) enables clinicians to make a distinction between distinct attachment dynamics. It is possible that a client is relatively secure in the knowledge that his or her partner is available and responsive if needed (i.e., the client is low in attachment-related anxiety), but that he or she characteristically relies upon distancing strategies in the relationship (i.e., the client is high on the avoidance dimension). If so, a treatment plan that focuses on altering the person's behavior and defensive styles may be more effective for promoting the well-being of the relationship than one that focuses on making the person feel more secure and confident. Existing categorical systems do not allow these kinds of distinctions to be made easily.

Summary

Self-report measures of adult attachment have evolved considerably over the past 20 years. Since Hazan and Shaver's (1987) landmark article, the field has moved from classifying people with respect to three categories to scaling people with respect to two dimensions. Although the dimensional system captures the same attachment patterns as the original categorical systems, it allows these patterns to be represented with a greater degree of specificity and fidelity than is possible with classificatory systems. Factor analyses of people's answers to attachment questions indicate that two key dimensions underlie the attachment patterns. The first, attachment-related anxiety, captures the extent to which people are insecure about their partners' availability, love, and responsiveness. The second, attachment-related avoidance, captures the strategies that people use for regulating attachment-related behavior, thought, and affect: Some people are comfortable opening up to others in intimate contexts, depending on others, and allowing others to depend on them; other people, in contrast, are more reserved and cautious, guarding themselves and their emotions. We contend that these two dimensions reflect variation in the basic functioning of the attachment system, and that clinical work can be enhanced by focusing on assessing change in a person's scores on these dimensions.

It is important to note that although self-report measures of adult attachment are commonly used in research, a great deal of work needs to be done before we fully understand what these scales measure. For example, it is not clear how well the two dimensions commonly studied in undergraduate college samples in the United States will be replicated in other cultures, and, indeed, whether the basic concepts will carry the same meaning from one culture to the next (see Onishi & Gjerde, 2002). Wei, Russell, Mallinckrodt, and Zakalik (2004) found that the factor structure of the ECR was similar across four American ethnic subcultures (i.e., African American, Asian American, Hispanic American, and European American), and that the dimensions were related to negative mood in similar ways in each, but it is possible that these dimensions have different meanings outside the United States. Moreover, there is still debate regarding the extent to which self-reports of attachment are related to the same kinds of constructs that are assessed with interview-based measures of attachment, such as the AAI (see Levy & Kelly, Chapter 6). Current research suggests that there is only a weak relationship between self-reported avoidance and dismissing attachment, as assessed with the AAI, but for the most part these two kinds of measures appear to tap different aspects of psychological functioning (see Roisman et al., 2007). Finally, we should note that these measures are designed to assess variation in the ways people experience and behave in close relationships; they are not used to determine whether a relationship qualifies as an attachment relationship. It is generally agreed that an attachment relationship is one in which one person uses the other as a safe haven and a secure base (see Hazan, Gur-Yaish, & Campa, 2004). There has been comparatively little research on how to assess whether a relationship qualifies as an attachment, but some preliminary measures have been created to do so. Interested readers should consult Hazan and Zeifman (1994), Fraley and Davis (1997), and Trinke and Barthlomew (1997) for examples of questions that can assist in identifying a current attachment figure. Some of these questions are included in the appendices of the book by Mikulincer and Shaver (2007). Another useful measure is Allen et al.'s (2001) Current Attachment Relationships questionnaire.

USING SELF-REPORTS IN CLINICAL PRACTICE

Why might it be valuable to use self-report measures of attachment in a clinical context? These measures now have a long history in the research arena, and it has been well demonstrated that variations in attachment style, as assessed with self-report measures, are associated with many phenomena of clinical interest. These include depressive symptoms (e.g., Hankin, Kassel, & Abela, 2005), susceptibility to symptoms of posttraumatic stress disorder (Fraley, Fazzari, Bonnano, & Dekel, 2006), antisocial behavior (Timmerman & Emmelkamp, 2006), suicidal tendencies (Martin, 1997), eating disorders (Troisi, Massaroni, & Cuzzolaro, 2005), personality disorders (Brennan & Shaver, 1998; Levy, Meehan, Weber, Reynoso, & Clarkin, 2005; Timmerman & Emmelkamp, 2006), alcoholism (Vungkhaching, Sher, Jackson, & Parra, 2004), and relationship dysfunction (Simpson et al., 1996). These studies suggest that assessing attachment constructs via self-reports should enable a clinician to gain insight into an aspect of the mind that has broad implications for adaptive and maladaptive patterns of thought, feelings, and behavior. Moreover, by using the two-dimensional system reviewed here, a clinician can hone in on some of the idiosyncratic ways in which a client's attachment system functions. It could be that if a client is highly anxious with respect to attachment issues (e.g., the availability and responsiveness of his or her partner), these insecurities will fuel many of the problems faced in his or her relationships. By assessing attachment patterns early in the therapeutic process, the clinician can gain insight into the unique ways in which the client approaches issues of attachment-related significance. Indeed, some clinicians have begun to use self-report measures to complement other assessments (e.g., Allen et al., 2001) and to inform treatment focus (e.g., Meyer & Pilkonis, 2002). (See Chs. 13–15 of Mikulincer & Shaver, 2007, for a more complete set of examples and references.)

Another reason for using self-reports to assess attachment is that they constitute a quick and inexpensive way to monitor changes in attachment patterns over time. Assessing attachment across sessions makes it possible to evaluate the effectiveness of the treatment plan and determine whether therapy is leading to the desired kinds of changes. In short, it can be valuable to assess attachment patterns in clinical contexts both for diagnostic purposes (e.g., identifying problem areas in a person's life) and for monitoring the effectiveness of therapies designed to alter a person's working models. This approach is consistent with the increasing emphasis on documenting treatment outcomes (Cone, 2001).

How should one go about assessing self-reported attachment patterns in a clinical context? The obvious way would be to administer a paper-and-pencil self-report instrument, such as the ECR or the ECR-R, to clients. (For clinicians interested in using self-reports in this fashion, detailed instructions on how to use and score the ECR-R, along with some nonpatient norms, are available at *www.psych.uiuc.edu/~rcfraley/measures/ecrr.htm*.) In short, one simply administers the questionnaire and then computes two scale scores, one for anxiety and one for avoidance, by averaging the responses to specific items. (Please note that some items require reverse keying, because high ratings reflect less anxiety or less avoidance.)

Unfortunately, administering self-reports in a standard questionnaire format is less than ideal for a number of reasons (e.g., the questionnaires have to be scored by hand, and clients who take questionnaire packets home may forget to complete them or bring them to the session). To make this process more practical, we have developed a Web-based assessment system called eSession. eSession can be used to assess and visualize a client's attachment organization across multiple relationships over time. These assessments can be used to understand what a client's attachment style is like in his or her romantic relationship, as well as in other relationships (e.g., relationships with parents, coworkers, friends); they can also reveal how current events and experiences in a client's life relate to changes in attachment-related anxiety and avoidance. The system offers an unprecedented opportunity to explore how the organization of a person's attachment system and the quality of his or her relationships (i.e., the structure of attachments in multiple relational domains) contribute to adaptive functioning. Of course, eSession can also be used for a simple, one-time assessment that immediately yields automatically computed scores on the two attachment dimensions.

In the sections that follow, we describe eSession, focusing on some pragmatic details, such as how to register a free eSession account and how to use it. Importantly, we also share some of the experiences we have had with using eSession in a therapeutic context. Finally, we highlight what we consider to be some of the unique advantages of this assessment system, as well as some directions for future developments. It is our hope that clinicians who are interested in assessing self-reported attachment patterns in their practices will be able to use eSession and to manage and interpret the resulting data in useful ways.

eSession's Measure of Attachment

eSession's measure of attachment is based on the Relationship Structures (RS) questionnaire—an inventory that was derived from the longer 36-item inventories commonly used in social-psychological attachment research (e.g., the ECR and the ECR-R). The RS is a 10-item measure that uses 6 statements designed to assess attachment-related avoidance and 4 statements designed to assess attachment-related anxiety. Unlike the ECR, which is oriented toward romantic relationships, the RS items are worded so as to be relevant to any relationship context, and the instructions are varied to tailor them to a specific context. In nonclinical research using the RS, we have found both scales to have high reliabilities (e.g., α's > .80) and to be related to a variety of outcomes, including behavioral outcomes, such as judgments regarding other people's emotional expressions (e.g., Fraley, Niedenthal, Marks, Brumbaugh, & Vicary, 2006).

How to Use eSession

If you are a psychotherapist, you can create a free account in eSession by visiting *www.yourpersonality.net/eSession/gettingstarted.htm*. You will be asked to enter your professional name (e.g., R. Chris Fraley) and your e-mail address, and to read and agree to the Terms of Service. You will also need to create a username and password that you can thereafter use to log into your account. Once your registration has been processed by eSession, you will be notified by e-mail. This process can take anywhere from 1 minute to several days, depending on server load.

Creating Client Accounts

Once you have registered your account successfully, you will be able to log in to eSession via the therapist login page at *www.yourpersonality.net/cgi-bin/eSession/clientlogin.pl*. After logging in, you will be taken to the main menu page of eSession. The left panel of the menu page lists your current clients and the dates you opened their accounts. The right panel provides you with various options, such as "View scatter analysis" and "View item responses for a client" (see Figure 7.2). To create a new account for one of your clients, choose the "Create new user" option. When the new page loads, you will need to do the following:

1. Enter your username and password (if your browser does not automatically store that information for you). This step is redundant, but offers an added measure of data security.
2. Choose a username and password for your client. You should select a username that does not include personally identifying information (e.g., names, Social Security numbers). You should keep a record of your clients' usernames and passwords in case they lose this information.
3. Enter the first name of your client's romantic partner (i.e., boyfriend, girlfriend, spouse), if relevant. For an added measure of data security, it is advisable to use initials.
4. Finally, nominate three individuals who play an important role in your client's life. When your client uses eSession, he or she will be asked attachment-related questions about these three people. If you have seen your client across several sessions in the past, it may be obvious which names to enter here. If not, you should consult with your client about the most significant people in his or her life.

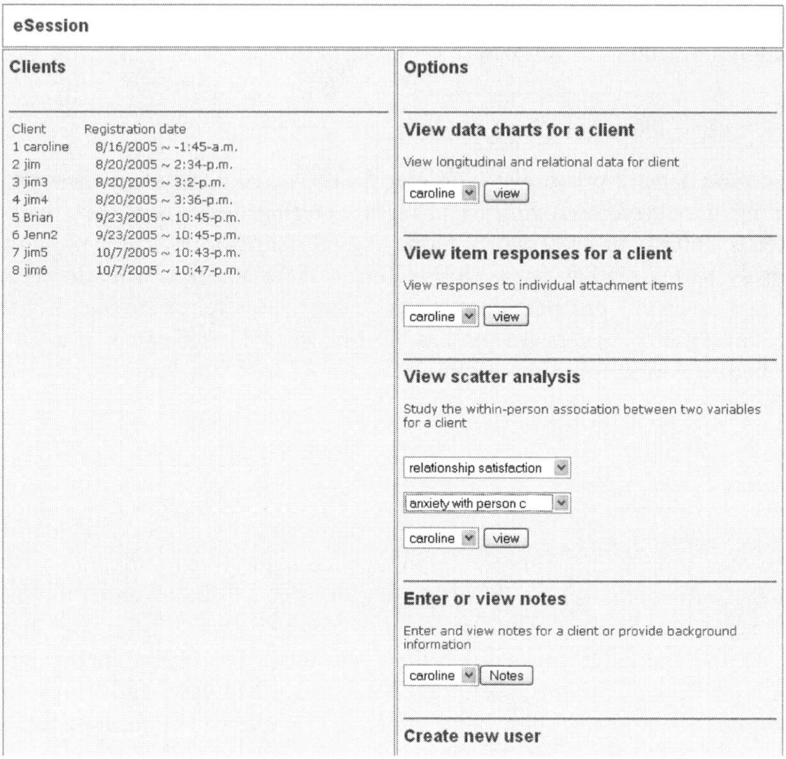

FIGURE 7.2. The main menu page in eSession.

Once you have submitted this information, the client account will be created. The next time you return to the main menu, you will see that client's username added to your registration list. You can create as many client accounts as needed; however, you can create only one account at a time.

Before creating a client account for use with a real client, we suggest that you create a fake or test client account, using your username with the word *test* at the end (e.g., *Fraleytest*). This way, you can log in to eSession as a client and see what the experience will be like from the client's point of view.

To make the most out of eSession, you will need to devote part of a counseling or therapy session to walking your client through the eSession process. Using your test account, you should show your client how to log in to eSession and how to enter responses. You will want to be able to answer any questions your client may have, and if you are familiar with the client side of eSession, you will be in a good position to answer those questions. The client web pages also contain a link to a tutorial. You might want to print a copy of that tutorial for your client to take home. It might even be valuable to write the client's username and password on that page, so that he or she has easy access to it.

Using eSession's Features

After one or more of your clients use eSession, you can view their data in the main menu. On the menu page, you have the following options:

- *"View data charts for a client."* This option allows you to view a large-scale summary of your client's attachment patterns over time. Specifically, this option will provide a graphic summary of your client's attachment patterns (or attachment styles) in each of four relationships: his or her romantic relationship and the other three relationships that you nominated when his or her account was created. This option will also show you some of the significant life events that were reported by the client, as well as charts that illustrate the client's relationship trajectory with respect to satisfaction and commitment. To view these charts, select the client of interest from the pull-down menu and click on the "View" button.
- *"View item responses for a client."* To view the actual answers the client provided to each attachment-related questionnaire item, select the client's username from the pull-down menu and click on "View." eSession will show you the client's response to each attachment item for each relationship and each session. Items that received extreme responses (e.g., answers of 6 or higher on a 1–7 scale measuring insecurity, after reverse scoring of the necessary items) will be highlighted. Depending on your therapeutic style, you may find it useful to follow up with your client on items with extreme responses. In our work, we have found it useful to ask clients why they gave extreme responses to certain items, and to use these discussions as springboards for exploring particular issues in the clients' lives.
- *"View scatter analysis."* As noted previously, most research on relational and clinical issues focuses on comparing variables across people rather than studying the association between variables within persons. The "View scatter analysis" option allows you to see how a client's scores correlate with one another across time. For example, by plotting depressive symptoms against relationship satisfaction, you can determine whether your client tends to experience increases in depressive symptoms on occasions in which his or her relationship is under duress. Some clients may show a strong coupling between certain variables, but others may not. By studying these within-person scatterplots, you should be able to identify some of the key factors that trigger certain emotional responses in your client.
- *"Enter or view notes."* eSession allows you to keep notes on your clients in a "blog-like" fashion. The notes feature of eSession allows you to enter any information you wish at any time and to save those notes in an organized manner. You will want to use this section to enter information

you deem of interest, such as presenting symptoms, basic demographics, treatment plans, or other information that is not specifically collected by eSession. eSession will automatically time- and date-stamp each entry.

A CASE STUDY IN eSESSION

In this section, we discuss a case study of a young European American woman, "Bridget." Although Bridget presented in the context of marital therapy, we focus for purposes of brevity on how eSession was used in conjunction with counseling to clarify and identify aspects of Bridget's attachment dynamics. Treatment was informed by the Gottman, Driver, and Tabares (2002) approach to marital work and by the assessment of attachment security.

Overview

Bridget, a 29-year-old pediatric nurse, entered counseling 2 years into her marriage. Her last argument with her husband, Samson, had escalated to an unprecedented level, including harsh name calling and potent threats to leave the relationship. The conflicts they were having caused them to distance themselves from one another, often withdrawing for days at a time. Their postconflict conclusions (e.g., "I can't live with this," and "This isn't who I married?") were adversely affecting their intimate lives, work performance, and mental health. Bridget thought that without counseling, these spats could result in the end of the marriage. She demanded that she and her husband attend treatment "or else."

At intake, Bridget was able to recall easily the reasons she had married Samson, and she perked up and laughed as she retrieved memories regarding their early romance. When the therapist asked, "On a 1–10 scale, where a 10 is 'I'd do anything required to save my marriage,' and a 1 is 'I'm not doing anything,' where do you stand?", she reported an 8. She was informed of the eSession project and was willing and interested to learn more about her attachment experiences.

Attachment History and Assessment

Bridget was the only child in an intact family. She began the discussion with the disclaimer that she always cries when she talks about her family. She recognized much greater closeness with her mother than her father, because her father worked a lot. There was very little open conflict in her family. When asked to select five adjectives or phrases to describe her childhood relationship with her mother, she chose "nurturing, interactive, loving, very communicative, and intentional." Bridget had ready access to salient memories that supported the adjectives she used. However, she would lay out a series of fragments of each recollection rather than coherently describing a particular event, suggesting a mild lack of coherence (see Levy & Kelly, Chapter 6, for a discussion of the importance of coherence in the AAI). For example, when asked if she could recall a specific episode that reflected her description of her mother as "loving," she responded: "She was always supportive of my sports events, came to every game. She was the coach, always involved and aware of where I was in my sports. And it wasn't that she wanted me to be in sports; she just knew I loved them." A similar kind of response was given with respect to the use of the descriptor "nurturing": "She has an ability to listen, to know when I need a hug; she could always give it to me. There were just so many times."

She described her father as "interactive, supportive, and humorous," but noted that there was "some tension" in the relationship. As with respect to her mother, Bridget's recollections regarding her father were a melding of events rather than specific episodes that fit the brief descriptors: "He was supportive of my grades, no matter what I got; he knew I pushed myself. He was proud of all my activities; he'd play blocks with me, take me fishing… "

Relationship Dynamics

During stressful times with her husband, Bridget would vacillate between attachment strategies: She might explode in anger and make contemptuous remarks (i.e., use hyperactivating strategies), or become uncommunicative and withdraw physically and sexually (i.e., use deactivating strategies). Both strategies seemed intended to punish Samson for failing to meet her needs, and to carry with them the hope that he might think twice about falling short in the future. When upset, Samson would place material issues (such as financial concerns) over his wife's feelings, or let his desire for orderliness and cleanliness eclipse his concern for Bridget's well-being. Bridget, in turn, would respond by absorbing herself in catastrophic, affect-laden conclusions, and eventually feel overwhelmed by despair. For example, when Samson chided her for spending "too much money," even though the purchases were modest, Bridget would conclude that she was not lovable enough to be worth modest pleasures; this would inevitably be followed by extreme extrapolations, such as "If I'm not worth it now, how can I expect him to want to stay with me in the long run?" Bridget's attachment strategies were also observable in sessions. She was often edgy and unpredictable; it was not uncommon for her to walk out in a fit or anger (only to return minutes later), to be caustically judgmental, or to become tearful and self-blaming.

eSession Analysis

Bridget was instructed to use eSession as "homework" between counseling sessions, and she completed it on five distinct occasions. In the sections that follow, we discuss the attachment patterns Bridget exhibited in her relationship with important people in her life, including Samson, and what those patterns might reveal about certain features of her psychological dynamics. For comparative purposes, we will reference her data against some norms we have collected, based on a diverse sample of nonclinical respondents who have completed the RS attachment questionnaire over the Internet. The descriptive statistics for those data (i.e., means and standard deviations) are reported in Tables 7.3 and 7.4 for women and men, respectively, of different ages.

Overview of the eSession Data

In Figure 7.3, we present a scatterplot of Bridget's attachment scores in each of three relationships (i.e., mother, father, and Samson) across the five assessments; the specific quantities are summarized in Table 7.5. Bridget reported a relatively secure relationship with her mother and Samson, but there was some variation in her attachment scores across time, particularly with respect to Samson (the standard deviation of her avoidance scores with Samson was over 6 times the standard deviation of her avoidance scores with her mother). This suggested that her experiences in her relationship with Samson had a measurable effect on her attachment-related thoughts and feelings.

Change over Time

Figure 7.4 illustrates the way in which Bridget's attachment scores changed over the course of counseling, as reflected in eSession. It is noteworthy that

TABLE 7.3. Means and Standard Deviations for Attachment-Related Anxiety and Avoidance among Women for Three Targets across Five Age Groups

	Age group				
Target	< 20 (*n* = 632)	20–30 (*n* = 1,315)	30–40 (*n* = 658)	40–50 (*n* = 441)	> 50 (*n* = 251)
Mother					
Anxiety	1.96 (1.44)	2.02 (1.48)	2.35 (1.69)	2.70 (1.86)	2.86 (1.92)
Avoidance	3.31 (1.71)	3.21 (1.69)	3.71 (1.80)	4.16 (1.81)	4.03 (1.89)
Father					
Anxiety	2.67 (1.64)	2.41 (1.80)	2.50 (1.78)	2.52 (1.75)	2.61 (1.83)
Avoidance	4.11 (1.69)	4.04 (1.75)	4.35 (1.77)	4.32 (1.81)	4.35 (1.80)
Partner					
Anxiety	2.92 (1.64)	3.20 (1.84)	3.13 (1.86)	3.05 (1.93)	2.83 (1.88)
Avoidance	2.06 (1.10)	2.35 (1.26)	2.59 (1.41)	2.76 (1.56)	2.77 (1.64)

TABLE 7.4. Means and Standard Deviations for Attachment-Related Anxiety and Avoidance among Men for Three Targets across Five Age Groups

	Age group				
Target	< 20 (n = 95)	20–30 (n = 256)	30–40 (n = 182)	40–50 (n = 139)	> 50 (n = 90)
Mother					
Anxiety	1.97 (1.46)	1.93 (1.52)	2.10 (1.47)	2.14 (1.49)	2.67 (1.64)
Avoidance	3.83 (1.69)	3.54 (1.48)	3.98 (1.70)	4.05 (1.66)	4.34 (1.51)
Father					
Anxiety	1.84 (1.10)	2.30 (1.66)	2.60 (1.68)	2.36 (1.52)	3.17 (1.80)
Avoidance	3.80 (1.56)	4.18 (1.68)	4.46 (1.62)	4.29 (1.62)	4.75 (1.57)
Partner					
Anxiety	2.47 (1.40)	2.84 (1.68)	2.88 (1.73)	2.71 (1.68)	2.51 (1.48)
Avoidance	1.99 (0.91)	2.39 (1.13)	2.57 (1.35)	2.71 (1.39)	2.68 (1.40)

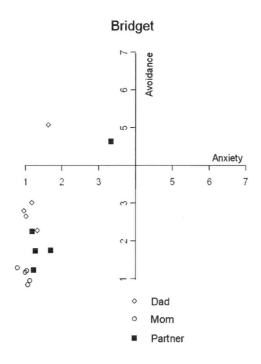

FIGURE 7.3. Attachment scores at different time points for Bridget's three major relationship partners. A random value (sampled from a random distribution with a mean of 0 and a standard deviation of 0.25) was added to each value to help separate some of the points more clearly in the figure. As such, some of the lower values appear as less than the minimum value of 1.

TABLE 7.5. Means and Standard Deviations for
Attachment-Related Anxiety and Avoidance for Bridget
across the Five eSessions

| | Bridget | |
Target	M	SD
Mother		
Anxiety	1.70	0.21
Avoidance	2.03	0.19
Father		
Anxiety	1.05	0.12
Avoidance	1.36	0.55
Partner		
Anxiety	1.75	0.87
Avoidance	2.33	1.37

Bridget's attachment scores varied a bit over time. With respect to her father, for example, she generally felt secure, but had a minor increase in avoidance at about the third session. She was highly secure in her relationship with her mother throughout the project. And although she was largely secure in the way she reported relating to Samson, on the fourth assessment she experienced a spike in insecurity. In the personal notes that she entered into eSession, she wrote the following regarding that occasion:

"We had our most extreme fight of our relationship. It was quite eye-opening about our personality differences. It was about something small, but the foundational issues were enormous. The gist was that the yogurt was left out all night by me, and when I found out I placed it in the garbage can. When Samson found it, I anticipated his reaction and told him that I didn't want to get into it. He got so upset because of the waste and not being able to vent and 'reprimand' me that he slammed the yogurt on the floor and kicked the garbage bag across the kitchen. ... The result of this fight: We spent Christmas separately."

This fight appears to have caused Bridget to feel substantially less secure in her relationship, as reflected in her eSession scores and in her corresponding behavior (she insisted on being apart over the holiday).

It is important to note that Bridget reported feeling relatively secure in her relationship with Samson from the beginning. As such, there was little reason to expect her to become much more secure over time. For the most part, their troubles seemed to stem from their styles of conflict and behavior, which were expected to be improved by counseling.

We also examined other aspects of Bridget's psychological dynamics as

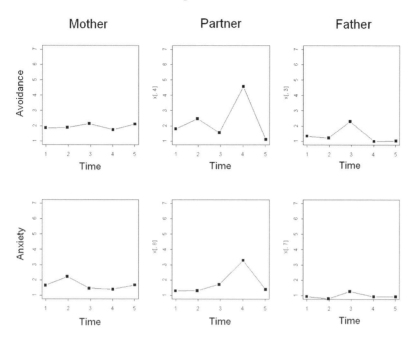

FIGURE 7.4. Bridget's attachment insecurity over time in regard to her three major relationship partners.

revealed by eSession data. For example, we studied the association between the negativity of her life events at about the time of each session and her perceptions of care and support from Samson. Her eSession data revealed a negative correlation between these variables. On occasions in which she felt that things were not going well, she also reported feeling unsupported by her partner. Although it is possible that the negative experiences were due in part to perceptions of a lack of support, this association nonetheless highlighted a potential problem in the functioning of their relationship. Ideally, perceptions of support should be higher during times of duress—a pattern that we observe in empirical data sets from less troubled samples.

FUTURE DEVELOPMENTS

In the few cases in which we have used eSession to date, we have found it to be a useful tool for assessing attachment-related variables. Moreover, our clients have enjoyed their experience with eSession and have reported that they find it useful. Nonetheless, eSession has some limitations in its present form. For example, the data analysis options that eSession currently offers are somewhat limited. It is our hope that we can expand those options as the program is developed further, and can allow clinicians to add their own questions or surveys to the assessment protocol. As we explored eSession, we observed that some of our clients wanted to see the graphs, not just receive summaries of them from their therapists. As currently configured, eSession allows only therapists to access the raw data and graphs, but there could be some utility in allowing clients to access this information themselves. Despite these limitations, we hope that eSession will be a useful application for clinicians who are interested in using self-reports of attachment in their clinical work.

RECOMMENDATIONS FOR FURTHER READING

Brennan, K. A., Clark, C. L., & Shaver, P. R. (1998). Self-report measurement of adult attachment: An integrative overview. In J. A. Simpson & W. S. Rholes (Eds.), *Attachment theory and close relationships* (pp. 46–76). New York: Guilford Press.—This breakthrough chapter established the now-accepted two-dimensional model of adult attachment, and includes the statistical basis for the ECR.

Hazan, C., & Shaver, P. R. (1987). Romantic love conceptualized as an attachment process. *Journal of Personality and Social Psychology, 52,* 511–524.—This landmark study was the first to empirically investigate John Bowlby and Mary Ainsworth's ideas as they might be applied to adults. The study contains the first self-report measure of adult attachment.

REFERENCES

Ainsworth, M. D. S., Blehar, M., Waters, E., & Wall, S. (1978). *Patterns of attachment: A psychological study of the Strange Situation.* Hillsdale, NJ: Erlbaum.

Allen, J. G., Huntoon, J., Fultz, J., Stein, H., Fonagy, P., & Evans, R. B. (2001). A model for brief assessment of attachment and its application to women in inpatient treatment for trauma-related psychiatric disorders. *Journal of Personality Assessment, 76,* 421–447.

Baldwin, M. W., & Fehr, B. (1995). On the instability of attachment style ratings. *Personal Relationships, 2,* 247–261.

Baldwin, M. W., Keelan, J. P. R., Fehr, B., Enns, V., & Koh-Rangarajoo, E. (1996). Social-cognitive conceptualization of attachment working models: Availability and accessibility effects. *Journal of Personality and Social Psychology, 71,* 94–109.

Bartholomew, K. (1990). Avoidance of intimacy: An attachment perspective. *Journal of Social and Personal Relationships, 7,* 147–178.

Bartholomew, K., & Horowitz, L. (1991). Attachment styles among young adults: A test of the four-category model. *Journal of Personality and Social Psychology, 61,* 226–245.

Bowlby, J. (1973). *Attachment and loss: Vol. 2. Separation: Anxiety and anger.* New York: Basic Books.

Bowlby, J. (1980). *Attachment and loss: Vol. 3. Loss: Sadness and depression.* New York: Basic Books.

Bowlby, J. (1982). *Attachment and loss: Vol. 1. Attachment* (2nd ed.). New York: Basic Books. (1st ed., 1969)

Brennan, K. A., Clark, C. L., & Shaver, P. R. (1998). Self-report measurement of adult attachment: An integrative overview. In J. A. Simpson & W. S. Rholes (Eds.), *Attachment theory and close relationships* (pp. 46–76). New York: Guilford Press.

Brennan, K. A., & Shaver, P. R. (1995). Dimensions of adult attachment, affect regulation and romantic relationship functioning. *Personality and Social Psychology Bulletin, 21,* 267–283.

Brennan, K. A., & Shaver, P. R. (1998). Attachment styles and personality disorders: Their connections to each other and to parental divorce, parental death, and perceptions of parental caregiving. *Journal of Personality, 66,* 835–878.

Carpenter, E. M., & Kirkpatrick, L. A. (1996). Attachment style and presence of a romantic partner as moderators of psychophysiological responses to a stressful laboratory situation. *Personal Relationships, 3,* 351–367.

Carnelley, K. B., Pietromonaco, P. R., & Jaffe, K. (1994). Depression, working models of others, and relationship functioning. *Journal of Personality and Social Psychology, 66,* 127–140.

Collins, N. L. (1996). Working models of attachment: Implications for explanation, emotion, and behavior. *Journal of Personality and Social Psychology, 71,* 810–832.

Collins, N. L., & Read, S. (1990). Adult attachment, working models and relationship quality in dating couples. *Journal of Personality and Social Psychology, 58,* 644–663.

Cone, J. D. (2000). *Evaluating outcomes: Empirical tools for effective practice.* Washington, DC: American Psychological Association.

Feeney, J. A., Noller, P., & Hanrahan, M. (1994). Assessing adult attachment. In M. B. Sperling & W. H. Berman (Eds.), *Attachment in adults: Clinical and developmental perspectives* (pp. 128–152). New York: Guilford Press.

Fraley, R. C., & Davis, K. E. (1997). Attachment formation and transfer in young adults' close friendships and romantic relationships. *Personal Relationships, 4,* 131–144.

Fraley, R. C., Fazzari, D. A., Bonanno, G. A., & Dekel, S. (2006). Attachment and psychological adaptation in high exposure World Trade Center survivors. *Personality and Social Psychology Bulletin, 32,* 538–551.

Fraley, R. C., Niedenthal, P. M., Marks, M. J., Brumbaugh, C. C., & Vicary, A. (2006). Adult attachment and the perception of emotional expressions: Probing the hyperactivating strategies underlying anxious attachment. *Journal of Personality, 74,* 1163–1190.

Fraley, R. C., & Shaver, P. R. (1998). Airport separations: A naturalistic study of adult attachment dynamics in separating couples. *Journal of Personality and Social Psychology, 75,* 1198–1212.

Fraley, R. C., & Shaver, P. R. (2000). Adult romantic attachment: Theoretical developments, emerging controversies, and unanswered questions. *Review of General Psychology, 4,* 132–154.

Fraley, R. C., & Spieker, S. J. (2003). Are infant attachment patterns continuously or categorically distributed?: A taxometric analysis of Strange Situation behavior. *Developmental Psychology, 39,* 387–404.

Fraley, R. C., & Waller, N. G. (1998). Adult attachment patterns: A test of the typological model. In J. A. Simpson & W. S. Rholes (Eds.), *Attachment theory and close relationships* (pp. 77–114). New York: Guilford Press.

Fraley, R. C., Waller, N. G., & Brennan, K. A. (2000). An item response theory analysis of self-report measures of adult attachment. *Journal of Personality and Social Psychology, 78,* 350–365.

Fuller, T. L., & Fincham, F. D. (1995). Attachment style in married couples: Relation to current marital functioning, stability over time, and method of assessment. *Personal Relationships, 2,* 17–34.

George, C., West, M., & Pettem, O. (1999). The Adult Attachment Projective: Disorganization of adult attachment at the level of representation. In J. Solomon & C. George (Eds.), *Attachment disorganization* (pp. 462–507). New York: Guilford Press.

Gottman, J. M., Driver, J., & Tabares, A. (2002). Building the sound marital house: An empirically derived couple therapy. In A. S. Gurman & N. S. Jacobson (Eds.), *Clinical handbook of couple therapy* (3rd ed., pp. 373–399). New York: Guilford Press.

Griffin, D. W., & Bartholomew, K. (1994a). Models of the self and other: Fundamental dimensions underlying measures of adult attachment. *Journal of Personality and Social Psychology, 67,* 430–445.

Griffin, D. W., & Bartholomew, K. (1994b). Metaphysics of measurement: The case of adult attachment. In K. Bartholomew & D. Perlman (Eds.), *Advances in personal relationships: Vol. 5. Attachment processes in adulthood* (pp. 17–52). London: Jessica Kingsley.

Hankin, B. L., Kassel, J. D., & Abela, J. R. Z. (2005). Adult attachment dimensions and specificity of emotional distress symptoms: Prospective investigations of cognitive risk and interpersonal stress generation as mediating mechanisms. *Personality and Social Psychology Bulletin, 31,* 136–151.

Hazan, C., & Shaver, P. R. (1987). Romantic love conceptualized as an attachment process. *Journal of Personality and Social Psychology, 52,* 511–524.

Hazan, C., & Shaver, P. R. (1990). Love and work: An attachment-theoretical perspective. *Journal of Personality and Social Psychology, 59,* 511–524.

Hazan, C., Gur-Yaish, N., & Campa, M. (2004). What does it mean to be attached? In W. S. Rholes & J. A. Simpson (Eds.), *Adult attachment: Theory, research, and clinical implications* (pp. 55–85). New York: Guilford Press.

Hazan, C., & Zeifman, D. (1994). Sex and the psychological tether. In K. Bartholomew & D. Perlman (Eds.), *Advances in personal relationships: Vol. 5. Attachment processes in adulthood* (pp. 151–178). London: Jessica Kingsley.

Klohnen, E. C., & John, O. P. (1998). Working models of attachment: A theory-based prototype approach. In J. A. Simpson & W. S. Rholes (Eds.), *Attachment theory and close relationships* (pp. 115–140). New York: Guilford Press.

Kobak, R. R., Cole, H. E., Ferenz-Gillies, R., Fleming, W. S., & Gamble, W. (1993). Attachment and emotion regulation during mother–teen problem solving: A control theory analysis. *Child Development, 64,* 231–245.

Lazarus, R. S., & Folkman, S. (1984). *Stress, appraisal, and coping.* New York: Springer.

Leary, T. (1957). *Interpersonal diagnosis of personality.* New York: Ronald Press.

Levy, K. N., Meehan, K. B., Weber, M., Reynoso, J., & Clarkin, J. F. (2005). Attachment and borderline personality disorder: Implications for psychotherapy. *Psychopathology, 38,* 64–74.

Levy, M. B., & Davis, K. E. (1988). Lovestyles and attachment styles compared: Their relations to each other and to various relationship characteristics. *Journal of Social and Personal Relationships, 5,* 439–471.

Main, M., Kaplan, N., & Cassidy, J. (1985). Security in infancy, childhood, and adulthood: A move to the level of representation. In I. Bretherton & E. Waters (Eds.), Growing points of attachment theory and research. *Monographs of the Society for Research in Child Development, 50*(1–2, Serial No. 209), 66–104.

Martin, K. M. (1997). Attachment style, depression, and loneliness in adolescent suicide attempters. *Dissertation Abstracts International, 57*(9), B.

Meehl, P. E., & Yonce, L. J. (1996). Taxometric analysis: II. Detecting taxonicity using covariance of two quantitative indicators in successive intervals of a third indicator (MAXCOV procedure). *Psychological Reports, 78,* 1091–1227.

Meyer, B., & Pilkonis, P. A. (2002). Attachment style. In J. C. Norcross (Ed.), *Psychotherapy relationships that work: Therapist contributions and responsiveness to patients* (pp. 367–382). London: Oxford University Press.

Mikulincer, M., & Shaver, P. R. (2007). *Attachment in adulthood: Structure, dynamics, and change.* New York: Guilford Press.

Onishi, M., & Gjerde, P. F. (2002). Attachment strategies in urban Japanese middle class couples: A cultural theme analysis of asymmetry in marital relationship. *Personal Relationships, 9,* 435–455.

Roisman, G. I., Fraley, R. C., Holland, A., Fortuna, K., Clausell, E., & Clarke, A. (2007). The Adult Attachment Interview and self-reports of attachment style: An empirical rapprochement. *Journal of Personality and Social Psychology, 92,* 678–697.

Scharfe, E., & Bartholomew, K. (1994). Reliability and stability of adult attachment patterns. *Personal Relationships, 1,* 23–43.

Shaver, P. R., Hazan, C., & Bradshaw, D. (1988). Love as attachment: The integration of three behavioral systems. In R. J. Sternberg & M. Barnes (Eds.), *The psychology of love* (pp. 68–99). New Haven, CT: Yale University Press.

Simpson, J. A. (1990). Influence of attachment styles on romantic relationships. *Journal of Personality and Social Psychology, 59,* 971–980.

Simpson, J. A., Rholes, W. S., & Nelligan, J. S. (1992). Support seeking and support giving within couples in an anxiety-provoking situation. *Journal of Personality and Social Psychology, 62,* 434–446.

Simpson, J. A., Rholes, W. S., & Phillips, D. (1996). Conflict in close relationships: An attachment perspective. *Journal of Personality and Social Psychology, 71,* 899–914.

Timmerman, I. G. H., & Emmelkamp, P. M.G. (2006). The relationship between attachment styles and Cluster B personality disorders in prisoners and forensic inpatients. *International Journal of Law and Psychiatry, 29,* 48–56.

Trinke, S. J., & Bartholomew, K. (1997). Hierarchies of attachment relationships in young adulthood. *Journal of Social and Personal Relationships, 14,* 603–625.

Troisi, A., Massaroni, P., & Cuzzolaro, M. (2005). Early separation anxiety and adult attachment style in women with eating disorders. *British Journal of Clinical Psychology, 44,* 89–97.

Vungkhanching, M., Sher, K. J., Jackson, K. M., & Parra, G. R. (2004). Relation of attachment style to family history of alcoholism and alcohol use disorders in early adulthood. *Drug and Alcohol Dependence, 75,* 47–53.

Waller, N. G., & Meehl, P. E. (1998). *Multivariate taxometric procedures: Distinguishing types from continua.* Newbury Park, CA: Sage.

Wei, M., Russell, D., Mallinckrodt, B., & Zakalik, R. (2004). Cultural equivalence of adult attachment across four ethnic groups: Factor structure, structured means, and associations with negative mood. *Journal of Counseling Psychology, 51,* 408–417.

Weinberger, D. A. (1995). The construct validity of the repressive coping style. In J. L. Singer (Ed.), *Repression and dissociation: Implications for personality theory, psychopathology, and health* (pp. 337–386). Chicago: University of Chicago Press.

8

Attachment Styles, the Rorschach, and the Thematic Apperception Test

Using Traditional Projective Measures to Assess Aspects of Attachment

Ety Berant

> As it turns out, Bowlby had thought that in one of the research projects his team was doing in London he would like to use the Rorschach test .... I thought that this was simply not a feasible thing to do. I kept using it as a clinical psychologist for diagnostic work. ... I have never really settled down to make a new system of analysis that would fit the attachment theory.
> —AINSWORTH (quoted in Rudnytsky, 1997, p. 387)

Traditional measures of personality assessment, such as the Rorschach Inkblot Test (Rorschach, 1921/1942) and the Thematic Apperception Test (TAT; Murray, 1936/1971), are used for the most part in clinical settings. They are typically administered at the beginning of therapy as part of personality assessment, to facilitate a clinician's understanding of a client's psychological state, self-perception, interpersonal relationships, and related psychodynamic processes. The Rorschach often circumvents the avoidance and guardedness displayed by certain clients in interviews and on self-report scales. The Rorschach's ambiguous stimuli force a client to rely on his or her internal store of associations, thereby decreasing the influence of social desirability and personal censorship. The TAT performs the same function by using vague pictures rather than inkblots to evoke partially subconscious motives and cognitive predispositions. Some of the motives are attachment-related, and some of the cognitive predispositions can be viewed as aspects of attachment-related *internal working models,* or IWMs (see Cobb & Davila, Chapter 9, this volume, for a discussion of IWMs).

Careful analysis of Rorschach and TAT responses enables a clinician to detect a client's coping strategies and defense mechanisms. Used in conjunction with attachment measures, such as the Experiences in Close Relationships (ECR) inventory (Brennan, Clark, & Shaver, 1998; see Fraley & Phillips, Chapter 7, this volume), the Rorschach and the TAT can enhance a clinician's understanding of attachment security and insecurity.

In this chapter, I discuss the value of using self-expressive (Ritzler, 2004) instruments in adult attachment research, and I review the growing literature on connections between these instruments and self-report measures of attachment insecurity.[1] To illustrate the combined use of self-expressive and self-report measures, I present the case of Y, who was in brief psychodynamic psychotherapy for 1 year.

SELF-EXPRESSIVE MEASURES AND ADULT ATTACHMENT

Although Bowlby (1969/1982, 1973, 1988) had intended attachment theory to be in part a revision or replacement of the then-reigning psychoanalytic paradigm, his fellow analysts often criticized the theory as not dynamic enough to capture the richness of a person's internal world, and not complex enough to characterize the interplay of subjective perceptions and reality (for a historical review, see Fonagy, 2001). Ironically, today Bowlby's theory is one of the most highly regarded psychodynamic theories.

A more recent version of the inadequate-depth argument is that self-report measures of adult attachment cannot plumb the unconscious (e.g., Crowell & Treboux, 1995; Jacobvitz, Curran, & Moller, 2002), because these measures elicit conscious, deliberate answers to explicit questions, are susceptible to censorship, and cannot tap the deep psychodynamic processes of interest to Bowlby (1969/1982) and to today's psychodynamically oriented clinicians. Many of these critics prefer the Adult Attachment Interview (AAI; George, Kaplan, & Main, 1984, 1985, 1996; see Levy & Kelly, Chapter 6, this volume), which they believe taps unconscious processes as revealed in patterns of discourse in oral narratives of childhood attachment experiences (Main, Kaplan, & Cassidy, 1980). A debate between Jacobvitz et al. (2002) and other users of the AAI on the one hand, and Shaver and Mikulincer (2002a, 2002b) on the other, was published in *Attachment & Human Development,* but the issues continue to be controversial.

In this chapter, I address some of these issues empirically by reporting associations between a self-report attachment measure (i.e., the ECR scale) and such self-expressive tools as the Rorschach, the TAT, and the Children's Apperception Test (CAT; Bellak & Bellak, 1949/1986). Several features of self-expressive instruments make them suitable and useful for probing attachment-related mental processes. First, self-expressive measures give clients free rein to describe their perceptions and associations, without the preimposed structure of a standard interview or the limited and closed-answer alternatives provided on a questionnaire. Second, self-expressive instruments have the potential to sidestep conscious attempts to distort or withhold information. Thus, studying the associations between self-expressive instruments and self-report attachment scales can clarify and expand upon our understanding of attachment styles, attachment-related coping strategies, subconscious motives, and mental organization.

THE RORSCHACH

The Rorschach brings unique strength to the examination of attachment processes. The Rorschach stimulus cards were created initially as follows: "[A] few inkblots are thrown on a piece of paper, the paper [is] folded, and the ink [is] spread between the two halves of the sheet" (Rorschach, 1921/1942, p. 15), resulting in mirror-image forms of a particular inkblot. Schachtel (1966) proposed that this symmetry opens a window into how the examinee perceives and understands relationships. The symmetry provokes examinees to imagine an interaction or relationship between two "figures," and so naturally provides insight into attachment-related dynamics. Specifically, symmetrical figures may give us some insight into the idiosyncratic activation of the attachment system, as well as the content and organization of IWMs. Another advantage of the Rorschach is that it provides an opportunity to observe subconscious processes in action as portrayed in the form and content of an examinee's response (Masling & Bornstein, 2005). This allows us to infer, for example, how individual differences in attachment security manifest themselves in the perception and processing of the external environment.

Given these advantages of the Rorschach, my colleagues and I (Berant, Mikulincer, Shaver, & Segal, 2005) thought that the Rorschach would be a useful tool to address the criticisms of self-report measures as shallow and unsophisticated. We (Berant et al., 2005; Berant & Wald, 2008) have found that assessments of attachment-related anxiety and avoidance with the ECR (in a nonpatient adult sample) were systematically associated with a finer-grained analysis of psychological functioning as reflected in Rorschach responses, and that the associations between the two instruments were consistent with attachment theory.

Findings Pertaining to Anxious Attachment

Self-reported anxious attachment on the ECR was associated with Rorschach scores in the emotional domain. First, high scores on attachment-related anxiety were significantly associated with the Afr Rorschach score, which is theorized to reflect an attraction to emotional situations (Weiner, 1998).

Second, attachment-related anxiety was significantly associated with CF, a Rorschach score thought to indicate loose regulation of emotional expression (Weiner, 1998). Third, people who scored high on anxious attachment gave more Rorschach responses indicating complex, ambivalent, and confused emotions and a crowding out of positive feelings by negative ones (Blends and Color Shading Blends, respectively; Weiner, 1998).

Taken together, this pattern of Rorschach responses implies that anxiously attached people are drawn to emotional intensity, despite the predictably high price they pay in terms of hurt feelings, confusion, and injuries to their self-esteem and sense of well-being. Their intense and richly variegated emotional life can be overwhelming and self-destructive because of the difficulties they have in controlling and modulating their emotions and soothing their hurt feelings (Cassidy, 1994; Shaver, Mikulincer, Lavy, & Cassidy, in press). Unregulated, intense negative emotional states often make for volatile interpersonal relations.

Anxiously attached individuals' tendency to give Color Shading Blend responses to the Rorschach fits with Mikulincer and Shaver's (2003) claim that hyperactivating attachment strategies produce a chaotic mental architecture pervaded by unregulated negative affect. Even after a positive mood induction in a laboratory, which causes secure individuals to become more mentally relaxed, expansive, and creative (Mikulincer & Sheffi, 2000), anxiously attached individuals actually became more cognitively constricted, as if thinking about positive experiences reminded them of previous potentially positive experiences that somehow ended painfully. Once attuned to the negative aspects and possibilities of otherwise positive experiences, these individuals succumb to a spreading of negative associations that precludes the sustained experience and psychological benefits of positive affect (Mikulincer & Shaver, 2003). In others words, anxiously attached individuals seem drawn to intense emotional experiences and memories like moths to a flame.

Following Schachtel's (1943) lead, Overton (2000) interpreted the meaning of CF responses in relational terms. She reasoned that CF responses reflect immature means of relating to others, which are manifested in difficulties differentiating between self and others and inaccurate perception of others' traits, attitudes, beliefs, and reactions. CF responses suggest a predominantly subjective orientation that is based mainly on emotional experiences ("How does this make me feel?", "His discomfort really makes me feel inadequate," "I'm really anxious in this situation, so she is too"). This interpretation fits with research indicating that anxiously attached people tend to minimize cognitive distance from others by creating an illusion of consensus (Mikulincer, Orbach, & Iavnieli, 1998) and inappropriately projecting their own traits onto others (Mikulincer & Horesh, 1999), perhaps partly as a way of promoting solidarity, if not actual fusion.

In our research, self-reports of attachment-related anxiety also converged with Rorschach scores reflecting current experiences of situational stressors (m) and a sense of helplessness (Y) (Exner & Erdberg, 2005; Weiner, 1998). (This association occurred even though participants in our study did not report having encountered a specific major stressor in recent months.) These findings are consistent with Mikulincer and Shaver's (2003) claim that anxiously attached individuals are frequently overwhelmed by feelings of distress, vulnerability, and helplessness. Moreover, according to Mikulincer (1998), this sense of helplessness is not just a reflection of difficulties in emotion regulation, but also an instrumental means of eliciting love and support—that is, a component of anxious individuals' hyperactivating strategies (see Shaver & Mikulincer, Chapter 2, this volume).

This line of theorizing is further supported by the tendency of highly anxious participants in our study to give Rorschach responses involving food. According to Exner (2000), food responses characterize people who chronically want others to contain them, direct them, and be tolerant of and compliant with their needs and demands.

The Rorschach also produced theoretically meaningful associations between attachment-related anxiety and vulnerable self-images. Anxiety was correlated with Rorschach scores thought to reflect a pessimistic view of the self (MOR; Exner & Erdberg, 2005; Weiner, 1998). This result fits with previous findings concerning anxiously attached individuals' low self-esteem and their focus on negative self-traits (e.g., Mikulincer, 1995).

We (Berant & Wald, 2008) enlarged this psychodynamic portrait of attachment-related anxiety by examining Rorschach indices of defense mechanisms, a firm but semipermeable self-boundary, and cognitive susceptibility to illogical reasoning. These variables were measured with several Rorschach scoring scales: Lerner's (1998) Defenses scale, Fisher and Cleveland's (1958) Barrier and Penetration scales, and Exner's (2005) thought disorder codes (CS, INC, and FAB). Findings indicated that attachment-related anxiety was associated with the use of projective identification, a sense of being easily affected, and a propensity toward cognitive slippage—all suggestive of the blurring of boundaries (Blatt & Ritzler, 1974).

These findings are consistent with previous research. Regarding the elements of projective identification, anxious individuals have been shown to perceive others (inaccurately) as similar to them (Mikulincer et al., 1998) and to project their own traits onto others (Mikulincer & Horesh, 1999). Fraley and Shaver (1997) also found that anxious adults were unable to screen out unwanted stimuli (thoughts about a painful relationship breakup); they were less able to suppress disturbing thoughts; and they continued to show high autonomic arousal (high skin conductance) after being asked to stop thinking about their breakups. (Both secure and avoidant individuals were able to think less about their breakups, and, in tandem, to lower their skin conductance levels back to normal.)

Taken together, our findings with the Rorschach fit with other research results showing that anxious individuals use hyperactivating attachment and emotion regulation strategies. They are prone to projective identification, less resistant to disturbing stimuli, and likely to combine objects' and people's traits illogically or unjustifiably. They amplify rather than down-regulate distress and are likely to be viewed by their adult attachment figures as exaggerative, intrusive, or manipulative. This pattern of interaction often increases the likelihood of their partners' distancing themselves, rejecting them, or leaving, which is precisely what the anxiously attached persons fear. In the language of ego psychology, anxious individuals have weaker ego functions (Bellak, Hurvich, & Gediman, 1973; Blanck & Blanck, 1979).

Clinical Implications

When treating anxiously attached persons, therapists should focus first on strengthening ego functions—that is, enhancing coping and emotion regulation—while expecting this work to be slow going, given the negative and pessimistic views anxious individuals tend to have of themselves and the frequency with which their negative feelings dominate their mood. This is an example of why it is necessary to customize treatment in order to facilitate the formation of a secure base. Just as security-enhancing parents help their young children cope effectively with emotions and stress, a therapist needs to provide adequate scaffolding and suggestions to help an anxious client find new strengths and better methods of handling unpleasant thoughts and feelings.

Findings Pertaining to Avoidant Attachment

Our study (Berant et al., 2005) also revealed that self-reports of attachment-related avoidance were associated with Rorschach scores theorized to reflect primary need states that are not being experienced in typical ways (low FM responses), a disengaged orientation to the world (high L score), and a maintenance of a grandiose self-façade (reflection and Cg responses).

Avoidant adults often resort to distraction and psychological distancing—defenses similar to those of the low-FM person described by Weiner (1998). He viewed people with low FM scores as rarely experiencing needs, rarely entertaining hopes and dreams, and usually remaining bland and unconcerned. The association between avoidant attachment and L scores fits with laboratory studies that have documented avoidant individuals' relative imperviousness to experimental inductions of either positive or negative affect (Mikulincer & Sheffi, 2000), as well as the boredom and distance they feel in their daily interactions with friends and romantic partners (Shaver & Hazan, 1993; Tidwell, Reis, & Shaver, 1996). This pattern of constrained feelings reflects the main goal of deactivating strategies—to block or dampen activation of the attachment system so as to avoid acute pain and distress caused by negative reactions from attachment figures (Cassidy & Kobak, 1988). (Like other forms of attachment insecurity, avoidance was probably a functional strategy in a nonoptimal caregiving situation earlier in life, but it is often dysfunctional when played out in an adult relationship.)

High scores on avoidant attachment were also associated with high reflection and Cg Rorschach scores, both thought to reflect an exaggerated sense of self-worth, the use of narcissistic defenses, and a tendency to maintain a veneer of self-confidence (Exner, 2000). These findings are consistent with Mikulincer and Shaver's (2003) assertion that avoidant individuals' perceptions of themselves as competent and powerful is a defensive façade that helps them handle distress and convince others that they do not need help or support. In experimental studies, avoidant individuals react to threatening situations by inflating their positive self-views, but this defense collapses when a cognitive or emotional load is imposed (Mikulincer, Dolev, & Shaver, 2004). The same thing seems to happen in real life, when stressors overwhelm avoidant defenses (Berant, Mikulincer, & Shaver, 2008).

When we (Berant & Wald, 2008) examined the contents of the reflection responses given by avoidant individuals, we noticed that none of the content responses referred to human beings. The bulk of the contents suggested grandiose or narcissistic themes—for example, "a Viking ship standing on a high spot," "a frog with wings," "a bird rising out of the water." The absence of human contents in the reflection responses points to avoidant individuals' low interest and low emotional investment in close relations. Interestingly, Weiner (1998) suggested that Cg responses also represent suspiciousness about others' good will, which causes a person to be less likely to reveal weakness to others.

Avoidant attachment was associated with devaluation of others as measured by Lerner's (1998) Rorschach-based Defenses scale (mentioned earlier). This suggests that avoidant individuals are likely to devalue others in order to preserve their preference for interpersonal distance and view themselves as strong and perfect. This finding dovetails with Mikulincer and Horesh's (1999) finding that avoidant people are likely to defensively project their own unwanted traits onto others, enabling them to enhance their own self-worth by downgrading others' abilities.

Clinical Implications

Because avoidant clients are likely to exaggerate views of themselves as capable and independent, therapists must tread delicately when attempting to challenge or disarm their defenses. By virtue of pursuing treatment, avoidant individuals are implicitly admitting some degree of need and inadequacy. But confronting their vulnerabilities too quickly is likely to provoke denial, minimization, or withdrawal. Similarly, therapists should consider temporarily modulating the depth of empathic reflections to sidestep the possibility of provoking resistance to feelings of neediness or weakness. Moreover, therapists should be prepared to receive regular doses of devaluation, as avoidant clients increasingly sense that they are becoming invested in the therapeutic relationship.

THE THEMATIC APPERCEPTION TEST

Another source for understanding attachment-related dynamics is the TAT (Murray, 1936/1971). TAT cards depict interpersonal situations or solitary protagonists. Although the cards were not designed specifically to elicit attachment themes, they were intended to arouse a wide variety of needs and feelings, and this makes it likely that they can reveal individual differences in attachment organization and dynamics.

A window into the object relations (i.e., attachment representations) of healthy nonpatient adolescents was provided by two unpublished studies. In the first, Gilad (2002) examined 58 nonpatient adolescents (male and female) ranging in age from 17 to 19 years ($M = 18$, $SD = 0.54$) living with their intact families in a large Israeli city. The adolescents completed the ECR and composed stories in response to TAT cards (1, 2, 3, 4, 6BM, 6GF, 7BM, and 7GF). The stories were then analyzed with the Social Cognition and Object Relations Scale (SCORS; Westen, Lohr, Silk, Kerber, & Goodrich, 1985). The components of the scale were devised to measure the developmental level of object relations of children and adults—by recording, for instance, the realization that a person may have multiple, partially contradictory traits (object complexity); the affective tone of the person's relationships (e.g., the extent to which the individual expects relationships to be destructive, harmful, or threatening as opposed to safe, nurturing, and rewarding); the degree of social understanding; and the emotional investment in others (e.g., the extent to which relationships with others are portrayed as ends rather than means, where relationships emphasize mutuality as opposed to need gratification).

The stories of anxiously attached adolescents displayed high levels of "object" (i.e., person) complexity, emotional investment in "objects," and social understanding tinged with negative affect. The stories of avoidantly attached adolescents were also characterized by negative affective tone, but they generated an almost opposite pattern of SCORS codes: lower object complexity, less emotional investment in the object, and lower social understanding. Like the Rorschach findings reviewed earlier, these results converge with predictions from attachment theory. The complex internal world of anxious individuals includes a desire to be caring, or see themselves as caring, and is colored by negative affect and expectancies of negative outcomes in relationships. The internal world of avoidant individuals, in contrast, is devoid of complexity and caring, yet ultimately is unable to protect against negative affect.

In the second unpublished study, we (Berant & Farber, 2007) tested 57 adolescents ranging in age from 15 to 18 years ($M = 16.5$, $SD = 0.87$) who were living in rural Israeli kibbutzim. (As in the previous study, people who were assessed as having mental health or medical problems were excluded from the testing.) Study participants completed the ECR and the Object Representation Inventory (Blatt, Chevron, Quinlan, & Wein, 1981), and they composed stories in response to the same TAT cards used in Gilad's study. In this sample, as in the former one, adolescents who scored higher on anxious attachment had a more negative affective tone and described their mothers in less benevolent terms, but in contrast to Gilad's city sample and our expectations, they displayed *lower* emotional investment in the object. Those who scored higher on avoidant attachment also described their mothers in less benevolent terms. The differences between the city and kibbutz samples are being pursued in follow-up studies.

THE CAT AND THE TRANSGENERATIONAL TRANSMISSION OF ATTACHMENT SECURITY

The findings discussed thus far have focused on the attachment dynamics of mentally and physically healthy individuals who were not necessarily undergoing any special stresses or difficulties. However, adult attachment researchers have also studied the role of attachment security in buffering individuals from intense stressors and the psychological maladjustment associated with being subjected to such stress (for a review, see Mikulincer & Shaver, 2007). This role is particularly important in the case of long-term, persistent stressors, such as chronic illness, and has been shown to be highly significant when an adult copes with the painful experience of raising a child who has a severe, life-threatening disease (e.g., Berant, Mikulincer, & Florian, 2001a, 2001b, 2003). In such cases, mothers bear the brunt of the coping burden (e.g., Cohn, 1996; Rae-Grant, 1985); hence their sense of attachment security is likely to affect both their own well-being and mental health, and the socioemotional development of their children.

The CAT (Bellak & Bellak, 1949/1986; see also Bellak & Abrams, 1997; Haworth, 1963) has led to new insights into the intergenerational transmission of psychological problems among children who suffer from congenital heart disease (CHD). We (Berant et al., 2008) followed up mothers in a 7-year longitudinal study of children with CHD, a condition that requires surgery or catheterization. We examined the long-term contribution of mothers' attachment insecurities to their own and their children's psychological functioning.

Sixty-three mothers of newborns with CHD participated in our three-wave study, beginning with the CHD diagnosis (T1), continuing through a time point 1 year later (T2), and ending 7 years later (T3). At T1, the mothers reported on their attachment style and mental health. At T2, mental health and marital satisfaction were assessed. At T3, participants completed the T2 measures again, and their children completed the CAT as an expressive measure of self-image, dominant affect, anxieties, and maternal perceptions. All along, we also considered the severity of each child's CHD.

Of special interest here are the results at T3. A mother's avoidant attachment score at the time of her child's birth and diagnosis (T1) was associated with a deterioration in both her mental health and her marriage over 7 years, and with the child's poorer self-image as indicated by the CAT, but only for children whose CHD was severe. In addition, the higher the mother's avoidance score was at T1, the less positive the child's dominant affect was in the stories he or she told at age 7. Interestingly, the higher the mother's attachment-related anxiety or avoidance was at the time of the child's diagnosis, the less positive the child's representation of the mother was in the CAT.

It is interesting that the detrimental effects of maternal avoidance were observed mainly in children who suffered from more severe, life-threatening CHD. When the illness was less severe and the children's lives were not endangered by cardiac problems, highly avoidant mothers and their children did not have notable psychological problems. But when the CHD was severe, which presumably increased the number of stressors on the mothers over the years, the more avoidant mothers had children with measurably damaged self-images.

Illustrative Responses

To illustrate the ways the children with CHD perceived their mothers and themselves, I present a selection of responses to the CAT and other self-expressive measures. The first story illustrates some of the CAT features associated with having an avoidantly attached mother. It is a 7-year-old girl's story, given in response to CAT Card 4.

> "The mother is in a big hurry to go to on a trip. She is not waiting for her elder child. The mother is angry at the elder son because he is not hurrying. The elder child is sad because his mother is not waiting for him. In the end they will go on the trip, but the child is sad because his mother was moving very fast and did not wait for him."

Here we see the unavailability and inattentiveness of the mother to her child's wishes and needs. Furthermore, the mother is not responsive to the child's signals of distress and sadness; on the contrary, she is angry with the child. This story corresponds to Ainsworth, Blehar, Waters, and Wall's (1978) description of unattentive maternal behaviors.

The following story illustrates some of the CAT features associated with having an anxiously attached mother. It is a 7-year-old boy's story given in response to CAT Card 1, which depicts a mother hen and her chicks sitting at a dining or kitchen table.

> "Here is a mother hen, and she prepared a meal for her chicks. They knocked on the table, and suddenly their mother disappeared. She disappeared to the sky; perhaps she died. The chicks couldn't eat because they didn't have a mother to feed them."

The mother's behavior in the story is remarkably like that of anxious-ambivalent children's mothers in Ainsworth et al.'s (1978) home observations. The mother is described as being inconsistently present for her children, despite her efforts to be nurturing (i.e., preparing food). When her chicks express (possible) impatience or a demand (rapping on the table), she disappears; the children are left alone, helpless, and unable to thrive.

Another story, given in response to another instrument, is also worth mentioning. As a warm-up for the CAT task, children were presented with Winnicott's (1971) interview technique, the Squiggle Game. In this procedure, the test administrator draws a random line drawing on a sheet of paper and invites the child to "turn it into something," and then the child makes a squiggle for the examiner to turn into something. Each makes a scribble on two separate sheets of paper, and the scribbles are then exchanged. Drawings are created based on each other's scribbles, and the test administrator then places the four pictures in a linear series and asks the child to tell a story about the series. Here is one 7-year-old boy's story (his mother scored high on attachment-related avoidance at the time of the child's diagnosis):

> "Once upon a time, there was a snail who did not know where to go, and he got lost in the forest and could not find his house. The snail could not find a place to sit or rest, and he walked and walked until he came to a place with sea lions. The snail asked them where he could rest, and the sea lions told him to rest under the snow. He tried it but felt too cold, so he went back to the forest and there met a fox. He asked the fox where he could rest, and the fox instructed the snail to rest behind a tree, but there the snail was bothered by the sun. Finally, he looked a bit more by himself and found a nice shady bush where he could rest and relax."

Not only is the advice the snail receives from the other animals unsuitable to the snail, but it suggests that the other animals are unable to tailor their suggestions to the snail's needs, so ultimately the snail must fend for himself. It is tempting to speculate that the ineptness of the other animals mirrors the inability of the storyteller's avoidant mother to provide sensitive and reassuring care. Indeed, the care provided may vacillate between extremes of coldness and demandingness (the "cold" and "hot" in the story). Analogously, the snail's solution, self-reliance, may reflect how the child has been made to adapt to his mother's caregiving style, in an example of the now well-documented intergenerational transmission of attachment patterns (Obegi, Morrison, & Shaver, 2004; for a review, see van IJzendoorn, 1995).

Clinical Implications

The CHD study alerts us to the importance of parental attachment insecurity when children face medical problems. The avoidant mothers in this study did not, on the surface, seem to be particularly vulnerable when they first gave birth to their children with CHD. It is unlikely that the physicians with whom they interacted would have noticed or encoded it. But they clearly suffered over the years when their children's difficulties could not be ignored or pushed out of mind.

It would be useful to assess such people's attachment orientations and coping strategies with an eye toward providing periodic advice or support. Avoidant individuals are not likely to ask for help even when they objectively need it, so special kinds of approaches may be necessary before help can be provided. Our study also suggests that the ill or disabled children of insecure, and especially avoidant, parents may need special support. For present purposes, however, the main point of discussing this study is that expressive measures administered to children can reveal attachment-related difficulties that might not be easy to assess in other ways. These measures are therefore likely to continue to be useful for clinicians who work with such children.

CLINICAL ILLUSTRATION

To illustrate the practical benefits of using self-report measures of adult attachment in conjunction with expressive measures, such as the Rorschach and TAT, I present the case of Y. Y referred himself to a public clinic where the fee is modest and clients are entitled to time-limited psychodynamic therapy (1 year, approximately 30–40 sessions). Most of the clients in the clinic are given personality assessments prior to the start of therapy and at the end of 1 year, to assist clinicians in monitoring treatment progress and in making recommendations about termination.

Y's chief complaints were emptiness and loneliness following a breakup initiated by his girlfriend. Twenty-six years old and a college graduate, he had recently began a job at a high-tech company. He was born in one of the Muslim countries in the former Soviet Union, and his family's finances were constantly strained throughout Y's childhood. His father, who owned an unsuccessful business, was described as dominant and aggressive. Y's mother, a kindergarten teacher, was described as submissive.

Y was the youngest of four siblings, one of whom he vividly remembered biting him on many occasions during childhood. He reported that his minority status as Jewish made him feel insecure. In his first years of school, he was a poor student, but at some point he decided to "take my fate into my own hands." He became the top student in his class and won several academic awards. At age 15, his family immigrated to Israel. Y graduated from high school and was drafted into the army, where he met his girlfriend. The girl came from the same background as Y, and their families knew each other. When he was 17, his father had a stroke and became paralyzed; 2 years later, the father died.

In the intake meeting, the psychologist was impressed with Y's sadness, and she worried about the risk of suicide. Y denied any suicidal thoughts or intentions, and said instead that he wanted to feel better and to "reformat" his personality. During the intake meeting, he was asked to provide some memories of his father and mother. Regarding his father, he said:

> "He used to drink alcoholic drinks and did not work too much. I felt deprived all the time, and he could not provide me with necessities, especially for school activities. I felt insecure, because my father was the one who was supposed to take care of all these matters. He used to hit my mother and all of us children."

Regarding his mother, he said:

> "I feel that she is not bad and not good; I don't love her or hate her. I feel sympathy for her because when my father hit her, she used to absorb the hitting in order for me not to be hurt. She is not friendly; she does not have good friends. She was very judgmental and woke me up every morning without a smile, which made me feel bad. But I also remember that when I was 9 she sent me to art and music lessons, using money that she earned."

Y clearly longed for emotional nurturance from both parents, but his needs were greeted with indifference, if not hostility. His remarks suggested that Y received little beyond the rudimentary elements of care. Y's wish for a maternal smile in the morning spoke to both her aloofness or insensitivity and Y's hunger for even the most modest signs of affection.

Y's ECR scores and Rorschach profile supported and clarified this clinical picture. Before his first session, Y completed the ECR and scored high on both the Anxiety (4.29 on a 7-point scale) and Avoidance (5.15) scales, suggesting a fearful-avoidant style in relationships (see Fraley & Phillips, Chapter 7, this volume, for a detailed description of the ECR). Y's Rorschach scores (see Figure 8.1) indicated that he had poor coping resources (EA = 5.5), which might have reflected his dispositional coping resources or his current sense of being overwhelmed with stressors. The ECR provided a general picture of someone with fears of intimacy and a propensity to withdraw, as well as a yearning for someone to lean on and depend upon. The Rorschach added some insight into the source of these qualities. His

Location features		Determinants		Contents		Approach	
		Blends	Single				
Zf	18	FMa.FC'	M 2	H	2	I	W,WS
ZSum	59	FMa.FC'	FM 5	(H)	2	II	WS,DW
Zest	59.5	Ma.CF	m 0	Hd	2	III	WS,D,Dd,D
		FMa.CF	FC 1	(Hd)	0	IV	W,W
W	12		CF 0	Hx	1	V	W
D	11		C 0	A	13	VI	D,W
W+D	23		Cn 0	(A)	3	VII	D,D,DS
(Wv)	0		FC' 1	Ad	0	VIII	WS,D,W
Dd	2		C'F 0	(Ad)	0	IX	W,DS
S	7		C' 0	An	0	X	DdS,D,D
			FT 1	Art	0		
			TF 0	Ay	2	Special Scores	
			T 0	Bl	0		
DQ			FV 1	Bt	2		Lv 1 Lv 2
+	6		VF 0	Cg	3	DV	2 x 1 0 x 2
O	19		V 0	Cl	0	INC	2 x 2 0 x 4
v/+	0		FY 1	Ex	0	DR	2 x 3 0 x 6
V	0		YF 0	Fd	0	FAB	1 x 4 0 x 7
			Y 0	Fi	0	ALOG	1 x 5
			Fr 0	Ge	0	CON	0 x 7
Form Quality			rF 0	Hh	1	Raw Sum 6	8
			FD 1	Ls	0	Wght Sum 6	21
	FQx	MQ W+D	F 8	Na	0		
+	0	0 0	(2) 7	Sc	3	AB 1	PER 1
O	10	1 10		Sx	0	AG 1	PSV 1
U	8	0 8		Xy	0	CP 0	GHR 2
–	7	2 5		Id	0	COP 2	PHR 2
none	0	0 0				MOR 1	AgC 5

Ratios, Percentages, and Derivations

Core Section

R	25	L	.47		
EB	3:2.5	EA	5.5	EBPer	N/A
eb	8:6	es	14	D	–3
		Adj es	14	Adj D	–3
FM	8	Sum C'	3	Sum T	1
m	0	Sum V	1	Sum Y	1

Cognitive Triad: Ideation, Mediation, Processing

Ideation

a:p	10:1	Sum6	8
Ma:Mp	2:1	L:v2	0
2AB+(Art+Ay)	4	WSum6	21
M–	2	M none	0
MOR	1		

Mediation

XA%	.72	P	4
WDA%	.78	X+%	.40
X–%	.28	Xu%	.32
S-frequency	2		

Processing

Zf	18	PSV	0
W:D:Dd	12:11:2	DQ+	6
W:M	12:3	DQv	0
Zd	–.5		

Affect

Sum C': WSum C	3:2.5	Pure C	0
Afr	.47	S	7
CP	0	Blends:R	4:25
FC:CF+C	1:2		

Self-perception

3r+(2)÷R	.28	An + Xy	0
Fr + rF	0	H:(H)+Hd+(Hd)	2:4
FD	1	MOR	1
Sum V	1		

Interpersonal Perception

COP	2	GHR:PHR	2:2
AG	1	Sum T	1
Food	0	a:p	10:1
Pure H	2	Human Cont	6
PER	1	Isolation Index	.08

PTI	2	HVI	NS
DEPI	5	OBS	0
CDI	2	SCON	5

FIGURE 8.1. Structural summary of Y's Rorschach at the beginning of treatment.

Rorschach responses suggested unmet needs for nurturance (FM = 8). Y felt like an intruder, a burden, another mouth to feed. His mother was busy trying to avoid her husband's wrath and could not provide Y with warmth, attention to his emotional needs, or support. As a result, he seemed not to have developed a sense of confidence or agency.

Translating this interpretation into practice, Y might be expected to wish for more warmth and containment from the therapist than was realistic (due to his high attachment-related anxiety), but at the same time he might be ambivalent or conflicted about expressing this wish (due to his high attachment-related avoidance). At times, he might demand more attention or session time (as is generally expected of anxious persons and high-FM persons). But even if his therapist tried to respond favorably to some of these wishes, his high avoidance might cause him to doubt her benevolence and acceptance of his needs. The therapist's reactions were compatible with these inferences. She perceived Y as having a constant "open mouth." At times, she felt she was facing a hungry but insatiable baby; at other times, Y attempted to disguise his needs and act indifferent to the therapist's efforts to soothe him and care for him.

For example, at times he arrived early at the clinic and demanded to be seen right away. On several occasions early in treatment, he asked, "Am I not good enough to be seen immediately?" Despite his angry and disapproving reactions, he continued to attend sessions. Eventually he exhausted his therapist to the point that she purposely did not schedule a client during the hour following Y's session; she needed time to recuperate. She said that the information provided by the ECR, Rorschach, and TAT (discussed later) assisted her in being with him without pushing him to acknowledge his neediness.

On the Rorschach, Y gave a high number of S responses (S = 7), which means that he utilized the white space of the cards to inform his responses. The S response is interpreted as an indication of anger, negativism, or dissatisfaction (Exner, 2000). Other Rorschach scholars (e.g., Merceron, Hussain, & Rossel, 1988; Smith, 1997) claim that a high number of S responses is characteristic of individuals who have experienced losses (real or symbolic) and are trying to fill the "void" with meaningful content. Integrating these conceptualizations, it seems that Y could be understood as angry and negativistic as a result of experiencing losses and the unresponsiveness of his parents during childhood.

Y's "oral aggressive" tendencies were also manifested in his responses to the Rorschach:

"Here is a huge animal, and its hands are coming to grab something. It can swallow things without chewing them. You can see its teeth and scary eyes. Its mouth is so big that it can swallow a whole mouse, and it does not have to cut it into pieces—everything is entering at once."
[Card III]

"Here is a bad bird that eats other smaller birds. Like the American emblem, it is like a big eagle. Here is the moment the bird gets down on its prey, and the legs are holding the prey so it won't be able to run away." [Card IV]

"A big animal from ancient times that eats only meat. It eats animals and human beings." [Card VI]

These responses suggest a desperate, insatiable appetite and the aggressive seizure of nourishment. Indeed, the therapist felt at times that she needed to protect herself from Y's demandingness. On rare occasions when the therapist did not comply with Y's requests for extra time, he would "punish" her in a way consistent with an avoidant approach to intimacy problems: not showing up for the next session, waiting for her to invite him to therapy, or claiming that he could manage on his own (despite contrary evidence).

Regarding Y's cognition, the Rorschach revealed a tendency toward rigid thinking (a:p = 10:1) across contexts, and substantial disordered thinking (WSum6 = 21), implying slippage into "primary-process" thinking. Exner (2004) has referred to the a:p ratio as measuring "the ability to change in therapy." Empirical studies also show that rigid thinking is characteristic of avoidant adults (Main, 1991; Mikulincer, 1997; Mikulincer & Shaver, 2003; Wallin, 2007). In supervision, Y's therapist was encouraged to repeat or revisit previous reflections and interpretations, and to do so with patience and compassion. In the context of Y's fearful-avoidant attachment style, his slow progress might be attributed to his rigid thinking processes rather than resistance to the therapy.

Another important issue was Y's tendency to perceive his environment in idiosyncratic ways (X+% = .40; P = 4; Xu% = .32), especially in affect-laden contexts (minus responses to colored cards). The emotional context of his distorted perceptions corresponds to the difficulty insecure individuals have in regulating their emotions. Another interesting finding was Y's two M– responses. An M– response indicates that the individual is not able to accurately read or infer the intentions or mental states of others (i.e., to mentalize; Fonagy, 1991; Fonagy, Gergely, Jurist, & Target, 2002). Informed by these findings, Y's therapist made a special effort to introduce alternative ways of perceiving interpersonal situations, although Y often declined to accept them. This fits with Bowlby's (1988) recommendation to encourage clients to discard outdated modes of thinking and replace them with more reality-based assessments.

The TAT cards offered another view into Y's world. His TAT stories underscored his yearning for a parental figure and secure base. In the following story excerpt, the lack of a secure base prevents the child from exploring:

"This child's problem is that he didn't have a teacher. That's why he couldn't learn to play the guitar." [Card 1]

Another TAT story demonstrates the absence of a secure base and the bitter price paid as a result:

"The man wants to propose to the woman. She will agree because she doesn't have a choice. She doesn't want him—she's in love with someone else—but he is financially supporting her. She doesn't have anywhere to turn. The man she loves doesn't have money, and this man is wealthy and will provide for her." [Card 6GF]

After 30 psychotherapy meetings, all three measures—the ECR, the Rorschach, and the TAT—showed evidence of Y's progress. On the ECR, his Anxiety score declined modestly (4.15), while his Avoidance score was substantially lower (3.43). The findings of the second Rorschach, administered after 30 sessions, converged with those of the ECR and offered further insight into the nature of the changes seen in the ECR (see Figure 8.2). Y's coping resources were improving (EA = 6.5); he also exhibited fewer indicators of anger and negativism (S = 4), and less yearning for nurturance (FM = 6). Interestingly, in contrast to the Rorschach administered before beginning therapy, there were now no Rorschach responses indicating oral aggressiveness. Although we cannot know which aspects of the treatment were transformative, it seems reasonable to assume that a contributing factor was the therapist's ability to provide support, gratify intimacy needs, and assist Y in reevaluating his past and current experiences. Progress of this nature probably assisted Y in relinquishing his highly avoidant and anxious strategies of attaining security.

The second Rorshach also indicated an improvement in Y's reality testing and conventional reality perception (X+% = .57), a decrease in individualistic ways of interpreting the world (Xu% = .19), and a drastic lowering of thinking errors (WSum 6 = 5). His thinking processes became flexible (a:p = 6:4), and his inner world became richer (the number of blends increased from 4 to 8). It is possible that the supporting and containing therapeutic relationship improved the ego functions of reality testing and thinking processes. A major improvement in thinking processes was also the disappearance of M– responses. This finding converges with evidence pointing to improved reflective functioning following 1 year of therapy (Levy et al., 2006). According to Fonagy, Steele, Steele, Moran, and Higgitt (1991), interactions with available and supportive attachment figures provide the capacity to understand and articulate emotional experiences and to integrate these experiences into the self-concept.

Y's second set of TAT stories demonstrated the beginning of internalization of a security-enhancing attachment figure. Consider the change in Y's response to Card 1:

Location features		Determinants		Contents		Approach	
		Blends	Single				
Zf	9	FMa.CF.VF	M 3	H	2	I	W,D,WS
ZSum	22.5	FMa.FY	FM 1	(H)	2	II	W,WS
Zest	27.5	FD.FC'	m 0	Hd	1	III	D,D,D
		FC'.FV	FC 1	(Hd)	1	IV	W
W	9	FMa.FV	CF 1	Hx	1	V	W
D	8	FMp.FY	C 0	A	13	VI	W
W+D	17	Mp.FY	Cn 0	(A)	0	VII	Dd,Dd,D,Dd
(Wv)	0	FMa.FT	FC' 1	Ad	0	VIII	D,D
Dd	4		C'F 0	(Ad)	0	IX	W,DS
S	4		C' 0	An	0	X	WS,D
			FT 1	Art	0		

		Special Scores			

DQ			FV 1	Bt	0		Lv 1	Lv 2
+	4		VF 0	Cg	0	DV	0 x 1	0 x 2
O	17		V 0	Cl	0	INC	1 x 2	0 x 4
v/+	0		FY 1	Ex	0	DR	1 x 3	0 x 6
V	0		YF 0	Fd	0	FAB	0 x 4	0 x 7
			Y 0	Fi	0	ALOG	0 x 5	
			Fr 0	Ge	0	CON	0 x 7	
	Form Quality		rF 0	Hh	1	Raw Sum 6	2	
			FD 1	Ls	0	Wght Sum 6	5	

	FQx	MQ	W+D	F 3	Na	0			
+	0	0	0	(2) 3	Sc	2	AB	0	PER 0
O	12	2	12		Sx	0	AG	3	PSV 0
U	4	2	3		Xy	0	CP	0	GHR 2
−	5	0	2		Id	0	COP	1	PHR 7
none	0	0	0				MOR	1	AgC 3

Ratios, Percentages, and Derivations

Core Section						Affect			
R	21	L	.16			Sum C': WSum C	3:2.5	Pure C	0
EB	4:2.5	EA	6.5	EBPer	N/A	Afr	.40	S	4
eb	6:12	es	18	D	−4	CP	0	Blends:R	9:21
		Adj es	15	Adj D	−2	FC:CF+C	1:2		
FM	6	Sum C'	3	Sum T	1				
m	0	Sum V	4	Sum Y	4	Self-perception			

Cognitive Triad: Ideation, Mediation, Processing					3r+(2)÷R	.14	An + Xy	0
					Fr + rF	0	H:(H)+Hd+(Hd)	2:4
	Ideation				FD	1	MOR	1
a:p	6:4	Sum6	2		Sum V	4		
Ma:Mp	2:2	L:v2	0					
2AB+(Art+Ay)	0	WSum6	5		Interpersonal Perception			
M−	0	M none	0					
MOR	1				COP	0	GHR:PHR	1:0
	Mediation				AG	3	Sum T	1
XA%	.76	P	4		Food	0	a:p	6:4
WDA%	.88	X+%	.57		Pure H	2	Human Cont	6
X−%	.24	Xu%	.19		PER	0	Isolation Index	.05
S-frequency	0							
	Processing							
Zf	9	PSV	0		PTI	0	HVI	NS
W:D:Dd	9:8:4	DQ+	4		DEPI	6	OBS	0
W:M	9:4	DQv	0		CDI	2	SCON	8
Zd	−.5							

FIGURE 8.2. Structural summary of Y's Rorschach after 1 year of therapy.

"He looks at the violin that reminds him of his past. Perhaps this is his father's violin. He remembers that his father used to play the violin. He decides that he will learn to play the violin. He wants to learn and practice."

Y's response to Card 6GF was similarly improved:

"Now I see this picture in a different light to last year. Here is a woman with a caring father. He is a supporting father who wants the best for his daughter. They are a wealthy family. The father is surprising his daughter, perhaps by suggesting that she meet someone who is suitable for her. The father is not pressuring her; he only wants her to consider this. He is a supportive father."

Finally, after 1 year of therapy, Y's descriptions were more balanced, inclusive, and detailed. Regarding his father, he said:

"He was the leader of the family. The whole family was afraid of him because he was strong. He hit me less than the others. He also loved me more than my brothers. When he became ill, it was hard for me, because he went from being a leader to being helpless. In the last years of his illness, when I used to wheel him around in the wheelchair, he had a helpless look in his eyes."

Regarding his mother, he said:

"When I think of her, I believe she was the underdog in the family. She went through many troubles. She used to take care of the whole family, and worried about our basic needs. When he [the father] became ill, she had to take care of him too. She never rested, nor did she have good days. I really should help her, watch over her, and support her. I remember how she bought me a bicycle with her money. Whatever my father did not give us, she tried to make up for it. I think that now I should return the favor."

The TAT stories and the descriptions of his parents illuminated the changes in Y's inner world. He now represented significant attachment figures as more available, more attentive, and more complex. He was now able to recall the trauma he experienced when his strong father became ill and helpless. He was exploring his parents' reality and their inner mental states. Perhaps due to the significant decrease in his attachment-related avoidance, he was experiencing pain in connection with memories of his parents. He was even willing to take the role of a mature and secure adult and help his mother. It seems that the therapy enabled him to explore his world, to perceive it more accurately, and to understand other people's mental states.

Following 1 year of therapy, therefore, Y appeared to be relinquishing his avoidant defenses; this allowed him to develop a more reality-oriented attitude, an improved ability to reflect upon himself and significant others, and a more complex and integrated perception of himself and his parents. However, these changes came with a price, in the form of an elevated Suicide Constellation Index. Since Y was less reserved and guarded, he was experiencing more pain and confronting feelings of being worthless and helpless ($V = 4$; $C' = 3$, $Y = 4$). Now that he did not have the protective shield of the avoidance, he was also experiencing emotional confusion (Color Shading Blend) and emotional pain (Shading Blend). Access to these agonizing feelings about his early relationships, though possibly helpful in processing his complex relations with his parents and coming into terms with them, also evoked a sense of loss and grief. For this reason, he was offered another year of therapy, which he accepted.

CONCLUSIONS

This chapter demonstrates that integrating information from self-report attachment scales and the traditional self-expressive tools (the Rorschach and the TAT) can assist the clinician in planning the therapy and "mapping" the "therapeutic journey." The resulting picture is more detailed, accurate, and deep, and it illustrates the particular feelings and thoughts a client may be experiencing in his or her relationships. The Rorschach and TAT can inform a therapist about subconscious aspects of a client's life, and in particular can draw the therapist's attention to dissociated or denied parts that the client is unable to disclose because they are too painful or distressing. These traditional tools help the therapist observe the roots of the client's withdrawal, guardedness, and pain, as well as feelings about the absence of protecting and attentive figures. The TAT stories can heighten the therapist's empathy toward the client by enabling the therapist to imagine, understand, and empathically resonate with the client's subjective experience. The data can cue the therapist regarding the specific therapeutic stance most likely to be in tune with a particular client's developmental needs, as well as warn the therapist regarding potentially "dangerous areas" and transference "traps."

The combined knowledge of a client's attachment style and his or her Rorschach and TAT profile is analogous to a highly detailed map given to a hiker entering a forest for the first time. A rudimentary map shows all the paths in the forest, but it does not show how the trees change color or how the quality of the light differs in relation to the sun's zenith or when it is cloudy, rainy, or windy. The Rorschach and TAT depict the delicate details, over and above the general map of attachment styles. An informative map such as this is a substantial help in the beginning of therapy, and also in the appraisal of the therapeutic progress.

The material in this chapter supports Shaver and Mikulincer's (2005) claim that research on adult attachment provides persuasive evidence for many of the unconscious processes discovered and described by psychodynamic clinicians. Clinicians can benefit from the growing research in attachment and traditional tools. Similarly, adult attachment researchers can profit from psychoanalytic insights. The integration of insights achieved in both fields has the potential to enrich both fields and lead to a more comprehensive and integrative understanding of clients.

NOTE

1. Another projective measure, which I have not yet used in my own work, is the Adult Attachment Projective (AAP; George & West, 2001, 2004). This promising measure uses TAT-like pictures to assess some of the same constructs assessed with the Adult Attachment Interview (AAI). Examples of the clinical use of the AAP can be found in Brisch (2002) and Finn (2007).

RECOMMENDATIONS FOR FURTHER READING

Berant, E., Mikulincer, M., Shaver, P. R., & Segal, Y. (2005). Rorschach correlates of self-reported attachment dimensions. Dynamic manifestations of hyperactivating and deactivating strategies. *Journal of Personality Assessment, 84,* 70–81.—This article examines the associations between attachment dimensions and Rorschach Comprehensive System scores.

Berant, E., Mikulincer, M., & Shaver, P. R. (2008). Mothers' attachment styles, their mental health, and their children's emotional vulnerabilities: A seven year study of children with congenital heart disease. *Journal of Personality Assessment, 76,* 31–65.—This article addresses the contribution of self-expressive tools such as CAT to the understanding of the psychodynamics of children of insecure mothers.

REFERENCES

Ainsworth, M. D. S., Blehar, M. C., Waters, E., & Wall, S. (1978). *Patterns of attachment: A psychological study of the Strange Situation.* Hillsdale, NJ: Erlbaum.

Bellak, L., & Abrams, D. M. (1997). *The Thematic Apperception Test, The Children's Apperception Test, and the Senior Apperception Technique in clinical use* (6th ed.). Boston: Allyn & Bacon.

Bellak, L., & Bellak, S. S. (1986). *Children's Apperception Test (CAT).* New York: CPS. (Original work published 1949)

Bellak, L., Hurvich, M., & Gediman, H. K. (1973). *Ego functions in schizophrenics, neurotics, and normals: A systematic study of conceptual, diagnostic, and therapeutic aspects.* New York: Wiley.

Berant, E., & Farber, J. (2007). *Kibbutz youth's choice of their accommodation:*

The contribution of attachment styles and mental representations. Unpublished manuscript, Bar-Ilan University, Ramat-Gan, Israel.

Berant, E., Mikulincer, M., & Florian, V. (2001a). The association of mothers' attachment styles and their psychological reactions to the diagnosis of infants' congenital heart disease. *Journal of Social and Clinical Psychology, 29,* 208–232.

Berant, E., Mikulincer, M., & Florian, V. (2001b). Attachment style and mental health: A 1-year follow-up study of mothers of infants with congenital heart disease. *Personality and Social Psychology Bulletin, 27,* 956–968.

Berant, E., Mikulincer, M., & Florian, V. (2003). Marital satisfaction among mothers of infants with congenital heart disease: The contribution of illness severity, attachment style, and the coping process. *Anxiety, Stress, and Coping, 16,* 397–415.

Berant, E., Mikulincer, M., & Shaver, P. R. (2008). Mothers' attachment styles, their mental health, and their children's emotional vulnerabilities: A seven year study of children with congenital heart disease. *Journal of Personality, 76,* 31–65.

Berant, E., Mikulincer, M., Shaver, P. R., & Segal, Y. (2005). Rorschach correlates of self-reported attachment dimensions: Dynamic manifestations of hyperactivating and deactivating strategies. *Journal of Personality Assessment, 84,* 70–81.

Berant, E., & Wald, Y. (2008). *Self-reported attachment patterns and Rorschach Barrier and Penetration scores and defense scale.* Manuscript submitted for publication.

Blanck, G., & Blanck, R. (1979). *Ego psychology II: Psychoanalytical developmental psychology.* New York: Columbia University Press.

Blatt, S. J., Chevron, E., Quinlan, D. M., & Wein, S. J. (1981). *The assessment of qualitative and structural dimensions of object representation.* Unpublished manuscript.

Blatt, S. J., & Ritzler, B. A. (1974). Thought disorders and boundary disturbances in psychosis. *Journal of Consulting and Clinical Psychology, 42,* 370–381.

Bowlby, J. (1973). *Attachment and loss: Vol. 2. Separation: Anxiety and anger.* New York: Basic Books.

Bowlby, J. (1982). *Attachment and loss: Vol. 1. Attachment* (2nd ed.). New York: Basic Books. (1st ed., 1969)

Bowlby, J. (1988). *A secure base: Clinical applications of attachment theory.* London: Routledge.

Brennan, K. A., Clark, C. L., & Shaver, P. R. (1998). Self-report measurement of adult attachment: An integrative overview. In J. A. Simpson & W. Rholes (Eds.), *Attachment theory and close relationships* (pp. 46–76). New York: Guilford Press.

Brisch, K. H. (2002). *Treating attachment disorders: From theory to therapy* (Translated by Kenneht Kronenberg) New York: Guilford Press

Cassidy, J. (1994). Emotion regulation: Influence of attachment relationships. In N. A. Fox (Ed.), The development of emotion regulation: Biological and behavioral considerations. *Monographs of the Society for Research in Child Development, 59*(2–3, Serial No. 240), 228–249.

Cassidy, J., & Kobak, R. R. (1988). Avoidance and its relationship with other defensive processes. In J. Belsky & T. Nezworski (Eds.), *Clinical implications of attachment* (pp. 300–323). Hillsdale, NJ: Erlbaum.

Cohn, J. K. (1996). An empirical study of parents' reaction to the diagnosis of congenital heart disease in infants. *Social Work in Health Care, 23,* 67–80.

Crowell, J. A., & Treboux, D. (1995). A review of adult attachment measures: Implications for theory and research. *Social Development, 4,* 294–327.

Exner, J. E., Jr. (2000). *Primer for Rorschach interpretation.* Asheville, NC: Rorschach Workshops.

Exner, J. E., Jr. (2004, August). *Rorschach interpretation workshop.* Presented at the University of Stockholm, Stockholm, Sweden.

Exner, J. E., Jr. (2005). *The Rorschach: A comprehensive system. Vol. 1: Basic foundations* (5th ed.). Hoboken, NJ: Wiley.

Exner, J. E., Jr., & Erdberg, P. (2005). *The Rorschach: A comprehensive system. Vol. 2: Advanced interpretation* (3rd ed.). Hoboken, NJ: Wiley.

Finn, S. E. (2007, March). *The use of the Adult Attachment Projective in psychotherapy—A symposium.* Society for Personality Assessment Annual Meeting, Washington, DC.

Fisher, S., & Cleveland, S. (1958). *Body image and personality.* New York: Van Nostrand.

Fonagy, P. (1991). Thinking about thinking: Some clinical and theoretical consideration in the treatment of borderline patient. *International Journal of Psycho-Analysis, 72,* 639–656.

Fonagy, P. (2001). *Attachment theory and psychoanalysis.* New York: Other Press.

Fonagy, P., Gergely, G., Jurist, E. J., & Target, M. (2002). *Affect regulation, mentalization, and the development of the self.* New York: Other Press.

Fonagy, P., Steele, M., Steele, H., Moran, G. S., & Higgitt, P. (1991). The capacity for understanding mental states: The reflective self in parent and child and its significance for security of attachment. *Infant Mental Health Journal, 12,* 201–218.

Fraley, R. C., & Shaver, P. R. (1997). Adult attachment and the suppression of unwanted thoughts. *Journal of Personality and Social Psychology, 73,* 1080–1091.

George, C., Kaplan, N., & Main, M. (1984). *Adult Attachment Interview protocol.* Unpublished manuscript, University of California, Berkeley.

George, C., Kaplan, N., & Main, M. (1985). *Adult Attachment Interview protocol* (2nd ed.). Unpublished manuscript, University of California, Berkeley.

George, C., Kaplan, N., & Main, M. (1996). *Adult Attachment Interview protocol* (3rd ed.). Unpublished manuscript, University of California, Berkeley.

George, C., & West, M. (2001). The development and preliminary validation of a new measure of adult attachment: The Adult Attachment Projective. *Attachment & Human Development, 3,* 55–86.

George, C., & West, M. (2004). The Adult Attachment Projective: Measuring individual differences in attachment security using projective methodology. In M. Herson (Series Ed.) & M. Hilsenroth & D. Segal (Vol. Eds.), *Comprehensive handbook of psychological assessment: Vol. 2. Personality assessment* (pp. 431–447). Hoboken, NJ: Wiley.

Gilad, G. (2002). *The integration of object relations theory and attachment theory: Object representations in the Thematic Apperception Test.* Unpublished master's thesis, Bar-Ilan University, Ramat-Gan, Israel.

Hazan, C., & Shaver, P. R. (1987). Romantic love conceptualized as an attachment process. *Journal of Personality and Social Psychology, 52,* 511–524.

Hesse, E. (1999). The Adult Attachment Interview: Historical and current perspectives. In J. Cassidy & P. R. Shaver (Eds.), *Handbook of attachment: Theory, research, and clinical applications* (pp. 395–433). New York: Guilford Press.

Haworth, M. R. (1963). A schedule for the analysis of CAT responses. *Journal of Projective Techniques and Personality Assessement, 27,* 181–184.

Jacobvitz, D., Curran, M., & Moller, N. (2002). Measurement of adult attachment: The place of self-report and interview methodologies. *Attachment & Human Development, 4,* 207–215.

Lerner, P. M. (1998). *Psychoanalytic perspectives on the Rorschach.* Hillsdale, NJ: Analytic Press.

Levy, K. N., Kelly, K. M., Meehan, K. B., Reynoso, J. S., Clarkin, J. F., Lenzenweger, M. F., et al. (2006). Change in attachment patterns and reflective function in the treatment of borderline personality disorder with transference focused psychotherapy. *Journal of Consulting and Clinical Psychology, 74,* 1027–1040.

Main, M. (1991). Metacognitive knowledge, metacognitive monitoring, and singular (coherent) vs. multiple (incoherent) model of attachment: Findings and directions for future research. In C. M. Parkes, J. Stevenson-Hinde, & P. Marris (Eds.), *Attachment across the life cycle* (pp. 127–159). London: Routledge.

Main, M., Kaplan, N., & Cassidy, J. (1985). Security in infancy, childhood, and adulthood: A move to the level of representation. In I. Bretherton & E. Waters (Eds.), Growing points of attachment theory and research. *Monographs of the Society for Research in Child Development, 50*(1–2, Serial No. 209), 66–104.

Masling, J. M., & Bornstein, R. F. (2005). Scoring the Rorschach: Retrospect and prospect. In R. F. Bornstein & J. M. Masling (Eds.), *Scoring the Rorschach: Seven validated systems* (pp. 1–25). Mahwah, NJ: Erlbaum.

Merceron, C., Hussain, O., & Rossel, F. (1988). A specific category of borderline conditions: Perverse personality organization and the Rorschach. In H. Lerner & P. Lerner (Eds.), *Primitive mental states and the Rorschach* (pp. 377–402). Madison, CT: International Universities Press.

Mikulincer, M. (1995). Attachment style and the mental representation of the self. *Journal of Personality and Social Psychology, 69,* 1203–1215.

Mikulincer, M. (1997). Adult attachment style and information processing: Individual differences in curiosity and cognitive closure. *Journal of Personality and Social Psychology, 72,* 1217–1230.

Mikulincer, M. (1998). Adult attachment style and affect regulation: Strategic variations in self-appraisals. *Journal of Personality and Social Psychology, 74,* 420–435.

Mikulincer, M., Dolev, T., & Shaver, P. R. (2004). Attachment-related strategies during thought suppression: Ironic rebounds and vulnerable self-representations. *Journal of Personality and Social Psychology, 87,* 940–956.

Mikulincer, M., & Horesh, N. (1999). Adult attachment style and the perception of others: The role of projective mechanisms. *Journal of Personality and Social Psychology, 76,* 1022–1034.

Mikulincer, M., Orbach, I., & Iavnieli, D., (1998). Adult attachment style and effect regulation: Strategic variations in subjective self-other similarity. *Journal of Personality and Social Psychology, 75,* 436–448.

Mikulincer, M., & Shaver, P. R. (2003). The attachment behavioral system in adulthood: Activation, psychodynamics, and interpersonal processes. In M. P. Zanna

(Ed.), *Advances in experimental social psychology* (Vol. 35, pp. 53–152). San Diego, CA: Academic Press.

Mikulincer, M., & Shaver, P. R. (2007). *Attachment in adulthood: Structure, dynamics, and change.* New York: Guilford Press.

Mikulincer, M., & Sheffi, E. (2000). Adult attachment style and cognitive reactions to positive affect: A test of mental categorization and creative problem solving. *Motivation and Emotion, 24,* 149–174.

Murray, H. A. (1971). *Thematic Apperception Test.* Cambridge, MA: Harvard Press. (Original work published 1936)

Obegi, J. H., Morrison, T. L., & Shaver, P. R. (2004). Exploring intergenerational transmission of attachment style in young female adults and their mothers. *Journal of Social and Personal Relationships, 21,* 625–638.

Overton, C. G. (2000). A relational interpretation of the Rorschach color determinants. *Journal of Personality Assessment, 75,* 426–448.

Rae-Grant, O. (1985). Psychological problems in medically ill children. *Pediatric Clinics of North America, 32,* 653–663.

Ritzler, B. A. (2004). Cultural applications of the Rorschach, Thematic Apperception Test, and figure drawings. In M. Herson (Series Ed.) & M. J. Hilsenroth & D. L. Segal (Vol. Eds.), *Comprehensive handbook of psychological assessment* (pp. 573–585). Hoboken, NJ: Wiley.

Rorschach, H. (1942). *Psychodiagnostics: A diagnostic test based on perception.* Bern, Switzerland: Hans Huber. (Original work published 1921)

Rudnytsky, P. L. (1997). The personal origins of attachment theory: An interview with Mary Salter Ainsworth. *Psychoanalytic Study of the Child, 52,* 386–405.

Schachtel, E. G. (1943). On color and affect. *Psychiatry, 6,* 393–409.

Schachtel, E. G. (1966). *Experimental foundation of Rorschach's test.* New York: Basic Books.

Shaver, P. R., & Hazan, C. (1993). Adult romantic attachment: Theory and evidence. In D. Perlman & W. Jones (Eds.), *Advances in personal relationships* (Vol. 4, pp. 29–70). London: Jessica Kingsley.

Shaver, P. R., & Mikulincer, M. (2002a). Attachment-related psychodynamics. *Attachment & Human Development, 4,* 133–161.

Shaver, P. R., & Mikulincer, M. (2002b). Dialogue on adult attachment: Diversity and integration. *Attachment & Human Development, 4,* 243–257.

Shaver, P. R., & Mikulincer, M. (2005). Attachment theory and research: Resurrection of the psychodynamic approach to personality. *Journal of Research in Personality, 39,* 22–45.

Shaver, P. R., Mikulincer, M., Lavy, S., & Cassidy, J. (in press). Understanding and altering hurt feelings: An attachment-theoretical perspective on the generation and regulation of emotions. In A. Vangelisti (Ed.), *Feeling hurt in close relationships.* New York: Cambridge University Press.

Smith, B. C. (1997). White bird: Flight from the terror of empty space. In J. R. Meloy, M. W. Acklin, C. B. Gacono, J. F. Murray, & C. A. Peterson (Eds.), *Contemporary Rorschach interpretation* (pp. 191–216). Mahwah, NJ: Erlbaum.

Tidwell, M. C. O., Reis, H. T., & Shaver, P. R. (1996). Attachment, attractiveness, and social interaction: A diary study. *Journal of Personality and Social Psychology, 71,* 729–745.

van IJzendoorn, M. H. (1995). Adult attachment representations, parental responsiveness, and infant attachment: A meta-analysis on the predictive validity of the Adult Attachment Interview. *Psychological Bulletin, 117,* 387–403.

Wallin, D. J. (2007). *Attachment in psychotherapy.* New York: Guilford Press.

Weiner, I. B. (1998). *Principles of Rorschach interpretation.* Mahwah, NJ: Erlbaum.

Westen, D., Lohr, N., Silk, K., Kerber, K., & Goodrich, S. (1985). *Social Cognition and Object Relations Scale (SCORS): Manual for coding TAT data.* Ann Arbor: University of Michigan.

Winnicott, D. W. (1971). *Therapeutic consultation in child psychiatry.* New York: Basic Books.

Part III
CLINICAL UTILITY

9

Internal Working Models and Change

Rebecca J. Cobb
Joanne Davila

Bowlby (1969/1982, 1988) developed attachment theory in part as a way to understand how individuals come to be at risk for mental health disorders and to guide treatment, but the pace at which his and others' (e.g., Ainsworth, Blehar, Waters, & Wall, 1978; Main, Kaplan, & Cassidy, 1985) ideas have been adopted by clinicians and tested in therapeutic settings with adults has been relatively slow. Given the elaboration of normative aspects of the theory, and the large body of literature devoted to individual differences in attachment security, the time seems ripe to consider how attachment theory can contribute to therapeutic work.

Although Bowlby (1969/1982, 1973, 1979, 1980, 1988) intended attachment theory to inform understanding and treatment of pathology, the theory is most clearly a description of normative relationship development and individual differences (for an overview, see Shaver & Mikulincer, Chapter 2, this volume). Attachment theory describes how and why humans develop and maintain close emotional bonds with others. A key concept of attachment theory is that on the basis of early attachment experiences, people develop *internal working models* (IWMs) of themselves and important others (Bowlby, 1969/1982, 1973, 1980). Broadly described, IWMs are defining beliefs about the self, others, and the relations between the two. They influence the meaning people ascribe to interpersonal experiences, and they influence thoughts, emotions, and behaviors in close relationships. IWMs are believed to be responsible for habitual patterns of responses in close relationships, known as adult attachment *orientations, styles,* or *pat-*

terns. In short, IWMs directly affect how people construe their social world, how their attachment desires and needs develop, and how they go about expressing and attempting to meet these desires and needs.

Our goals in this chapter are to consider theoretical and empirical knowledge about IWMs, and to discuss how change in IWMs can be accomplished in treatment. We begin with a theoretical overview of the origins, components, and structure of IWMs. We then describe theories of change in IWMs, with a discussion of current empirical support for change and stability in IWMs. Building upon this basic research, we discuss general therapeutic change principles and attachment-specific therapeutic considerations. We do not propose new techniques; rather, we suggest how therapists can use attachment theory and the IWM concept to conceptualize and accomplish change in therapy.

IWMs AND ADULT ATTACHMENT PATTERNS

Bowlby (1969/1982, 1973, 1988) conceptualized IWMs as cognitive representations of the world and important figures in it, such as the self and attachment figures.[1] Repeated interactions between an infant and his or her caregiver(s) give rise to expectations and beliefs about the self and the attachment figure(s), and these expectations and beliefs become internalized as parts of the attachment behavioral system. With repeated activation, the models become habitual and generalized, and they operate largely unconsciously on thoughts, emotions, and behavior. Individuals who experience attachment figures as available, sensitive, and appropriately responsive develop a model of others that is generally positive. They expect others to be available and willing to provide support to restore a sense of felt security during times of emotional distress (e.g., Bowlby, 1969/1982, 1988). A complementary model of the self as worthy of assistance, affection, and love is expected to develop out of those same interactions (Bowlby, 1969/1982, 1988). Positive models of self and others reflect attachment security, and negative models of the self and/or others reflect insecurity. Research has linked secure models of the self to self-worth, social confidence, interpersonal orientation, and assertiveness (Collins & Read, 1990), coherent narratives of attachment relationship histories (Crowell & Treboux, 1995; Main et al., 1985), and integrated and complex self-knowledge (Mikulincer, 1995).

Components of IWMs

Extending and refining Bowlby's ideas, Collins and Read (1994) proposed four components of IWMs: (1) memories of attachment-related experiences; (2) beliefs, attitudes, and expectations about the self and others; (3) attachment goals and needs; and (4) plans and behavioral strategies to achieve attachment goals. Each component is related to individual differences in attachment security in childhood (e.g., Ainsworth et al., 1978; Egeland & Farber, 1984; Vaughn, Egeland, Sroufe, & Waters, 1979) and adulthood (e.g., Bartholomew & Horowitz, 1991; Hazan & Shaver, 1987; Kirkpatrick & Hazan, 1994; Kobak & Hazan, 1991; Mikulincer & Shaver, 2004; Simpson, Rholes, Oriña, & Grich, 2002).

Adult attachment researchers generally conceptualize attachment security of IWMs in terms of two dimensions: *anxiety* and *avoidance* (e.g., Brennan, Clark, & Shaver, 1998). Anxiety refers to worry and concern about the availability and willingness of others to meet attachment needs. Anxiety is characterized by a low threshold for activation of the attachment system, fears about the worthiness of the self in relation to others, and the use of hyperactivating strategies (e.g., excessive proximity seeking) to manage distress. Avoidance refers to discomfort with intimacy and use of deactivating strategies (e.g., avoidance of proximity seeking) to deal with threats to security. The intersection of these theoretically independent dimensions defines four adult attachment prototypes: *secure, fearful, preoccupied,* and *dismissing* (Bartholomew & Horowitz, 1991). Secure individuals are low in anxiety and avoidance, whereas fearful individuals are high on both dimensions. Preoccupied (ambivalent) individuals are high in anxiety and low in avoidance, and dismissing individuals exhibit the opposite configuration. Generally, a person is expected to be most consistent with one prototype, but it is possible to exhibit behavior characteristic of other prototypes in different attachment relationships.

Attachment-related memories are thought to derive from real experiences with attachment figures and from individuals' interpretations of those experiences. There are individual differences in the content and accessibility of attachment-related memories (e.g., Hazan & Shaver, 1987; Hesse, 1999; Mikulincer & Orbach, 1995). For example, secure individuals are more likely to recall positive experiences with attachment figures (content), such as seeking a parent when upset and being comforted by a parent's reassurance; they are also likely to retain access to and cogently process negative memories (accessibility). Avoidant (especially dismissing) individuals may defensively describe relationships with parents as generally positive, but when pushed for specifics, they are likely to describe attachment figures as rejecting or unavailable when needed. They also have difficulty accessing negative emotional memories and appear to underreport their intensity. Descriptions of parents as inconsistent in their availability, or descriptions of parent–child relationships characterized by role reversal, are likely to be given by anxious (especially preoccupied) individuals. They have difficulty distancing themselves from and remaining emotionally regulated in the face of negative memories. The depth and richness with which individuals describe attachment-related memories are likely to differ according to level of security. Secure individuals tend to have a more coherent and richer set of memories and to recall more affect-laden memories than less secure individuals do (e.g., Fraley, Garner, & Shaver, 2000; Mikulincer & Orbach, 1995).

Attachment-related memories are manifested in the way individuals think about the world. Complex sets of expectations, which may be either general or specific to certain kinds of relationships or to certain individuals, are developed on the basis of attachment experiences and memories of such experiences. For example, secure individuals may believe that others can be relied upon and expect that if others are sought out, they will provide support and reassurance when needed. Avoidant individuals may believe that others are not accepting and may expect them to be disapproving and rejecting, whereas anxious individuals may believe that they are worthy only when others shower them with attention and love. Individuals also build impressions of their own self-efficacy in the face of attachment-related distress (e.g., separation from an attachment figure; Mikulincer & Shaver, 2004). Successful early negotiations with parents about attachment-related needs and threats result in self-descriptors such as *confident, competent,* and *strong,* whereas negotiations marred by insensitivity or unresponsiveness are likely to result in self-derogation or self-doubt. These ideas and beliefs are fundamental to the way individuals construe and respond to the people to whom they become attached.

The overarching goal of the attachment system is to maintain a sense of felt security. But the complex sets of memories, beliefs, expectations, and attitudes that compose the IWMs give rise to a host of specific goals in the service of fostering a sense of security, such as increasing intimacy or feelings of comfort, gaining proximity to an attachment figure, or reducing distressing emotions. Specific attachment goals differ according to attachment pattern. Anxious individuals are oriented toward goals of intimacy, but their lack of self-confidence and worries about rejection motivate them to seek unrealistic levels of proximity, emotional closeness, and support from others. In contrast, avoidant individuals are more likely to maintain emotional distance from others in the service of their goal of self-reliance (or, in the case of fearful individuals, their goal of avoiding rejection). Secure individuals are likely to be balanced in their attachment goals; their desire for intimacy and closeness is balanced with a desire to rely on inner resources and to maintain a sense of autonomy.

Plans and behavioral strategies are developed to meet attachment-related goals and needs. Strategies may be ways of coping with challenging experiences, regulating attachment emotions (e.g., anxiety), or seeking comfort from others. Secure individuals show the most diverse and flexible strategies—for example, relying on the self or directly requesting support as appropriate when experiencing distress. Insecure individuals are more likely to utilize indirect strategies that are less effective in communicating their needs to others. Anxious individuals may be overreliant on others and become angry when attachment needs are not met. Avoidant individuals are likely to use escape strategies to minimize the effects of attachment-related anxiety.

Multiple IWMs

Although typical patterns of thinking and behaving in close relationships are expected to arise from IWMs, people may shift strategies or exhibit inconsistent attachment-related beliefs across time or across relationships. A source of these differences may be multiple IWMs. Bowlby (1969/1982) originally suggested that multiple models may develop in childhood, and this is consistent with recent theorizing (e.g., Collins, Guichard, Ford, & Feeney, 2004; Mikulincer & Shaver, 2004) and empirical evidence (Overall, Fletcher, & Friesen, 2003; Trinke & Bartholomew, 1997). Indeed, people's adult attachment patterns do not necessarily map directly onto their infant–parent attachment patterns. As depicted in Figure 9.1, multiple models are understood as existing in a hierarchical nested structure: Relationship-specific models (e.g., of mother, father, a romantic partner) are nested within domains (e.g., friends, family, romantic partners), which in turn are nested within an overarching general model (Collins et al., 2004). The IWMs are not expected to be static, and the forces causing change within the hierarchy are likely to be bidirectional. Early in life, general models are abstracted from relationship-specific models developed in the context of child–caregiver relationships. Later, subordinate models (e.g., relationship-specific models) are based partly on the superordinate IWMs and partly on experience with particular relationship partners. Hence new subordinate models offer opportunities for updating and increasing the complexity of general models.

Bowlby (1969/1982, 1988) and others (Collins et al., 2004; Mikulincer & Shaver, 2004) have also noted that multiple IWMs may not be consistent or compatible with each other. Thus models both within and across different levels of the hierarchy may differ in degree of security. The hierarchy of IWMs mirrors the various levels of security clients may exhibit across their personal relationships. Some relationships may be characterized by mutual respect for attachment needs, while others may exhibit emotional overinvolvement or distance indicative of insecurity.

STABILITY AND CHANGE OF IWMs

Bowlby expected IWMs to be relatively enduring, stable, and self-perpetuating. He attributed their stability to at least three sources: (1) continuity in caregiving and interpersonal environments; (2) the creation of relationship dynamics that confirm models; and (3) the operation of cognitive biases that maintain current IWMs (Bowlby, 1969/1982, 1988). Stability of IWMs is

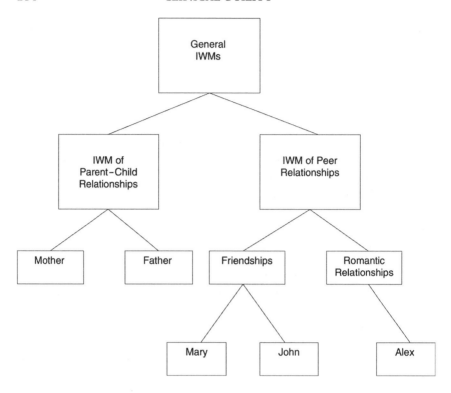

FIGURE 9.1. Collins and Read's (1994) hierarchical conceptualization of the structure of IWMs. This figure provides a heuristic tool to understand multiple models; however, consideration of attachment security as a dimensional construct is more in keeping with current research on and theory about the complexity of human experience (see Fraley & Phillips, Chapter 7, this volume). From Collins and Read (1994). Reprinted with permission of Kim Bartholomew.

important for maintaining some continuity in interactions with others, but stability of insecure models is undesirable.

Bowlby (1969/1982, 1988) believed that IWMs must be kept up to date to allow for accurate expectations and predictions in relationships and to be applicable across situations. Updating may occur gradually, with the incorporation of new information, and will result in the development of increasingly complex and comprehensive IWMs. IWMs are expected to be most flexible and open to change in the individual's formative years, but to become less modifiable with age, especially if similar experiences of insecurity occur repeatedly. For example, research suggests that optimal updating is less likely among insecure individuals, who are more apt to cling to obsolete descriptions of partners even in the face of new information (e.g., Mikulincer & Arad, 1999).

Bowlby (1988) also suggested that more rapid change in IWMs could occur under certain circumstances, most notably during major life transitions (e.g., losing an attachment figure or entering therapy). He believed that individuals are set on a developmental trajectory by their early experiences, and they will tend to continue along that trajectory unless some event or set of circumstances causes a directional shift. A shift may move individuals in the direction of increasing or decreasing security of IWMs. This process has been conceptualized as a transactional model (Fraley & Brumbaugh, 2004). Existing IWMs influence the kinds of caregiving environment encouraged or selected by the individual, and the caregiving environment acts on the individual to either maintain stability or bring about instability in attachment models. Thus previous experiences that give rise to particular IWMs influence the quality of current and new relationships, but the individual does not merely impose his or her own expectations and beliefs on the social environment. In each new relationship, a dynamic is created based on how others react and interact, and this may alter existing IWMs.

THEORETICAL MODELS OF ATTACHMENT CHANGE

Life Stress Model

Change in attachment security can be explained by a number of possible theoretical models (Davila & Cobb, 2004). The life stress model is consistent with Bowlby's (1969/1982) proposition that change is most likely during shifts in the interpersonal environment. This is clearly supported by early research on the stability of infant attachment patterns (e.g., Egeland & Farber, 1984; Egeland & Sroufe, 1981; Vaughn et al., 1979). Stability was associated with continuity in the quality of care, and infants were more likely to shift from secure to insecure when the caregiving environment was disrupted (e.g., by increased life stress for mothers, mother–infant separations, and changes in mothers' living arrangements). In longitudinal studies that followed infants all the way to early adulthood, individuals who experienced the most adverse life events (e.g., parental loss, abuse) also showed the most instability in attachment security (Waters, Merrick, Treboux, Crowell, & Albersheim, 2000; Weinfield, Sroufe, & Egeland, 2000). For example, infants classified as secure in Ainsworth's Strange Situation had a 66% chance of being labeled insecure as young adults with the Adult Attachment Interview if they had experienced one or more negative life events (Waters et al., 2000).

Research on change in adult attachment provides mixed support for the life stress model. Specific life events do not consistently lead to changes in security (e.g., Baldwin & Fehr, 1995; Davila & Cobb, 2003, 2004; Davila & Sargent, 2003; Kirkpatrick & Hazan, 1994; Scharfe & Bartholomew, 1995). However, change may be effected by the meaning people ascribe to events, rather than by the events themselves. In other words, changes in adult attachment are likely to be mediated by cognitive and emotional processes associated with life circumstances, rather than the objective features of the circumstances (e.g., Bowlby, 1988; Davila & Sargent, 2003).

Clinicians are certain to be familiar with situations in which clients have unique and intense cognitive and emotional reactions to life circumstances that may seem to have little to do with the situations themselves, or that may seem to the clients or therapists to be disproportionate to these situations. Indeed, these cognitive and emotional experiences are very much at the heart of therapeutic work. From a variety of clinical perspectives, the manner in which clients view their life experiences is considered an important determinant of subsequent emotions and behaviors. And treatment is often designed to help people develop a new meaning or a new understanding of earlier experiences, or to provide people with new experiences that they can use to change cognitive and emotional functioning.

Social-Cognitive Model

Although people are considered to have one dominant IWM, subordinate models in the IWM hierarchy can occasionally take precedence and thus have a powerful impact on behavior. The social-cognitive model proposes that temporary changes in attachment security are the result of interpersonal circumstances that increase the availability of one model over others (Baldwin & Fehr, 1995; Baldwin, Keelan, Fehr, Enns, & Koh-Rangarajoo, 1996). Thus the availability of IWMs of varying security differs across time and contexts. A number of findings support this model (e.g., Baldwin et al., 1996, Study 3). In addition, changes in how people perceive their relationships and themselves, even daily, are associated with fluctuations in how secure they feel (e.g., Davila & Sargent, 2003).

Again, clinicians have surely noticed such fluctuations in clients, for better and for worse. In different states of mind, clients may report different thoughts and feelings about their circumstances. In addition, as clients begin to develop new ways of viewing and experiencing themselves and their lives, they can still revert to old views when under stress or when faced with something that reminds them of past experiences. It is often a goal (and a challenge) in treatment to help clients form and maintain healthier IWMs.

Individual-Difference Model

The individual-difference model proposes that there are individual differences in the degree to which IWMs are vulnerable to change (Davila, Burge, & Hammen, 1997; Davila & Cobb, 2003). This model differs from the previous two, in that it describes a pathological vulnerability to change as opposed to normative change. Individuals with histories of adverse interpersonal experiences, life stressors, and psychopathology may have unclear

IWMs. The lack of clarity ultimately leads to instability in self-reports of attachment security, because such individuals experience frequent, transient fluctuations in their views of self and others. Because they do not experience continuity in their IWMs, they are likely to have extreme difficulty functioning in relationships. Their expectations and thoughts about relationships, as well as their behavioral and emotional responses, will vary; this produces chaotic and confusing interpersonal experiences. This is not a linear model of change in the underlying cognitive structures; rather, it reflects the shifting nature of IWMs in vulnerable individuals.

Perhaps the best example of this process is the case of borderline personality pathology, although the model can also apply to less extreme forms of lack of clarity about self and others. When clients are uncertain about who they or others are, it can cause frequent and sometimes intense shifts in how the clients feel. The shifts can be extreme and far from reality-based, and therapy is often directed at helping such clients develop more integrated and balanced views.

Empirical Evidence of Change in IWMs

The bulk of research on stability and change in attachment models documents change as it occurs naturally, and supports all three of the models described here (e.g., Davila et al., 1997; Davila & Cobb, 2003, 2004; Hamilton, 2000; Scharfe, 2003). However, there is a growing body of research on evoked changes in attachment security.[2] By *evoked changes*, we mean changes brought about by therapeutic interventions; such interventions may or may not be guided by attachment theory but may have consequences for individual security (see Davila & Levy, 2006). For example, a number of interventions aimed at improving mother–child interactions have resulted in increased child security (Hoffman, Marvin, Cooper, & Powell, 2006; Lieberman, Weston, & Pawl, 1991; Toth, Cicchetti, & Rogosch, 2006; van Zeijl et al., 2006). And changes in aspects of adult attachment have been shown in response to individual and group psychotherapy (Levy et al., 2006; Travis, Bliwise, Binder, & Horne-Moyer, 2001; see Mikulincer & Shaver, 2007, Chs. 14 and 15, for a review).

Although there is relatively little work on evoked changes in adult attachment security or IWMs, the concepts of attachment theory have been used to guide the development of therapeutic approaches, and this is particularly true for work with couples and families (e.g., see Clulow, 2001, and Johnson & Whiffen, 2003). According to attachment theory, psychopathology stems in part from IWMs that are applied rigidly or that are incoherent and unintegrated—either of which may result in maladaptive behavior, especially when potentiated by unfavorable life events (Bowlby, 1969/1982, 1973, 1988). These IWMs may be understandable consequences of difficult attachment relationship histories, but they are maladaptive when applied to current relationships. The goal of therapy is to revise inadequate models or replace insecure models with more secure ones.

IWMs IN THERAPY

When clinicians conceptualize and organize interventions, it may be useful to focus specifically on changes in IWMs. Many of the concepts discussed here will be familiar to proponents of various schools of therapy. We are not proposing that therapists change their methods of working with clients, but rather that they change the lens through which they understand the development of a client's problems, needs, and motives, and adopt a new perspective on the mechanisms and goals of change in therapy.

Traditionally, attachment theory concepts have been most embraced by therapists with a psychodynamic perspective, because they already think about how early relationship experiences shape mental representations and current relationship dynamics. Moreover, consistent with an attachment-theoretical view, in contemporary relational psychodynamic models (e.g., Messer & Warren, 1995) psychopathology is thought to manifest itself mainly in repetitive maladaptive interpersonal patterns. However, IWMs are conceptualized in terms of cognition, affect, and behavior, so they can be relevant to a variety of therapeutic approaches. Rather than describing how to incorporate an attachment perspective into specific types of therapy (readers can consult Chapters 14 through 17 of the present volume for examples), we discuss the general principles proposed by Bowlby (1988) and how these principles are relevant to change in psychotherapy.

Goldfried and colleagues (e.g., Goldfried & Davila, 2005; Goldfried, 1980) proposed five components of treatment that are required to effect change in any therapy: (1) fostering positive expectancies for change (e.g., assisting the client in being motivated to change); (2) fostering an optimal therapeutic alliance (e.g., developing an empathic bond between the client and the therapist, and agreeing on treatment goals and strategies); (3) increasing awareness (e.g., about thoughts, feelings, behavior); (4) fostering corrective experiences (e.g., helping the client engage in new behavior and experience it differently); and (5) helping the client engage in continued reality testing (e.g., generalizing the work to other domains). As we describe below, Bowlby's therapeutic principles fit well within these general efforts to create change.

Bowlby (1988) proposed five therapeutic tasks with the explicit goal of increasing security (i.e., increasing the salience and availability of secure IWMs). The first task is to provide a secure base for the client from which to explore past and present attachment experiences. This is predicated on the creation of a good working alliance (*fostering an optimal therapeutic alliance*). Provision of a secure base allows the client to explore cognitive, behavioral, and affective components of relevant attachment bonds (*increas-*

ing awareness). This is critically important, because insecure individuals are unlikely to seek information about themselves or their relationships if it is threatening to attachment security.

The second task is to assist the client in exploring current attachment relationships and perceptions, biases, and expectations about self and others (*increasing awareness*). The importance of this task is highlighted by research on the construal and memory biases of IWMs, which may operate to selectively direct attention, information processing, and memory for information consistent with existing models (see Collins et al., 2004, for a review). Clients will need assistance with attending to all aspects of their experience, so that revision of IWMs is possible. Likewise, the relatively unconscious nature of IWMs may necessitate input from an observer to bring previously unrecognized aspects of IWMs to light.

Indeed, much of what is contained in IWMs may exist and operate outside of consciousness. As such, therapists need to focus not only on promoting change in consciously held beliefs about current relationships, but also on highlighting aspects of models of which clients are unaware. People with insecure attachments may recognize some aspects of their maladaptive models, but there will likely be much that they do not recognize, including many untested assumptions, cut-off emotions, and self-defeating behaviors.

Bowlby (1988) assumed that IWMs will affect a client's feelings about and expectations and perceptions of the therapist. Thus the third task is to explore the therapeutic relationship. Examination of the client–therapist relationship may provide a window into the nature and operation of clients' IWMs. The therapy relationship will allow observation and processing of emotional reactions and cognitive appraisals as they occur in the moment; it will also be a source of new attachment experiences, and will provide a place to perhaps try new attachment behavioral strategies that are more effective in meeting attachment needs (*fostering a corrective experience*). Thus change in attachment structures comes not just through cognitive exploration of attachment relationships within and outside therapy, but also through creation of a new (and, one hopes, secure) attachment bond in the therapeutic relationship.

The fourth task is to explore and understand how past situations, experiences, and relationships have produced current cognition, affect, and behavior (*increasing awareness*). This involves examination of not only how important figures in childhood responded to and interacted with the client, but also what attachment figures may have said. This task requires that the client and therapist trace the developmental roots of IWMs. The goal is to understand how the demands of the past shaped attachment beliefs, behaviors, and emotional responses to allow the individual to function in a less than optimal caregiving environment.

Exploration of developmental roots and function of existing IWMs will help the client recognize that current mental models of self and other may not be functional, accurate, or appropriate in the present interpersonal context. This is the fifth task in therapy—to recognize the inaccurate elements of IWMs that are no longer tenable (*helping the client engage in continued reality testing*). Once clients appreciate that their current models may be maladaptive and unsuited to current circumstances, they may be able to consider alternative models that will allow them "to feel, to think, and to act in new ways" (Bowlby, 1988, p. 139).

The progression in therapy through these five tasks is not expected to be sequential; nor is it expected that each task will be fully accomplished before moving on to the next. Bowlby (1988) envisioned the therapist as working on these interrelated tasks throughout therapy, but with the primary goal being provision of a secure base from which the client can begin to explore IWMs.

Specific Mechanisms of Change in IWMs

The tasks outlined by Bowlby provide a starting point for thinking about change in IWMs and are consistent with the principles that foster change in therapy. However, there are some specific issues to consider in the therapeutic context. Bowlby (1973, 1988) stated that if the presenting problems are attachment issues, then there is a need not just for cognitive restructuring, but also for emotional and interpersonal change. This implies that change can be targeted at different levels—behavioral, cognitive, or emotional— depending on the needs of the client and the therapeutic approach.

Attachment Behavioral Strategies

Attachment behavioral strategies are patterns of behavior enacted to meet attachment-related goals. Attachment goals and behavioral strategies are expected to derive either directly or indirectly from IWMs (Bowlby, 1969/1982; Collins et al., 2004). Some behavioral responses to activation of the attachment system may be so automatic and overlearned that there is little conscious cognitive–affective mediation. Other behavioral strategies may be mediated by cognitive–affective aspects of IWMs. Regardless of the pathway by which IWMs affect behavior, it is clear that individuals' responses to others in attachment-relevant situations have consequences for the quality of those interactions (e.g., Cobb, Davila, & Bradbury, 2001; Feeney & Collins, 2004; Pietromonaco, Greenwood, & Barrett, 2004; Simpson et al., 2002).

To begin changing existing behavioral strategies, the therapist must identify and focus on what attachment strategies the client is currently using (e.g., hyperactivating or deactivating). For example, does the client avoid others when feeling anxious? Does the client show excessive help seeking and clinginess? Once the pattern of behavioral strategies is revealed, the client can be encouraged to explore alternative, more adaptive plans to meet attachment goals and needs. If a client has a relationship in which he or she holds relatively more secure relationship-specific IWMs, adaptive strategies used in that relationship can be explored, strengthened, and applied in other relationship contexts. If the client has few or no adaptive behavioral strategies in his or her repertoire, new behavioral patterns will have to be explored in the context of therapy and then applied in other relationships. A good working alliance and the client's cooperation in trying these behavioral experiments, is necessary. With encouragement, clients may try new ways of dealing with attachment issues—in other words, replacing maladaptive attachment strategies with adaptive (i.e., secure) ones. The goal of these behavioral experiments is repeated successful meeting of attachment needs to reinforce the use and automaticity of more secure behavioral strategies.

As an example, we can consider the case of distressed couple relationships, in which maladaptive attachment behaviors often occur. In a distressed relationship, one or both individuals often feel that the security of attachment to the partner is threatened (e.g., one partner may threaten to reject or leave the other). In attempting to restore felt security, partners may engage in strategies that are ultimately maladaptive and that further threaten the relationship. For example, a person with a preoccupied pattern will often deal with the attachment threat by using hyperactivating strategies. He or she may excessively seek reassurance (e.g., constantly asking, "Do you love me? Will you stay with me?") or seek more than the usual amount of proximity (e.g., wanting to be with the partner constantly, wanting to know where the partner is and what the partner is doing at all times). Although the intent is to gain reassurance, it often engenders frustration and annoyance in the partner, who may interpret the behavior as a lack of trust and a threat to normative autonomy. Consequently, the partner may express frustration, which only heightens rather than lessens the person's attachment anxiety. In such a case, the clinician can assist the couple in delineating the behavioral cycle, highlight each partner's attachment-related feelings and needs, and (in particular) underscore the desired and actual consequences of the behavior. New behavioral strategies will then need to be collaboratively designed and tried out to allow the partners to observe the new consequences. This approach is characteristic of the emotionally focused therapy for couples developed by Johnson (2004; see also Johnson, Chapter 16, this volume).

Cognitive Components

Although enacting new attachment behavioral strategies that elicit different and reinforcing responses from others can result in changed IWMs, it may also be necessary to assist the client in directly restructuring the content of the IWMs and associated cognitive processes. Distortions may exist in the content of IWMs, and memory and construal biases may operate to preserve the current status of IWMs. Thus assisting clients to process information and experiences that are not consistent with existing models will be particularly important, because IWMs are apt to operate in a self-confirming manner (Bowlby, 1969/1982, 1973).

For example, existing IWMs affect allocation of attentional resources, information encoding, memory, attributions, and perceptions in interpersonal situations (e.g., Collins, 1996; Feeney & Cassidy, 2003; Fraley et al.,, 2000; Fraley & Shaver, 1997; Gallo & Smith, 2001; Mikulincer, 1997; see Collins et al., 2004, for a review). Therefore, insecure individuals will have more difficulty regulating attention in attachment-relevant situations (e.g., Fraley et al., 2000; Fraley & Shaver, 1997; Mikulincer, 1997), and anxious individuals may be hypervigilant to threat cues (Baldwin & Kay, 2003). Avoidant individuals attend less to elements of emotional events, which limits encoding of attachment-relevant experiences (Fraley et al., 2000). And over time, people appear to reconstruct their memories of attachment experiences to confirm existing models (Feeney & Cassidy, 2003; Mikulincer & Arad, 1997). When working with a client who is exhibiting distorted cognitive processing, a therapist may find it necessary to educate the client about common cognitive biases and help the client identify his or her typical biases (e.g., selective attention). This work can include standard cognitive therapy procedures. Alternatively, narrative approaches may be used to redress the rigid or impoverished stories insecure individuals have constructed over time about themselves and their attachment figures (Holmes, 2001).

Cognitive work that draws attention to and restructures clients' distorted perceptions of self and others will allow reshaping of IWMs and help clients to view themselves and others in a more secure manner. Typical maladaptive cognitions characteristic of attachment insecurity include "I'm not worthy," "I'm unlovable," and "People can't be trusted." Following from Bowlby's therapeutic tasks, the goal is to assist the client in making these aspects of IWMs accessible for updating and revision. In sum, identifying maladaptive thoughts and schemas, followed by questioning the evidence for them and replacing them with more realistic, adaptive thoughts, can be an important part of attachment-oriented therapy.

Affect

Although IWMs were originally described as primarily cognitive models (because Bowlby was a professional friend of Jean Piaget, and because he was affected by early cybernetic control theories and the beginning of what was eventually called the "cognitive revolution" in psychology), IWMs are now recognized to be heavily affect-laden (e.g., Collins et al., 2004). Consideration of emotional experience is necessary, because emotion is an important organizing feature of experience in close relationships (Johnson

& Whiffen, 2003), and a main function of the attachment behavior system is to regulate emotional distress.

Attachment-related emotion regulation may be maladaptive in several ways. First, individuals whose IWMs are characterized by fears of abandonment and low self-worth may use hyperactivating strategies when faced with a threat to security. That is, they may focus on their negative emotion, do things that will increase it (e.g., ruminate), and be unable to calm or soothe themselves. Helping such individuals learn to tolerate distress and regulate feelings more successfully may be necessary. Mindfulness-based approaches, such as those used in dialectical behavior therapy (Linehan, 1993), can be useful strategies to accomplish this task.

Individuals whose IWMs are characterized by lack of trust in the availability of others and consequent avoidance of intimacy may use deactivating strategies when faced with a threat to security. They may ignore, suppress, or deny negative emotion—especially feelings of vulnerability. Such individuals may therefore need assistance in identifying and experiencing emotions that have been cut off. This may be particularly difficult clinical work. Defenses involving deactivating strategies tend to be quite strong, and such a client may have little motivation for change. Treatment may need to proceed slowly, and a strong, trusting therapeutic relationship may be necessary before emotional awareness and expression can be tolerated.

Another common problem arises when secondary emotions replace primary ones in reaction to attachment threats. From an attachment perspective, the primary emotions elicited are fear and anxiety. However, for a variety of reasons (e.g., those feelings are too threatening or they leave a person feeling too vulnerable), secondary emotions may take precedence. Thus the client may express secondary emotions, such as anger or frustration, rather than the primary ones. These secondary emotions may be thought of as distorted attachment signals (e.g., Kobak & Hazan, 1991; Kobak, Ruckdeschel, & Hazan, 1994). In therapy, it may be useful to help clients become more aware of, and to foster the experience and expression of, primary emotions. This may be done a number of ways, including through careful processing of the attachment threats and the clients' reactions to these; through acceptance-based interventions that help clients become less judgmental about their emotional reactions; and through emotionally focused or experiential strategies (e.g., Elliott, Watson, Goldman, & Greenberg, 2004; Johnson, 2002).

As noted, the choice of technique in therapy will depend on the therapist's case conceptualization and theoretical orientation. The therapies mentioned here are only samples of applicable approaches. The process of changing IWMs may be accomplished by focusing simultaneously on the three domains of behavior, affect, and cognition, or the therapist may choose to give one domain a more central focus. However, as with the five therapeutic tasks outlined by Bowlby, interventions addressing change in any component of IWMs may be inextricably linked to the other components. Also, change in any component of IWMs may result in changes in the other components.

CONSIDERATION OF THE THEORETICAL
MODELS OF CHANGE IN THERAPY

Earlier in the chapter, we described three models of change in attachment security: the life stress model, the social-cognitive model, and the individual-difference model. Change in IWMs through a focus on behavior, cognitions, and affects can be understood through the lens of each of these models, and all three may contribute to conceptualizing change during treatment.

The life stress model suggests that important life events or changes in interpersonal circumstances may be related to change in IWMs. However, the direction of change may depend on the meaning ascribed by individuals to the events. Thus it will be important for therapists to help clients explore the meaning of events in their lives that are relevant to attachment issues (e.g., interpersonal loss, relationship transitions, or threats to relationship integrity). For example, a client who comes to therapy following a relationship breakup or divorce may experience stronger feelings of insecurity or of security, depending on how the loss is construed and processed. Although a relationship loss may initially reinforce insecurity and negative IWMs, security may be fostered by helping clients explore what they have learned from the experience, and even how they may have grown or potentially could grow in response to the loss.

As previously noted, the social-cognitive model proposes that various attachment-related IWMs may be more or less salient at different times and in different circumstances. Thus one goal in therapy would be exploring contradictions in IWMs and increasing the salience and chronicity of activation of alternate secure models (although if none exist, they must first be formed, perhaps through the therapeutic relationship). The meaning and interpretation of the events, and the individual's subsequent response (both affective and behavioral), must be highlighted and discussed. Over time, and with repeated reinforcement of these more secure models, old insecure models should be rendered less chronically activated and accessible. One example of such a process is a client's application of a model of a prior relationship to a current one for which it is not appropriate. For instance, a female client may have had an insecure relationship with her father, reflected by a lack of trust in him and uncertainty about his availability. She may currently be in a generally secure and satisfying relationship with a male partner. However, in times of stress, this client may view her partner through the lens of the IWM of her father and behave toward her partner as if he were her father, resulting in a distorted view of her current experiences. Therapy may focus on helping the client distinguish between IWMs of her father and her partner, identify times when she is most likely to apply the inappropriate IWM, and develop strategies to help her view the reality of the situation with her partner.

The individual-difference model suggests that apparent change in consciously held aspects of attachment models is a reflection of instability and incoherence in IWMs. Such incoherence and instability are often manifested in rapidly changing thoughts and feelings about the self and other people (in extreme cases, splitting), emotional reactivity, and problems with self-identity. Clients may report awareness of confusion arising from conflicting feelings about or views of themselves. Or these conflicts may be acted out emotionally and behaviorally in an unconscious manner. Thus helping clients develop a more coherent, positive, and stable sense of the self and other people will be necessary. This calls for exploration of current IWMs to identify sources of contradiction or incompatibility. Attention to emotion, including awareness, acceptance, and expression, will be important, as will the development of a secure therapeutic alliance in which the therapist can provide support and validation for the client's developing sense of self.

ADDITIONAL CONSIDERATIONS
FOR FOCUSING ON IWMs IN THERAPY

Although attachment theory and the IWM concept clearly provide a useful framework for clinicians, there are several issues and cautions to be considered. One of the main therapeutic tasks described by Bowlby (1988) and thought to form the foundation of work on IWMs and attachment change is the development of the secure base in therapy. The question of what constitutes a true attachment relationship is an important one that is currently unresolved, although most scholars would agree that it includes secure-base functions and the presence of mourning in the face of loss (e.g., Hazan, Gur-Yaish, & Campa, 2004; Trinke & Bartholomew, 1997). Moreover, the developmental timeline of the appearance of attachment functions in close relationships is not known. In the current climate of managed care, where short-term therapy is increasingly valued, whether the therapeutic relationship can truly develop as an attachment relationship in a short period is debatable. This empirical question remains to be explored. However, research on the therapeutic alliance clearly shows that a collaborative working alliance can be developed even in the context of short-term therapy (Crits-Christoph & Connolly, 1999), and this may be sufficient to support clients' exploration of attachment issues. (For a review of these and other issues, see Farber & Metzger, Chapter 3, this volume.)

Even if the client develops a secure attachment bond to the therapist, other factors must be considered in the change process. Empirical evidence suggests that relatively insecure individuals are less cognitively open and flexible (e.g., Kobak & Hazan, 1991). A defining feature of security is having flexible IWMs that are perhaps more accessible for revision (Bowlby, 1988; Kobak & Hazan, 1991). What makes an individual secure is the ability to respond to changing interpersonal environments by adjusting IWMs to create action plans that best meet attachment needs, and to accommodate new information about attachment figures as it becomes available. Individuals with relatively insecure models are at a disadvantage, because their models may be more rigid (Bowlby, 1973, 1988), and because cognitive biases will operate to exclude information that would allow revision (e.g., Collins et al., 2004). Thus individuals who have IWMs most in need of revision may be the ones least able to accomplish it.

Also hindering exploration of attachment IWMs in therapy is the largely unconscious nature of the models. Bowlby (1969/1982) and others (e.g., Main et al., 1985) have made it clear that IWMs develop out of real experiences, but that expectations and perceptions based on these experiences are abstracted into structures that often operate automatically and may not be readily accessible to conscious appraisal (Bowlby, 1969/1982; Main et al., 1985). This poses a problem for the therapist: How can these unconscious processes become the focus of conscious attention? Individuals may be more or less able to expose their models to conscious processing, but to effect change, the models must be made explicit and conscious so that checking, revision, or extension can be accomplished.

Another problem for the therapist is deciding how to evaluate and measure IWMs for the purposes of developing treatment and monitoring therapy outcome. Questions to consider are (1) whether change is occurring in conscious or unconscious aspects of the models, (2) at what level of the model hierarchy change is occurring, and (3) what the best indicators of change in IWMs may be. Because IWMs cannot be directly observed, either therapists can use self-reports (which may be limited by reporting biases), or they may infer the nature of IWMs from clients' affect, behavior, and cognitions in the context of the therapeutic relationship and other attachment relationships (Westen, Nakash, Thomas, & Bradley, 2006). The therapist may attend to the coherence, complexity, sophistication, and integration of clients' narrative descriptions of themselves and others in their social worlds, and specifically attend to their descriptions of relationships with relevant attachment figures. (See Chapters 6 through 8, this volume, for discussions of how to assess attachment security.)

A related difficulty is that, as therapists, we are used to thinking about types of people and diagnostic categories. Thinking about prototypes or categories of attachment, therefore, may be more familiar than thinking about dimensions of attachment; however, it is important to recognize the dimensions (see Fraley & Phillips, Chapter 7) and also to recognize that people may hold multiple IWMs that operate in different circumstances. Although there is no one answer to questions about how to conceptualize IWMs and change for every client, the choices therapists make to observe and evaluate change must be guided by a clear conception of the kinds of change they are working toward. For example, for some clients it may be appropriate to work toward a relatively full shift in attachment pattern from insecure to secure. For other clients, it may be more appropriate to expect only a change from highly anxious to less anxious. For some clients, these changes may be necessary in only one problematic relationship; for other clients, changes may be necessary in multiple relationships.

The definition and scope of IWMs constitute another issue that scholars have identified as problematic and that has implications for change. Some scholars argue that IWMs are poorly defined, abstract concepts that have been conceptualized too broadly (e.g., Thompson & Raikes, 2003). In addition, they suggest that IWMs have not been clearly linked to existing models of cognitive development or aspects of cognitive processing, and some argue that IWMs have been overapplied in explanations of interpersonal phenomena (Thompson & Raikes, 2003). Given this, the warning for clinicians is to be careful about interpreting all behavior and all relationships in the context of attachment theory. At its narrowest conceptualization, the attachment behavioral system may be most relevant in intimate relationships and in times of stress—for example, when a person is ill, tired, or facing a threat to security, and is, therefore, in need of assistance in regulating distress (Bowlby, 1969/1982). Furthermore, Bowlby and others (Feeney & Collins, 2004; Hazan & Diamond, 2000) have postulated that other behavioral systems (e.g., caregiving and sexual mating) influence behavior, cognition, and affect in close relationships. Thus the attachment behavioral system is not the only system playing a role in individual dynamics and the dynamics of close relationships.

CONCLUSIONS

Clearly, there are important gaps in our understanding of the nature and function of IWMs and the processes by which they change. However, it is also clear that attachment theory and the IWM concept have important implications for understanding and fostering change in psychotherapy. As Bowlby (1988) noted, attachment theory holds great promise to inform our interventions with couples, families, and individuals, and we can hope to see this promise fulfilled in coming years. To that end, we have discussed some of the theoretical and empirical bases for conceptualizing attachment change in general and particularly in therapy. Although many of the suggestions in this chapter will not be new to practicing clinicians, we have provided some of the research findings relevant to using the IWM construct in therapy, and shown how this perspective may fit with and inform therapists' goals and orientation in treatment. We hope that in doing so, we have challenged therapists to think about treatment and change from an attachment perspective. Bowlby suggested that people are happiest when life is a series of successful excursions, short and long, from a secure base. By approaching therapy from an attachment perspective, we may begin to help people achieve this goal.

ACKNOWLEDGMENTS

Preparation of this chapter was supported by Social Sciences and Humanities Research Council of Canada Research Grant No. 410-2005-0829 to Rebecca J. Cobb and by National Institute of Mental Health Grant No. R01 MH063904-1A2 to Joanne Davila.

NOTES

1. The term *internal working models* (IWMs) may be used interchangeably with *representational models, models of self and other, attachment models, attachment representations,* and *attachment schemas.* Most readers will realize that the idea that early interactions are encoded in cognitive representations is not unique to attachment theory. Constructs from other clinical theories that overlap with but are not identical to IWMs include *core beliefs* and *schemas* from cognitive theory, *cyclical maladaptive patterns* in interpersonal theory, and *object relations* in psychoanalytic theory.
2. See Bakermans-Kranenburg, van IJzendoorn, and Juffer (2003) for a review of early interventions to enhance infant attachment security.

RECOMMENDATIONS FOR FURTHER READING

Collins, N. L., Guichard, A. C., Ford, M. B., & Feeney, B. C. (2004). Working models of attachment: New developments and emerging themes. In W. S. Rholes & J. A. Simpson (Eds.), *Adult attachment: Theory, research, and clinical implications* (pp. 196–239). New York: Guilford Press.—This chapter provides a more in depth discussion of the components of IWMs.

Davila, J., & Cobb, R. J. (2004). Predictors of change in attachment security during adulthood. In W. S. Rholes & J. A. Simpson (Eds.), *Adult attachment: Theory, research, and clinical implications* (pp. 133–156). New York: Guilford Press.— This chapter provides more detailed information about theory and research on attachment stability and change.

REFERENCES

Ainsworth, M. D. S., Blehar, M. C., Waters, E., & Wall, S. (1978). *Patterns of attachment: A psychological study of the Strange Situation.* Hillsdale, NJ: Erlbaum.

Bakermans-Kranenburg, M. J., van IJzendoorn, M. H., & Juffer, F. (2003). Less is more: Meta-analyses of sensitivity and attachment interventions in early childhood. *Psychological Bulletin, 129,* 195–215.

Baldwin, M. W., & Fehr, B. (1995). On the instability of attachment style ratings. *Personal Relationships, 2,* 247–261.

Baldwin, M. W., & Kay, A. C. (2003). Adult attachment and the inhibition of rejection. *Journal of Social and Clinical Psychology, 22,* 275–293.

Baldwin, M. W., Keelan, J. P. R., Fehr, B., Enns, V., & Koh-Rangarajoo, E. (1996). Social-cognitive conceptualization of attachment working models: Availability and accessibility effects. *Journal of Personality and Social Psychology, 71,* 94–109.

Bartholomew, K. (1990). Avoidance of intimacy: An attachment perspective. *Journal of Social and Personal Relationships, 7,* 147–178.

Bartholomew, K., & Horowitz, L. M. (1991). Attachment styles among young adults: A test of a four-category model. *Journal of Personality and Social Psychology, 61,* 226–244.

Bowlby, J. (1973). *Attachment and loss: Vol. 2. Separation: Anxiety and anger.* New York: Basic Books.

Bowlby, J. (1979). *The making and breaking of affectional bonds.* London: Tavistock.

Bowlby, J. (1980). *Attachment and loss: Vol. 3. Loss: Sadness and depression.* New York: Basic Books.

Bowlby, J. (1982). *Attachment and loss: Vol. 1. Attachment* (2nd ed.). New York: Basic Books. (1st ed., 1969)

Bowlby, J. (1988). *A secure base: Parent–child attachment and healthy human development.* London: Routledge.

Brennan, K. A., Clark, C. L., & Shaver, P. R. (1998). Self-report measurement of adult attachment: An integrative overview. In J. A. Simpson & W. S. Rholes (Eds.), *Attachment theory and close relationships* (pp. 46–76). New York: Guilford Press.

Clulow, C. (2001). *Adult attachment and couple psychotherapy: The 'secure base' in practice and research.* London: Brunner-Routledge.

Cobb, R. J., Davila, J., & Bradbury, T. N. (2001). Attachment security and marital satisfaction: The role of positive perceptions and social support. *Personality and Social Psychology Bulletin, 27,* 1131–1143.

Collins, N. L. (1996). Working models of attachment: Implications for explanation, emotion, and behavior. *Journal of Personality and Social Psychology, 71,* 810–832.

Collins, N. L., Guichard, A. C., Ford, M. B., & Feeney, B. C. (2004). Working models of attachment: New developments and emerging themes. In W. S. Rholes & J. A. Simpson (Eds.), *Adult attachment: Theory, research, and clinical implications* (pp. 196–239). New York: Guilford Press.

Collins, N. L., & Read, S. J. (1990). Adult attachment, working models, and relationship quality in dating couples. *Journal of Personality and Social Psychology, 58,* 644–663.

Collins, N. L., & Read, S. J. (1994). Cognitive representations of attachment: The structure and function of working models. In K. Bartholomew & D. Perlman (Eds.), *Advances in personal relationships: Vol. 5. Attachment processes in adulthood* (pp. 53–90). London: Jessica Kingsley.

Crits-Christoph, P., & Connolly, M. B. (1999). Alliance and technique in short-term dynamic therapy. *Clinical Psychology Review, 19,* 687–704.

Crowell, J. A., & Treboux, D. (1995). A review of adult attachment measures: Implications for theory and research. *Social Development, 4,* 294–327.

Davila, J., Burge, D., & Hammen, C. (1997). Why does attachment style change? *Journal of Personality and Social Psychology, 73,* 826–838.

Davila, J., & Cobb, R. J. (2003). Predicting change in self-reported and interviewer-assessed adult attachment: Tests of the individual difference and life stress models of attachment change. *Personality and Social Psychology Bulletin, 29,* 859–870.

Davila, J., & Cobb, R. J. (2004). Predictors of change in attachment security during adulthood. In W. S. Rholes & J. A. Simpson (Eds.), *Adult attachment: Theory, research, and clinical implications* (pp. 133–156). New York: Guilford Press.

Davila, J., & Levy, K. N. (2006). Introduction to the special section on attachment theory and psychotherapy. *Journal of Consulting and Clinical Psychology, 74,* 989–993.

Davila, J., & Sargent, E. (2003). The meaning of life (events) predicts changes in attachment security. *Personality and Social Psychology Bulletin, 29,* 1383–1395.

Egeland, B., & Farber, E. A. (1984). Infant–mother attachment: Factors related to its development and changes over time. *Child Development, 55,* 753–771.

Egeland, B., & Sroufe, L. A. (1981). Attachment and early maltreatment. *Child Development, 52,* 44–52.

Elliott, R., Watson, J. C., Goldman, R. N., & Greenberg, L. S. (2004). *Learning emotion-focused therapy: The process-experiential approach to change.* Washington, DC: American Psychological Association.

Feeney, B. C., & Cassidy, J. (2003). Reconstructive memory related to adolescent–parent conflict interactions: The influence of attachment–related representations on immediate perceptions and changes in perceptions over time. *Journal of Personality and Social Psychology, 85,* 945–955.

Feeney, B. C., & Collins, N. L. (2004). Interpersonal safe haven and secure base caregiving processes in adulthood. In W. S. Rholes & J. A. Simpson (Eds.), *Adult attachment: Theory, research, and clinical implications* (pp. 300–338). New York: Guilford Press.

Fraley, R. C., & Brumbaugh, C. C. (2004). A dynamical systems approach to conceptualizing and studying stability and change in attachment security. In W. S. Rholes & J. A. Simpson (Eds.), *Adult attachment: Theory, research, and clinical implications* (pp. 86–132). New York: Guilford Press.

Fraley, R. C., Garner, J. P., & Shaver, P. R. (2000). Adult attachment and the defensive regulation of attention and memory: Examining the role of preemptive and postemptive defensive processes. *Journal of Personality and Social Psychology, 79,* 816–826.

Fraley, R. C., & Shaver, P. R. (1997). Adult attachment and the suppression of unwanted thoughts. *Journal of Personality and Social Psychology, 73,* 1080–1091.

Gallo, L. C., & Smith, T. W. (2001). Attachment style in marriage: Adjustment and responses to interaction. *Journal of Social and Personal Relationships, 18,* 263–289.

Goldfried, M. R. (1980). Toward the delineation of therapeutic change principles. *American Psychologist, 35,* 991–999.

Goldfried, M. R., & Davila, J. (2005). The role of relationship and technique in therapeutic change. *Psychotherapy: Theory, Research, Practice, Training, 42,* 421–430.

Hamilton, C. E. (2000). Continuity and discontinuity of attachment from infancy through adolescence. *Child Development, 71,* 690–694.

Hazan, C., & Diamond, L. M. (2000). The place of attachment in human mating. *Review of General Psychology, 4,* 186–204.

Hazan, C., Gur-Yaish, N., & Campa, M. (2004). What does it mean to be attached? In W. S. Rholes & J. A. Simpson (Eds.), *Adult attachment: Theory, research, and clinical implications.* (pp. 55–85). New York: Guilford Press.

Hazan, C., & Shaver, P. R. (1987). Romantic love conceptualized as an attachment process. *Journal of Personality and Social Psychology, 52,* 511–524.

Hesse, E. (1999). The Adult Attachment Interview: Historical and current perspectives. In J. Cassidy & P. R. Shaver (Eds.), *Handbook of attachment: Theory, research, and clinical applications.* (pp. 395–433). New York: Guilford Press.

Hoffman, K., Marvin, R., Cooper, G., & Powell, B. (2006). Changing toddlers' and preschoolers' attachment classifications: The Circle of Security intervention. *Journal of Consulting and Clinical Psychology, 74,* 1017–1026.

Holmes, J. (2001). *The search for the secure base: Attachment theory and psychotherapy.* Hove, UK: Brunner-Routledge.

Johnson, S. M. (2002). *Emotionally focused couple therapy with trauma survivors: Strengthening attachment bonds.* New York: Guilford Press.

Johnson, S. M. (2004). *The practice of emotionally focused couple therapy: Creating connection* (2nd ed.). New York: Brunner-Routledge.

Johnson, S. M., & Whiffen, V. E. (Eds.). (2003). *Attachment processes in couple and family therapy.* New York: Guilford Press.

Kirkpatrick, L. A., & Hazan, C. (1994). Attachment styles and close relationships: A four-year prospective study. *Personal Relationships, 1,* 123–142.

Kobak, R. R., & Hazan, C. (1991). Attachment in marriage: Effects of security and accuracy of working models. *Journal of Personality and Social Psychology, 60,* 861–869.

Kobak, R., Ruckdeschel, K., & Hazan, C. (1994). From symptom to signal: An attachment view of emotion in marital therapy. In S. M. Johnson & L. S. Greenberg (Eds.), *The heart of the matter: Perspectives on emotion in marital therapy* (pp. 46–71). New York: Brunner/Mazel.

Levy, K. N., Kelly, K. M., Meehan, K. B., Reynoso, J. S., Clarkin, J. F., & Kernberg, O. F. (2006). Change in attachment organization during the treatment of borderline personality disorder. *Journal of Consulting and Clinical Psychology, 74,* 1027–1040.

Lieberman, A. F., Weston, D. R., & Pawl, J. H. (1991). Preventive intervention and outcome with anxiously attached dyads. *Child Development, 62,* 199–209.

Linehan, M. M. (1993). *Skills training manual for treating borderline personality disorder.* New York: Guilford Press.

Main, M., Kaplan, N., & Cassidy, J. (1985). Security in infancy, childhood, and adulthood: A move to the level of representation. In I. Bretherton & E. Waters (Eds.), Growing points of attachment theory and research. *Monographs of the Society for Research in Child Development, 50*(1–2, Serial No. 209), 66–104.

Messer, S. B., & Warren, C. S. (1995). *Models of brief psychodynamic therapy: A comparative approach.* New York: Guilford Press.

Mikulincer, M. (1995). Attachment style and the mental representation of the self. *Journal of Personality and Social Psychology, 69,* 1203–1215.

Mikulincer, M. (1997). Adult attachment style and information processing: Individual differences in curiosity and cognitive closure. *Journal of Personality and Social Psychology, 72,* 1217–1230.

Mikulincer, M., & Arad, D. (1999). Attachment working models and cognitive openness in close relationships: A test of chronic and temporary accessibility effects. *Journal of Personality and Social Psychology, 77,* 710–725.

Mikulincer, M., & Orbach, I. (1995). Attachment styles and repressive defensiveness: The accessibility and architecture of affective memories. *Journal of Personality and Social Psychology, 68,* 917–925.

Mikulincer, M., & Shaver, P. R. (2004). Security-based self-representations in adulthood: contents and process. In W. S. Rholes & J. A. Simpson (Eds.), *Adult attachment: Theory, research, and clinical implications* (pp. 159–195). New York: Guilford Press.

Mikulincer, M., & Shaver, P. R. (2007). *Attachment in adulthood: Structure, dynamics, and change.* New York: Guilford Press.

Overall, N. C., Fletcher, G. J. O., & Friesen, M. D. (2003). Mapping the intimate relationship mind: Comparisons between three models of attachment representations. *Personality and Social Psychology Bulletin, 29,* 1479–1493.

Pietromonaco, P. R., Greenwood, D., & Barrett, L. F. (2004). Conflict in adult close relationships: An attachment perspective. In W. S. Rholes & J. A. Simpson (Eds.), *Adult attachment: Theory, research, and clinical implications* (pp. 267–299). New York: Guilford Press.

Scharfe, E. (2003). Stability and change of attachment representations from cradle to grave. In S. M. Johnson & V. E. Whiffen (Eds.), *Attachment processes in couple and family therapy* (pp. 64–84). New York: Guilford Press.

Scharfe, E., & Bartholomew, K. (1995). Accommodation and attachment representations in young couples. *Journal of Social and Personal Relationships, 12,* 389–401.

Simpson, J. A., Rholes, W. S., Oriña, M. M., & Grich, J. (2002). Working models of attachment, support giving, and support seeking in a stressful situation. *Personality and Social Psychology Bulletin, 28,* 598–608.

Thompson, R. A., & Raikes, H. A. (2003). Toward the next quarter-century: Conceptual and methodological challenges for attachment theory. *Development and Psychopathology, 15,* 691–718.

Toth, S., Cicchetti, D., & Rogosch, F. (2006). The efficacy of toddler–parent psychotherapy to reorganize attachment in the young offspring of mothers with major depressive disorder: A randomized preventive trial. *Journal of Consulting and Clinical Psychology, 74,* 1006–1016.

Travis, L. A., Bliwise, N. G., Binder, J. L., & Horne-Moyer, H. L. (2001). Changes in clients' attachment styles over the course of time-limited dynamic psychotherapy. *Psychotherapy: Theory, Research, Practice, Training, 38,* 149–159.

Trinke, S. J., & Bartholomew, K. (1997). Hierarchies of attachment relationships in young adulthood. *Journal of Social and Personal Relationships, 14,* 603–625.

van Zeijl, J., Mesman, J., van IJzendoorn, M. H., Bakermans-Kranenburg, M. J., Juffer, F., Stolk, M. N., et al. (2006). Attachment-based intervention for enhancing sensitive discipline in mothers of 1- to 3-year-old children at risk for externalizing behavior problems: A randomized controlled trial. *Journal of Consulting and Clinical Psychology, 74,* 994–1005.

Vaughn, B. E., Egeland, B. R., Sroufe, L. A., & Waters, E. (1979). Individual differences in infant–mother attachment at twelve and eighteen months: Stability and change in families under stress. *Child Development, 50,* 971–975.

Waters, E., Merrick, S., Treboux, D., Crowell, J., & Albersheim, L. (2000). Attachment security in infancy and early adulthood: A twenty-year longitudinal study. *Child Development, 71,* 684–689.

Weinfield, N. S., Sroufe, L. A., & Egeland, B. (2000). Attachment from infancy to early adulthood in a high-risk sample: Continuity, discontinuity, and their correlates. *Child Development, 71,* 695–702.

Westen, D., Nakash, O., Thomas, C., & Bradley, R. (2006). Clinical assessment of attachment patterns and personality disorder in adolescents and adults. *Journal of Consulting and Clinical Psychology, 74,* 1065–1085.

10

An Attachment Approach to Adult Psychotherapy

Brent Mallinckrodt
Katherine Daly
Chia-Chih D. C. Wang

Our assignment in this chapter was to explain how an attachment-oriented therapist might approach the tasks involved in psychotherapy, basing the approach whenever possible on the research literature generated by attachment theory. In reviewing this literature from a clinical perspective, we encountered a fundamental tension between science and practice. Empirical research is incremental, and those who seek to further a scientific understanding of psychotherapy are cautious about interpreting the findings of any particular study. This stance is in keeping with the scientific tradition of null hypothesis testing, in which a group difference or the effect of a variable is presumed not to exist unless there is quite convincing evidence to the contrary. Because of the considerable negative consequences of concluding that an effect exists when in fact it does not, researchers impose a high standard of proof when interpreting their results. Setting a .05 or .01 level for a Type I error is comparable to the legal standard of proof "beyond a reasonable doubt" used in criminal cases, where the negative consequences of convicting an innocent defendant are considered far more serious than those of exonerating a defendant who has committed a crime.

A review of adult attachment research (Meyer & Pilkonis, 2001) led the American Psychological Association's Division 29 (Psychotherapy) Task Force on Psychotherapy Relationships to conclude that evidence is "insufficient to make a clear judgment" about specific recommendations regarding psychotherapy relationships based on clients' attachment style (Ackerman et al., 2001, p. 496). From a "beyond a reasonable doubt" standpoint, this conclusion is probably still warranted today and probably reflects the fact that research on attachment and adult psychotherapy is still nascent.

However, appropriate scientific caution does not release therapists from their obligation to make tough decisions. Although we ourselves (the authors of this chapter) are researchers, we are also practitioners who work with adult outpatients suffering considerable emotional distress resulting from interpersonal problems. Like any practitioner reading this chapter, we have been faced with on the spot demands in a session to make a clinical decision. Often such decisions take the form of either–or dilemmas that are not amenable to the .05 level of certainty. For example, when a client we have been seeing weekly asks for a second session later the same week, the request must either be granted or denied. When a client's disclosure prompts our own feeling of deep empathic sadness, we must decide to make a self-disclosure of this feeling or to let the moment pass. In making these choices, we are especially mindful of the ethical imperative to "above all, do no harm," but we are still faced with the question of whether granting the request for an extra session or making the self-disclosure is likely to be helpful or harmful.

This chapter is written for practitioners whose work with adult outpatients requires them to make choices like these. For them the standard of proof is not "beyond a reasonable doubt," but rather "based on the evidence, which course of action is the best?" To continue with the legal analogy, in civil cases the standard of proof is the "preponderance of the evidence"; that is, given competing versions of events, which among these is the most likely explanation for the observed facts? Often some doubt remains about the chosen version, but after careful consideration, one interpretation is judged to be more plausible than any other. Because therapists make clinical decisions based on the most reasonable interpretation of the evidence, even though they are not certain beyond a doubt, we have also adopted a "preponderance of the evidence" standard in reviewing literature for this chapter. After considering the available evidence, we draw conclusions that, from our perspective, are the most reasonable interpretations of the data. We hope that therapists reading this chapter will find our recommendations helpful, but it is important to remember that there are alternative interpretations of the literature.

A few other caveats are in order. Although the literature on attachment is large, we focus on empirical studies of relatively high-functioning adult clients and, for studies of nonclient samples, on the laboratory and correlational studies that are most directly relevant for psychotherapy processes. We use the term *client* in preference to *patient*, and focus on psychotherapy with relatively high-functioning adult outpatients whose presenting problems include maladaptive patterns of behavior in interpersonal relationships. These patterns need not be the primary presenting problem—indeed, some clients may not list improving their interpersonal relationships among their goals for therapy—but key features of the problem suggest that (1) maladaptive interpersonal patterns significantly contribute to a client's predicament, and (2) adult attachment theory offers a useful framework for case conceptualization and treatment of these maladaptive patterns. Excellent resources have recently become available for readers interested in the applications of attachment theory to clients with pervasive and more debilitating personality disorders than the populations we consider in this chapter (Bateman & Fonagy, 2003; Clarkin & Posner, 2005; Holmes, 2005).

Finally, as we prepared this chapter, two of us were engaged in a qualitative study, informed by the methodology of grounded theory (Charmaz, 2006; Glasser & Strauss, 1967), of how expert therapists use attachment theory in their work with the kinds of clients on whom we focus here. To supplement our review of the quantitative empirical literature, we summarize some of the results of this qualitative study (Daly & Mallinckrodt, 2008). A few words about the methodology are in order.

We began by preparing two case descriptions based on the items from the Avoidance and Anxiety subscales of the Experiences in Close Relationships inventory (Brennan, Clark, & Shaver, 1998). A narrative describing each client was presented in terms reflecting how an intake interviewer might describe a client with a high self-report score on the Avoidance subscale (client "R") or a high score on the Anxiety subscale (client "J"): for example, "R is very uncomfortable opening up to others on a deep personal level, and finds it equally uncomfortable when others begin to get too close.... " or "J has always feared abandonment in relationships and usually experiences a lot of anxiety even at the slightest sign of rejection or loss.... " To avoid adding an extra layer of complexity and length to the interviews, therapists were not asked how they might work with a client scoring high on both Avoidance and Anxiety. Neither vignette made reference to the gender of the client, thus freeing the therapists to "adapt the scenario to the circumstances you experience most frequently in your practice."

Therapists were presented with written copies of both case descriptions and informed they should assume that neither client had experienced sexual or physical abuse, that neither had any organic neurological problems, and that neither had any history or current pattern of substance abuse. They were further told to assume that couple therapy was not an option, that the romantic partners of each clients had been persons of the opposite sex of the clients, and that the clients would finance their own therapy up to a limit of 20 sessions. No preauthorization from an insurance provider would be necessary.

Therapists known to one of us (Brent Mallinckrodt) were contacted in three communities: a large city on the East Coast, and two midsized cities each containing a large university, one in the Midwest and one on the West Coast. The therapists contacted in each community were asked to nominate colleagues whom they considered experts in working with adult outpatients who have problems in close personal relationships. Interviews were then conducted with those therapists who had been nominated as experts by two or more of their colleagues. At the conclusion of the interview, each expert was also asked to nominate colleagues, using the same criteria by which they had been nominated. A total of 12 interviews were completed, transcribed, and analyzed by our qualitative research team.

The clinically rich and informative accounts provided by these expert therapists have been enormously helpful—not only as sources of data in themselves about how they conceptualize cases and work with adult clients who manifest problems with either anxious or avoidant attachment, but also in helping us organize the other literature we reviewed. The interviews generated a total of 96 themes that were classified into eight higher-order categories: (1) conceptualization, (2) client defenses, (3) managing therapeutic boundaries, (4) markers of progress, (5) transference and therapist nontransference reactions, (6) individual interventions, (7) corrective relational patterns, and (8) internal representations and models.

Our interviews suggest that expert therapists think in terms of an initial *engagement* phase of therapy in which they simultaneously gather data and conceptualize a client, while at the same time systematically tailoring the psychotherapy relationship to engage this particular client in therapy. Ideally, this initial phase leads to a *working* phase after certain *transition markers* become evident. The working phase must be followed with careful attention to the dynamics of *termination*. Many readers will recognize similarities in overall sequence of these stages to psychodynamic models of therapy process (e.g., Goldman & Milman, 1978; Weiner, 1998), even though the content differs. In the remainder of this chapter, we use the process model suggested by our interviews—conceptualization, engagement, transition markers, working phase, and termination—to organize our research review and present some of the preliminary findings of our own qualitative study.

CONCEPTUALIZATION

One of the most helpful schemes for conceptualizing relatively high-functioning adults with interpersonal problems is the model of attachment system activation and associated affect regulation strategies proposed by Mikulincer, Shaver, and Pereg (2003; for an overview, see Shaver & Mikulincer, Chapter 2, this volume). According to the model, when adults perceive a sufficiently great threat, their attachment system is activated in much the same way as in infancy. However, adults have a longer history of developmental experiences that influence the next stage of the process—namely, a determination of whether an attachment figure is available and likely to be responsive. If the answer to these questions is "yes," adults will use *security-based* strategies to seek comfort and emotional proximity with an attachment figure. However, adults who appraise their social environment as lacking in available and responsive attachment figures experience a heightened sense of distress and will engage in one of two possible secondary strategies. Those who anticipate that proximity seeking, if exaggerated, may result in at least some measure of felt security are likely to engage in a *hyperactivating* secondary attachment strategy, whereas those who believe that proximity seeking is at best useless and at worst likely to lead to further emotional injury engage in a *deactivating* secondary attachment strategy.

Although these three reactions may be specific, to some degree, to a particular caregiver or situation (especially early in development), Mikulincer et al. (2003) describe a range of mechanisms that tend to ingrain these patterns by early adulthood as habitual, trait-like dispositions. For example, processes of selective attention and increasingly inflexible working models of self and others serve to harden attachment activation patterns that had greater plasticity early in development. In concrete terms, this means that therapists can expect clients to predominantly employ one of these strategies or a mix of the secondary strategies, corresponding to four broadly different types of adult attachment styles, each with a different ingrained pattern of attachment, affect regulation style, and potential vulnerability to a different set of interpersonal problems. (For an in-depth review of each style, see Lopez, Chapter 5, this volume.)

Most important, each attachment strategy requires a different engagement approach in order to lay the foundation for a working alliance that will eventually lead to therapeutic change. Clients who rely predominantly on security-based strategies generally present the fewest challenges for therapists, because they have developed relatively optimistic expectations of self-efficacy and others' responsiveness in the face of distress, and they come to therapy with considerable capacity for affect regulation and for self-reflection that bodes well for therapeutic change (Fonagy, Gergely, Jurist, & Target, 2002). We do not discuss these clients in great detail, because they have developed a capacity for secure attachment to others and to a therapist that presents relatively fewer challenges than the two types of clients on whom we focus.

Clients who rely on hyperactivating strategies present formidable challenges. In Mikulincer et al.'s (2003) model, these individuals have negative beliefs about their ability to cope with distress and expect that others will be inconsistently responsive and available. They tend to score relatively high on self-report measures of anxious attachment. Anxious attachment is associated with rumination and exaggerated appraisal of perceived threat, intense reactions to stressful events, and pervasive fears of abandonment (Mikulincer & Florian, 1998). Experimental research suggests that persons with high attachment anxiety are unable to suppress painful thoughts of separation, even when explicitly instructed to do so, and instead become more alert to their self-perceived weaknesses (Mikulincer, Dolev, & Shaver, 2004). Studies of undergraduates report that the positive association between anxious attachment and self-reported symptoms of distress is mediated by a low capacity for self-reinforcement and a high need for reassurance from others (Wei, Mallinckrodt, Larson, & Zakalik, 2005), emotional reactivity (Wei, Vogel, Ku, & Zakalik, 2005), alexithymia (i.e., low emotional awareness), and the perception of low self-efficacy in social relationships (Mallinckrodt & Wei, 2005).

Clients who rely on deactivating strategies present equally formidable challenges, but of a different nature. Mikulincer et al. (2003) describe these individuals as tending to inflate their self-esteem defensively in the face of attachment threats and to avoid interactions that might involve intimacy or dependency. Under conditions of perceived threat, their secondary strategy involves both conscious and unconscious efforts to suppress attachment-related thoughts and feelings in an effort to avoid heightened distress. These individuals have relatively high scores on self-report measures of avoidant attachment. Studies based on self-reports of undergraduates have found that the association between attachment-related avoidance and self-reported symptoms of distress is mediated by the tendency to suppress emotional experience (Wei, Vogel, et al., 2005).

Experimental studies suggest that persons with high attachment avoidance do not initially encode into memory attachment-related material as well as others, although their rate of forgetting material once it is encoded is no higher than that for nonavoidant persons (Fraley, Garner, & Shaver, 2000). Experimental research also suggests that avoidant individuals are actually able to reduce physiological arousal when they suppress thoughts of attachment, rather than merely masking distress or denying it in self-reports (Fraley & Shaver, 1997). However, more recent experimental research suggests that the capacity to suppress thoughts about a previous painful separation tends to break down when cognitive resources are otherwise taxed, resulting in a rebound of suppressed thoughts about separation and heightened access to negative self-evaluations (Mikulincer et al., 2004). Avoidant individuals also have a tendency to project unwanted self-traits onto others (Mikulincer & Horesh, 1999). Similar to the self-reports of persons scoring high on attachment-related anxiety, avoidant individuals' self-reports of distress tend to be mediated by alexithymia (i.e., low emotional awareness) and the perception of low self-efficacy in social relationships (Mallinckrodt & Wei, 2005).

Although there is now a considerable body of experimental and correlational research to differentiate the three variations in attachment activation described by Mikulincer et al. (2003) in the general population, much less is known about how clients might exhibit these strategies in the initial sessions of psychotherapy. However, some indication may be found in the factor analysis that Mallinckrodt, Gantt, and Coble (1995) used to develop the 36-item Client Attachment to Therapist Scale (CATS). In this study of over 130 clients, three factors emerged that appear to parallel the security-based, hyperactivating, and deactivating strategies described in research with nonclients. The highest-loading five items from each subscale are shown in Table 10.1.

The first factor comprises perceptions of the therapist as supportive, responsive, and dependable, and as providing a secure base for exploration. The second CATS factor taps clients' reluctance to self-disclose; perceptions of the therapist as disapproving and easily rejecting; and negative "self-conscious" feelings about therapy, including shame and humiliation (Lewis & Wolan Sullivan, 2005). These client characteristics are consistent with the research literature on individuals who rely on deactivating attachment strategies. The third CATS factor involves clients' wishes for boundary-crossing merger or constant contact with the therapist, which seem quite compatible with the strong dependency needs of clients who rely on hyperactivating attachment strategies.

Studies of clients have shown that the CATS subscales are significantly associated with the working alliance and with clients' self-reports of their object relations capacity (Mallinckrodt et al., 1995; Mallinckrodt, Porter, & Kivlighan, 2005). A study using the CATS with 51 client–therapist dyads reported that clients' memories of fathers as inconsistent were positively associated with scores on the Preoccupied/Merger subscale, whereas memories of mothers as cold were positively associated with scores on the Avoidant-Fearful subscale. Therapists' perceptions of negative client transference were positively associated with scores on both the Secure and the Preoccupied/Merger CATS subscales (Woodhouse, Schlosser, Crook, Ligiero, & Gelso, 2003). The authors interpreted the somewhat surprising find-

---

TABLE 10.1. Selected Items of the Client Attachment to Therapist Scale (CATS)

Factor 1: Secure
1. I don't get enough emotional support from my counselor.*
2. My counselor is sensitive to my needs.
3. My counselor is dependable.
4. I feel that somehow things will work out OK for me when I am with my counselor.
5. My counselor isn't giving me enough attention.*

Factor 2: Avoidant-Fearful
6. I think my counselor disapproves of me.
7. Talking over my problems with my counselor makes me feel ashamed or foolish.
8. I know I could tell my counselor anything and s/he would not reject me.*
9. I don't like to share my feelings with my counselor.
10. I feel humiliated in my counseling sessions.

Factor 3: Preoccupied/Merger
11. I yearn to be "at one" with my counselor.
12. I wish my counselor could be with me on a daily basis.
13. I would like my counselor to feel closer to me.
14. I'd like to know more about my counselor as a person.
15. I think about calling my counselor at home.

Note. Adapted from Mallinckrodt, Gantt, and Coble (1995). Copyright 1995 by the American Psychological Association. Adapted by permission. * indicates a reverse-keyed item.

ing of a connection between the Secure subscale and negative transference as perhaps indicating that a certain degree of attachment security may be necessary for clients to express their negative feelings of transference.

Whether or not the expert therapists we interviewed (Daly & Mallinckrodt, 2008) explicitly used terms derived from the CATS, most conceptualized clients' initial presentations with regard to hyperactivation or deactivation of their attachment systems. Another concept discussed explicitly by most of these therapists (and implied by the others) was the concept of engagement and alliance formation as a corrective emotional experience. They described their primary goals for the engagement phase of therapy as beginning the process of helping a client form a secure attachment that he or she had rarely, if ever, known previously. This secure attachment could then become the basis for a transformative experience of psychotherapeutic change. These experts described their work in terms of continually monitoring and managing what we term *therapeutic distance* in their unfolding relationship with a client. Although not all of the 12 clinicians used this phrase, each described some variation of the concept. Some described it with such terms as *level of intimacy, self-disclosure, gratification of needs, boundaries,* or *depth* of the work.

Embodied in the concept of decreasing therapeutic distance is the notion of increasing transparency and disclosure—from both client and therapist—and strengthening the bond aspect of the working alliance. Clients who seek very low levels of therapeutic distance tend to have high dependency needs, a limited capacity to function autonomously, and a tendency to push limits and cross appropriate boundaries in the relationship. Thus it is apparent that the construct of therapeutic distance, as described by the expert therapists interviewed in the Daly and Mallinckrodt (2008) study, is composed of a mixture of component strands with positive and negative valence. More importantly, for each client there is an optimal therapeutic distance that characterizes healthy functioning in the psychotherapy relationship, as well as a level of therapeutic distance that the client initially seeks to establish in the early sessions but is typically not the level the therapist views as ultimately optimal.

For clients who employ security-based strategies, the levels of initial and optimal therapeutic distance are not far apart. Generally, therapists and clients in these dyads are able to enter a mutual partnership indicative of a secure attachment and are able to close the gap between initial and ideal distance relatively quickly. However, clients who employ hyperactivating strategies begin therapy with a desire for much less therapeutic distance than is optimal, whereas clients who employ deactivating strategies seek to maintain far more therapeutic distance than is ideal. For both kinds of clients, the gap between the initial level of therapeutic distance and the optimal level is very wide indeed. Furthermore, because a secure client–therapist attachment is difficult to establish, the process of closing this gap is often long and difficult.

Thus the process of change described by the experts we interviewed (Daly & Mallinckrodt, 2008) requires that therapists (1) continually monitor the therapeutic distance sought by a given client; (2) recognize the optimal distance in the psychotherapy relationship that would represent a corrective emotional experience for this client; and, finally, (3) engage in an active and carefully planned effort to manage the psychotherapy relationship so as to close the gap between 1 and 2. At each stage, this process is informed by attachment theory, especially by an understanding of the dynamics of attachment hyperactivation and deactivation. In Figure 10.1 we have summarized our view of this process, gleaned from a review of the empirical literature and from the Daly and Mallinckrodt (2008) interviews with expert therapists.

Clients with high attachment-related anxiety have a strong tendency to hyperactivate their attachment systems. In the initial sessions, they seek to shrink therapeutic distance to a degree that is much closer than optimal. The tendency of some of these clients to push boundaries in the engagement phase of therapy is represented in the upper left-hand portion of Figure 10.1 by placing the "C" symbol for these clients immediately adjacent (or even intruding across) the vertical line indicating the midpoint of optimal therapeutic distance. In these circumstances, if a therapist insists on maintaining his or her share of the optimal therapeutic distance, indicated by the "X" on the continuum, few hyperactivating clients are able to tolerate the resulting frustration. Instead, an expert therapist takes deliberate steps to reduce ther-

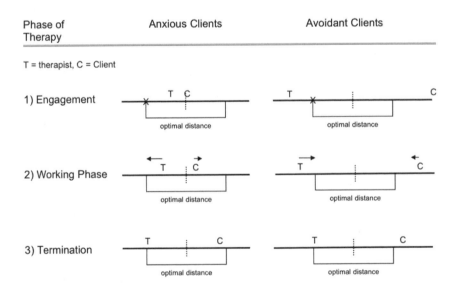

FIGURE 10.1. The process of change in therapy from an attachment-theoretical perspective.

apeutic distance in the early work, symbolized by the right-pointing arrow. The "T" indicates the therapist's initial stance, which involves gratifying some client needs in the early sessions and establishing a closeness that the therapist knows would not be optimal in the long term but is necessary at the outset to engage an anxiously attached client.

Once these clients have been sufficiently engaged, the beginnings of an increasingly secure psychotherapeutic attachment emerge. Transitional markers make their appearance, signaling that therapists can begin the working phase by gradually increasing their portion of the therapeutic distance (left-pointing arrow). Ideally, clients respond with a reciprocal—though usually somewhat lesser—increase in their own contribution to the therapeutic distance (smaller right-pointing arrow). Rarely is the work as smooth as the middle section of Figure 10.1 implies. Anxious clients, fearing abandonment, often make bids to close therapeutic distance. New stresses in their lives precipitate setbacks. Therapists may need to reverse course temporarily. However, when things go well, the process of change generally follows the pattern of gradually increasing therapeutic distance as shown in Figure 10.1. The prospect of termination presents a fresh set of challenges, but ideally when the work is finished, the therapist can consistently maintain an optimal level of therapeutic distance. The "C" for anxious clients is shown slightly inboard of the optimal distance at termination, to represent an acknowledgment that these clients may always retain some tendency toward hyperactivation and anxious attachment.

For clients with a highly avoidant attachment style, who have a strong tendency to deactivate their attachment systems, the right-hand column of Figure 10.1 depicts the usual process. Initially, these clients seek to maintain a much greater therapeutic distance than would be optimal. A therapist who insists on maintaining an optimal distance ("X" on the continuum) early in treatment will create considerable discomfort in these clients. (Note the paradox: The optimal therapeutic distance tends to produce tension and discomfort in avoidant clients, whereas it tends to produce frustration for anxious clients.) To engage clients who tend to deactivate their attachment systems, a therapist must take an initial stance that is more distant than will ultimately be best (left-pointing arrow). After these clients are sufficiently engaged and transitional markers appear, the working phase involves a gradual approach by the therapist that narrows the therapeutic distance. Ideally, the clients reciprocate, although their approach is not likely to match the therapist's in magnitude. Again, the process is by no means a smooth one and may contain a number of approaches and retreats. Ultimately, at termination, the therapist has narrowed the gap so that his or her contribution to the relationship is optimal, although these clients may always function at a distance slightly outside the optimal range, indicating a tendency toward avoidance and deactivation that is never entirely relinquished.

Research investigating the match of client and therapist attachment style provides some support for the model shown in Figure 10.1. A study that categorized 27 outpatients with fairly severe psychopathology and their 18 case managers along dimensions of secure–insecure strategies and preoccupied–dismissing (i.e., hyperactivating–deactivating) strategies also coded the case managers' interventions in terms of depth and responsiveness to clients' dependency needs (Dozier, Cue, & Barnett, 1994). Case managers' insecurity interacted with client attachment strategy, such that insecure, but not secure, managers tended to react with greater depth of intervention as client hyperactivation increased. However, the generalizability of these results is limited because these case managers included seven with only bachelor's-level training, seven who had earned a master's degree in social work or a related field, and four who were working toward a master's degree. It is also not clear whether inferences to other types of psychotherapy can be drawn from the case management interventions examined in this study.

A second study of 21 somewhat more experienced case managers and similar outpatient clients assessed participants on similar dimensions (Tyrrell, Dozier, Teague, & Fallott, 1999). Results suggested that client and case manager deactivation interacted, such that less deactivating case managers formed stronger working alliances with more deactivating clients.

These findings have been interpreted as suggesting that therapists whose own attachment style is noncomplementary to that of their clients have a natural inclination toward providing the type of corrective emotional experience that is best for clients with either attachment-related anxiety or avoidance. Writers have speculated about the benefits of matching clients to therapists on the basis of dissimilar attachment styles (Bernier & Dozier, 2002). We suspect that practical difficulties will prevent this suggestion from ever being widely implemented; more importantly, however, the model we have described suggests that different types of relationships are needed to facilitate change at different points in therapy. For example, even though clients with high attachment-related anxiety may ultimately benefit from interacting with a therapist who resists their bids to become enmeshed, in the initial sessions it will be necessary to gratify some of these needs for proximity. Matching this client with a therapist whose own attachment-related avoidance makes establishing distance easier may not be the best way to facilitate initial engagement.

Instead, our reading of the empirical literature and our synthesis of the Daly and Mallinckrodt (2008) interviews suggests that expert therapists—whatever their own attachment tendencies—have an especially high capacity for flexibility in the relationship conditions they offer to clients. They are able to adjust the "thermostat" of therapeutic distance through a wide range, as the needs of a particular client dictate. Whether attempting to foster more or less distance, they are able to maintain a consistently high level of genuineness through a flexible range of relationships—a quality Lazarus (1993) has termed "being an authentic chameleon (p. 404)." This allows them to work effectively with both hyperactivating and deactivating clients, although, interestingly, many of the expert therapists expressed a preference for working with one type over the other.

We are aware that thus far, our discussion of client conceptualization and the presentation of our theoretical model have remained at a highly abstract level. In the next sections, we discuss concretely what therapists do to increase or decrease therapeutic distance as they engage, enter the working phase, and terminate therapy with clients who have strong tendencies toward either attachment system hyperactivation or deactivation. Fortunately, the therapists we interviewed shared a great deal of their hard-won clinical wisdom.

ENGAGEMENT

The expert therapists in the Daly and Mallinckrodt (2008) interviews emphasized the importance of initially engaging clients with high attachment-related anxiety by "giving more" than they might with other clients. Hyperactivating clients require reassurance and repeated evidence of the therapist's positive regard. Clients' anxiety may be alleviated by therapists' disclosing about their experience of a session and feelings toward the clients. As clients begin to divulge more aspects of themselves that are shameful or unacceptable, it becomes especially important for therapists to reassure them that these disclosures strengthen rather than weaken the developing relationship. Several therapists revealed that they typically set less strict boundaries—but boundaries nonetheless—in the initial sessions with these clients. The therapists sense that these clients are less able to tolerate a level of withholding that would be appropriate for other clients, and at a point later in therapy will be more appropriate for these clients as well.

Therapists were quick to add that any decision to gratify these clients' needs must be carefully considered and may well represent the beginnings of a "slippery slope" that will need to be halted with stricter limit setting later in the work. Therapists acknowledged that in these early sessions, they may well be colluding in clients' maladaptive patterns of managing anxiety. However, some degree of collusion is necessary until such clients develop alternative, more adaptive ways of regulating affect and meeting their own needs. The expert therapists spoke in terms of building a "temporary bridge," and of "intentionally" rather than impulsively deciding to grant the implicit request of these clients for a decrease in therapeutic distance.

Expert clinicians emphasized that the initial engagement phase of therapy is crucial precisely because the diminished capacity for secure attachment (i.e., having access to and using security-based strategies) in both hyperactivating and deactivating clients is fundamental to their interpersonal problems, and at the same time presents considerable obstacles to forming a productive working alliance. Many of our expert informants spoke of how they monitored the initial sessions for signs of how clients might be projecting onto the relationship expectations developed from their earlier interactions with attachment figures. Some therapists believed that this tendency requires early and frequent discussions about the relationship as a way to promote engagement, especially with clients who manifest high attachment-related anxiety.

Discussions of how these clients feel toward the therapist and about the relationship serve to engage clients, particularly if they are also invited to reveal any disappointments about the therapist or fears of rejection in these early sessions. Several therapists mentioned that anxious clients tend to be relatively easier to engage in the beginning, but may pose greater challenges later, when their idealization of the therapist is inevitably shattered. Discussing negative feelings toward the therapist in the early sessions tends to blunt idealization and sets the stage for a crucial task that is to follow—namely, working through feelings of frustration and disappointment with the therapist as well as other attachment figures. Many anxious clients find consistency and some level of structure in a session reassuring; for example, a therapist could begin each session with a similar opening question, as well as ending each session in a consistent way (perhaps taking a few minutes to ask clients about their experience of the previous hour).

Many expert therapists believe that one of the most powerful tools for engaging clients with high attachment-related anxiety is for a therapist to directly solicit any negative feelings a client harbors toward the therapist or about something that has happened in a session. Because of their developmental history, hyperactivating clients fear that any criticism of an attachment figure risks the dissolution of the relationship. Thus therapists who solicit criticism and respond nondefensively in ways that validate such clients' feelings can create a powerful corrective experience. Clients learn more adaptive and direct ways of handling relationship setbacks and conflict. They also develop a stronger sense that the psychotherapy relationship is not as fragile as they feared. In other words, open dialogues are opportunities for clients to experiment with a security-based strategy for dealing with negative feelings. However, many clients with high attachment-related anxiety will require considerable encouragement and coaching to express any negative feelings toward a therapist. Thus therapists need to be especially vigilant for nonverbal as well as verbal indications that a client is displeased with the ongoing process.

These moments can be acknowledged with a process comment, or a statement of curiosity from the therapist about what the observed behavior may signify. For example, one therapist discussed how he approaches this issue:

> "It needs to be discussed much more openly with a client like J, compared to others—because [clients like J] will say they forgive, but they will hold onto it. It might be okay at the moment, but it almost inevitably, with patients as vulnerable as J, leads to them thinking that I don't

care about them and occasional thoughts of quitting therapy. It surprised me that it was not in your vignette that J has had many therapists because no one is quite good enough. This is just like her relationships; she always needs a therapist, but no work is ever going to be good enough. So we need to constantly be talking about how we are doing. I'm encouraging her to tell me when she thinks I've screwed up, when she thinks I haven't been sensitive enough. We need to continually talk about how things are going between us."

Many of the therapists felt that overt client resistance, such as canceling an appointment or arriving late for a session, provides an invitation for open dialogue regarding the client's reaction to the therapist. A gentle, nonblaming exploration of the meaning of this behavior promotes engagement and makes it less likely that the pattern will be repeated. The following excerpt illustrates what this might look like:

"I think if R and I had a really deep session and [in the next session] R no-showed, I would call ... and say, 'I noticed you didn't come in. What's up?' I would process that with [R] and try and make [R] feel safe enough to come back in. But I would [also] try to prevent that in the session by being connected when the client is feeling vulnerable."

Therapists reported using such interventions to encourage engagement with clients who were high in either attachment-related anxiety or avoidance, although they reported implementing them at different paces, depending on the clients' attachment styles. A tactic for promoting safety and engagement that may be particularly useful for avoidant clients is to allow them considerable control of the topics discussed in early sessions; this may serve to protect them from feeling overwhelmed or pressured to disclose to an extent that might otherwise risk premature termination. Some therapists expressed reticence about proceeding too quickly with initiating open dialogue about the therapeutic relationship with clients high in avoidance. The following excerpt underscores some of the concerns most frequently expressed:

"I guess I would be concerned about not invading him [R]. It would be easy to invade his space, but it is also a delicate balance because you don't want to be avoidant yourself, because then you just have an avoidant pair. So I would want to be trying to move in, but be empathically aware of when I'm going too far."

Establishing rapport and promoting engagement must be a gradual process for avoidant clients, because a distinguishing feature of their attachment style is discomfort with closeness and with the intimacy that effective therapy requires. Another therapist commented:

"They're uncomfortable opening up and unable to depend on someone. In a sense, their very issue is what's going to happen in therapy—if therapy goes right. They're going to open up to me; they're going to feel deeply connected; at some stage in therapy they're going to feel dependent. And so the tricky thing is to not push that too fast, I think, because that could scare them away."

Avoidant clients may find talking about emotions and relationship issues a rather aversive experience. Therapists described increasing engagement with avoidant clients by continually monitoring signs of anxiety or discomfort, and by being sensitive to indications that a client was reaching the limits of her or his tolerance for decreased therapeutic distance. When this limit is approached, therapists spoke of "slowing the pace." In early sessions therapists often permitted the dialogue to remain superficial or intellectualized, thus allowing clients to retain a sense of safety. Consider this example:

"I can think of clients I've worked with who are avoidant, and their avoidance is manifested partly through intellectualization as a defense. These are people who live in their heads. ... one of the ways of engaging them is to do a little bit of that. Maybe talk about things that are intellectual. If they're talking about philosophy, rather than move away from this because you're being too intellectualized, maybe doing a little bit of that. I think this creates a rapport that you are in a 'similar enough tribe,' if you will. It's sort of sidling up to the patient to an extent, and that could be engaging. Now, if you go too far, then you've lost the game, I think."

Another example of a tactic that therapists endorsed for engaging both hyperactivating and deactivating clients—but one that required more gradual pacing for deactivating clients—was the practice of involving them in a spirit of mutual curiosity about the clients' history, feelings, and sources of motivation. Here is an example:

"I try to engage them in being curious about themselves. Then we can start to connect around the curiosity about him, my curiosity and interest and his, in a way that can begin to allow him to absorb himself."

Other therapists spoke about developing a mutual collaboration with the client to join forces to work at defeating the client's pain. One therapist explained:

"For me, the metaphor is sort of like the suicidal client. If clients tell you they're suicidal, then there's a small piece of them that wants you to stop them, and so [I focus on connecting] to that part. [For a client with attachment problems,] there's a huge part … that wants to depend on someone, that wants a relationship, that wants to feel safe in a relationship—or else [the client] would not be coming into therapy about this. So I would really work hard to access that part of what has been painful for the person in this pattern, and really try to talk to and reach the part that wants things to be different."

Presenting a client with the metaphor of fighting as allies against his or her pain can be useful, because the client is invited to become an active collaborator in the change process. In addition, this collaboration early in the work establishes a pattern quite different from anything the client may have known. Adults with either anxious or avoidant attachment patterns often have a history with caregivers who were unavailable, inconsistent, or hurtful in some way. Thus, if a therapist is perceived as a person who is genuinely concerned about a client's well-being, allying and empathizing with the client can be a healing experience. Another way of looking at the "fighting as allies" metaphor is that the client is invited to connect with a painful past experience but—unlike in the past—to use more security-based strategies to process the experience and regulate affect.

Instillation of hope is another intervention used to promote engagement by the therapists we interviewed (Daly & Mallinckrodt, 2008). Helping clients envision what they would like to see change and how relationships could potentially look different following therapy is a powerful incentive that can increase engagement. This may enable a therapist to connect with the part of a client that is in pain and wants to experience closeness with others or wants to feel comfortable alone. Some therapists reported using more tangible means of expressing their belief that change is possible—for instance, drawing a continuum on a 3 × 5 note card that depicts a beginning with the client's current issues and an endpoint of what he or she would like to achieve. This emphasis in the early sessions on eventual outcomes is another way that therapists can engage clients by showing a high level of interest and an eagerness to help clients achieve desired goals. Emphasizing final goals may be especially important for avoidant clients, because this concrete conversation in the beginning of therapy paves the way for subsequent discussions of the more abstract (and frightening) session-level tasks that will be necessary to achieve these goals.

Finally, a crucial aspect of the engagement process (and subsequent phases of therapy), according to the experts interviewed in the Daly and Mallinckrodt (2008) study, is a therapist's capacity to manage the strong affective reactions that hyperactivating or deactivating clients can engender, together with the strong "pulls" these clients exert to replicate dysfunctional interpersonal patterns. Slade (1999) has speculated that avoidant clients deny the therapist a meaningful personal connection, just as they were once denied closeness and intimacy in their own childhood. The "impermeability" of the narratives that avoidant clients tell about their relationships, their rigid inflexibility, their interpersonal aloofness, and their rejection of bids for empathic connection leave the therapist "caught in the same barren landscape" as the clients, and left feeling much as the clients once felt as children: "angry, unacknowledged, silly, and inept" (p. 588). In contrast, hyperactivating clients can focus tremendous energy on efforts to have the therapist take care of them and ease their sense of emotional confusion. Because a true mutual collaboration is all but impossible in the early sessions with these clients, their overwhelming dependency leaves the therapist feeling much the way the clients felt as children: swamped, angry, helpless, confused, and dysregulated" (p. 588).

Not surprisingly, then, expert therapists reported intense countertransference to clients high in either attachment-related anxiety or avoidance. Frustration and boredom emerged as examples of fairly frequent reactions to avoidant clients. As one therapist explained:

"I have to watch out for feeling really frustrated and becoming disengaged from the work. You know, chatting and abstract disclosures are difficult to engage with—they are too far away. And his presentation may keep me away from the interesting stuff, so I may even experience boredom."

On the other hand, many therapists asserted that it was relatively easy for them to empathize and connect with avoidant clients, because they conceptualized the avoidant clients they work with as more closely resembling the fearful attachment style (high in both attachment-related anxiety and avoidance) than the dismissing style (high in avoidance but low in anxiety). Thus therapists were able to concentrate on the part of avoidant clients that deeply yearns for a real connection, despite the fear of rejection or hurt typical of previous relationships. The following excerpt captures this kind of reaction:

"My countertransference is very maternal. This is a very wonderful client for me to work with, because it is very clean and clear to understand what the person needs. There is a lot of tenderness in my work with this kind of client."

Frustration was a common response that emerged in therapists' work with clients high in attachment-related anxiety. One therapist noted:

"It frustrates me, but I understand that this is the nature of the work. They are not frustrating me out of any sense of meanness. They have been terribly hurt early in life and are always testing the world to see who else is going to hurt them."

Unlike reactions to clients high in avoidance, where the relationship evolves at a slower pace that can produce boredom, therapists said they often felt the need to brace themselves for the intensity of relationships with clients high in anxiety. Many therapists underscored the importance of knowing themselves and their boundaries so that they did not react with anger to the incessant demands of anxious clients. One therapist explained how she responds to the intensity of an anxious client:

> "I think J would come to really be intense with me and have our relationship be really, really, really important, and I would have to not be afraid of that. I would have to be able to engage and really connect, but not merge and keep my own boundaries. And let them know I really do care. I really would have to be one of the people who fill their hole. I mean, we talk about 're-parenting' sometimes in therapy. I think there may be a stage where J wants me to fill his hole, and I'd have to not run away from that. I'd have to really stay okay with that. And know that it was part of the process and not be freaked out by it."

TRANSITION MARKERS

Engagement involves the gradual development of a sufficiently firm therapeutic alliance to allow the difficult work of change to begin. As the engagement phase comes to a close, the avoidant/deactivating client's fears of intimacy and vulnerability in the therapeutic relationship, and the anxious/hyperactivating client's fears of the therapist's abandonment and rejection, have been sufficiently contained for a new phase of the therapy to begin. The expert therapists we interviewed (Daly & Mallinckrodt, 2008) described beginning the process depicted in the middle row of Figure 10.1—namely, developing a closer relationship with avoidant clients, or introducing more distance and insisting on a more autonomous relationship with anxious clients. But how do therapists know when to safely begin this new phase of the work? In our interviews, the expert therapists described the emergence of signals that indicated when each type of client was now ready for this more intensive phase of therapy. We term these signals *transition markers*.

Therapists stressed the idiosyncratic nature of transition markers, but nevertheless four general themes cut across the interviews: (1) The client makes a commitment to change; (2) the client reports some behavioral change outside sessions; (3) the client develops tolerance for deeper and more intense affect in sessions; and (4) the client evinces a capacity to "do the work of therapy." With regard to the first theme, from a stages-of-change standpoint (Prochaska & DiClemente, 1983), the client has moved from the stage of *precontemplation* or *contemplation* to the *preparation* stage, which features a firm commitment to change; also, although there is as yet little movement toward achieving the primary goals, some of the component changes required for these larger goals have begun to occur. From the standpoint of the working alliance, the bond has been reasonably established, and there is initial agreement about the goals and tasks of therapy (Gelso & Carter, 1994).

With regard to changes outside of therapy, clients high in attachment-related anxiety report an increase in their ability to regulate affect independently of the therapist, an increasing repertoire of self-soothing skills, and at least some increase in autonomous coping ability. One therapist explained:

> "You're feeling a good bond with the person, a good alliance, a real relationship. And the person is at work—not that he has good feelings towards everything or you, but he's working on understanding and invested in understanding. So it's two things: the person doing the work of therapy, which from my vantage point concerns the patient's understanding, and outside of treatment it involves changing behavior and feeling better."

Among the in-session transition markers mentioned by therapists is an increase in clients' ability to experience and effectively process more intense affect in the session. For avoidant clients, this may take the form of a willingness to approach feelings and allow an experience of affect instead of only an intellectualized examination. Conversely, for anxious clients, the intense experience of affect is coupled with a decreased fear of being overwhelmed and an increased capacity for insight and introspection.

Another sign of progress that many therapists mentioned is evidence that a client is emotionally affected by a therapist—for example, a negative reaction, such as feeling rejected or angered by the therapist's absence. Evidence of positive influence includes reports of feeling comforted between sessions or recalling an in-session experience or something the therapist has said. Of course, a client's disclosures of a therapist's influence present new opportunities to discuss the therapy relationship, how it is evolving, and what it has come to mean for both client and therapist.

Examples of demonstrating an ability to do the work of therapy include an avoidant client's capacity to engage in a sustained discussion about the ongoing therapy relationship—even occasionally initiating such a discussion, or speculating about the possibility that patterns occurring with significant others might also be influencing the relationship with the therapist. Such discussions may come more naturally to clients high in attachment-related anxiety, because they are preoccupied by their relationship to the therapist. However, therapists observed that the capacity to engage in more productive introspection develops for both anxious and avoidant clients only after they have developed more effective affect regulation skills. Fonagy et al. (2002) have described a cluster of skills they term the capacity to *mentalize* (see Jurist & Meehan, Chapter 4, this volume). At the core of these skills is a self-reflective capacity to understand one's own behavior and the behavior of others in terms of changing mental states. This capacity allows clients to understand the sources of their own motives in interpersonal transactions and to reliably predict others' reactions. Mentalizing is developed through secure attachment early in life and is a key to effective affect regulation (Fonagy et al., 2002). Clients who demonstrate some capacity for mentalizing signal that they may be ready to enter a more difficult phase of therapy.

Some of our expert therapists spoke of testing clients to assess their capacity for doing the work of therapy. For example, because anxious clients frequently externalize and are so focused on having their needs met by others, they tend to overlook their own role in maintaining painful interactions. Therapists may redirect the focus of these clients' stories back to themselves, to assess their willingness to self-reflect and accept some responsibility for the pattern. Similarly, therapists can test the willingness of avoidant clients to work with affect by assessing their reaction to an empathic reflection of feeling or asking the clients to imagine the feelings that motivate the behavior of important others in their lives. If, rather than immediately dismissing the redirection, a client tentatively accepts the reflection and elaborates on it, this could be taken as a signal that more in-depth affective work may be possible.

Taken together, these transition markers can be considered indicators that a secure therapeutic attachment is in the making. Bowlby (1988, p. 71) placed particular emphasis on the therapist's serving as a secure base as a requisite for successful therapy. He stressed that perceived threat is incompatible with exploration for both infants and adults. However, when a sufficiently secure therapeutic attachment has been formed, an adult client is able to use the presence of the therapist and the comparative safety of the session to quell perceptions of threat. Bowlby believed that under these conditions clients can examine and eventually integrate previously warded-off experiences, which include unresolved past traumatic events, but also feelings in the here and now about the therapist. Although few of the experts interviewed by Daly and Mallinckrodt (2008) explicitly mentioned the term *secure base,* it is clear that the transition markers they described are evidence, in attachment-theoretical terms, that the client has begun to use the therapist as (1) a valued target for proximity seeking, (2) a safe haven when threats are perceived, and (3) a secure base for exploration. (See also Farber & Metzger, Chapter 3, this volume.)

At least 4 of the 14 items of the CATS Secure subscale tap the secure-base aspect of the relationship: "I feel that somehow things will work out OK for me when I am with my counselor," "My counselor helps me to look closely at the frightening or troubling things that have happened to me," "My counselor is a comforting presence to me when I am upset," and "I know my counselor will understand the things that bother me" (Mallinckrodt et al., 1995, p. 317). Client scores on the secure subscale between the 4th and 8th sessions of 12-session time-limited therapy were strongly and positively associated with depth of exploration in a session (Mallinckrodt et al., 2005), providing support for Bowlby's conclusions about the value of the therapist as a secure base for clients' exploration. Perhaps scores on the CATS Secure subscale above a minimum threshold, or simply clients' general agreement with the four items that assess secure-base perceptions of the therapist, could be taken as an additional indicator that the working phase of the therapy can begin.

WORKING PHASE

In her seminal chapter on attachment and psychotherapy, Slade (1999) wrote that attachment theory "*informs* rather than *defines* intervention and clinical thinking" (p. 577; emphasis in original) and that a manualized attachment-based therapy for individual psychotherapy with adults does not yet exist. We interpret this comment as suggesting that a "cookbook" list of techniques and proscriptive directives is not likely to emerge from the application of attachment theory to psychotherapy. However, instead of a definitive series of linked statements (e.g., "If the client does X, the therapist should respond with Y"), attachment theory can provide a rich description of a range of options that are likely to be effective. In this sense the guidance offered by attachment theory to therapists is more like a jazz chord progression than a musical score for a chamber quartet.

Thus it is perhaps not surprising that the remarkable agreement we (Daly & Mallinckrodt, 2008) observed in expert therapists' descriptions of conceptualization and engagement disappeared in these clinicians' idiosyncratic descriptions of treatment interventions and specific techniques. Indeed, although the therapists described in detail how concepts from attachment theory guide the formation of their relationships with clients, many of the 12 experts interviewed were reluctant to describe any specific techniques they use in the working phase. Some of them felt that the individual circumstances of each client render meaningless any discussion of techniques that should be used with a hypothetical "typical" client with an anxious or avoidant attachment style. Therefore, readers seeking a guide for "what to do when with whom" may be disappointed in this section.

However, a clear theme that emerged throughout the interviews was the idea that at least a minimal level of security in the client–therapist attachment is a necessary precursor for implementing techniques at this stage. Furthermore, work to deepen and broaden the quality of therapeutic attachment was viewed by many experts as a core component of facilitating change. Therapists described how in the working phase they gradually withdraw the considerable amount of direct support they have been providing to anxious clients in the engagement phase.

For example, whereas a therapist may have initially responded to clients in emotional crisis with a very problem-focused, highly directive intervention, in the working phase the same therapist may begin by asking clients in crisis to first generate their own possibilities for a solution. For clients high in attachment-related anxiety, careful monitoring of their fears of abandonment and tolerance for frustration is necessary. Like withdrawing control rods from a nuclear reactor, a precipitous movement could result in "meltdown," whereas gradual increments of withdrawal lead to clients' steadily growing confidence in their ability to function more autonomously. In contrast to this process of slowly fostering more self-reliance for anxious clients, therapists described the working phase with clients who exhibit high attachment-related avoidance as involving gradual insistence on reducing therapeutic distance—that is, insisting on less superficiality and less intellectualization, together with more in-session emotional experience and discussion of affect. Careful monitoring of these clients' tolerance for vulnerability and fears of intimacy is required. Gradual increments of emotional connection with the therapist lead to the clients' steadily growing capacity for mutually satisfying relationships with others.

In essence, an important goal for the working phase for both types of clients—and the chief goal for some therapists we (Daly & Mallinckrodt, 2008) interviewed—is to develop a secure attachment in which clients are able to meet their needs consistently through security-based strategies of attachment, rather than relying on either hyperactivating or deactivating strategies to regulate affect or meet their interpersonal needs (Mikulincer et al., 2003). This is the core feature of the corrective emotional experience. Students who are first exposed to these concepts often question how a corrective emotional experience in only one relatively temporary relationship, even when this relationship is the most secure possible attachment to a therapist, can overcome hundreds of negative interactions with others and decades of time that have solidified maladaptive patterns in a client. When teaching beginning practicum students, one of us (Brent Mallinckrodt) uses the following allegory to illustrate:

> "Once there was a starving peasant who passed a large gnarled tree on her way to work in the fields each day. One evening on her way home, in hunger and desperation, she reached up and thrust her hand deep into a hollow high up in this tree. The recess was so high and so deep that she could not see what lay inside, but she had caught a whiff of something sweet, and so great was her hunger that her need overcame her fear. To her great dismay, as she reached inside, her hand was stabbed with painful splinters. The next evening, still driven by hunger, she again desperately groped in the hollow recess for anything that might sustain her. This time her hand was pierced by thorns. On the next occasion she was stung by bees. After dozens of similar painful and disappointing encounters, what impression would the peasant form about this tree? About all hollow trees? If this were her only experience, it would certainly be understandable if she concluded that such trees are dangerous and should be always be avoided.
>
> "But consider how the outcome would be different if, on what she vowed would be her last attempt, she reached into the hollow this

time slowly and carefully, and on this occasion she discovered the bees' honey and was neither stung nor injured in any way. Wouldn't just this one countervailing experience completely change her thinking about the tree and about the possibilities of trying yet again? Even if she were stung or occasionally injured on subsequent tries, her *conception* of the tree would be changed forever. She might even learn the patience to consistently reach inside slowly. She might teach herself how to avoid bees by using a ladder and a torch to see more clearly inside and dislodge them with smoke. In time, she might even seek out other hollow trees, trusting in her ability to cope with the dangers in order to reap the rewards."

Such is the power of the corrective experience of secure attachment with a therapist to provide a single countervailing example that begins to break up clients' monolithic negative thinking about attachment and rigid patterns of interacting with others.

The interviewed therapists emphasized that the process of building a secure therapeutic relationship is not linear. Many described the unavoidable rough patches of alliance breaches and repairs in the struggle to form a secure attachment with these clients as an essential part of the process of change itself. Research suggests that strains in the relationship are inevitably brought about when therapists initially fail to respond as clients had hoped, but that these alliance ruptures can be repaired by validating clients' feelings of hurt and disappointment, and by responding nondefensively and effectively to these secondary reactions. Such repairs may even leave the relationship stronger, or in attachment terms "more secure," than before (Safran & Muran, 1996; Safran, Muran, Samstag, & Stevens, 2001).

In addition to establishing a secure attachment and healing inevitable alliance ruptures, more recent research suggests other possible goals for the working phase of therapy, based on a study of variables that mediate the relationship between attachment anxiety or avoidance and psychological distress. It must be stressed that this relatively new area of research has only examined *statistical mediation*—that is, circumstances in which a significant proportion of the association between an attachment variable X and an indicator of symptoms or distress Y can be accounted for by an intervening mediating variable M that is associated with both X and Y. In theory, X causes M, and M in turn causes Y; in practice, because most of these studies collect data at only one time point, these strong causal inferences cannot be fully supported. However, findings of statistical mediation suggest at least potential targets for intervention.

Among the mediators identified so far, this correlational research suggests that persons with high attachment-related anxiety may be helped by interventions that reduce their need for reassurance from others (Wei, Mallinckrodt, et al., 2005) and their tendency toward high emotional reactivity (Wei, Vogel, et al., 2005). This research also suggests that avoidant persons may be helped by interventions that reduce their tendency to cut off emotional experience (Wei, Vogel, et al., 2005). Finally, these studies suggest that both avoidant and anxious individuals may be helped by interventions that reduce maladaptive perfectionism (Wei, Heppner, Russell, & Young, 2006; Wei, Mallinckrodt, Russell, & Abraham, 2004), increase the capacity for self-reinforcement (Wei, Mallinckrodt, et al., 2005), increase emotional self-awareness and a sense of self-efficacy in close relationships (Mallinckrodt & Wei, 2005), and enhance the ability to cope with distress (Wei, Heppner, & Mallinckrodt, 2003).

Some of the pioneering research on attachment and psychotherapy investigated the connection between attachment styles and responses to treatment. Horowitz, Rosenberg, and Bartholomew (1993) used the interpersonal circumplex, formed by the two orthogonal dimensions of dominance versus submissiveness and hostility versus affiliation, to characterize presenting problems of outpatients in brief therapy. An analysis of these interpersonal problems suggested that clients in the dominant/hostile quadrant of the circumplex were the least likely to show improvement in 20-session time-limited treatment. Furthermore, outpatients classified as dismissing in attachment style tended to report interpersonal problems centered in this portion of the circumplex. However, Fonagy et al. (1996) reported that in a sample of inpatients with fairly severe personality disorders, those with a dismissing attachment style tended to respond best to treatment that averaged over 9 months of inpatient hospitalization. A post hoc analysis of archival videotapes used observers to classify the attachment styles of 29 clients who received up to 25 sessions of outpatient therapy (Travis, Binder, Bliwise, & Horne-Moyer, 2001). Results suggested a significant shift from insecure to secure attachment style over the course of therapy. Attachment security did not predict better therapeutic outcomes as measured by the Symptom Checklist 90, although improvement in scores on the Global Assessment Scale did differ by attachment type. In a study of interpersonal psychotherapy Cyranowski et al. (2002) found that clients with secure attachment tended to recover from a depressive episode more quickly than clients with a fearful style did. Unfortunately, this small number of studies is as yet insufficient to guide therapists in confidently determining which specific variables may be productive targets of intervention to reduce clients' attachment-related anxiety or avoidance.

TERMINATION

From an attachment perspective, the nature of terminating a therapeutic relationship represents the loss of and separation from an attachment figure (the therapist). The client may perceive this as the end of a stable, safe, and nurturing relationship that he or she has come to rely upon for proximity, comfort, and security. The anticipated loss of a therapeutic relationship is likely to result in feelings of grief and anxiety. In addition, clients anticipate that after termination they will need to face challenges and difficulties on their own, and this may be an additional source of considerable anxiety (Webb, 1985). For most clients, especially those who have experienced losses of significant others or unresolved issues connected with previous relationship endings, the grief, anxiety, and vulnerability they experience when ending work with their therapists are likely to activate some of their previous maladaptive patterns (Bembry & Ericson, 1999).

Paradoxically, the more secure a client's attachment to a therapist has been, the more grief and overwhelming affect he or she may experience as termination nears. This may especially be the case for clients who experience the therapist as their first truly secure adult attachment figure. Under the best of circumstances, even when the work has been quite successful, therapists should anticipate the reemergence of some vestige of the clients' previous hyperactivating or deactivating secondary strategy. Clearly, termination must be approached with great care and skill. However, like all crises, termination holds the potential for considerable client growth as well as potential setbacks.

Because there is always a foreseeable ending for every therapeutic relationship, we believe that, conceptually, all of the work throughout the process should be viewed in terms of preparation for a successful termination. The general task for the termination is to create a more effective, more positive ending experience than the problematic endings the client has experienced in the past. Several of the interviewed therapists emphasized that clients must be prepared for termination from the very beginning of therapy. The following excerpt captures this idea:

> "Even in the beginning, I'm talking about the end. Sometimes my first assignment is to have clients imagine that they have just successfully completed therapy, and then I have them make a list of the ways they are different. I ask them to be specific. I think it works great, because it gives people hope and lets clients know that I believe they can change."

The highly intimate and temporary nature of the therapeutic relationship poses the risk of recapitulating painful experiences of abandonment for clients high in attachment-related anxiety, and risks confirming the belief of clients high in attachment-related avoidance that close attachments are not worth the risk. Such a damaging ending might unravel much of the gains of the previous therapeutic work.

Although some aspects of termination may be applied more generally, therapists can anticipate that reactions to termination will differ substantially between anxious and avoidant clients, just as individuals with these patterns form attachments differently. The therapists we interviewed (Daly & Mallinckrodt, 2008) connected early interactions with caregivers to the strategies children adopted, whether hyperactivating or deactivating, and subsequently related these strategies to relationship functioning in adulthood. Therapists should be keenly aware of any reemergence of the behaviors associated with hyperactivating and deactivating strategies when termination is approaching. After all, these are the coping mechanisms clients developed early in life to help them deal with separation and unmet needs, and they may resurface as the clients are faced with the challenge of the end of the therapeutic relationship.

According to our interviewees, avoidant clients may display a wide array of behaviors as termination nears, such as pulling away from the therapist, minimizing the importance of the relationship, acting critical toward the therapist, and responding negatively to gestures of warmth or empathy. It may be useful to encourage avoidant clients to revisit how they developed these strategies. For instance, a common antecedent may be a parent who was harsh and punitive in response to the expression of emotion. Some therapists find it helpful to reiterate that this relationship is different from the earlier relationship(s), and that expressions of sadness, grief, and anger are appropriate reactions to the loss of an important relationship. Therapists may model such reactions by disclosing their sadness over losing a meaningful relationship with the clients. Reflecting on the clients' growth in terms of their increased receptiveness to connection with others may be comforting, because it instills hope and reaffirms that meaningful connections are worthwhile despite the risk, investment, and sometimes pain inherent in close relationships.

When therapists are preparing anxiously attached clients for termination, a different set of reactions can be expected. These clients have learned to exaggerate their responses in order to increase the likelihood of a desired response, so they may become demanding, unstable, or angry in response to termination. Therapists will want to distinguish the relationship termination from previous endings that were probably traumatic for the clients. In addition, a therapist may want to highlight how a client has changed since the earlier losses. Adopting an empowering and affirming stance that the client has the resilience to continue making positive changes without the assistance of the therapist may help an anxious client to feel more stable. Reframing termination as a change in the relationship, but not an end to the care the therapist feels for the client, may be needed for such a client. Some interviewed therapists reported that they offer a more gradual termination, leaving the possibility of returning to therapy open for their clients. For clients high in attachment-related anxiety, who have often experienced abandonment by attachment figures, this might be yet another way to demonstrate how the therapeutic relationship is different and that endings need not be abrupt or devastating, but can gradually wane over time as the clients develop the skills necessary to function autonomously. The following excerpt illustrates this point:

"When I terminate, it usually starts with meeting once every 2 weeks, then once a month, but I suggest, 'Come back in 2 months and tell me how you're doing.' It's totally what they want, but it's nice to be able to say that if it doesn't feel better, [they can] come back. 'I'm here in town, so if it starts acting up again, come back in.' So it's more of that family doc kind of model. 'This is just a resource in your life now, and I won't ever turn you away.'"

Given the histories of abandonment and mistrust experienced by anxious clients, it is important to prepare them for the end of therapy from the earliest sessions. Talking about the eventual ending provides clients with information and opportunities to process their concerns with their therapist. This also opens a dialogue that is germane to a client's core issues, increasing the possibility for the client to improve in this area and learn to cope with his or her reaction to loss and the absence of important figures. One therapist explained:

"At some point as we get closer and have worries about losing our relationship and having serious feelings, we would talk about that. That's okay if they have concerns about that. I won't try to do things to make that not happen, because that's a growth opportunity for us to find out what their underlying needs are and what's driving it, and this is how we're going to help them get what they need."

For avoidant clients, this discussion should probably be postponed until they show evidence of more comfort in talking about the therapy relationship. However, once these discussions have begun, it is important not to delay introducing the topic of the relationship ending. As clients begin to recognize maladaptive patterns in their relationships, they can be helped to anticipate their own strong reactions as termination nears.

For example, after anxious clients have recognized how their pattern of hyperactivation is manifested with others, the therapist might ask, "How do you suppose your pattern might show up as our work together nears an end?" Similarly, after avoidant clients recognize their deactivating patterns, a therapist might ask them to speculate about how they might be tempted to pull back in the last weeks of working together. Anticipating these patterns makes it less likely that they will be manifested in an unmanageable way during the actual termination phase.

Assuming that a client has been carefully prepared for termination throughout treatment, once the therapist assesses that the client is ready for the work to end (or external events mandate the termination), it is critical to allow the client adequate time to resolve the conflict of separation/individuation associated with the termination. There are no clear guidelines for how many sessions will be sufficient, because of the idiosyncratic attachment needs of each client. However, inexperienced therapists often underestimate how much time will be needed. Thus the halfway point of the work may not be too early for a discussion of termination. It is important to recognize that discussions of the relationship ending need not occupy an entire session. As the termination date nears, these discussions can become more frequent and may occupy a proportionately larger part of the session.

When the therapist and the client agree upon a specific date for the final session, this helps provide needed structure and a clear timeline for a successful termination (Teyber, 2006). Other techniques, such as counting down the number of sessions left for counseling and repeatedly initiating a "check-in" for the client to express any feelings or emotions associated with the upcoming ending, may also be helpful. Forced termination may result in clients' regression and should be handled with extra caution and care (Anthony & Pagano, 1998; Teyber, 2006; Ward, 1984). If the therapist needs to terminate because of external constraints, time limits, or other extratherapeutic reasons, it is important to acknowledge the reasons and the unfinished counseling work, and to invite clients to talk about their emotions and reactions in response to this abrupt ending.

Clients who perceive the termination as a loss or threat are likely to feel angry and abandoned, and to use denial or other defense mechanisms to cope with the anticipated anxiety (Siebold, 1991). It is critical for the therapist to communicate acceptance and validation of clients' feelings in a nondefensive manner. One of our interviewed therapists stated:

> "I would prepare them for termination, and want to walk through that with them, so they don't experience me as abandoning them. There are memories and internal thoughts that I hope to leave them with, so that they don't feel so alone."

Clients are more likely to perceive the termination as a positive transition if the therapist empowers them by allowing adequate time to process their feelings and giving them maximal control and choices during the termination process (Baum, 2005). Therapists can facilitate the process by guiding clients to directly express the emotions aroused by the upcoming termination, and by encouraging them to explore their previous experience of ending relationships, together with the meanings they attach to such endings (Shefler, 2000). Many clients with insecure attachment styles may hold a false expectation that the therapist will not end the treatment if he or she "really cares about me" (Youngren, Alonso, & Nahum, 2000). This belief is likely to be manifested during the termination process. It is important to help clients to understand and accept that termination of a relationship is an inevitable part of life, and that learning to simultaneously separate from and remain connected to significant others is a lifelong task (Teyber, 2006).

Therapists can help to reframe the termination as an opportunity for growth, and as yet another corrective emotional experience that helps to increase clients' confidence and self-efficacy in managing other losses and relationship endings in the future (Baum, 2005; Teyber, 2006). Termination can be described to clients as an opportunity to integrate and consolidate their learning from the previous weeks of therapy, as well as serving as a safe environment to practice the new interpersonal patterns they have developed (Anthony & Pagano, 1998). In addition, the therapist may discuss the meaning and feelings associated with the completion of a meaningful life-enhancing task, what it means to become more independent and autonomous after the termination, and possible ways to celebrate this accomplishment. The goals of a successful termination can be defined as part of a meaningful relationship with a therapist that comes to an end with more closure and resolution than clients have typically experienced. In the terms of the model proposed by Mikulincer et al. (2003), security-based strategies predominate in a successful therapeutic termination, and neither hyperactivation nor deactivation is much in evidence as a secondary strategy. Although clients will feel grief and loss with regard to this ending, and perhaps considerable anger toward the therapist as well, the differences from what happened following previous endings are that clients have ideally developed newfound skills to cope with this affect, and are given an opportunity to process and integrate their reactions. As a result, they leave therapy free to enter new attachment relationships relatively unencumbered by unresolved feelings from a previous ending, and perhaps with greater confidence in their ability to experience closure. For many clients, this will be a new experience of freedom.

Therapists can bring about this type of termination in the last sessions by inviting clients to review and revisit significant topics discussed previously, and to synthesize what they have learned about themselves and about relationships to form a hopeful perspective for the future. A therapist may invite clients to describe a few "critical moments" that occurred during the counseling process—moments at which the clients felt inspired, gained a new insight, or experienced unusual emotional arousal (Ward, 1984). It may be useful to ask clients to examine past endings and to extract the common features of the "best and worst good-byes." With these insights, clients can be encouraged to actively bring about the best features and avoid the worst features of other endings, thereby taking more control of this ending. Clients can be encouraged to identify what they liked best about their relationship with the therapist, and then develop strategies to cultivate these features in other existing relationships, or to seek out new connections in which these relationship qualities can be developed. For many clients, interpersonal group therapy (with a different therapist as facilitator) may provide an ideal opportunity to consolidate skills and continue growth.

Finally, therapists' continued transparency and genuineness through the termination process can be very beneficial to clients. Therapists can share their genuine joy and pleasure at the clients' progress and improvement, as well as their feelings of sadness and loss at the ending of this relationship. Clients should not leave their final session without a clear understanding of whether a therapist will be available to work with them in the future, and/

or what types of future contact with the therapist (or other therapists at the agency) will be possible.

CONCLUSIONS

We have reviewed studies from a broad range of disciplines (including counseling, clinical, social, and developmental psychology) that represent the growing body of research using attachment theory to gain a better understanding of how adult clients change in psychotherapy. A theme that has emerged from these diverse lines of research is the importance of the psychotherapy relationship as a primary catalyst for change. We now have a fairly detailed understanding from laboratory and correlational research of the maladaptive patterns of interaction and affect regulation difficulties experienced by adults with attachment-related avoidance and/or anxiety. This research has identified a growing number of variables that appear to mediate the associations between anxious or avoidant attachment styles and symptoms of distress in nonclinical samples. Relatively less is known about how these patterns manifest themselves in psychotherapy, but a coherent picture is beginning to emerge.

This research suggests that skillful therapists are able to build a psycho-therapy relationship that provides a secure base and safe haven for clients. Secure attachment to a therapist provides a corrective emotional experi-ence through which a client eventually comes to rely more on security-based strategies to regulate affect, and develops more effective social competencies to form satisfying attachments with others (Mallinckrodt, 2001). A crucial element of this corrective experience appears to be the therapist's deliberate regulation of emotional distance in the psychotherapy relationship, so that clients' initial needs (for close involvement in the case of anxious clients, and for distance in the case of avoidant clients) are met sufficiently to engage the clients in therapy. At the close of this initial engagement phase, transitional markers appear, signaling that the working alliance is sufficiently strong and the therapeutic attachment is sufficiently secure to permit more intensive work to commence. Some of the most important of these transition markers may be the first appearance of a client's capacity for productive introspec-tion about relationships, the arousal of intense affect, and the capacity to reflect in the therapy hour about the client–therapist relationship.

In the working phase, the therapist gradually begins to insist on more intimacy from avoidant clients and more independence from anxious ones. This regulation of therapeutic distance fosters a new kind of corrective expe-rience, in which clients eventually develop more reliable capacities for affect regulation and secure attachment to people outside therapy. Therapists nominated by their peers as experts in working with adult interpersonal problems report that this working phase of therapy poses significant chal-lenges and requires continual monitoring of a client's level of engagement, anxiety, and frustration, as the relationship is gradually shifted from the level of distance a client prefers to the level of distance a therapist believes is optimal (Daly & Mallinckrodt, 2008). Even when (and perhaps *especially* when) the engagement and working phases have been successful, termination of the psychotherapy relationship poses fresh challenges—not least because it represents the ending, or mental reorganization and internalization, of a very significant attachment for many clients.

Although it is encouraging to see the growing number of studies of clients in therapy that extend what has been learned from experimental and correlational studies with nonclinical samples, we still need to know much more about the session-by-session interactions between client and therapist that serve to build a secure base in psychotherapy (Bowlby, 1988). We also need to know more about how this base of attachment security facilitates lasting change in adult clients with interpersonal problems. This may be the greatest challenge for the next generation of attachment and psychotherapy researchers.

RECOMMENDATIONS FOR FURTHER READING

Bowlby, J. (1990). *A secure base: Parent–child attachment and healthy human development*. New York: Basic Books.—This book is a collection of Bowlby's lectures and some previously published papers covering a diverse range of topics. It provides an excellent summary of his thinking about attachment theory in the last years of his life. Ch. 8, "Attachment, Communication and the Therapeutic Process," is of particular interest to psychotherapists.

Cassidy, J., & Shaver, P. R. (Eds.). (2008). *Handbook of attachment: Theory, research, and clinical applications* (2nd ed.). New York: Guilford Press.—A comprehensive resource, and one of the best single general references about research and applications of attachment theory.

Fonagy, P., Gergely, G., Jurist, E. L., & Target, M. (2002). *Affect regulation, mentalization, and the development of the self*. New York: Other Press.—This book places special emphasis on the role of childhood attachment in the development of capacities necessary for healthy adult emotional functioning.

Mallinckrodt, B. (2001). Interpersonal processes, attachment, and development of social competencies in individual and group psychotherapy. In B. R. Sarason & S. Duck (Eds.), *Personal relationships: Implications for clinical and community psychology* (pp. 89–117). New York: Wiley.—This chapter reviews empirical research supporting a theoretical model of how insecure forms of attachment in childhood lead to deficits in critical adult social competencies, which in turn create vulnerabilities to the kinds of interpersonal problems clients typically present in psychotherapy. The struggle to form a productive working alliance helps clients to develop these social competencies. The model is also applied to the change process in interpersonal group therapy.

Meyer, B., & Pilkonis, P. A. (2001). Attachment style. *Psychotherapy: Theory, Research, Practice, Training, 38*, 466–472.—A review of attachment research that has special relevance for the psychotherapy relationship.

Mikulincer, M., & Shaver, P. R. (2007). *Attachment in adulthood: Structure, dynamics, and change.* New York: Guilford Press.—A comprehensive review of the latest research applying attachment theory to the understanding of adult close relationships. It contains chapters on psychopathology and psychotherapy.

REFERENCES

Ackerman, S. J., Benjamin, L. S., Beutler, L. E., Gelso, C. J., Goldfried, M. R., Hill, C., et al. (2001). Empirically supported therapy relationships: Conclusions and recommendations of the Division 29 Task Force. *Psychotherapy, Theory, Research, Practice, Training, 38,* 495–497.

Anthony, S., & Pagano, G. (1998). The therapeutic potential for growth during the termination process. *Clinical Social Work Journal, 26,* 281–296.

Bateman, A. W., & Fonagy, P. (2003). Development of an attachment-based treatment program for borderline personality disorder. *Bulletin of the Menninger Clinic, 67,* 187–211.

Baum, N. (2005). Correlates of clients' emotional and behavioral responses to treatment termination. *Clinical Social Work Journal, 33,* 309–326.

Bembry, J. X., & Ericson, C. (1999). Therapeutic termination with the early adolescent who has experienced multiple losses. *Child and Adolescent Social Work Journal, 16,* 177–189.

Bernier, A., & Dozier, M. (2002). The client–counselor match and the corrective emotional experience: Evidence from interpersonal and attachment research. *Psychotherapy: Theory, Research, Practice, Training, 39,* 32–43.

Brennan, K. A., Clark, C. L., & Shaver, P. R. (1998). Self-report measurement of adult attachment: An integrative overview. In J. A. Simpson & W. S. Rholes (Eds.), *Attachment theory and close relationships* (pp. 46–76). New York: Guilford Press.

Bowlby, J. (1988). *A secure base: Parent–child attachment and healthy human development.* New York: Basic Books.

Charmaz, K. (2006). Constructing grounded theory: A practical guide through qualitative analysis. Thousand Oaks, CA: Sage.

Clarkin, J. F., & Posner, M. (2005). Defining the mechanisms of borderline personality disorder. *Psychopathology, 38,* 56–63.

Cyranowski, J. M., Bookwala, J., Feske, U., Houck, P., Pilkonis, P., Kostelnik, B., et al. (2002). Adult attachment profiles, interpersonal difficulties, and response to interpersonal psychotherapy in women with recurrent major depression. *Journal of Social and Clinical Psychology, 21,* 191–217.

Daly, K. D., & Mallinckrodt, B. (2008). *Experienced therapists' approaches to psychotherapy for adults with attachment avoidance or attachment anxiety.* Manuscript submitted for publication.

Dozier, M., Cue, K. L., & Barnett, L. (1994). Clinicians as caregivers: Role of attachment organization in treatment. *Journal of Consulting and Clinical Psychology, 62,* 793–800.

Fonagy, P., Gergely, G., Jurist, E. L., & Target, M. (2002). *Affect regulation, mentalization, and the development of the self.* New York: Other Press.

Fonagy, P., Leigh, T., Steele, J., Steele, H., Kennedy, R., Mattoon, G., et al. (1996).

The relation of attachment status, psychiatric classification, and response to psychotherapy. *Journal of Consulting and Clinical Psychology, 64,* 22–31.

Fraley, R. C., Garner, J. P., & Shaver, P. R. (2000). Adult attachment and the defensive regulation of attention and memory: Examining the role of preemptive and postemptive defensive processes. *Journal of Personality and Social Psychology, 79,* 816–826.

Fraley, R. C., & Shaver, P. R. (1997). Adult attachment and the suppression of unwanted thoughts. *Journal of Personality and Social Psychology, 73,* 1080–1091.

Gelso, C. J., & Carter, J. A. (1994). Components of the psychotherapy relationship: Their interaction and unfolding during treatment. *Journal of Counseling Psychology, 41,* 296–306.

Glasser, B., & Strauss A. (1967). *The discovery of grounded theory.* Chicago: Aldine.

Goldman, G. D., & Milman, D. S. (Eds.). (1978). *Psychoanalytic psychotherapy.* Reading, MA: Addison-Wesley.

Holmes, J. (2005). Disorganized attachment and borderline personality disorder: A clinical perspective. *Archives of Psychiatry and Psychotherapy, 7,* 51–61.

Horowitz, L. M., Rosenberg, S. E., & Bartholomew, K. (1993). Interpersonal problems, attachment styles, and outcome in brief dynamic psychotherapy. *Journal of Consulting and Clinical Psychology, 61,* 549–560.

Lazarus, A. A. (1993). Tailoring the therapeutic relationship or being an authentic chameleon. *Psychotherapy, 30,* 404–416.

Lewis, M., & Wolan Sullivan, M. (2005). The development of self-conscious emotions. In A. J. Elliot & C. S. Dweck (Eds.), *Handbook of competence and motivation* (pp. 185–201). New York: Guilford Press.

Mallinckrodt, B. (2001). Interpersonal processes, attachment, and development of social competencies in individual and group psychotherapy. In B. R. Sarason & S. Duck (Eds.), *Personal relationships: Implications for clinical and community psychology* (pp. 89–117). New York: Wiley.

Mallinckrodt, B., Gantt, D. L., & Coble, H. M. (1995). Attachment patterns in the psychotherapy relationship: Development of the Client Attachment to Therapist Scale. *Journal of Counseling Psychology, 42,* 307–317.

Mallinckrodt, B., Porter, M. J., & Kivlighan, D. M. Jr. (2005). Client attachment to therapist, depth of in-session exploration, and object relations in brief psychotherapy. *Psychotherapy: Theory, Research, Practice, Training, 42,* 85–100.

Mallinckrodt, B., & Wei, M. (2005). Attachment, social competencies, social support and psychological distress. *Journal of Counseling Psychology, 42,* 358–367.

Meyer, B., & Pilkonis, P. A. (2001). Attachment style. *Psychotherapy: Theory, Research, Practice, Training, 38,* 466–472.

Mikulincer, M., Dolev, T., & Shaver, P. R. (2004). Attachment-related strategies during thought suppression: Ironic rebounds and vulnerable self-representations. *Journal of Personality and Social Psychology, 87,* 940–956.

Mikulincer, M., & Florian, V. (1998). The relationship between adult attachment styles and emotional and cognitive reactions to stressful events. In J. A. Simpson & W. S. Rholes (Eds.), *Attachment theory and close relationships* (pp. 143–165). New York: Guilford Press.

Mikulincer, M., & Horesh, N. (1999). Adult attachment style and the perception of others: The role of projective mechanisms. *Journal of Personality and Social Psychology, 76,* 1022–1034.

Mikulincer, M., Shaver, P. R., & Pereg, D. (2003). Attachment theory and affect regulation: The dynamics, development, and cognitive consequences of attachment-related strategies. *Motivation and Emotion, 27,* 77–102.

Prochaska, J. O., & DiClemente, C. C. (1983). Stages and processes of self-change in smoking: Toward an integrative model of change. *Journal of Consulting and Clinical Psychology, 51,* 390–395.

Safran, J. D., & Muran, J. C. (1996). The resolution of ruptures in the therapeutic alliance. *Journal of Consulting and Clinical Psychology, 64,* 447–458.

Safran, J. D., Muran, J. C., Samstag, L. W., & Stevens, C. (2001). Repairing alliance ruptures. *Psychotherapy, 38,* 406–412.

Shefler, G. (2000). Time-limited psychotherapy with adolescents. *Journal of Psychotherapy Practice and Research, 9,* 88–99.

Siebold, C. (1991). Termination: When the therapist leaves. *Clinical Social Work Journal, 19,* 191–204.

Slade, A. (1999). Attachment theory and research: Implications for the theory and practice of individual psychotherapy with adults. In J. Cassidy & P. R. Shaver (Eds.), *Handbook of attachment: Theory, research, and clinical applications* (pp. 575–594). New York: Guilford Press.

Travis, L. A., Binder, J. L., Bliwise, N. G., & Horne-Moyer, H. L. (2001). Changes in clients' attachment styles over the course of time-limited dynamic psychotherapy. *Psychotherapy, Theory, Research, Practice, Training, 38,* 149–159.

Teyber, E. (2006). *Interpersonal process in therapy: An integrative model* (5th ed.). Belmont, CA: Thomson Brooks/Cole.

Tyrrell, C. L., Dozier, M., Teague, G. B., & Fallott, R. D. (1999). Effective treatment relationships for persons with serious psychiatric disorders: The importance of attachment states of mind. *Journal of Consulting and Clinical Psychology, 67,* 725–733.

Ward, D. E. (1984). Termination of individual counseling: Concepts and strategies. *Journal of Counseling and Development, 63,* 21–25.

Webb, N. B. (1985). A crisis intervention perspective on the termination process. *Clinical Social Work Journal, 13,* 329–340.

Wei, M., Heppner, P. P., & Mallinckrodt, B. (2003). Perceived coping as a mediator between attachment and psychological distress: A structural equation modeling approach. *Journal of Counseling Psychology, 50,* 438–447.

Wei, M., Heppner, P. P., Russell, D. W., & Young, S. K. (2006). Maladaptive perfectionism and ineffective coping as mediators between attachment and future depression: A prospective analysis. *Journal of Counseling Psychology, 53,* 67–79.

Wei, M., Mallinckrodt, B., Larson, L. M., & Zakalik, R. A. (2005). Adult attachment, depressive symptoms, and validation from self versus others. *Journal of Counseling Psychology, 52,* 368–377.

Wei, M., Mallinckrodt, B., Russell, D. W., & Abraham, T. (2004). Maladaptive perfectionism as a mediator and moderator of attachment and depressive mood. *Journal of Counseling Psychology, 51,* 201–212.

Wei, M., Vogel, D. L., Ku, T.-Y., & Zakalik, R. A. (2005). Adult attachment, affect regulation, negative mood, and interpersonal problems: The mediating roles of emotional reactivity and emotional cutoff. *Journal of Counseling Psychology,* 52, 14–24.

Weiner, I. B. (1998). *Principles of psychotherapy.* New York: Wiley.

Woodhouse, S., Schlosser, L. Z., Crook, R. E., Ligiero, D. P., & Gelso, C. J. (2003). Client attachment to therapist: Relations to transference and client recollections of parental caregiving. *Journal of Counseling Psychology, 50,* 395–408.

Youngren, V. R., Alonso, A., & Nahum, J. P. (2000). When goodbye precedes hello: A premature termination. *Harvard Review of Psychiatry, 8,* 25–35.

11

Transference and Attachment

Rami Tolmacz

What are transferences? They are the new editions or facsimiles
of the tendencies and phantasies which are aroused and made
conscious during the progress of the analysis; but they have this
peculiarity, which is characteristic of their species, that they replace
some earlier person by the person of the physician.
                                    —FREUD (1905/1953, p. 116)

Once the importance of transference material is recognized, indeed,
some model of this kind is forced upon us; and from Freud onwards
some such model is present in the thinking of all practicing analysts.
The issue, therefore, is not whether this type of model [attachment
theory] is useful but whether it is used as a supplement to a
psychical energy model or as a replacement of it.
                                    —BOWLBY (1969/1982, p. 17)

Since the inception of psychoanalysis, *transference* has been one of its most
central concepts. Partly a product of internalization and partly a reflection
of assessments and expectations, it forms an integral part of typical functioning, contributes to the development of psychopathology, and is considered a vital component of the therapeutic process. However, despite the
consensus regarding the importance of transference, and the widespread
belief that its analysis must constitute a major part of any psychoanalytic
technique (Greenson, 1967), serious and enduring disputes over its nature
and function have denied us a comprehensive and standard explanation of
transference in therapy (Abend, 1992). Consequently, the communicative
value of the term has dwindled, while theories have proliferated (Shane,
Shane, & Gales, 1997; Westen & Gabbard, 2002).
　　For many years, attachment theory was given the "cold shoulder" by the
psychoanalytic establishment—a consequence of the bitter rivalry between
Kleinian and Freudian factions in the 1950s. Since the 1980s, there has been

a discernible shift: Considerable efforts have been made to bridge the gap between attachment theory and psychoanalysis (e.g., Cortina & Marrone, 2003). In this spirit, I review psychoanalytic and attachment-based views of transference. I discuss two emerging trends of thought with regard to transference, review relevant research, and share case material illustrating transferential themes that may typify clients with various forms of insecurity.

TRANSFERENCE: MAJOR AREAS
OF AGREEMENT AND DISAGREEMENT

Since Freud's (1905/1953, 1912a/1958, 1912b/1958) early ideas about transference, the concept has evolved considerably (for a review, see Esman, 1990). Today, discussions in the psychoanalytic literature on transference center on several controversies: (1) the main content of the transference (e.g., the centrality of Oedipal wishes vs. desires for a relationship) and the main developmental stages in which it arises; (2) transference as a fantasy-based distortion of the past vis-à-vis an accurate look at the past; and (3) transference as a distorted view of the therapist versus transference as a consequence of selective attention and extreme sensitivity to the therapist's behavior. Along with these disputes, there are also several points of unanimity:

1. *The origins of transference.* All psychoanalytic theories share the view that we approach new people by following patterns of interpersonal relations that, to a large extent, stem from internalization of interactions between our desires or basic needs and events in our surroundings, especially those connected to relationships with significant figures. In other words, we all transfer aspects of earlier relationships to later ones (Westen & Gabbard, 2002).

2. *The mechanism of transference.* Psychoanalytic theorists seem to agree that the mechanism underlying transference involves reactivating memories of the emotional outcomes of encounters between our basic motivations and our surroundings, mainly early in life.

3. *The ubiquity of transference.* Even though the term *transference* is frequently used in the context of the client–therapist relationship, Freud, like other theorists, maintained that it is applicable to close relationships in general, especially those involving authority figures. Transference may involve various emotions directed toward various people. Moreover, one person may be the object of several completely different transferences.

4. *The conscious component of transference.* Identifying the content of transference is a complex task, partly because many elements of relational schemas are unconscious. The standard therapeutic process attempts to make these relational schemas conscious. In this regard, it is worth noting that researchers who have used the Core Conflictual Relationship Theme

(CCRT) method (Luborsky & Crits-Christoph, 1998), a tool widely used to assess the content of transference, have found that people repeat basic, identifiable themes throughout their narratives of relationships.

ATTACHMENT AND TRANSFERENCE:
PRELIMINARY COMMENTS

Because attachment theory assumes that existing representations are carried from one relationship to the next, the concept of transference is easily integrated into it. The theory proposes its own version of how early experiences affect future attitudes and interpersonal interactions. The theoretical and empirical focus of attachment theory is on the formation of *internal working models* (IWMs), which stem from encounters between an individual's basic needs and motivations and the way caregivers respond to these needs (for a review of IWMs, see Cobb & Davila, Chapter 9, this volume). Although attachments and transferences involve strong emotions, we must be aware of their fundamental difference: Whereas attachment is an enduring social bond, the need for which exists from "cradle to grave" (Bowlby 1969/1982, p. 172), transference is an idiosyncratic way of perceiving and relating, determined largely by early relations; it often attests to the disturbances characterizing these early relations, and reveals the specific IWMs of the individual. Although attachment theory was initially based primarily on observations of children and ethological research, in recent decades it has been heavily influenced by research in the neurosciences, especially studies of memory and affect regulation. Because transference is based on memory mechanisms and is emotionally charged (i.e., related to affect regulation), it is not surprising that there has been a renewed focus on transference and its role in the therapeutic process.

In the literature on attachment and psychotherapy, I believe we can now discern two trends of thought with regard to transference. For the sake of convenience, I refer to the first trend as the *conservative* or *traditional* approach, and the second as the *revisionist* or *theory-of-mind* approach. The conservative approach focuses primarily on unconscious representations of the self, the object, and the relationship between the two as manifested in therapy through the transference. A major therapeutic task, according to this conception, is to bring those representations to consciousness by promoting insight through interpretation. In keeping with Santayana's (1905/1998) adage that those who cannot remember the past are condemned to repeat it, the conservative approach attempts to reconstruct the past in order to avoid a repetition of problematic relationships and behaviors. In contrast, the revisionist approach focuses more on prerepresentational information that is inaccessible to the conscious mind. Consequently, the therapeutic process places less emphasis on interpretation and on reconstructing the past, and focuses instead on promoting affect regulation and developing ego functions. Proponents of this approach take a strong interest in findings from the neurosciences. In other words, whereas the conservative approach focuses on the characteristics of the displaced material (i.e., on the distortion of the "picture received"), the revisionist approach focuses primarily on the factors underlying the distortion (i.e., the "characteristics of the lens"). This situation has considerable theoretical ramifications, as I will discuss later. Generally speaking, most clients will benefit from some combination of both approaches, though theoretically some clients may do better with one or the other approach.

THE CONSERVATIVE APPROACH

The conservative approach to attachment and psychotherapy understands transference in a unique manner because of several factors: its concept of motivation, its IWM-based understanding of the nature of the inner world, its ideas about the origins of experiences (reality vs. fantasy), and the therapeutic process that it proposes. Each of these is discussed below, together with the conservative view of how therapists' attachment patterns affect countertransference.

Theory of Motivation

> ... there are certain other features of the approach that do differ from
> Freud's. Of these by far the main one concerns the theory of motivation.
> —BOWLBY (1969/1982, p. 13)

Motivation in attachment theory differs in two critical ways from motivation in classical psychoanalytic theory. First, Bowlby's thinking was pluralistic: He proposed the existence of several motivational systems that interact with one another. In particular, Bowlby emphasized the *attachment behavioral system,* a system designed to improve the infant's chances of survival. The functioning of this system has a major impact on the exploratory motivational system. The main idea here, as discussed by Ainsworth, Blehar, Waters, and Wall (1978), is that confidence in the availability and responsiveness of attachment figures promotes exploration of unfamiliar situations, and eventually a balance between leaning on others and using personal resources to cope with challenging circumstances. In addition, attachment theory proposes the existence of the caregiving, affiliation, and sexual mating systems. Thus Bowlby proposed a less economical model than Freud's.

The second important difference is in the status accorded to sex and aggression. Attachment theory's emphasis on attachment and exploration as motivational systems minimizes the importance of sexuality and aggression, which are at the heart of classical theory. In viewing aggression as a response to the frustration of attachment needs, attachment theory differs from both the Freudian and Kleinian versions of classical psychoanalysis. In contrast to aggression, sexuality is given the status of a drive. However, whereas Freud (1920/1955) related the sexual libido to an entire spectrum of attitudes and behaviors, including friendship, love, humanism, and cultural interest, Bowlby viewed it as just one of several behavioral systems. This is why, from the perspective of attachment theory, the main focus of therapy is on threats to security, the emotional reaction to these experienced threats, and the way the client copes with this reaction, rather than on sexuality, aggression, and their derivatives.

It is worth noting that an increasing number of studies are currently focusing on behavioral systems other than attachment. As knowledge about the functioning of these systems increases, we can expect it to be reflected in the emphasis given to these systems in the analysis of transference phenomena. For example, we will be better able to discern components of caregiving, and affiliation in the transference alongside the component of attachment. The social-cognitive model of the transference lends support to this view, as, according to this model, transference is perceived as a manifestation of the reactivation of an individual's various behavioral systems (Andersen & Chen, 2002).

Finally, though we all share the same behavioral systems, early interactions with our caregivers will determine, to a large extent, the specific ways in which they will be experienced and expressed in different situations. This is why the specific quality and content of the transference will be highly dependent on a client's specific attachment style. For example, as a result of their experiences with inconsistently responsive caregivers, persons with a preoccupied style will be prone to feelings of vulnerability in relation to therapists and will be especially watchful of the ways therapists respond to their needs. During sessions, preoccupied clients tend to be hypervigilant to cues of threat and will often cope by using hyperactivating strategies. On the other hand, clients with a dismissing style will exhibit little interest in becoming attached to or in revealing private feelings to therapists. In addition, they will attend less to emotional events and use deactivating strategies to deal with threats to security (for a review of hyperactivating and deactivating strategies, see Shaver & Mikulincer, Chapter 2, this volume). Finally, disorganized clients will exhibit a rather stormy and chaotic attachment to therapists, characterized by unpredictable ways of relating and severe difficulties with self-soothing.

Internal Working Models

... the concept of transference implies, first, that the analyst in his caretaking relationship to the patient is being assimilated to some pre-existing (and perhaps unconscious) model that the patient has of how any caretaker might be expected to relate to him, and, second, that the patient's pre-existing model of caretakers has not yet been accommodated—namely, is not yet

modified—to take account of how the analyst has actually behaved and still
is behaving in relation to him.
—BOWLBY (1973, p. 206)

Now that I have discussed the characteristics of the material transferred, according to classical attachment theory, I turn to the mechanism of transference proposed by the theory. Like many psychoanalytic theories, attachment theory needed to account for the existence of repetitive attitudes and behavioral patterns in relationships, especially pathological ones. Bowlby (1969/1982) proposed that these phenomena result from the internalization of experience. According to his theory, behaviors, emotions, and cognitive assessments combine to create models of the self based on the degree of security with and the accessibility of attachment figures. Bowlby's proposed mechanism of IWMs was based partly on Piaget's (1955) concept of *cognitive schemas* (or inner maps). People assimilate new experiences and relationships within their existing models, which is why change is so difficult. IWMs of attachment include representations of the self, representations of the other, the expected relationship between them, and the emotions associated with them. The perceptions of the self and the other are interdependent, and, insofar as a child can trust an attachment figure and his or her attention to the child's needs and communications, a positive self-perception develops. In contrast, if children feel abandoned or if their attachment figures have difficulty relating appropriately to their needs, the children develop a perception of themselves as unworthy of love and a perception of others as untrustworthy (Cortina & Liotti, 2005). This characterization of IWMs highlights the similarity between them and the concept of transference. Indeed, Bowlby (1973, 1979, 1988) explicitly wrote about transference in the therapeutic relationship and the importance of understanding transference in terms of clients' IWMs of attachment. Similarly, he regarded transference as "forecasts" clients make about psychotherapists. The forecasts are based on IWMs that do not necessarily apply to the clients' current relationships with the therapists (Woodhouse, Schlosser, Crook, Ligiéro, & Gelso, 2003).

Bowlby (1969/1982) also recognized that people may hold multiple IWMs relating to different attachment figures, and that the respective contents of these models may be incompatible. He argued that his hypothesis that multiple models are highly influential, but partially or completely unconscious, was merely a different version of Freud's thinking about a dynamic unconscious. The idea of multiple IWMs is also shared by the social-cognitive model of transference, according to which people hold idiographic knowledge about several significant others and behave differently depending on which representation of these others is triggered (Andersen & Chen, 2002).

Reality versus Fantasy

The third aspect of the conservative attachment-based view of transference concerns the role of actual experience. Bowlby (1973) postulated that the expectations of others that children build are "tolerably accurate reflections" (p. 202) of their early experiences with caregivers.

There is symbolism in the fact that Bowlby (who had Melanie Klein as a supervisor and Joan Riviere as his analyst) was vehement about the importance of reality in the development of internal representations, and that he minimized the role of fantasy and unconscious desires. The tendency to perceive transference as a fairly accurate reflection of an individual's significant experiences is unquestionably one of the most important contributions of attachment theory with respect to the sources of psychopathology and transference patterns. However, several scholars doubt the accuracy of this assertion. Gullestad (2001), for example, argues that attachment theory may create an artificial antagonism between real experience and personal constructions of meaning—that is, between reality and fantasy. Eagle (1997) also questions Bowlby's assumption, arguing that because of an infant's cognitive immaturity, which may distort his or her perception and understanding of a caregiver's behavior, it is unreasonable to assume that there will be a simple, direct relationship between the content of IWMs and the caregiver's behavior. Furthermore, innate differences in abilities such as self-soothing capacity make it inevitable that different infants will experience similar caregiver behaviors differently. Mikulincer and Shaver (2003) support this view, claiming that attachment insecurity leads to distortions of the situation as well as of the attachment figure's nonverbal behavior. Similarly, Noller (2005) has suggested that attachment style acts like a filter, "distorting both encoding and decoding processes" (p. 171).

The Therapeutic Process: Studies Examining the Relationship between Clients' Attachment Styles and Transference

One of the unique aspects of attachment theory is the empirical evidence upon which the theory is based and its contribution to the reassessment of the transference in the therapeutic meeting. Although several methods of assessing transference have been developed, little empirical research has been done regarding the phenomenon of transference (Gelso & Hayes, 1998). Recently, several empirical studies have been conducted from the perspective of attachment theory, and those have made a substantial contribution to our understanding of transference in therapeutic settings.

Interested in identifying attachment patterns in psychotherapy, Mallinckrodt, Gantt, and Coble (1995) developed the Client Attachment to Therapist Scale (CATS) and found that to a large extent, attachment to the therapist reflected the four-category model of adult attachment suggested by Bartholomew and Horowitz (1991). For example, clients scoring high on the Secure subscale of the CATS perceived their therapists as emotionally accepting and responsive, and as promoting a secure base from which they could observe threatening aspects of their emotional experiences. These clients also tended to describe themselves in a positive and competent manner. On the other hand, clients who received high scores on the Preoccupied/Merger subscale expressed a wish to dissolve the therapeutic boundaries between themselves and their therapists. They desired more contact with their therapists, hoped that they were the therapists' favorite clients, and wanted to be friends with their therapists outside of sessions. Clients who received high scores on the Avoidant-Fearful subscale reported a lack of trust in their therapists and feared rejection. These clients had a negative perception of themselves, as well as a negative and somewhat ambivalent perception of the therapists; therefore, it is not surprising that although they strongly desired contact, these clients demonstrated the worst therapeutic alliances, and it is doubtful to what extent they were able to sustain therapy.

In another study that examined the relation between clients' attachment to their therapists and the therapists' perception of the transference, Woodhouse et al. (2003) found a positive correlation between Preoccupied/Merger scores on the CATS and the amount of negative transference. This finding is consistent with the claim made by Slade (1999) that preoccupied clients tend to have transferences characterized by rage and to perceive their therapists as insufficiently available or helpful. However, Woodhouse et al. (2003) also found that clients who felt secure with their therapists tended to have high levels of negative transference. This finding is not necessarily surprising; as the researchers put it, "when the therapist can function as a secure base, it may be that deeper, and perhaps more difficult material can come into the work" (p. 404). Mohr, Gelso, and Hill (2005) have found links between attachment styles and therapeutic dynamics. Their findings indicate that from the very first therapy meeting, fearfully attached clients, compared to other clients, reported that their sessions were less smooth and meaningful. Thus therapists may find fearful clients more challenging to work with, and find themselves more susceptible to negative countertransference reactions; both reactions may leave fearful clients feeling more uncomfortable and even less helped.

In a study of the relationship between attachment patterns and transferential themes, as reflected in the CCRT method, Waldinger et al. (2003) found that persons with dismissing states of mind, as assessed by the Adult Attachment Interview (AAI; George, Kaplan, & Main, 1984, 1985, 1996), were more likely to express wishes for autonomy in their CCRT narratives than were persons classified as either secure or preoccupied. The results of this study support the idea that different levels of emphasis on the desire for autonomy may reflect differences in attachment figures' sensitivity to attachment needs and how these experiences were encoded in IWMs. It is interesting that the various AAI classifications did not differ in terms of the frequency of closeness themes in their relationship narratives.

The Therapeutic Process: Therapists' Attachment Styles
and Countertransference

Over the years, the concept of *countertransference* has not received the attention it deserves in attachment theory, either theoretically or empirically. Presumably, one of the primary reasons for this has to do with the long years of "drought" in addressing the clinical aspects of the theory. Furthermore, the main therapeutic objective posed by Bowlby (1988) is that the therapist acts as an attachment figure who serves as a secure base for clients, enabling them to explore their own personal history and its effect on their perceptions of themselves and significant others. As such, the therapist's inner world is perceived as relevant only insofar as it makes it difficult for the therapist to be available and responsive to clients. Nonetheless, as the psychotherapeutic aspects of the theory have gained attention, researchers have examined the impact of therapists' attachment styles on countertransferential feelings and behaviors.

In a recent study, Martin, Buchheim, Berger, and Strauss (2007) found that a vignette of a secure client evoked the friendliest and the least hostile responses from therapist trainees and medical students; a vignette of a dismissing client evoked the least friendly and most hostile feelings; and a vignette of an enmeshed client evoked responses that fell in between. Several studies also examined the interaction of therapists' and clients' attachment style in producing countertransference behaviors. For instance, Mohr et al. (2005) found that dismissing therapist trainees were rated by their supervisors as more likely to engage in negative countertransference behaviors overall, and especially when the trainees' clients were preoccupied. Similarly, preoccupied trainees were most likely to be rated as engaging in negative countertransference behaviors when their clients were dismissing.

Dozier and Tyrrell (1998) examined the relationship between therapists' attachment styles and their therapeutic interventions, and found that therapists' attachment styles were associated with distinct methods of intervention for clients with different attachment styles. Specifically, case managers with a secure style were seen as being better able than those with an insecure style to respond appropriately to clients' basic needs, regardless of their clients' attachment styles. The researchers' impression was that secure therapists could make better use of countertransference, because they were capable of reflecting on what the clients brought up and of providing noncomplementary feedback. In contrast, case managers with insecure attachment styles were more likely to intervene in a way that matched the clients' expectations based on their past experience. Specifically, case managers who tended more toward a preoccupied style intervened more intensively than those with a somewhat dismissing style.

In a survey study, Leiper and Casares (2000) examined the extent to which therapists' attachment style was related to experiences of difficulties and reward they reported in their work and to their level of work satisfaction. Their findings were consistent with those of Dozier and Tyrrell (1998): The results indicated that insecure therapists tended to experience more difficulties in the therapeutic encounter, to feel less rewarded and less supported, and to attribute their difficulty to themselves. These findings suggest that therapists' attachment styles may have a significant impact on their responses to clients and on the risk of manifestations of *complementary* countertransference (where there is an unhealthy "fit" between the therapist and the client, in which the former is induced to enact some aspects of the latter's pathology), as opposed to *concordant* countertransference (in which the therapist resonates more empathically with the client's unconscious needs; Racker, 1968).

Linking countertransference only with therapists' attachment styles runs the risk of a limited view of the transference–countertransference relationship, however. With countertransference, as with transference, it is valuable to examine the reactivation of the various behavioral systems. The Leiper and Casares study (2000) made a major contribution regarding the caregiving system, as these authors found that compulsive patterns of caregiving and care seeking were not clearly linked to any of the attachment styles. The significance of these findings is that it invites us to address the role of the behavioral system of caregiving in a more fundamental manner, going beyond the effect of attachment styles on this system.

THE REVISIONIST APPROACH

> But if psychoanalysis is to rest on its past accomplishments, it must
> remain, as Jonathan Lear and others have argued, a philosophy of mind,
> and the psychoanalytic literature—from Freud to Hartmann to Erikson to
> Winnicott—must be read as modern philosophical or poetic text alongside
> Plato, Shakespeare, Kant, Schopenhauer, Nietzsche, and Proust.
> —KANDEL (1999, p. 507)

For many years, analyzing and interpreting the content of transference formed the heart of the analytic process. This approach tends to lead researchers to focus on the cognitive content of IWMs, and so to ask "what" questions: What do individuals desire? What response do they expect from others? What are their characteristic ways of relating? In view of new findings—some from the field of therapy, some from psychological research, some from the natural sciences, and some from the interfaces between these (e.g., neuropsychology)—this therapeutic approach, which is aligned with what I have termed the conservative approach, is being reexamined.

Increasingly, researchers are also asking "how" questions in addition to the "what" questions. In addition to the displacement of certain content from previous experiences, researchers are examining the transfer of qualities of mental responses (ways of coping with stressful situations, levels of attention, and processing methods). These qualities seem to have a strong impact on the nature of relationships and expectations, and, along with other changes, constitute the focus of the revisionist approach to transference. The AAI, created by George et al. (1984, 1985, 1996), is the flagship instrument in this approach (for an in-depth review of the AAI, see Levy & Kelly, Chapter 6, this volume). The AAI is original in that its scoring system (Main & Goldwyn, 1984; Main, Goldwyn, & Hesse, 2003) is based on the form and structure of the subject's narrative as well as its content. The focus is on such parameters as coherence, degree of detail, processing, and balance in describing previous relationships. The AAI's coding system captures what Holmes (2001) calls *narrative competence*. Proceeding from the idea that early attachments are related to narrative style, Holmes has described the three narrative patterns that correspond with the three insecure AAI classifications (dismissing, preoccupied, and unresolved/disorganized): "clinging to rigid stories, overwhelmed by unstoried experience, or being unable to find a narrative strong enough to contain traumatic pain" (p. 88). Thus, whereas people with a secure state of mind with respect to attachment present highly coherent narratives, in which positive memories are supported by evidence and attachment relationships are appreciated, people with insecure states of mind have difficulty integrating memories experiences with their meaning. More specifically, persons classified as dismissing demonstrate avoidance by denying memories and by idealizing or devaluing (or both) previous relationships. People classified as preoccupied tend to have narratives in which they are confused, angry, or passive in their relationships with attachment figures, and often complain of having been hurt as children. Finally, people classified as unresolved/disorganized demonstrate a significant degree of disorganization in their narratives about attachment relationships (Fonagy, 1999).

The development of the AAI paved the way for researchers to investigate the quality of metacognitive functioning. As part of this trend, leading scholars (e.g., Fonagy, Gergely, Jurist, & Target, 2002; Liotti, 1999; Lyons-Ruth, 1999) have examined the degree to which early attachments affect an adult's *reflective functioning* and the degree to which reflective functioning may predict the development of psychopathology. Reflective functioning involves the ability to reflect on one's own mental states, such as thoughts and feelings, and those of others (for a discussion of reflective functioning, see Jurist & Meehan, Chapter 4, this volume). To a large extent, its development depends on the degree to which mental states were represented appropriately in the caregiver's mind, as manifested in the caregiver's expressions, way of relating, and responses to the infant (Eagle, 2003). Not surprisingly, parents with a good ability to mentalize are more likely to raise securely attached children (Fonagy, Steele, Steele, Higgitt, & Target, 1994; Slade, Belsky, Aber, & Phelps, 1999).

Using research on the relationship between attachment and the development of ego functions, Fonagy and Target (1996) have proposed the *interpersonal interpretive mechanism* (IIM) model. According to this model, early attachments are significant because they exert a major influence on the infant's capacity to assess their interpersonal environment. Fonagy and Target have proposed three factors that can mediate the relationship between the quality of early attachment experience and the sophistication of this capacity: stress regulation, attention regulation, and mentalization. We currently have a significant amount of empirical evidence suggesting that a secure attachment in early childhood is closely related to the development of a broad spectrum of abilities that are dependent on an IIM, including exploration, linguistic ability, ego stability, tolerance for frustration, and curiosity. According to Fonagy et al. (2002), early experiences do not determine the nature of representations of other–self relationships. Rather, the healthy or deficient development of a mental system that can be used to represent object relations, to function in stressful situations, and to process emotionally charged social interactions appropriately is what shapes mental models. In their opinion, focusing exclusively on the connection between the quality of attachment and representations of relationships reduces the importance of attachment to mental development. Early relationships are primarily important, not because they determine the IWMs that will oversee future relationships, but due to their role in developing brain regulation mechanisms and ensuring the strength or quality of these mechanisms that shape future social functioning.

Thus, individuals with secure attachments in childhood develop a good ability to reflect on their own and others' complex, distinct inner states, which in turn enables them to maintain fruitful interpersonal relationships. In contrast, insecure attachments result in a vulnerability to social influence and difficulties in preserving a clear distinction between self and other, which lead to the activation of defense mechanisms. For instance, one might deliberately strengthen one's representation of oneself relative to one's representation of the other, as in the avoidant attachment style. Another method of defense is based on empowering representations of the other, as in the anxious-ambivalent attachment style. Finally, in situations in which the attachment pattern led to a major failure of the IIM, as in the disorganized attachment pattern, there is a fundamental difficulty in differentiating between representations of the other's thoughts and desires and one's own.

The revisionist or theory-of-mind approach has major ramifications for our understanding of, and attitude toward, the mechanism of transference. According to this approach, in therapy, clients do not simply apply learned expectations based on their internalized other–self representations; they rely on their IIMs in order to respond in various situations and process emotionally charged social interactions. In other words, they transfer their mental systems when they interact with the therapist. For example, a client with disorganized attachment may transfer poor reflective capacity, difficulties with self-soothing skills, and a tendency to use projective identifications, alongside specific beliefs he or she holds about the therapist (e.g., the therapist's untrustworthiness). On the other hand, a client with a preoccupied style will transfer his or her hyperactivation strategies and difficulties in regulating attention.

Memory

Needless to say, transference depends on memory. Changes in our understanding of memory have led to new views about the nature of transference. Neuropsychological research in the second half of the 20th century suggests that memory is composed of different systems that are grouped into two main categories: *declarative (explicit) memory*, which can be divided into *episodic memory* and *semantic memory*, and *procedural (implicit) memory*, which can be divided into *emotional memory* and *nonassociative learning* (Squire, 1993). Crittenden (1990) noted that these memory systems have distinct courses of development. Procedural memory develops first; evidence suggests that it already exists in the first months of life. Throughout life, much of our daily activity relies on procedural memory.

The declarative and procedural memory systems also differ in the way memories are encoded and processed, in their accessibility, and in the regions of the limbic system with which they are associated. Whereas declarative memory is particularly associated with the hippocampus and other structures (such as the temporal lobes), procedural memory is associated with the amygdala, basal ganglia, and cerebellum, among others. Nevertheless, a single event will generally be perceived by both systems, meaning that their activity entails a great deal of overlap. Both systems are required for various learning experiences, and they may even influence each other (Kandel, 1999).

When we can say what, when, where, and why something occurs, we are in the realm of declarative memory (Talvitie & Ihanus, 2002). This kind of memory involves conscious retrieval of information about the past. As stated above, declarative memory is composed of episodic memory and semantic memory. Episodic memory is recall for events that can be situated in space and time; it consists of personal, situation-specific memories that enter the mind sequentially as verbally or visually encoded anecdotes or vignettes. Semantic memory represents the meaning of a given event and the aggregate of concepts and contexts underlying our knowledge (categories, facts, assumptions, etc.). Repressed memories are the domain of declarative memory; various techniques have been developed to restore them to consciousness, where they can be reevaluated on the basis of new information or from a new perspective. In this sense, they conform to the first of Freud's three definitions of the unconscious as presented in his later writings—the dynamic or repressed unconscious. This unconscious is referred to in the classical psychoanalytic literature as "*the* unconscious" (Kandel, 1999).

In contrast, procedural memory consists of behavioral patterns that appear consistently in certain situations. It relates to the "how" component of behavior (e.g., knowing how to ride a bicycle). This memory is devoid of verbal content, so it cannot be made conscious; yet it can influence the way we interpret and respond to events. Thus there is a fundamental difference between repressed declarative memories, which have been encoded in a verbal format, and procedural memories, which cannot be retrieved or represented verbally. In this context, Fonagy (1999) quotes Sandler and Joffe (1969), who argued that procedural memories of one's experiences vis-à-vis others are intrinsically unknowable.

Whereas Bowlby (1980) described two memory types relevant to attachment (episodic and semantic), Crittenden (1990) pointed out the connection between attachment patterns and procedural memory. Indeed, many components that underlie the unique way each of us faces attachment situations are within the realm of this memory system. The distinction between procedural and declarative memory is very relevant to the issue of IWMs. Whereas the content of our reflections (including their meanings and our insights into them) constitutes the declarative portion of our IWMs, the various ways in which we approach and function in an interaction constitute procedural memory.

I believe that transference can be conceptualized as the activation of both declarative memory and procedural memory in the context of emotionally significant interpersonal situations (the importance of the procedural component of transference and IWMs is discussed by Lyons-Ruth, 1999, and Eagle, 2003). Although Morgan et al. (1998) have claimed that implicit relational knowledge is a general principle of relating and that transference is frequently associated with therapeutic relationships and psychopathology, it seems that this distinction is unnecessary. The procedural component also deserves the status of a component of transference, even if it has qualities other than those attributed to transference in the conservative approach, which places more emphasis on the declarative and semantic aspects. This viewpoint is held by Cortina and Marrone (2003), who define transference as "implicit and unconscious (occasionally explicit and conscious) expectations, attributions, beliefs and attitudes that are embodied as internal working models (IWMs) of self and others" (p. 29).

The way these two sources of transference (implicit and explicit memory) interact may dictate the synchronicity of the material transferred. For example, a history of traumatic attachments is liable to lead to salient asynchrony, due to the opposite effects of high levels of cortisol secretion on explicit and implicit memory. In such a case, the traumatized person remembers "too much" in terms of implicit memory (i.e., becomes very emotional, hyperaroused, and hypervigilant), but remembers "too little" in terms of declarative memory (i.e., tends to suffer from different kinds of amnesia). As the IIM is employing implicit memory, which is itself influenced by the quality of early attachments, it is no wonder why individuals with different attachment styles may experience and encode the aspects of the same situation in different ways. Since secure clients have well-functioning IIMs, they will be able to encode the declarative aspects of the situation in a coherent ways. Thus it is likely that the contents of declarative and procedural memories will be synchronized. In contrast, dismissing clients, for example, may poorly encode painful events into declarative memory, leading them to claim (accurately) that they do not remember special difficulties in their early childhood. Yet their unconscious reactions to these events may be encoded quite well into procedural memory. The result is that two pivotal memory systems contain conflicting information—a situation that could compromise the functioning of dismissing clients' IIMs.

Therapeutic Implications

It is impossible to think about psychoanalytically oriented therapy without considering memory. Our concepts of the unconscious assume that data have been entered into our minds and stored there over the years, and our ideas about bringing unconscious material to awareness rely on that material's being verbally encoded and accessible. As a result, intervention has been aimed chiefly at reconstructing unconscious memories and mitigating harmful transferences. The idea of two different kinds of transference rooted in different memory systems has major implications for how the therapeutic process is conceptualized. First, if we assume that the interplay between early attachments and developing mental systems (the IIM) yields various qualities of mental functioning that influence interpersonal perception and behavior, than we must admit that our current conceptualizations of transference are inadequate. Gaps in the ability to reflect on an event (in terms of being aware of our own and others' feelings and thoughts), and differences in emotional engagement (e.g., over- or underinvolvement) with past or current events, are likely to have a major impact on memory encoding, and in turn on subsequent expectations and perceptions. (As noted above, this is something familiar to anyone working with clients who have experienced traumatic incidents, especially attachment-related trauma.) From this standpoint, Bowlby seems to have overstated the degree of accuracy of transferred material. An approach that gives pride of place to implicit knowledge requires reexamining basic assumptions and techniques in psychoanalysis.

One of the salient figures in this area is Stern, who, together with his associates, has linked developmental issues and implicit memories with a new way of understanding the therapeutic process (Stern et al., 1998). Stern (1998) has also proposed that "schemes of ways of being-with-another" (p. 303) are developed before explicit memory systems are in place. Implicit memories, then, are the building blocks of IWMs. Unconscious schemes define the "how" of interpersonal behavior that is expressed in the course of therapy (e.g., the manner, rhythm, and intonation of speech). They attest to elements of a particular client's procedural knowledge. According to Stern, moments in therapy that are ripe for change ("now moments," as he calls them) come up unintentionally. Interventions during such moments can undermine a client's ordinary manner of interacting. If we treat manifestations of transference as opportunities to reassess implicit knowledge about relationships or automatic ways of relating, then we have an opportunity for a new intersubjective context (a "specific moment of meeting") that can facilitate change in implicit knowledge.

What is important for our purposes is that this process does not require interpretation; nor does it even have to be verbal. Fonagy (2003) has explained this idea well, arguing that the main aspect of therapy is not the lifting of repression, but rather the change that occurs in implicit memory and alters the procedures used by individuals in their relationships. Similarly, Morgan et al. (1998) have argued that therapy involves more than just semantic knowledge, and therefore that change can occur to a large extent without interpretation and insight. In their opinion, it is more important that clients develop new ways of relating to themselves and others than it is to facilitate insight. In other words, the goal is to acquire more flexible ways of being and behaving (i.e., implicit relational knowledge that weakens old patterns of relating to others and creates new, more flexible, and more adaptive responses). For example, therapists may aim to improve their clients' reflective capacities and ability to regulate stress, thus reducing the likelihood of projective identification. The assessment of clients' attachment styles may give therapists some idea about particular weaknesses in the clients' IIMs, and therefore about the most effective ways of working with them. Generally speaking, the more disorganized a client's attachment, the more the therapist must struggle with projective identification and deal with implicit knowledge. Secure clients, on the other hand, will probably benefit from a more or less exclusive focus on problematic declarative memories.

CLINICAL ILLUSTRATIONS

I now share two case illustrations of the way the transference relationship in therapy reflects an individual's IWMs in accordance with both the conservative and the revisionist (or theory-of-mind) approaches.

The Dismissing Attachment Style

In general, dismissing clients attempt to reduce the importance of their relational experiences. Often they rely on denial in order to deal with their conflicts and feelings. In the therapeutic encounter, they may minimize the impact or importance of the therapist's remarks and insist that they have no difficulty with breaks in the treatment, such as vacations. Because these individuals tend to deny difficulties in relationships, it is no wonder that they tend not to seek treatment, and that even when they do come for therapy they tend to devaluate it and shorten its duration. Many of them approach therapy at the insistence of others, such as family members and partners. In other cases, they may come to treatment because of difficulties arising from feelings of emptiness or difficulties regarding their performance on a professional level. It is important for the therapist to understand that everything about this style indicates an attempt to defend against the pain that arises in response to experiences of rejection, and that it is not necessarily an expression of a basic lack of interest in attachment.

The Case of Ben

Ben, a computer professional in his 30s, sought therapy because of difficulty in conducting himself professionally at work and ambivalence about his choice of career. In his day-to-day life, Ben had only a few friendships, and these were characterized by rigidity, alienation, and sometimes even detachment. Every time he felt he was treated unfairly—a feeling that he reported often and that appeared in his dreams—he would quarrel with his peers and criticize them severely. Ben explained that even if his response was inappropriate, it was the only one he could imagine.

Several months into treatment, I realized I had only a very vague portrait of Ben's growing up and his relationships with immediate family members. Ben rarely mentioned his early childhood, usually stating that he simply did not remember significant events from his past. Against the backdrop of this pattern, the following description from his childhood stood out: After his father suspected him of stealing something from his mother's purse, he threw Ben against the wall, while his mother, who was present at the scene, prevented the grandmother from protecting Ben. Another important event Ben described was that when he was approximately 20 years old, he shared his homosexual preferences with his parents; they responded by breaking off all contact with him for several years. In fact, it was not long before he began therapy that he resumed his relationship with them, and then only in a very limited way. These descriptions could, of course, help to explain a habit he had developed over the years: Very often he would look away from the person he was talking to, scuttling a basic attachment behavior—mutual gaze.

With me, Ben maintained a guarded attitude, sometimes using dark humor. In general, it seemed as if therapy was first and foremost a logical service for him, intended to help him conduct himself differently and advise him about the direction he should take in his life. In addition, I could occasionally feel rather detached during sessions; this gave rise to an uncomfortable feeling of having lost contact with Ben, and anxiety that I might not succeed in renewing contact and that we would remain in an embarrassing state of alienation. Alongside this feeling (which might be understood as a concordant countertransference), I was aware of Ben's tendency to avert his eyes or rub them repeatedly, as if exposed to a strong glare that was making it difficult for him to sustain eye contact. Thus it was palpable that for Ben, much of our dialogue was accompanied by discomfort with respect to closeness. Similarly, during many sessions I felt tired and impatient or found myself calculating the time remaining in session. Only gradually were we able to understand that his gaze aversion was a strategy intended to reinstate a feeling of power or punish others; the basic function of the gaze as a way to make contact was converted into a means to protect himself and deter others from being intimate. Emotional events, such as the birth of a son or severe distress regarding his relationship with his son's mother, were so perfunctorily addressed that it was as if any sensitive participation on my part was out of place. In fact, in times of significant emotional strain in Ben's life, he was likely to cancel a meeting, as if to say that things were difficult enough for him and he did not need any additional burden. Thus it came as no surprise when Ben suggested, after feeling an improvement in his functioning and mood, that perhaps it was now possible to decrease the frequency of our meetings.

The Preoccupied Attachment Style

Preoccupied individuals tend to be extremely preoccupied with their attachment figures. Their expressions of need are laced with anger and suspicion. They tend to ruminate on their past and their relationships with their caregivers in a way that is somewhat confused. When preoccupied adults seek treatment, they give their therapists a great deal of attention, and show intense feelings overlain with neediness and fear in relation to their place in their therapists' world in general and in relation to their therapists' other clients in particular. Thus they may be very concerned with what their therapists really think, feel, and mean, all of which suggests extreme cautiousness about trusting caregivers. This is perhaps why preoccupied clients tend to be hypervigilant about what they perceive as threatening cues and will often deal with them by using hyperactivating strategies. They may therefore vacillate between anger and suspicion on the one hand, and yearning for the physical presence of their therapists and hanging on their every word on the other hand.

The Case of Dan

Dan, a computer professional in his 20s, sought therapy due to his difficulty persevering in romantic relationships. Early in romances, he would be enthusiastic and indulgent, all along fearing that his new partner would discover something unlikable about him and lose interest. Dan was alert to hints of boredom or criticism—a certain word in a text message on his cell phone, or an intonation that he experienced as lacking enthusiasm—and to prevent these, he made an enormous effort to be an ideal partner. He felt a great deal of pressure to keep his affect bright and confident, certain that if his partner were to detect his anxiety or need for her presence and her reassurance, she would quickly discard him. If after several months Dan's fears did not materialize, a new, almost opposite pattern would appear: Apparently more confident in his partner's commitment, Dan would begin to feel harshly critical of her. Shortly afterward, he would decide that the relationship was not right for him and end it in a way that usually took his partner completely by surprise. Thus Dan played out the complementary roles of anxious attachment: the intense pursuer of closeness and the unpredictable rejecter.

Dan was the firstborn son of an emotionally labile mother with hypomanic tendencies who was essentially unavailable to meet Dan's needs. Dan was a particularly sensitive child, and his mother dismissed his many wishes for contact with her by complimenting him on being a wonderful child and ignoring anything about him that was inconsistent with this picture. Dan began to feel that his mother was a perfect being, that their rare moments of meeting were precious to him, and that achieving proximity to her depended on avoiding doing or saying anything that might decrease his attractiveness to her. Thus Dan left childhood not only idealizing his mother, but harboring the misperception that submerging attachment needs and being outwardly compliant and cheerful were the only ways to win and maintain affection from intimate others, as well as to avoid sadness and loneliness. Moreover, he seemed to believe that when affection did arrive, it was untrustworthy and invariably conditional, and therefore unlikely to endure over the long run. To put it another way, Dan's longing was eventually overtaken by a pessimism that suffocated his passionate interest. Indeed, research indicates that people with anxious styles have greater difficulty compromising when choosing a partner than people with other attachment styles do (Tolmacz, 2004).

Although at the outset it seemed that this pattern was exclusive to Dan's relationships with women, it quickly manifested itself in the therapeutic encounter. For a long period of time, Dan also idealized me. When he entered the room, he was quick to position his seat so that he was directly opposite me. He gazed at me intensely as if vigilantly monitoring my availability and references to him. Dan also checked the clock in my office often, and when I brought this to his attention, he confessed that from our first meeting he was preoccupied by how much time he had left in each session. At the end of the session, Dan made a point of inquiring about my feelings toward him: Was I happy the session was over? Would I now remove my therapeutic mask to reveal the naked truth—namely, my impatience for and lack of interest in him? Occasionally, when he felt criticized by a girlfriend or coworker, he wanted to see how I perceived the goings-on that he described. In these cases, as well as in other circumstances, the suspicion lurking behind the idealization was apparent: Did I really respect him? Was I even on his side?

As the therapy progressed, Dan's devaluative tendencies surfaced. Sometimes he accused me of being jealous of his many romantic conquests. At other times he felt that we were not going deeply enough into his issues, and that perhaps another, more expensive therapy would do so and therefore benefit him more. In other words, my acceptance of and investment in him were, like those of the previous women in his life, rewarded with a disdain that seemed intended to protect his vulnerability to feeling worthless and rejected. Inevitably, Dan's bold criticisms gave way to great anxiety: Now that he had expressed doubt in my ability, I must surely no longer wish to treat him—or, worse, might feel the need to seek revenge.

CONCLUSIONS

Although attachment theory is relatively young, observing transference through its lens yields two conceptions, which I have termed the *conservative* and *revisionist* approaches. However, because attachment theory is based on bold ideas and strong empirical support, these conceptions do not necessarily threaten the coherence of the theory. Trying to fuse the two approaches is, in my opinion, a worthy challenge, but it is negligible compared with trying to integrate the results of this attempt with major analytical approaches. Indeed, I have mentioned at the beginning of this chapter that much-needed work is now being done to bridge the gap between attachment theory and psychoanalysis. The findings regarding separate memory systems, and the implications of these findings for a new understanding of transference, pose a major challenge to these efforts. Since transference is linked with the most basic building blocks of theories of psychopathology and psychotherapy, these reflections on the nature of transference provide us with completely new ways of understanding the therapeutic process. If autobiographical memory is activated secondary to procedural memory, we must test the hypothesis of attachment theory regarding the ability of IWMs to give us reasonably accurate information about an individual's personal history. Even more significantly, it will be necessary to continue exploring the function of making repressed material conscious in the therapeutic process. However, especially now, when we appear to have strayed far from the basic concepts of transference—so far, in fact, that it seems impossible to bridge the gaps—we may turn to Freud:

> The deficiencies in our description would probably vanish if we were already in a position to replace the psychological terms with physiological or chemical ones. ... We may expect [physiology and chemistry] to give the most surprising information and we cannot guess what answers it will return

in a few dozen years of questions we have put to it. They may be of a kind
that will blow away the whole of our artificial structure of hypothesis.
                                              —FREUD (1920/1955, p. 60)

RECOMMENDATIONS FOR FURTHER READING

Dozier, M., & Tyrrell, C. (1998). The role of attachment in therapeutic relationships. In J. A. Simpson & W. S. Rholes (Eds.), *Attachment theory and close
relationships* (pp. 221–248). New York: Guilford Press.—Dozier and Tyrrell
outline the therapist's critical role, from an attachment perspective, in facilitating therapeutic change. They also review research implicating transference and
individual differences in attachment security, in both clients and therapists, in
shaping therapeutic process and outcome.
Fonagy, P., Gergely, G., Jurist, E., & Target, M. (2002). *Affect regulation, mentalization, and the development of the self*. New York: Other Press.—In this
book, Fonagy and colleagues give a comprehensive overview of mentalization,
its development, and its clinical implications.
Gullestad, S. E. (2001). Attachment theory and psychoanalysis: Controversial issues.
Scandinavian Psychoanalytical Review, 24, 3–16.—This paper outlines current
issues in integrating attachment and psychoanalytic concepts.
Stern, D. N. (1998). The process of therapeutic change involving implicit knowledge: Some implications of developmental observations for adult psychotherapy. *Infant Mental Health Journal, 19*, 300–308.—Stern provides an in-depth
discussion of the role of implicit knowledge in therapeutic change, and defines
moments of meeting—in his view, the most essential process in bringing about
changes in implicit memory.

REFERENCES

Abend, S. M. (1992). An inquiry into the fate of the transference in psychoanalysis.
Journal of the American Psychoanalytic Association, 41, 627–651.
Ainsworth, M. D. S., Blehar, M. C., Waters, E., & Wall, S. (1978). *Patterns of attach-
ment: A psychological study of the Strange Situation*. Hillsdale, NJ: Erlbaum.
Andersen, S .M., & Chen, S. (2002). The relational self: An interpersonal social-
cognitive theory. *Psychological Review, 109*, 619–645.
Bartholomew, K., & Horowitz, L. M. (1991). Attachment styles among young
adults: A test of a four-category model. *Journal of Personality and Social Psy-
chology, 61*, 226–244.
Bowlby, J. (1973). *Attachment and loss: Vol. 2. Separation: Anxiety and anger*. New
York: Basic Books.
Bowlby, J. (1979). *The making and breaking of affectional bonds*. London: Tavis-
tock.
Bowlby, J. (1980). *Attachment and loss: Vol. 3. Loss: Sadness and depression*. New
York: Basic Books.
Bowlby, J. (1982). *Attachment and loss: Vol. 1. Attachment* (2nd ed.). New York:
Basic Books. (1st ed., 1969)

Bowlby, J. (1988). *A secure base: Clinical applications of attachment theory.* London: Routledge.

Cortina, M., & Liotti, G. (2005, June 11). *Building on attachment theory: Toward a multimotivational and intersubjective model of human nature.* Paper presented at the annual meeting of the Rappaport–Klein Study Group, Austen Riggs Center, Stockbridge, Massachusetts.

Cortina, M., & Marrone, M. (2003). Attachment theory, transference, and the psychoanalytic process. In M. Cortina & M. Marrone (Eds.), *Attachment theory and the psychoanalytic process* (pp. 27–41). London: Whurr.

Crittenden, P. (1990). Internal representational models of attachment relationships. *Infant Mental Health Journal, 11,* 259–277.

Dozier, M., & Tyrrell, C. (1998). The role of attachment in therapeutic relationships. In J. A. Simpson & W. S. Rholes (Eds.) *Attachment theory and close relationships* (pp. 221–248). New York: Guilford Press.

Eagle, M. (1997). Attachment and psychoanalysis. *British Journal of Medical Psychology, 70,* 217–229.

Eagle, M. (2003). Clinical implications of attachment theory. *Psychoanalytic Inquiry, 23,* 27–53.

Esman, A. H. (Ed.). (1990). *Essential papers on transference.* New York: New York University Press.

Fonagy, P. (1999). Memory and therapeutic action. *International Journal of Psycho-Analysis, 80,* 215–223.

Fonagy, P. (2003). Repression, transference and reconstruction: Rejoinder to Harold Blum. *International Journal of Psycho-Analysis, 84,* 503–509.

Fonagy, P., Gergely, G., Jurist, E., & Target, M. (2002). *Affect regulation, mentalization, and the development of the self.* New York: Other Press.

Fonagy, P., Steele, M., Steele, H., Higgitt, A., & Target, M. (1994). The theory and practice of resilience. *Journal of Child Psychology and Psychiatry, 35,* 231–257.

Fonagy, P., & Target, M. (1996). Playing with reality: I. Theory of mind and the normal development of psychic reality. *International Journal of Psycho-Analysis, 77,* 217–233.

Freud, S. (1953). Fragment of an analysis of a case of hysteria. In J. Strachey (Ed. & Trans.), *The standard edition of the complete psychological works of Sigmund Freud* (Vol. 7, pp. 3–122). London: Hogarth Press. (Original work published 1905)

Freud, S. (1955). Beyond the pleasure principle. In J. Strachey (Ed. & Trans.), *The standard edition of the complete psychological works of Sigmund Freud* (Vol. 18, pp. 3–64). London: Hogarth Press. (Original work published 1920)

Freud, S. (1958). The dynamics of transference. In J. Strachey (Ed. & Trans.), *The standard edition of the complete psychological works of Sigmund Freud* (Vol. 12, pp. 97–108). London: Hogarth Press. (Original work published 1912a)

Freud, S. (1958). Recommendations to physicians practicing psycho-analysis. In J. Strachey (Ed. & Trans.), *The standard edition of the complete psychological works of Sigmund Freud* (Vol. 12, pp. 109–120). London: Hogarth Press. (Original work published 1912b)

Gabbard, G. O., & Westen, D. (2003). Rethinking therapeutic action. *International Journal of Psycho-Analysis, 84,* 823–841.

Gelso, C. J., & Hayes, J. A. (1998). *The psychotherapy relationship*. New York: Wiley.

George, C., Kaplan, N., & Main, M. (1984). *Adult Attachment Interview protocol*. Unpublished manuscript, University of California, Berkeley.

George, C., Kaplan, N., & Main, M. (1985). *Adult Attachment Interview protocol* (2nd ed.). Unpublished manuscript, University of California, Berkeley.

George, C., Kaplan, N., & Main, M. (1996). *Adult Attachment Interview protocol* (3rd ed.). Unpublished manuscript, University of California, Berkeley.

Greenson, R. (1967). *The technique and practice of psychoanalysis* (Vol. 1). New York: International Universities Press.

Gullestad, S. E. (2001). Attachment theory and psychoanalysis: Controversial issues. *Scandinavian Psychoanalytical Review, 24,* 3–16.

Holmes, J. (2001). *The search for the secure base: Attachment theory and psychotherapy*. Hove, UK: Brunner-Routledge.

Kandel, E. R. (1999). Biology and the future of psychoanalysis: A new intellectual framework for psychiatry revisited. *American Journal of Psychiatry, 156,* 505–524.

Leiper, R., & Casares, P. (2000). An investigation of the attachment organization of clinical psychologists and its relationship to clinical practice. *British Journal of Medical Psychology, 73,* 449–464.

Liotti, G. (1999). Understanding dissociative processes: The contribution of attachment theory. *Psychoanalytic Inquiry, 19,* 757–783.

Luborsky, L., & Crits-Christoph, P. (1998). *Understanding transference: The core conflictual relationship theme method* (2nd ed.). Washington, DC: American Psychological Association.

Lyons-Ruth, K. (1999). The two-person unconscious: Intersubjective dialogue, enactive relational representation, and the emergence of new forms of relational organization. *Psychoanalytic Inquiry, 19,* 576–617.

Main, M., & Goldwyn, R. (1984). *Adult attachment scoring and classification system*. Unpublished manuscript, University of California, Berkeley.

Main, M., Goldwyn, R., & Hesse, E. (2003) *Adult attachment scoring and classification system*. Unpublished manuscript, University of California, Berkeley.

Mallinckrodt, B., Gantt, D. L., & Coble, H. M. (1995). Attachment patterns in the psychotherapy relationship: Development of the Client Attachment to Therapist Scale. *Journal of Counseling Psychology, 42,* 307–317.

Martin, A., Buchheim, A., Berger, U., & Strauss, B. (2007). The impact of attachment organization on potential countertransference reactions. *Psychotherapy Research, 17,* 46–48.

Mikulincer, M., & Shaver, P. R. (2003). The attachment behavioral system in adulthood: Activation, psychodynamics and interpersonal processes. In M. Zanna (Ed.), *Advances in experimental social psychology* (Vol. 35, pp. 53–152). San Diego, CA: Academic Press.

Mohr, J. J., Gelso, C. J., & Hill, C. E. (2005). Client and counselor trainee attachment as predictors of session evaluation and countertransference behavior in first counseling sessions. *Journal of Counseling Psychology, 52,* 298–309.

Morgan, A., Bruschweiler-Stern, N., Harrison, A., Lyons-Ruth, K., Nahum, J., Sander, L., et al. (1998). Moving along to things left undone. *Infant Mental Health Journal, 19,* 324–332.

Noller, P. (2005). Attachment insecurity as a filter in the decoding and encoding of nonverbal behavior in close relationships. *Journal of Nonverbal Behavior, 29,* 171–176.

Piaget, J. (1955). *The construction of reality in the child.* London: Routledge & Kegan Paul.

Racker, H. (1968). *Transference and countertransference.* New York: International Universities Press.

Sandler, J., & Joffe, W. G. (1969). Towards a basic psychoanalytic model. *International Journal of Psycho-Analysis, 5,* 79–90.

Santayana, G. (1998). *Life of reason.* Amherst, NY: Prometheus Books. (Original work published 1905)

Shane, M., Shane, E., & Gales, M. (1997). *Intimate attachments.* New York: Guilford Press.

Slade, A. (1999). Representation, symbolization, and affect regulation in concomitant treatment of a mother and child: Attachment theory and child psychotherapy. *Psychoanalytic Inquiry, 19,* 797–830.

Slade, A., Belsky, J., Aber, J. L., & Phelps, J. L. (1999). Mothers' representations of their relationships with their toddlers: Links to adult attachment and observed mothering. *Developmental Psychology, 35,* 611–619.

Squire, L. R. (1993). The organization of declarative and nondeclarative memory. In T. Ono, M. Fukuda, L. R. Squire, M. E. Raichle, & D. I. Perrett (Eds.), *Brain mechanisms of perception and memory: From neuron to behavior* (pp. 219–227). New York: Oxford University Press.

Stern, D. N. (1998). The process of therapeutic change involving implicit knowledge: Some implications of developmental observations for adult psychotherapy. *Infant Mental Health Journal, 19,* 300–308.

Stern, D. N., Sander, L.,W., Nahum, J. P., Harrison, A. M., Lyons-Ruth, K., Morgan, A.C., et al. (1998). Noninterpretive mechanisms in psychoanalytic psychotherapy: The "something more" than interpretation. *International Journal of Psycho-Analysis, 79,* 903–921.

Talvitie, V., & Ihanus, J. (2002). The repressed and implicit knowledge. *International Journal of Psycho-Analysis, 83,* 1311–1323.

Tolmacz, R. (2004). Attachment style and willingness to compromise when choosing a mate. *Journal of Social and Personal Relationships, 21,* 267–272.

Waldinger, R. J., Seiman, E. L., Gerber, A. J., Leim, J. H., Allen, J. P., & Hauser, S. T. (2003). Attachment and core relational themes: Wishes for autonomy and closeness in the narratives of securely and insecurely attached adults. *Psychotherapy Research, 13*(1), 77–98.

Westen, D., & Gabbard, G. O. (2002). Developments in cognitive neuroscience: I. Conflict, compromise, and connectionism. *Journal of the American Psychoanalytic Association, 50,* 53–98.

Woodhouse, S. S., Schlosser, L. Z., Crook, R. E., Ligiéro, D. P., & Gelso, C. J. (2003).: Client attachment to the therapist: Relations to transference and client recollections of parental caregiving. *Journal of Counseling Psychology, 50,* 395–408.

12

Attachment-Related Defensive Processes

Mario Mikulincer
Phillip R. Shaver
Jude Cassidy
Ety Berant

The concept of psychological defense has been important to psychology ever since Breuer and Freud (1895/1955) first explained how repression works: "The basis for repression ... can only be a feeling of unpleasure, the incompatibility between the single idea that is repressed and the dominant mass of ideas constituting the ego" (p. 116). Breuer and Freud went on to say that "when this process occurs for the first time there comes into being a nucleus and center of crystallization for the formation of a psychical group divorced from the ego—a group around which everything which would imply an acceptance of the incompatible idea subsequently collects" (p. 123).

Almost 110 years later, we (Mikulincer, Dolev, & Shaver, 2004) conducted two experiments in which college students with an avoidant attachment style were encouraged to think about painful breakups of romantic relationships, then not to think about them, and then to name the colors in which various words (presented one at a time on a computer screen) were typed. When not further burdened cognitively or emotionally, avoidant individuals were able to name the colors in which breakup-related words appeared, and they also showed signs (slower reaction times) of having activated mental representations of their own self-nominated laudable traits (measured a month earlier). When burdened by a cognitive load (remembering a seven-digit number), however, avoidant participants became relatively slow at naming the colors in which breakup-related words and their own self-nominated *negative* traits were printed. In other words, avoidant individuals used some combination of unconscious (repression) or conscious censoring (suppression) and self-image inflation to ward off painful thoughts of rejection and abandonment, but these defenses were defeated by an interfering cognitive load.

These studies, and hundreds of others, both classic and recent (many of them reviewed by Hentschel, Smith, Draguns, & Ehlers, 2004), indicate that (1) Breuer and Freud were right in believing that the human mind is capable of repressing unpleasant thoughts (including thoughts about relationship losses and negative self-traits); (2) at least sometimes (e.g., when rejection experiences and negative self-traits are associatively linked in memory), repression involves "a psychical group" of related mental representations (or a neural network, as Freud, a neurologist, might also have conceptualized such psychical groups); (3) repression requires mental effort (*psychic energy,* in Freud's terms); and (4) the concept of *defense* is alive and well in present-day psychology, despite having been criticized over the decades.

These points could be made just as well by focusing on the Adult Attachment Interview (AAI; George, Kaplan, & Main, 1984, 1985, 1996; described by Hesse, 1999, 2008), which classifies people as secure, dismissing of, or preoccupied with attachment on the basis of a clinical interview about childhood relationships with parents and other attachment figures. People classified as secure in the AAI show a current valuing of attachment; have ready access to attachment-related memories from childhood; and can articulate them in a coherent, organized, and thoughtful way to an interviewer. People classified as dismissing of attachment seem to maintain defensive mental barriers to such memories and are unwilling or unable to recall and describe them to an interviewer. People classified as preoccupied with attachment seem to be enmeshed in strong and poorly regulated feelings about childhood relationships with attachment figures, making it difficult for them to explain their troubled histories coherently to an interviewer.

The term *defense* was quite familiar and acceptable to Bowlby (1980), a psychoanalyst and the founder of attachment theory. It has not, however, seemed completely acceptable to many research psychologists since Bowlby's time, so it is continually being resurrected under apparently less threatening (i.e., less psychodynamic) names such as *coping* strategies (e.g., Lazarus & Folkman, 1984) and strategies of *affect regulation* or *emotion regulation* (e.g., Gross, 2007). We have used all three terms—*defense, coping,* and *emotion regulation*—in our own writings (e.g., Cassidy, 1994; Mikulincer & Shaver, 2007; Shaver & Mikulincer, 2007) and do not shy away from any of them here. In line with what all of these concepts have in common, we consider defenses to be mental mechanisms aimed at adaptation and self-regulation—a view shared by psychoanalytic writers (e.g., McWilliams, 1994).

What is being defended against in a particular case may be as different as potentially uncontrollable impulses (which Freud viewed as instinctive, but which may arise from almost any motive, wish, or desire); a feeling of falling apart under stress (losing the coherence and solidity of the sense of self); negative emotions (e.g., anxiety, shame, guilt, fear, anger); and unacceptable thoughts about the self (e.g., about one's own mortality, mistakes, personal weaknesses, or social unacceptability) and others (e.g., about another person's indifference, rejecting behavior, or threats of abandonment). Although threatening experiences have been conceptualized in many ways—for example, as threatening one's life, one's self-control, one's social acceptance, one's self-image, or one's sense of coherence and consistency (Cramer, 2006)—all of the conceptualizations are compatible with the claim that they involve "a feeling of unpleasure [attributable to] the incompatibility between the single idea that is repressed and the dominant mass of ideas constituting the ego" (Breuer & Freud, 1895/1955, p. 116).

Our goals in the present chapter are to summarize what attachment researchers have discovered about defenses and their use by people with different attachment styles or states of mind regarding attachment. We begin with a review of ideas and empirical findings concerning the forces against which people with different attachment patterns typically defend. That is, we deal with the pain and distress that the unavailability, nonresponsiveness, or loss of an attachment figure can cause, and the different forms this pain and distress can take in people with anxious and avoidant attachment styles. We then review theoretical ideas and empirical findings concerning the goals and the cognitive, affective, and behavioral mechanisms involved in avoidant and anxious defenses. We also present clinical examples showing how particular kinds of attachment-related defenses are manifested in clinical settings. Finally, we briefly discuss the special case of disorganized attachment in infancy and unresolved or unclassifiable attachment in adulthood—the attachment patterns that appear to be most strongly linked with serious psychopathology (e.g., Carlson, 1998).

WHAT IS DEFENDED AGAINST?:
ATTACHMENT-RELATED SOURCES OF PAIN AND DISTRESS

According to attachment theory (Bowlby, 1969/1982, 1973, 1980), the unavailability or nonoptimal responsiveness of a primary attachment figure in times of need, as well as the resulting disruption of one's sense of safety, security, and protection, is a major source of psychological suffering. When an attachment figure proves to be uninterested, unavailable, unempathic, unhelpful, or even frightening, a person in need fails to regulate the distress that has activated his or her attachment system (due, e.g., to an unexpected loud noise in infancy, an insulting comment by an elementary school teacher in childhood, the breakup of a romantic relationship in adolescence, or a miscarriage or serious physical illness in adulthood), and the distress is exacerbated by frustration of the person's attachment needs and the rejection of his or her efforts to seek love, understanding, comfort, and protection. As a result, the person not only feels vulnerable and anxious while trying to handle the threatening experience without the assistance of what Bowlby called a "stronger and wiser" attachment figure; the person also feels rejected and demeaned or humiliated. This complex of feelings, or state of mind, can take at least two organized forms (Ainsworth, Blehar, Waters, & Wall, 1978; Main & Solomon, 1990; Mikulincer, Shaver, & Pereg, 2003) or be seriously disorganized.

In one organized state of mind, attention is focused mainly on the ways in which one's bids for proximity and support fail to achieve a positive interpersonal result (closeness, love, comfort), and instead typically result in a negative outcome (inattention, rejection, anger, disdain, abuse) for showing vulnerability or need. In such cases, reliance on an attachment figure, and involvement in a dependent or interdependent relationship more generally, is construed as frustrating, demeaning, and painful. Under these conditions, a person may decide, consciously or unconsciously, to rely on him- or herself—becoming what Bowlby (1969/1982) called compulsively self-reliant, and what others have called *dismissive of attachment* or simply *avoidant* (of intimacy, closeness, and interdependence). We (Mikulincer & Shaver, 2007; Cassidy & Kobak, 1988; see also Main, 1981) conceptualize this stance in terms of deactivation of the attachment system. Anything that would normally activate the system, such as physical or psychological threats to the self, feelings of vulnerability, or wishes for an attachment figure's protection or support, is defended against, suppressed, countered with narcissistic self-enhancement, or denied (as we found in the experiments mentioned earlier; Mikulincer et al., 2004).

The other organized state of mind that can develop in response to unreliable or unresponsive care includes ineffective regulation of distress and construing oneself as inadequately supported, insufficiently loved, vulnerable to uncontrollable threats, and improperly or unfairly treated. In this state of mind, attention is focused on one's own vulnerability and inadequacy in the threatening situation, which can be momentarily accepted ("I'm hopelessly alone," "I'm worthless") and/or raged against ("He's never there for me," "She promised me this would never happen"). This state of mind encourages anxiety, rumination, catastrophizing, jealousy, and envy, and can lead to increased efforts to capture a relationship partner's attention and loyalty (by acting seductive, being coy, or submitting to otherwise undesirable requests) and/or to attempts to coerce the partner into behaving more supportively (by making demands, expressing strong negative feelings, denigrating rivals, or spying on the partner). Ainsworth et al. (1978) identified one group of infants who displayed both of these kinds of behavior (strong proximity seeking and angry contact resistance) following a brief laboratory separation from the parent; these infants were initially labeled *anxious-ambivalent*. In adults, this state of mind is what Main and her colleagues (e.g., Main, Kaplan, & Cassidy, 1985) called *enmeshed and preoccupied with attachment,* and what we call, more simply, *anxious attach-*

ment. Theoretically, this state involves hyperactivation of the attachment system (Cassidy & Berlin, 1994; Main, 1990; Mikulincer & Shaver, 2007).

Although these two states of mind, avoidance and anxiety, are related, both being due to insecurity caused by an attachment figure's unavailability or unreliability, their relative strength may vary across situations, relationships, and individuals. Mikulincer et al. (2003) summarized the broad array of internal and external factors that contribute to the relative strength of each of the states of mind. The avoidant stance is encouraged by (1) consistent inattention, rejection, or angry disapproval on the part of an attachment figure in response to a person's bids for proximity and support; (2) threats of punishment or rejection if the person makes a bid for proximity, intimacy, or protection; (3) traumatic or abusive experiences during proximity-seeking efforts; and (4) explicit or implicit encouragement on the part of an attachment figure for one's greater self-reliance and suppression of expressions of need or vulnerability.

The anxious stance or state of mind is encouraged by (1) unreliable care, which is sometimes affectionate and at other times neglectful; (2) intrusive care that is more related to the caregiver's own needs and anxieties than to the needs of the attached individual; (3) care that discourages the acquisition of self-regulation skills and, directly or indirectly, punishes a person for attempting to function independently; (4) comments that emphasize a person's helplessness, incompetence, or weakness when trying to operate autonomously; and (5) traumatic or abusive experiences endured when one is separated from attachment figures. This kind of treatment causes a person to feel ambivalent because, on the one hand, relying on the attachment figure is awkward, discomforting, and sometimes annoying, but on the other hand, trying to care for oneself can seem dangerous or hopeless and therefore daunting. This kind of care may encourage a person to verbalize neediness and protest temporary abandonment (real or imagined), because making noise has sometimes recaptured a neglectful or self-preoccupied caregiver's attention. This encourages inauthentic emotionality—a form of behavior that can be humorous or endearing, but that can also seem dishonest and become exhausting for anyone who tries to respond helpfully to it.

The most insecure state of mind, *disorganized attachment,* seems to stem from experiences with an attachment figure who was either seriously abusive, frightened, or frightening when a person sought proximity and safety from the attachment figure (Hesse & Main, 2006; Main & Hesse, 1990; Main & Solomon, 1990). These experiences turn what should have been a safe haven and secure base into a source of threat, causing all organized attachment strategies to break down. Thus the individual's biologically based tendency to turn to an attachment figure in times of trouble is countered by the biologically based tendency to turn away from threat, and the individual is literally stuck. In childhood, these incompatible tendencies lead to unusual behavior—lying down on the floor in the midst of seeking proximity, veering off course when approaching the parent and going under a table, backing away from the parent while in obvious distress, or freezing. In adulthood, the equivalent state can involve odd beliefs, dissociative states, extreme lack of trust in others, and (when the person is discussing loss or trauma in the AAI) a lack of monitoring of discourse or reasoning.

The different insecure states of mind have implications for the kinds of defensive behavior a person is likely to exhibit. Individuals who score high on avoidant attachment tend to be vigilant about becoming needy, intimate, dependent, or emotional; they deny vulnerability, emphasize their personal strengths, avoid threats, and resist becoming dependent on anyone. Individuals who score high on anxious attachment, in contrast, tend to be vigilant about possible neglect, rejection, or abandonment, and to be hypersensitive to signs of danger and lack of care. This can cause them either to act out noisily and intrusively, or to comply submissively with relationship partners' requests. If necessary to gain support, they will admit (and perhaps even exaggerate) their own weaknesses and vulnerabilities, criticize themselves, and attempt to remake themselves (e.g., by undergoing cosmetic surgery; Davis & Vernon, 2002). That is, whereas avoidantly attached people are worried about intimacy, engulfment, and interdependence, anxiously attached people are worried about separation, abandonment, isolation, and interpersonal distance.

Although not all aspects of this theoretical analysis of defenses have been empirically tested, there is good evidence that avoidant people are intimacy-averse. Self-reported avoidant attachment is associated with higher scores on fear-of-intimacy scales (e.g., Doi & Thelen, 1993; Greenfield & Thelen, 1997; Hudson & Ward, 1997), with placing relationship partners at a greater distance from one's "core self" (Rowe & Carnelley, 2005), and with actually increasing physical distance from others, even in fairly simple settings (Kaitz, Bar-Haim, Lehrer, & Grossman, 2004). Kaitz et al. (2004), for example, used a stop-distance research paradigm in which people rated their level of discomfort as an experimenter moved toward them. They also assessed the physical distance freely chosen by participants when seated facing an experimenter and talking about personal issues. More avoidant people were less comfortable with physical proximity, disliked having the experimenter move into their personal space, and sat significantly further away from the experimenter when given that option. Dismissingly avoidant attachment, as measured with the AAI (Hesse, 1999), involves conversational tactics designed to maintain distance from the interviewer, such as not answering questions, engaging in long pauses, and failing to provide details necessary for the interviewer to understand the speaker's history.

Regarding anxious attachment, several studies have shown that anxious adults score higher than average on rejection sensitivity (e.g., Downey & Feldman, 1996; Taubman-Ben-Ari, Findler, & Mikulincer, 2002), are quicker to recognize rejection-related words in lexical decision tasks (Baldwin & Kay, 2003; Baldwin & Meunier, 1999), and have difficulty inhibiting thoughts of rejection (Baldwin & Kay, 2003; Baldwin & Meunier, 1999). Baldwin and Kay (2003) exposed people to sounds (pure tones) paired with rejecting (frowning) or accepting (smiling) faces, and then administered a lexical decision task in which rejection-related words were paired with each of the tones. Nonanxious (i.e., relatively secure) adults were slower to react to rejection-related words when they were paired with rejection tones (as compared to acceptance tones), but anxious people reacted faster to these words even in the presence of the acceptance tone. That is, anxious people were so sensitive to rejection-related cues that they were unable to dispense with worries about rejection even in accepting contexts.

In another series of experiments, Mikulincer, Florian, Birnbaum, and Malishkevich (2002) obtained indirect support for the idea that anxiously attached people construe an attachment figure's unavailability as a sign of their own helplessness and vulnerability. Participants were asked to imagine being separated from a loved one and then to perform a word completion task that measured the accessibility of death-related thoughts. Those who scored higher on attachment anxiety reacted to separation reminders with more death-related thoughts. This tendency was particularly strong when the imagined separation was long-lasting or final. In other words, for anxious individuals, social or psychological separation evoked thoughts of death. This finding is especially interesting in light of Bowlby's (1969/1982) theoretical speculation that the attachment system emerged during evolution because it protected primates (especially infants, but adults as well) from predation, dangerous accidents, and attacks by hostile others. In other words, seeking protection from attachment figures may have been motivated by fear of injury and death, and being rejected or abandoned by attachment figures might have accurately foreshadowed premature death.

This mental equating of separation and death was also noted by Hart, Shaver, and Goldenberg (2005), who examined defensive reactions to separation and reminders of death. American undergraduates were asked to think about their own death, separation from a close relationship partner, or a neutral control theme, and then to report their attitudes toward the writer of a pro-American essay provided by the experimenter. People who scored relatively high on attachment-related anxiety or avoidance rated the pro-American writer more favorably in the death-primed condition than in the control condition—the typical defensive reaction to mortality salience (Pyszczynski, Greenberg, & Solomon, 1999). However, anxious individuals, but not avoidant ones, also reacted more favorably to the pro-American writer in the separation-primed condition. In other words, anxious people showed the same defensive reaction (ethnocentric pro-Americanism) to reminders of death and separation.

Although anxiously attached adults are unusually afraid of losing a relationship partner, research has shown that they suffer from ambivalence or conflict between approach and avoidance relational tendencies (e.g., Maio, Fincham, & Lycett, 2000). On the one hand, they are highly motivated to gain a partner's attention and love. On the other hand, they suffer from intense fear of rejection and harbor serious doubts about their ability to gain a partner's love. These fears and insecurities can cause anxious individuals to restrain their approach tendencies when they sense a possibility of disapproval or rejection. Being caught in an approach–avoidance conflict, they are likely to ruminate obsessively about how to react in social situations, thereby interfering with adaptive social behavior. Studies show that anxiously attached people make important mistakes in the social realm—at times failing to explain their needs and wishes clearly because they fear disapproval, which can make them vulnerable to unwanted sexual experiences and hurt feelings (e.g., Davis, Shaver, & Vernon, 2004; Shaver, Mikulincer, Lavy, & Cassidy, in press); and at other times effusively or intrusively expressing their needs and fears to relationship partners (e.g., Mikulincer & Nachshon, 1991), which can lead to rejection or partner withdrawal. Moreover, these individuals have difficulties both initiating new relationships that might be highly rewarding (e.g., Bartz & Lydon, 2006), and being able to end troubled or abusive relationships decisively (e.g., Davila & Bradbury, 2001).

AVOIDANT ATTACHMENT AND DEFENSE: COGNITIVE, AFFECTIVE, AND BEHAVIORAL MECHANISMS

Theoretically, the main goal of avoidant defenses is to protect a person from experiencing or expressing feelings or needs that would activate the attachment system and increase the possibility of feeling vulnerable or worthy of rejection or abandonment. The avoidant person's motto seems to be "I would rather handle stresses and distress myself than be humiliated or thrown off guard by having someone reject my bids for help or protection." Intrapsychically, avoidant defenses involve three main self-protective maneuvers. The first is to block awareness of, or cognitive access to, any emotion, thought, image, fantasy, or memory that might activate the attachment system and cause a wish or desire to seek help or support from an unresponsive attachment figure. A second protective maneuver is to maintain an exaggerated sense of self-worth and entitlement while warding off any emotion, thought, image, fantasy, or memory that implies personal weakness, imperfection, vulnerability, or need. This makes it less likely that a person will be tempted to rely on others for comfort, protection, or support. Along with this strategy comes the third: devaluing others and looking down on them. By means of what social psychologists call *downward social comparison*, a person can view him- or herself as better, stronger, and wiser than others, and hence as not needing anyone else's love or assistance.

Suppression of Attachment-Related Emotions, Thoughts, and Memories

There is ample evidence for this conceptualization of avoidant people's defenses. For example, Mikulincer and Orbach (1995) conducted a series of experiments on emotional memories, asking participants to recall early childhood experiences of anger, sadness, anxiety, or happiness, and to rate the intensity of those focal emotions and any associated emotions for each recalled event. Avoidant individuals proved to have relatively poor access (longer recall latencies) to sad and anxious memories. Moreover, they rated focal emotions (e.g., sadness when asked to retrieve a sad memory) and nonfocal emotions (e.g., anger when retrieving a sad memory) as less intense than the emotions recalled by less avoidant, more secure individuals.

Fraley and Shaver (1997) obtained related evidence in a study of thought suppression. Participants wrote continuously about whatever thoughts and feelings came to mind while they were attempting not to think about a romantic partner's leaving them for someone else. Avoidance was associated with the ability to suppress separation-related thoughts, as indicated by less frequent thoughts of loss following the suppression task and lower skin conductance (autonomic arousal) during the task. A subsequent study used functional magnetic resonance imaging to observe brain processes during this same suppression task (Gillath, Bunge, Shaver, Wendelken, & Mikulincer, 2005) and found that avoidance was associated with a particular pattern of activation and deactivation in brain regions involved in suppression.

In two other experiments, mentioned earlier, we (Mikulincer et al., 2004) replicated and extended Fraley and Shaver's (1997) findings by using a Stroop color-naming task to measure the cognitive accessibility of previously suppressed thoughts about a painful separation. Avoidant individuals were able to suppress thoughts related to the breakup, and they seemed to do this in conjunction with bringing to mind some of their own positive qualities (assessed uniquely for each participant). However, their ability to maintain this defensive stance was disrupted when a cognitive load (remembering a seven-digit number) was added to the experimental task. Under this high cognitive load, avoidant individuals suddenly became hypersensitive to thoughts of separation and to their own undesirable traits. That is, the suppressed material resurfaced in experience and behavior when a high cognitive demand was imposed, indicating that avoidant defenses require cognitive work. Studies showing that avoidant people do sometimes experience strong negative emotions in response to chronic, uncontrollable, and severely distressing events also suggest a breakdown of defenses when the mental load includes not just cognitive processes but intense stress (e.g., Berant, Mikulincer, & Florian, 2001; Berant, Mikulincer, & Shaver, 2008).

Avoidant people's defenses are also evident in studies examining the coherence between self-reports of subjective experience and less conscious, more automatic indicators of thoughts and emotions. For example, Mikulincer, Florian, and Tolmacz (1990) found that avoidant individuals scored relatively low on an explicit self-report measure of death anxiety, but their fear of death was revealed in stories written in response to cards of the Thematic Apperception Test (Murray, 1936/1971) suggesting death or loss. Mikulincer (1998a) also found that avoidant people, as compared with secure ones, reacted to anger-eliciting events with lower levels of self-reported anger but higher levels of physiological arousal (heart rate). Other studies have found that avoidant people express relatively few negative feelings about their parents during the AAI, but show high levels of physiological arousal (heightened skin conductance) and more intense facial expressions of anger and sadness when thinking about these relationships (e.g., Dozier & Kobak, 1992; Roisman, Tsai, & Chiang, 2004; Zimmermann, Wulf, & Grossmann, 1997).

Self-Enhancement

With regard to avoidant individuals' fears of feeling vulnerable and dependent on others' kindness or assistance, causing them defensively to inflate their positive self-views, Gjerde, Onishi, and Carlson (2004) found that people classified as avoidant in a Romantic Attachment Interview (similar to the AAI) scored higher than secure people on an index of self-enhancement. (In particular, avoidant people described themselves on the Q-set items in significantly more favorable ways than trained observers described them—something that did not happen with more secure individuals.) Similar positively biased self-appraisals were also noted by Mikulincer (1995). Whereas secure people had ready access to both positive and negative self-attributes in a Stroop color-naming task, as well as to a highly integrated self-concept in a trait-sorting task, avoidant people's organizations of their own attributes seemed defensive. They could quickly access positive but not negative self-attributes, and their organization of these attributes was poor. This poor self-integration has also been documented in the form of positive associations between avoidant attachment and reliance on *splitting* defenses—that is, attempts to protect desirable aspects of the self by detaching them from the undesirable aspects (Lopez, 2001; Lopez, Fuendeling, Thomas, & Sagula, 1997).

Two experimental studies further corroborated avoidant people's attempts to bolster their self-image when threatened (Hart et al., 2005; Mikulincer, 1998b). Study participants were exposed to various kinds of threatening or neutral information, and self-appraisals were recorded both explicitly and via subtler techniques, such as reaction times for trait recognition. Across the various studies, avoidant people appraised themselves more positively (according to both explicit and implicit measures) after threatening as compared with neutral manipulations. Interestingly, secure individuals' self-appraisals did not differ across neutral and threatening conditions, suggesting that they do not need or rely on avoidant defenses.

A study using the AAI with college students also indicated a connection between avoidance and inflation of self-views. Despite the fact that, compared to secure students, dismissing students were rated by peers as having lower ego resilience, higher anxiety, and higher hostility, the dismissing students did not view themselves as lower on perceived self-competence and distress (Kobak & Sceery, 1988). This is consistent with avoidant adults' responses to the Rorschach test. We (Berant, Mikulincer, Shaver, & Segal, 2005) found that more avoidant adults were more likely to give responses indicating a tendency to hide behind a façade and maintain a grandiose, inflated self-image.

Devaluation of Others

As mentioned, avoidant defenses encourage negative views of other people, diverting attention away from others' positive traits, intentions, and relational behaviors. As a result, genuine signals of a partner's support and love can be missed; even when noted, they can be easily forgotten and remain inaccessible when the relationship partner is appraised later. Moreover, avoidant people's tendency to suppress negative self-aspects, coupled with their preference for emotional and cognitive distance from others, can encourage projection of the suppressed material onto relationship partners. This projection can then reinforce avoidant people's sense of their own uniqueness and value, while enabling them to cast aspersions on others.

There is evidence that avoidant people hold negative views of human nature in general, and negative views of relationship partners in particular (see Mikulincer & Shaver, 2007, for a review). Moreover, Zhang and Hazan (2002) found that these negative views are very stable and difficult to refute: Avoidant participants in their study needed (requested) more behavioral evidence to decide that others possessed positive traits or that their possession of negative traits was disconfirmed. There is also evidence that more avoidant people exaggerate dissimilarities between themselves and others, exhibiting what social psychologists call a *false-distinctiveness bias* (e.g., Gabriel, Carvallo, Dean, Tippin, & Renaud, 2005; Mikulincer, Orbach, & Iavnieli, 1998). Mikulincer et al. (1998) found that avoidant people reacted to threats by generating a self-description that was more dissimilar to a partner's self-description and by forgetting more of the traits they shared with the partner.

Following up these studies, Mikulincer and Horesh (1999) examined the projective mechanisms involved in avoidant people's devaluation of others. In the first of two study sessions, each participant generated traits for the actual self and for an unwanted self. In the second session, they formed impressions of hypothetical people, had their ability to retrieve memories of actual familiar people assessed, and drew inferences about the qualities of various hypothetical people. As expected, avoidant participants projected their own unwanted traits onto others. That is, they tended to perceive in others the very traits they had listed as ones they did not like in themselves. Moreover, they easily retrieved examples of known individuals whose traits resembled those of their unwanted selves, and they made faulty inferences that traits taken from their unwanted selves were among the features of a target person they heard about whose description included traits resembling those of the unwanted selves. These perceptual distortions fit the clinical definition of *defensive projection* (Freud, 1915/1957).

It is interesting to note that Kobak and Sceery (1988), whose AAI study of first-year college students making the transition from home to college found that peers rated dismissing students as more hostile than other students, speculated that this hostility (which contains an implicit devaluing of others) serves the defensive function of *displacement,* as direct hostility to rejecting parents could threaten the attachment relationship. The authors noted that "displacement of this hostility to peer contexts may have short-term adaptive value in terms of avoiding conflict in the parent–child relationship" (p. 143).

Avoidant Defenses in Psychotherapy Settings

Avoidant people's defensive exclusion of attachment- and distress-related thoughts and feelings, as well as their tendency to enhance their self-views and devalue other people, can obviously affect therapeutic processes such as the formation of a working alliance, transference, and resistance to therapeutic interventions. Avoidant clients' devaluation of others, dismissal of attachment needs, and reluctance to engage in self-disclosure interferes with establishing the kind of alliance that enables a therapist and client to work together to achieve therapeutic goals (e.g., Bordin, 1979; Gelso & Hayes, 1998). Avoidant clients' compulsive self-reliance and grandiosity work against Bordin's (1979) *goal* and *task* components of a working alliance, which require some acceptance of a therapist's suggestions about the aims of therapy. These clients' attempts to remain emotionally uninvolved also thwart a therapist's goal of establishing trust and a strong emotional bond (Bordin's *bond* component of the working alliance).

These claims about the ways in which avoidant attachment can interfere with the therapeutic process are supported by research. Dolan, Arnkoff, and Glass (1993) found that therapists of more avoidant clients reported less client–therapist agreement about the goals of therapy by the third therapeutic session. Satterfield and Lyddon (1995, 1998), Kivlighan, Patton, and Foote (1998), and Parish and Eagle (2003) found that more avoidant clients reported weaker alliances and more problems in establishing an emotional bond with their therapists during the initial therapy sessions (but see Reis & Grenyer, 2004, for a failure to find an association between self-reports of avoidant attachment and ratings of the working alliance in a sample of clients suffering from major depression.) Kanninen, Salo, and Punamaki (2000) assessed attachment patterns (with an interview based on the AAI) and the quality of the working alliance at the beginning, in the middle, and at the end of therapy among Palestinian former political prisoners, finding that avoidant clients reported a deteriorating alliance toward the end of therapy. (Perhaps avoidant defenses become more active and detrimental at the end of therapy, when painful issues of separation come to the fore.) In a sample of adults in treatment for serious psychopathological disorders, avoidance assessed with AAI Q-sort ratings was associated with lower likelihood of seeking and accepting treatment, less self-disclosure within treatment, and not using treatment services well (Dozier, 1990). Moreover, in an experimental study of clinical clients and their case managers who were given an interpersonal problem-solving task, Dozier, Lomax, Tyrrell, and Lee (2001) found that Q-sort ratings of clients' AAI avoidance were linked with more client time spent off task.

Clients' avoidant defenses and transference reactions can evoke particular kinds of reactions from therapists. For example, avoidant clients' rejection of therapeutic interventions that require emotional expression and disclosure of vulnerabilities can cause a therapist to use more rational and cognitive techniques (i.e., to intellectualize), which may not get to the heart of the clients' problems (Lyddon & Satterfield, 1994). A therapist who is not sufficiently cognizant of these avoidant defenses may use task-based interventions that do not challenge the defenses, but instead reinforce maladaptive relational patterns. In support of this view, Hardy et al. (1999) content-analyzed transcripts of therapy sessions and found that therapists tended to respond to avoidant clients by offering cognitive interpretations rather than reflecting on the clients' emotions and concerns (see also Dozier et al., 2001, for a clinical vignette illustrating this therapeutic tendency).

Avoidant people's tendency to devalue potentially "stronger and wiser" caregivers and reject other people's assistance may also make them unlikely to seek therapy in the first place. For example, Lopez, Melendez, Sauer, Berger, and Wyssmann (1998) found that more avoidant undergraduates were less willing to seek therapy and had more negative attitudes toward therapy. Similarly, Riggs, Jacobvitz, and Hazen (2002) assessed people's exposure to psychotherapy in a sample of middle-class women and found that women with a dismissing (i.e., avoidant) state of mind with respect to attachment (assessed with the AAI) were less likely than secure women ever to have been in therapy. Tasca et al. (2006) also found that higher scores on a self-report measure of avoidant attachment were associated with dropping out of cognitive-behavioral therapy for eating disorders.

A Clinical Example

Sam was a bright 30-year-old client who, characteristically for an avoidant person, devoted the first few therapy sessions to debating whether his therapist was smart enough to help him. At first his conclusion was negative, but he was sufficiently unhappy with his life to continue therapy anyway. It is possible that viewing the therapist as not smart enough for him—an example of dismissing and devaluing others—transformed the therapist into a less threatening person. Sam was especially dismissing and devaluing when he most needed help. Eventually, however, he developed enough trust to tell the therapist about times when he felt needy and unhappy about being alone.

Sam was the youngest of three siblings. Their mother suffered pregnancy complications with all of them, and their father was a busy businessman, who was himself the son of a self-sufficient and rarely available lawyer. A few months after beginning therapy, Sam entered a short story competition. The outcome was to be published in the daily newspaper that Sam knew his therapist read. He came into a session and asked whether he could look at the paper to see if he had won. He also said he knew that he must have lost, because someone from the paper usually telephoned the winner. The therapist decided to show him the paper, because she felt he did not want to be alone while feeling rejected. He opened the paper and confirmed that, indeed, he had not won. The therapist looked at him and asked how he felt. Sam reacted with a series of deactivating manuevers. He first said that he did not "feel anything." He then began to intellectualize and read to the therapist the criteria for winning. He said the stories had to convey a social message and not address personal issues, as his had done. He said that because he had dared to write about personal issues, he was bound to be rejected. Next, Sam abruptly changed the subject and stated he would no longer bring dreams to the therapist, because she was more interested in his dreams than in him. Despite this statement, he asked the therapist about a weak woman who appeared in one of his dreams the previous week; before she could reply, Sam complained that voices on the therapist's answering machine in the next room kept him from concentrating. Sam appeared to feel that the safety or comfort of the session was breached, and he used this interruption to avoid further reflection about his dream. Everything that happened in that session seemed to be colored by Sam's having lost the short story contest, which caused him to feel weak and insecure in ways he could not discuss directly.

On many occasions Sam indicated his self-sufficiency and others' painful devaluation of him only indirectly. For example, on one very hot day he came into the therapy session perspiring and asked whether he could have something cold to drink. The therapist offered him a glass of water. He tasted it and said it smelled bad. The therapist thought to herself, "Whenever he's needy, he has to devalue me." Nevertheless, she decided that voicing this interpretation might cause Sam to withdraw, so she exchanged the water for some juice, which he liked. From then on, the therapist always poured him some juice before his arrival, and Sam typically came in and said, "Oh, here's my juice." At one meeting, however, the therapist happened to have a different kind of juice, which Sam said he didn't like. As if to communicate his self-sufficiency, he came to the next session with a can of energy drink. This was just one of many examples of Sam's discomfort with relying on or collaborating with others, including the therapist, who tried to be responsive to his requests without incurring shame or communicating rejection.

Approximately 2 years into therapy, Sam attempted to get closer to his father and invited him to join him at a pub. The father at first declined the offer. After Sam and the therapist discussed the matter in several therapy sessions, Sam told his father how disappointed he felt, and the father replied, "I'm surprised. I thought I was the last person you'd be interested in spending time with." This is a good example of avoidance occurring across generations—a difficult pattern to break if neither party is willing to express needs and feelings. In this case, therapy was essential for changing the pattern.

ANXIOUS ATTACHMENT AND DEFENSE: COGNITIVE, AFFECTIVE, AND BEHAVIORAL MECHANISMS

As explained earlier, anxiously attached people view experiences of attachment figures' unavailability as a sign of their own deficiencies, helplessness, and unlovability. As a result, they often try mightily to avoid being alone or without the support of a relationship partner. They may prefer to remain in a frustrating relationship with an unreliable or insufficiently available and responsive partner, or even an abusive and violent partner, rather than be alone. At the interpersonal level, anxious defenses are rooted in hyperactivation of attachment needs and a wish for not only proximity and safety but even merger with a safety provider (Hazan & Shaver, 1987). Anxiously attached people are overly dependent on relationship partners, overly eager to coerce or cajole signals of acceptance and loyalty, and quick to express distress and anger if these exaggerated needs are not met by relationship partners (see Mikulincer & Shaver, 2007, for a review). At a deeper, intrapsychic level, their main goal may be to avoid fully experiencing their inability to count on anyone to love and protect them. Yalom (1980) identified this as a dread of existential isolation—the awareness that one can never fully share subjective experiences with others and can never fully appreciate or understand other people's subjectivity, despite intense desires for connection, solidarity, and intimacy. More secure individuals can accept their individuation, but they probably also have a deep feeling of connectedness based on previous secure relationships (Mikulincer & Shaver, 2007).

Amplification of Distress

The wish to feel more central to a relationship partner's attention and concern can cause anxiously attached individuals to exaggerate their expression of needs, pains, and frustrations. They are likely to be highly expressive, prone to rumination, sensitive to slights, envious, angry, and jealous. They can be either demanding or self-deprecating, depending on which stance seems more likely to garner the desired affection and support. However, their agitation and intensity, their self-preoccupation and intrusiveness, are often likely to produce exactly the opposite of what they want from relationship partners. At times, their noisy concerns may seem less than justified or less than authentic, perhaps partly because the *Sturm und Drang* constitute a defensive maneuver to avoid directly experiencing an even deeper sense of insufficiency and isolation.

This kind of emotionality runs counter to most discussions of defenses viewed in terms of emotion regulation, because the literature on emotion regulation (e.g., Gross, 2007) usually stresses *down*-regulation of negative emotions. In the case of anxiously attached persons, however, *regulation* can also mean histrionic intensification, which has been inadvertently rewarded in prior relationships by gaining the attention of an otherwise unreliable caregiver. As Cassidy (1994) has explained with reference to anxious attachment in children,

> The negative emotionality of the insecure/ambivalent child may be exaggerated and chronic because the child recognizes that to relax and allow herself to be soothed by the presence of an attachment figure is to run the risk of then losing contact with the inconsistently available parent. One reasonable strategy involves fearfulness in response to relatively benign stimuli. Through exaggerated fearfulness, the infant increases the likelihood of gaining the attention of a frequently unavailable caregiver should true danger arise. (p. 241)

This *up*-regulation of distress encourages catastrophic appraisals, amplification of threats, pessimistic beliefs about one's ability to manage distress, and attribution of threats to uncontrollable causes and global personal inadequacies (see Mikulincer & Shaver, 2007, for an extensive review of findings regarding this self-defeating attribution pattern). It also involves paying close attention to internal signs of insecurity, anxiety, or distress; engaging in what Lazarus and Folkman (1984) called *emotion-focused coping*; and ruminating on actual and potential threats. An additional paradoxical strategy is to intensify negative emotions by adopting a counterphobic, self-endangering stance toward threats, or making self-defeating decisions and taking ineffective courses of action that end in failure. These strategies create a self-amplifying cycle of distress, which Main (1990) described (with reference to the AAI) as involving high levels of anxiety, preoccupation, confusion, unresolved anger, and incoherence.

For anxiously attached people, histrionics may seem to have two beneficial effects. First, they sometimes elicit the desired attention, care, and love from others, which is theoretically the reason the anxious strategy was adopted in the first place. But there may be a second, less obvious benefit:

The hubbub and distraction generated by strident, impulsive expressions of pain, need, and anger may direct attention and energy away from a deeper problem: sensing oneself as not very substantial at all and not worthy of anyone's care. Agitating and grabbing someone's attention are at least likely to make *something* happen, and even if that something is unpleasant, it may feel better than nothing—that is, better than existential isolation and worthlessness.

Several studies have shown that attachment-related anxiety is associated with distress-intensifying appraisals of threatening situations—appraising threats as extreme and one's coping resources to deal with the threats as deficient (e.g., Berant et al., 2001; Birnbaum, Orr, Mikulincer, & Florian, 1997; Cozzarelli, Sumer, & Major, 1998). Anxious attachment is also associated with less positive expectations regarding the regulation of negative moods (e.g., Creasey, 2002; Creasey & Ladd, 2004), lower confidence in one's ability to solve life problems, and pessimistic self-defeating attitudes (e.g., Berant et al., 2005; Wei, Heppner, & Mallinckrodt, 2003). Researchers who assessed emotion-focused coping (e.g., wishful thinking, self-blame, rumination) consistently found it to be associated with anxious attachment (e.g., Berant et al., 2001; Mikulincer & Florian, 1995; Scharf, Mayseless, & Kivenson-Baron, 2004). Anxiously attached people tend to direct their attention toward their own distress rather than focusing on possible solutions to the problem at hand. Such individuals also intensify death concerns and keep death-related thoughts active in working memory (e.g., Mikulincer & Florian, 2000; Mikulincer et al., 1990). That is, anxious attachment is associated with a heightened fear of death and heightened accessibility of death-related thoughts even when no death reminder is present.

Anxiously attached individuals' intensification of negative emotions has also been noted with respect to their experiences of anger and jealousy. Mikulincer (1998a) reported that such people's recollections of anger-provoking experiences included an uncontrollable flood of angry feelings, persistent rumination on these feelings, and sadness and despair following conflicts. Guerrero (1998) and Sharpsteen and Kirkpatrick (1997) found that anxiously attached people tended to experience jealousy in intense ways, allowing it to ignite other negative emotions and overwhelm their thought processes. Specifically, these people experienced fear, guilt, shame, sadness, and anger during jealousy-eliciting events, and reported high levels of suspicion and worries during these events. This far-reaching spread of negative emotions was also evident in Mikulincer and Orbach's (1995) study of emotional memories. In this study (briefly described earlier), anxious people had rapid access to sad and anxious memories and they reported experiencing very intense focal *and* nonfocal emotions when asked to remember examples of anxiety, sadness, and anger. In other words, anxious people exhibited a rapid and extensive spread of activation among negative memories.

Researchers have also reported evidence of anxiously attached people's tendency to exaggerate expressions of negative mental states. For example, Magai, Hunziker, Mesias, and Culver (2000) found that such people were more expressive of negative emotions (based on coding facial expressions) during an emotion-induction procedure, and Roisman et al. (2004) obtained similar findings when anxious people talked (in the AAI) about their relationships with their mothers during childhood. A similar negative bias in facial expressions was noted by Sonnby-Borgstrom and Jonsson (2003), who presented people with pictures of happy and angry faces and assessed the activity of smile and frown muscles. More anxiously attached people had more active frown muscles while watching either happy or angry faces, implying a heightened tonic expression of negative emotions. Pietromonaco and Barrett (1997) found, in a daily diary study, that anxious people made global assessments of negative affect that were exaggerated compared to the specific negative affect they reported on a daily basis. Moreover, the Rorschach scores of anxious people indicate that their positive feelings tend to be pushed aside by negative ones, which seem to cause emotional confusion (Berant et al., 2005).

Anxious Self-Devaluation

Anxiously attached people, who strive to gain a partner's love, esteem, and protection while doubting their deservingness and efficacy, constantly reinforce the cognitive accessibility of negative self-representations. Moreover, their awkward, sometimes desperate attempts to gain proximity to a relationship partner end up reinforcing the negative self-image, because such people often present themselves in degrading, childish, or excessively needy ways in an effort to elicit compassion and support. Mikulincer (1998b) found that anxiously attached people tended to make more negative self-appraisals in threatening than in neutral conditions. Of great interest is his finding that this tendency could be reduced by a message that broke the likely connection between self-devaluation and others' supportive responses ("Findings show that people who hold a balanced self-view and can acknowledge both strong and weak self-aspects tend to elicit others' affection and support"), implying that anxious people usually denigrate themselves overtly to gain other people's sympathy, approval, and support. If this tactic is expected to fail, it is not as readily used. Anxious self-devaluation has also been noted in anxiously attached people's self-derogating forms of humor—for example, "I will often try to make people like or accept me more by saying something funny about my own weaknesses or faults" (e.g., Kazarian & Martin, 2004). A related self-devaluation tendency seems to be responsible for anxious individuals' tendency to seek for more negative than positive feedback from relationship partners (e.g., Brennan & Bosson, 1998; similar findings emerged from a reanalysis of data presented in Cassidy, Ziv, Mehta, & Feeney, 2003).

Poor Self–Other Differentiation

Anxiously attached persons' defenses intensify the desire for close proximity to, and even merger or fusion with, relationship partners as a means of avoiding the painful awareness of existential isolation. This tendency can encourage such people to project their own qualities onto relationship partners, creating an illusory sense of similarity and union, and blurring boundaries between self and other. In support of this idea, Mikulincer et al. (1998) and Lopez (2001) found that anxiously attached individuals were more likely than secure ones to perceive others as similar to themselves and to show a false-consensus bias in both trait and opinion descriptions. Mikulincer et al. (1998) also found that such people were likely to handle threats by generating a self-description that was more similar to a partner's description and by recalling more partner traits that they shared.

In a series of experiments described earlier, Mikulincer and Horesh (1999) found that anxiously attached people (as compared with secure ones) tended to project their traits onto others. That is, they perceived in an unfamiliar person traits characteristic of themselves, easily retrieved an example of a known person whose traits resembled their own, and made faulty inferences that traits taken from their own self-descriptions were found among qualities said to be self-descriptive by another person. In other words, it seems that anxious people's intense desire for closeness causes them to engage in what Klein (1940) called *projective identification*—projection of one's own traits onto others as a means of blurring self–other boundaries and defending against threats of distinctness, separation, or isolation.

Anxious Defenses in Psychotherapy

Anxiously attached people's heightened need for others' proximity and support, their self-devaluation, and their tendency to intensify distressing thoughts and emotions can obviously affect the quality of the working alliance with a therapist and a client's transference reactions. Although such clients' desire for merger and consensus may cause them to agree readily with the therapist about the goals and tasks of therapy, their hunger for attention, care, and love, and their exaggerated reactions to others' signals of disapproval, rejection, or criticism, can increase the frequency and intensity of ruptures in the alliance throughout therapy. As in other close relationships, an anxious client's relationship with a therapist can be so emotionally turbulent that it interferes with therapeutic success. In support of this view, Mallinckrodt, Coble, and Gantt (1995) found that more anxiously attached clients scored lower on self-reports of a good working alliance. Moreover, Kanninen et al. (2000) found that anxiously attached clients reported a poor alliance in the middle phase of therapy, but a strong alliance in later phases.

Interestingly, therapists' own anxious attachment style has been found to impair the quality of the working alliance with clients. For example, Sauer, Lopez, and Gormley (2003) found that anxiously attached therapists had adverse effects on clients' feelings about the working alliance after four and seven therapeutic sessions. Similarly, Black, Hardy, Turpin, and Parry (2005) found that anxiously attached therapists reported weaker alliances and more therapeutic difficulties (e.g., being "unable to comprehend the essence of a client's problem") than secure therapists did. However, it is important to note that Ligiero and Gelso (2002) found no significant association between therapists' anxious attachment and quality of the working alliance, so this matter deserves further study.

Rubino, Barker, Roth, and Fearon (2000) found that therapists were more emotionally involved with anxiously attached clients and reacted more empathically to them than to less anxious clients. Woodhouse, Schlosser, Crook, Ligiero, and Gelso (2003) found that anxious clients "tend to vacillate between a desire to cope with a lowered sense of self-worth by wishing to merge with the other (who is perceived as being unrealistically good) and feelings of anger at the other for not being available or understanding enough" (p. 398). (Again, this is very reminiscent of Ainsworth et al.'s [1978] label for anxiously attached infants: *anxious-ambivalent*.) As a result, their transferences are likely to include unrealistic hopes, frustration, rage, and perceptions of the therapist as inadequately supportive. Indeed, Woodhouse et al. (2003) found that more anxiously attached clients were rated by their therapists as displaying higher levels of negative transference (suspiciousness, annoyance). In addition, these transference demands seemed to elicit in therapists particular feelings and reactions aimed at assuaging such clients' exaggerated expressions of distress, vulnerability, and helplessness even during initial therapy sessions. A problem for therapists, therefore, is to avoid being pulled into an anxious client's insatiable needs and strongly ambivalent reactions.

A Clinical Example

Ruth was a 40-year-old woman who had married 2 years before entering therapy and was the mother of a 6-month-old baby. She was the sixth of nine siblings whose mother was widowed when Ruth was 10 years old. Her father suffered from a chronic disease for some years before his death and could not provide for the family, so the mother worked as a nanny for other children. When she returned home from her job, she was so tired that she was unable to pay much attention to her own children. Ruth said, "She did not see me even at arm's length." She complained bitterly that her mother was so busy with being a great mother figure to the children she took care of that she did not have energy to take care of her own children.

As an adult, Ruth suffered from temper tantrums, which can be viewed as similar to the angry protest exhibited by anxiously attached babies in Ainsworth's Strange Situation (Ainsworth et al., 1978). The tantrums occurred when Ruth felt that her husband was not sufficiently attentive or appreciative. For example, they went to a lecture together, and he didn't hold her hand. The lecturer was an attractive woman, and this made Ruth so jealous that she provoked an argument with her husband. What was meant to be a pleasant time together became an interpersonal disaster, causing Ruth to feel even less secure in her relationship with her husband.

Two months after the birth of her son, Ruth wanted to reciprocate her husband's desire to resume physical intimacy. However, she was certain that her physical appearance (she had not yet returned to her prepregnancy weight) repelled him and that his requests were not genuine. She was sure he would reject her because of her "appalling, fat, and disgustingly big stomach." Physical contact did not resume until her son was 6 months old, even though a number of clinical sessions were dedicated to examining her perceptions. Talking about this in therapy reminded her that she never felt good enough for her mother, and she worried that her mother preferred the "well-behaved" children she was taking care of for pay. These feelings were not completely irrational, because the mother used to say that if Ruth and her siblings didn't behave, they would be sent away to a boarding school financed by the government.

Ruth was troubled with a doubt common among anxiously attached adults: She could not believe that her husband's requests and actions were sincere or that his intentions were good. For example, she could not accept his affection at face value; she always worried that he was trying to get something from her. At Ruth's request, the therapist met with her husband twice. In these meetings, the husband relayed that he could not understand Ruth's temper tantrums and felt helpless when faced with her rage and sorrow. He added that he loved her very much and did not want the relationship to fail; he had tears in his eyes as he said this.

Ruth's case exemplifies what can happen when a child lacks a secure base in childhood—partly because of objective hardships and difficulties in a family, partly because of maternal threats of abandonment. This kind of anxious attachment leads to a combination of anxiety and anger, exaggerated demands for attention, care, and self–other merger that are difficult for well-intentioned relationship partners and therapists to overcome.

DISORGANIZED ATTACHMENT AND UNRESOLVED TRAUMAS AND LOSSES: THE BREAKDOWN OF DEFENSE

Disorganized attachment reflects an individual's failure to develop a single organized attachment strategy (either secure or insecure and, if insecure, either anxious or avoidant) in response to the caregiving environment, presumably because the caregiving was so threatening or chaotic that no single behavioral strategy was effective. This is in direct contrast to avoidant and anxious attachment. The organized pattern of avoidance is thought to arise when an infant who faces consistent rejection engages cognition, affect, and behavior in an organized way to minimize activation of attachment behavior, and so maintains sufficient proximity to the attachment figure while avoiding the rebuff that accompanies direct attachment bids. The organized pattern of anxious ambivalence is thought to arise when an infant who faces intermittent responsiveness engages cognition, affect, and behavior to heighten activation of the attachment system, and so increase the likelihood of access to the attachment figure if needed. Both of these organized insecure patterns have been referred to as *protective strategies,* devised to ensure access to the caregiver if needed.

When the caregiver him- or herself is the source of threat, neither strategy can prove effective, and elements of disorganization appear. The infant typically appears disorganized or disoriented, or combines or alternates attachment patterns. The notion that these disorganized attachment behaviors reflect the lack of an effective attachment strategy for regaining a sense of security in the face of stress has gained support from studies relating attachment disorganization to elevated cortisol secretion after exposure to brief stressors (Hertsgaard, Gunnar, Erickson, & Nachmias, 1995; Spangler & Grossmann, 1993). By early childhood, disorganized attachment behavior takes on the appearance of controlling behavior directed toward the parent (e.g., role reversal; Main & Cassidy, 1988).

In adolescence and adulthood, the AAI reveals two groups of people whose narratives parallel the behavior of disorganized infants, in that they too fail to demonstrate a single attachment organization. One group, in which a participant reveals different states of mind during different parts of the interview, is called the insecure *cannot classify* group. This pattern is surely familiar to clinicians who observe a client spend most of a therapy session with anxious or angry complaints about the thoughtlessness of a close relationship partner, only to end the session with a dismissing, avoidant statement about not caring at all about the treatment received. Another group of adults who fail to demonstrate a single organized attachment pattern are those with an *unresolved/disorganized* state of mind. These adults, most frequently identified as the parents of disorganized infants (Solomon & George, 1999), receive the unresolved classification when they demonstrate a brief lapse in the monitoring of discourse or reasoning (i.e., become disorganized; Main, 1995) while discussing loss or trauma. These lapses are thought to reflect temporary alterations in typical states of consciousness. Both the cannot classify and the unresolved groups are thought to reflect cases in which the "working" strategy has broken down (Main, 1995).

We agree with Main's (1995) characterization of disorganized behavior as reflecting the lack of an organized defense. In her words, "Defense, of course, is organized. Disorganized/disoriented behavior is not defensive in the traditional sense, and, indeed, Freud conceptualized disorganization as the state to which defense is the alternative" (p. 461). Yet the lack of organization in the AAI typically occurs in the context of some organized attachment strategy. In the cannot classify category, the individual may, for instance, alternate between avoidant and preoccupied strategies. In the unresolved category, the brief lapses in monitoring of reasoning or discourse can occur within the context of any predominantly underlying state of mind (e.g., a person can be classified as *unresolved/avoidant* or *unresolved/preoccupied*). The relative influence on functioning of the underlying organized state(s) of mind versus the disorganized elements (e.g., the lapses of monitoring and reasoning leading to the unresolved classification) is as yet unknown, and understanding the contribution of each will require extensive research. For instance, is the functioning of an individual classified as unresolved/avoidant different from an individual classified as avoidant? If so, how? What aspects of functioning reflect the avoidant strategy, and which the lack of resolution of trauma or loss? Does the functioning of an individual classified as unresolved/avoidant differ from that of an individual classified as unresolved/preoccupied?

Adults whose AAI narratives lack an organized state of mind with respect to attachment—those who fall into the unresolved and cannot classify groups—are at increased risk for psychopathology. There is evidence that both unresolved and cannot classify AAI attachment categories are overrepresented in clinical populations (van IJzendoorn & Bakermans-Kranenburg, 1996). For instance, in one study of psychiatric inpatients, 77% were placed in the unresolved group, as opposed to 7% of control participants; more specifically, 86% of patients with anxiety disorders and 88% of patients with borderline personality disorder were in the unresolved group (Fonagy et al., 1996; see also Hesse & van IJzendoorn, 1999, for evidence that unresolved status is associated with an increased tendency toward absorption, one of the characteristics of dissociative states). Moreover, there is emerging evidence that the most serious psychological disturbances are characterized by a relatively high proportion of individuals in the cannot classify group: 26% of young adults who had been previously psychiatrically hospitalized, as compared to 7% of nonhospitalized control participants (Allen, Hauser, & Borman-Spurrell, 1996); 37% of maritally violent men, as opposed to 10% of nonviolent men (Holtzworth-Munroe, Stuart, & Hutchinson, 1996); and 27% of male prisoners in a Dutch psychiatric prison for inmates who had committed serious crimes (van IJzendoorn et al., 1997).

THE IMPORTANCE OF INDUCED OR ENHANCED SECURITY IN DEALING CLINICALLY WITH DEFENSES

In Chapter 2, two of us (Shaver & Mikulincer) have described the *broaden-and-build* cycle of attachment security and the positive effects of warm and supportive interactions with available, sensitive, and responsive attachment figures on mental representations of the self and others, interpersonal behavior, affect regulation, mental health, and adjustment. In addition, we have emphasized that the sense of attachment security allows people to soften or let down their psychological defenses. Mental representations related to secure relationships and current feelings of attachment security reduce what Higgins (1998) has called a *prevention* motivational orientation, which focuses on the need for safety and the avoidance of negative, painful experiences. Dropping this prevention orientation and embracing a *promotion* orientation makes it less necessary to employ the deactivating and hyperactivating defenses we have described in the present chapter. Securely attached people generally feel sufficiently safe and protected without having to activate defenses. Moreover, they can interact with other people in a confident and open way, without worrying about being abandoned, engulfed, or controlled by others.

To characterize how attachment security relates to both mental health and lack of defensiveness, we (Mikulincer & Shaver, 2005) have proposed a two-level model of psychological defenses. At the primary level, we view interactions with security-enhancing attachment figures as natural contributors to a solid and stable psychological foundation. At this level, representations of attachment security can maintain emotional stability and effective functioning without reality-distorting defenses. Securely attached people maintain an authentic sense of worth and efficacy, while feeling safe and protected by actual attachment figures and mental representations of interactions with such figures.

A second level of defenses is required when a person fails to form secure attachments and is unable to build a secure psychological foundation that facilitates accurate, undistorted perception of internal and external events. For an insecurely attached person, many everyday experiences threaten the sense of safety and raise doubts about his or her tenuous hold on life, identity, and knowledge of the world. At this level, a prevention orientation and the use of deactivating and hyperactivating defenses can at times compensate for the absence of attachment security, create a semblance or façade of self-esteem and self-efficacy, and contribute to a degree of adjustment. At other times, when the level of stress is great, these defenses are likely to break down or be overwhelmed. As we have explained throughout this chapter, the notion of a second level of defenses is equally applicable to avoidant and anxious people. Although defensiveness is most evident in avoidant people, who engage frequently in defensive self-enhancement and repressive coping, the alternative anxious, hyperactivating strategies can also serve defensive functions and may sometimes provide a degree of adjustment.

We expect, and have explored the possibility experimentally, that exposing insecurely attached people to actual or symbolic interactions with security-enhancing attachment figures will allow them momentarily to reduce their deactivating or hyperactivating defenses and to explore their negative feelings in a more constructive way. This fits with Bowlby's (1988) notion of the therapist as a secure base, who needs to be an available, sensitive, and responsive figure for his or her clients; to infuse them with a sense of attachment security; and to help them explore their dysfunctional mental representations of self and others and their maladjusted patterns of interpersonal behavior. But these positive effects of an attachment figure's availability are not confined to client–therapist relations. They also occur within relational contexts in which an actual relationship partner's supportive behaviors are clear-cut, personally significant, and repeated over time and situations. Such behavior on the part of a romantic partner, friend, teacher, manager, or leader may counteract an insecure person's dispositional tendencies to doubt the availability and responsiveness of social interaction partners, and therefore may set in motion a broaden-and-build cycle of attachment security and reduce attachment-related defenses. In other words, a relationship partner who acts as a reliable secure base can help an insecure person function less defensively.

Although less stable and pervasive, doses of security can also be induced by the experimental priming of thoughts about available and supportive attachment figures, and this bolstered sense of security can renew one's broaden-and-build cycle of personal growth. In support of this view, we (Shaver et al., in press) found that experimentally activating security-enhancing mental representations reduced the strength of both deactivating and hyperactivating defenses when people were recalling painful experiences of a close relationship partner hurting their feelings. Specifically, participants completed the Experiences in Close Relationships (ECR) inventory (Brennan, Clark, & Shaver, 1998), tapping dispositional attachment-related anxiety and avoidance, and then wrote a description of an incident in which a close relationship partner hurt their feelings. The participants next completed a short computerized task in which they were repeatedly exposed subliminally (for 22 milliseconds) to either a security-enhancing prime (one of three words: *love, secure,* or *affection*) or a neutral prime (one of three words: *lamp, staple,* or *building*). Immediately after the priming trials, participants were asked to think again about the hurtful event they had described earlier and to rate how hurtful this kind of event would be for them if it happened again: how rejected they would feel, how the event would cause them to feel about themselves on a list of positive and negative self-relevant adjectives, and how much each of nine action descriptions fit the way they would react to the hurtful event (e.g., defensive and hostile reactions, constructive reactions, and crying).

In the neutral priming condition, the findings revealed the typical deactivating and hyperactivating defenses of avoidantly and anxiously attached people, respectively (e.g., Feeney, 2005). Specifically, avoidant attachment scores on the ECR were associated with less negative appraisals of the hurtful event, less intense feelings of rejection, less crying, and stronger defensive/hostile reactions. These findings fit previous results indicating that avoidant people tend to adopt deactivating defenses and then dismiss hurtful events, inhibit expressions of distress, and react hostilely to hurtful partners. Moreover, in the neutral priming condition, attachment anxiety was significantly associated with more intense feelings of rejection, more crying, and more negative emotions. These results are compatible with those from previous studies showing anxiously attached persons' reliance on hyperactivating defenses—distress intensification and overt expression of the negative feelings. However, the parallel associations for both attachment-related anxiety and avoidance were dramatically reduced (most of them approached zero) in the security-priming condition. In other words, as expected, security priming buffered the tendency of avoidant people to rely on deactivating defenses and the tendency of anxious people to cope badly with a hurtful event and to express vulnerability. In other studies (e.g., Mikulincer & Shaver, 2001; Mikulincer, Shaver, Gillath, & Nitzberg, 2005), we have found that similar priming procedures, which can be administered subliminally or supraliminally with similar effects, reduce defensive ingroup–outgroup prejudice and increase compassion and altruism. These findings suggest that clinically supported increases in security may have a broad range of beneficial personal and social effects.

Our preliminary study of hurt feelings supports the hypothesized role played by attachment security in reducing defensiveness. When a person is already secure, because of a security-bolstering attachment history, he or she can deal more constructively with pain and distress. When a person has experienced a history of unreliable, unpredictable attachment figures and has become dispositionally anxious as a result, he or she is likely to rely on hyperactivating defenses when coping with stress and distress. But this habitual response can be notably reduced by a brief, simple, unconscious augmentation of felt security. When a person has dealt with cool, consistently unsupportive attachment figures and has thereby developed a defensively avoidant pattern of relating to others, he or she is somewhat protected from inner pain and distress, but at the expense of rigid, distorting defenses and interpersonal distance. This protective armor can be at least temporarily softened by an infusion of felt security. Therefore, it seems that even a small subliminal security boost can allow an avoidant person to become more open to inner pain (Cassidy, 2004), which can then be addressed clinically.

CONCLUSIONS

Ever since Freud, defenses have been an important issue in psychodynamic therapy. As other modes of therapy have arisen (e.g., behavior therapy, cognitive-behavioral therapy, drug therapy), however, the importance of defenses has been challenged, along with projective measures of defenses such as the Rorschach (e.g., Wood, Nezworski, Lilienfeld, & Garb, 2003). Attachment theory, which is a branch of psychodynamic theory, includes the concept of defense and takes it seriously. Moreover, research inspired by the theory, including studies based on the Rorschach and other projective tests (e.g., Berant et al., 2005; Mikulincer et al., 1990), strongly supports the existence of defenses and their systematic links with attachment processes. Clinical assessments aimed at informing attachment-related therapy should consider a client's defenses, and therapists should be aware of the importance of providing a secure base for clients without accidentally and inappropriately strengthening dysfunctional defenses. Research conducted to date suggests that clients with different attachment patterns will present different kinds of defenses and difficulties for therapists. Keeping abreast of research on attachment issues in clinical settings should make it increasingly easier to soften the defenses and reduce associated personal and interpersonal difficulties.

RECOMMENDATIONS FOR FURTHER READING

Cassidy, J., & Shaver, P. R. (Eds.). (2008). *Handbook of attachment: Theory, research, and clinical applications* (2nd ed.). New York: Guilford Press.—The second edition of this handbook summarizes classic and recent contributions to attachment theory, and provides up-to-date reviews of many basic and applied research areas influenced by the theory.

Mikulincer, M., & Shaver, P. R. (2007). *Attachment in adulthood: Structure, dynamics, and change.* New York: Guilford Press.—This book summarizes research on adult attachment and contains an in-depth discussion of ideas and findings mentioned in this chapter.

REFERENCES

Ainsworth, M. D. S., Blehar, M., Waters, E., & Wall, S. (1978). *Patterns of attachment: A psychological study of the Strange Situation.* Hillsdale, NJ: Erlbaum.

Allen, J. P., Hauser, S. T., & Borman-Spurrell, E. (1996). Attachment theory as a framework for understanding sequelae of severe adolescent psychopathology: An eleven-year follow-up study. *Journal of Clinical and Counseling Psychology, 64,* 254–263.

Baldwin, M. W., & Kay, A. C. (2003). Adult attachment and the inhibition of rejection. *Journal of Social and Clinical Psychology, 22,* 275–293.

Baldwin, M. W., & Meunier, J. (1999). The cued activation of attachment relational schemas. *Social Cognition, 17,* 209–227.

Bartz, J. A., & Lydon, J. E. (2006). Navigating the interdependence dilemma: Attachment goals and the use of communal norms with potential close others. *Journal of Personality and Social Psychology, 91,* 77–96.

Berant, E., Mikulincer, M., & Florian, V. (2001). Attachment style and mental health: A 1-year follow-up study of mothers of infants with congenital heart disease. *Personality and Social Psychology Bulletin, 27,* 956–968.

Berant, E., Mikulincer, M., & Shaver, P. R. (2008). Attachment style, mental health, and intergenerational transmission of emotional problems: A seven-year study of mothers of children with congenital heart disease. *Journal of Personality, 76,* 31–66.

Berant, E., Mikulincer, M., Shaver, P. R., & Segal, Y. (2005). Rorschach correlates of self-reported attachment dimensions: Dynamic manifestations of hyperactivating and deactivating strategies. *Journal of Personality Assessment, 84,* 70–81.

Birnbaum, G. E., Orr, I., Mikulincer, M., & Florian, V. (1997). When marriage breaks up: Does attachment style contribute to coping and mental health? *Journal of Social and Personal Relationships, 14,* 643–654.

Black, S., Hardy, G., Turpin, G., & Parry, G. (2005). Self-reported attachment styles and therapeutic orientation of therapists and their relationship with reported general alliance quality and problems in therapy. *Psychology and Psychotherapy, 78,* 363–377.

Bordin, E. S. (1979). The generalizability of the psychoanalytic concept of the working alliance. *Psychotherapy, 16,* 252–260.

Bowlby, J. (1973). *Attachment and loss: Vol. 2. Separation: Anxiety and anger.* New York: Basic Books.

Bowlby, J. (1980). *Attachment and loss: Vol. 3. Loss: Sadness and depression.* New York: Basic Books.

Bowlby, J. (1982). *Attachment and loss: Vol. 1. Attachment* (2nd ed.). New York: Basic Books. (1st ed., 1969)

Bowlby, J. (1988). *A secure base: Clinical applications of attachment theory.* London: Routledge.

Brennan, K. A., & Bosson, J. K. (1998). Attachment-style differences in attitudes toward and reactions to feedback from romantic partners: An exploration of the relational bases of self-esteem. *Personality and Social Psychology Bulletin, 24,* 699–714.

Brennan, K. A., Clark, C. L., & Shaver, P. R. (1998). Self-report measurement of adult romantic attachment: An integrative overview. In J. A. Simpson & W. S. Rholes (Eds.), *Attachment theory and close relationships* (pp. 46–76). New York: Guilford Press.

Breuer, J., & Freud, S. (1955). Studies on hysteria. In J. Strachey (Ed. & Trans.), *The standard edition of the complete psychological works of Sigmund Freud* (Vol. 2, pp. 1–305). London: Hogarth Press. (Original work published 1895)

Carlson, E. A. (1998). A prospective longitudinal study of attachment disorganization/disorientation. *Child Development, 69,* 1107–1128.

Cassidy, J. (1994). Emotion regulation: Influences of attachment relationships. In N. Fox (Ed.), The development of emotion regulation: Biological and behavioral considerations. *Monographs of the Society for Research in Child Development, 59*(2–3, Serial No. 240), 228–249.

Cassidy, J. (2004). *Remaining open to the pain.* Invited address at a research conference on attachment, University of California, Davis.

Cassidy, J., & Berlin, L. J. (1994). The insecure/ambivalent pattern of attachment: Theory and research. *Child Development, 65,* 971–981.

Cassidy, J., & Kobak, R. R. (1988). Avoidance and its relationship with other defensive processes. In J. Belsky & T. Nezworski (Eds.), *Clinical implications of attachment* (pp. 300–323). Hillsdale, NJ: Erlbaum.

Cassidy, J., Ziv, Y., Mehta, T. G., & Feeney, B. C. (2003). Feedback seeking in children and adolescents: Associations with self-perceptions, attachment representations, and depression. *Child Development, 74,* 612–628.

Cozzarelli, C., Sumer, N., & Major, B. (1998). Mental models of attachment and coping with abortion. *Journal of Personality and Social Psychology, 74,* 453–467.

Cramer, P. (2006). *Protecting the self: Defense mechanisms in action.* New York: Guilford Press.

Creasey, G. (2002). Psychological distress in college-aged women: Links with unresolved/preoccupied attachment status and the mediating role of negative mood regulation expectancies. *Attachment & Human Development, 4,* 261–277.

Creasey, G., & Ladd, A. (2004). Negative mood regulation expectancies and conflict behaviors in late adolescent college student romantic relationships: The moderating role of generalized attachment representations. *Journal of Research on Adolescence, 14,* 235–255.

Davila, J., & Bradbury, T. N. (2001). Attachment insecurity and the distinction between unhappy spouses who do and do not divorce. *Journal of Family Psychology, 15,* 371–393.

Davis, D., Shaver, P. R., & Vernon, M. L. (2004). Attachment style and subjective motivations for sex. *Personality and Social Psychology Bulletin, 30,* 1076–1090.

Davis, D., & Vernon, M. L. (2002). Sculpting the body beautiful: Attachment style, neuroticism, and use of cosmetic surgeries. *Sex Roles, 47,* 129–138.

Doi, S. C., & Thelen, M. H. (1993). The Fear-of-Intimacy Scale: Replication and extension. *Psychological Assessment, 5,* 377–383.

Dolan, R. T., Arnkoff, D. B., & Glass, C. R. (1993). Client attachment style and the psychotherapist's interpersonal stance. *Psychotherapy, 30,* 408–412.

Downey, G., & Feldman, S. I. (1996). Implications of rejection sensitivity for intimate relationships. *Journal of Personality and Social Psychology, 70,* 1327–1343.

Dozier, M. (1990). Attachment organization and treatment use for adults with serious psychopathological disorders. *Development and Psychopathology, 2,* 47–60.

Dozier, M., & Kobak, R. (1992). Psychophysiology in attachment interviews: Converging evidence for deactivating strategies. *Child Development, 63,* 1473–1480.

Dozier, M., Lomax, L., Tyrrell, C., & Lee, S. (2001). The challenge of treatment for clients with dismissing states of mind. *Attachment & Human Development, 3,* 62–76.

Feeney, J. A. (2005). Hurt feelings in couple relationships: Exploring the role of attachment and perceptions of personal injury. *Personal Relationships, 12,* 253–271.

Fonagy, P., Leigh, T., Steele, M., Steele, H., Kennedy, R., Mattoon, G., et al. (1996). The relation of attachment status, psychiatric classification, and response to psychotherapy. *Journal of Consulting and Clinical Psychology, 64,* 22–31.

Fraley, R. C., & Shaver, P. R. (1997). Adult attachment and the suppression of unwanted thoughts. *Journal of Personality and Social Psychology, 73,* 1080–1091.

Freud, S. (1957). Instincts and their vicissitudes. In J. Strachey (Ed. & Trans.), *The standard edition of the complete psychological works of Sigmund Freud* (Vol. 14, pp. 109–140). London: Hogarth Press. (Original work published 1915)

Gabriel, S., Carvallo, M., Dean, K. K., Tippin, B., & Renaud, J. (2005). How I see me depends on how I see we: The role of attachment style in social comparison. *Personality and Social Psychology Bulletin, 31,* 1561–1572.

Gelso, C. J., & Hayes, J. A. (1998). *The psychotherapy relationship: Theory, research, and practice.* New York: Wiley.

George, C., Kaplan, N., & Main, M. (1984). *Adult Attachment Interview protocol.* Unpublished manuscript, University of California, Berkeley.

George, C., Kaplan, N., & Main, M. (1985). *Adult Attachment Interview protocol* (2nd ed.). Unpublished manuscript, University of California, Berkeley.

George, C., Kaplan, N., & Main, M. (1996). *Adult Attachment Interview protocol* (3rd ed.). Unpublished manuscript, University of California, Berkeley.

Gillath, O., Bunge, S. A., Shaver, P. R., Wendelken, C., & Mikulincer, M. (2005). Attachment-style differences in the ability to suppress negative thoughts: Exploring the neural correlates. *NeuroImage, 28,* 835–847.

Gjerde, P. F., Onishi, M., & Carlson, K. S. (2004). Personality characteristics associated with romantic attachment: A comparison of interview and self-report methodologies. *Personality and Social Psychology Bulletin, 30,* 1402–1415.

Greenfield, S., & Thelen, M. (1997). Validation of the Fear of Intimacy Scale with a lesbian and gay male population. *Journal of Social and Personal Relationships, 14.* 707–716.

Gross, J. J. (Ed.). (2007). *Handbook of emotion regulation.* New York: Guilford Press.

Guerrero, L. K. (1998). Attachment-style differences in the experience and expression of romantic jealousy. *Personal Relationships, 5,* 273–291.

Hardy, G. E., Aldridge, J., Davidson, C., Rowe, C., Reilly, S., & Shapiro, D. A. (1999). Therapist responsiveness to client attachment styles and issues observed in client-identified significant events in psychodynamic-interpersonal psychotherapy. *Psychotherapy Research, 9,* 36–53.

Hart, J. J., Shaver, P. R., & Goldenberg, J. L. (2005). Attachment, self-esteem, worldviews, and terror management: Evidence for a tripartite security system. *Journal of Personality and Social Psychology, 88,* 999–1013.

Hazan, C., & Shaver, P. R. (1987). Romantic love conceptualized as an attachment process. *Journal of Personality and Social Psychology, 52,* 511–524.

Hentschel, U., Smith, G., Draguns, J. G., & Ehlers, W. (Eds.). (2004). *Defense mechanisms: Theoretical, research, and clinical perspectives.* Amsterdam: Elsevier.

Hertsgaard, L., Gunnar, M., Erickson, M. F., & Nachmias, M. (1995). Adrenocortical responses to the Strange Situation in infants with disorganized/disoriented attachment relationships. *Child Development, 66,* 1100–1106.

Hesse, E. (1999). The Adult Attachment Interview: Historical and current perspectives. In J. Cassidy & P. R. Shaver (Eds.), *Handbook of attachment: Theory, research, and clinical applications* (pp. 395–433). New York: Guilford Press.

Hesse, E. (2008). The Adult Attachment Interview: Protocol, method of analysis, and empirical studies. In J. Cassidy & P. R. Shaver (Eds.), *Handbook of attachment: Theory, research, and clinical applications* (2nd ed., pp. 552–598). New York: Guilford Press.

Hesse, E., & Main, M. (2006). Frightened, threatening, and dissociative parental behavior in low-risk samples: Description, discussion, and interpretations. *Development and Psychopathology, 18,* 309–343.

Hesse, E., & van IJzendoorn, M. (1999). Propensities towards absorption are related to lapses in the monitoring of reasoning or discourse during the Adult Attachment Interview: A preliminary investigation. *Attachment & Human Development, 1,* 67–91.

Higgins, E. T. (1998). Promotion and prevention: Regulatory focus as a motivational principle. In M. P. Zanna (Ed.), *Advances in experimental social psychology* (Vol. 30, pp. 1–46). San Diego, CA: Academic Press.

Holtzworth-Munroe, A., Stuart, G. L., & Hutchinson, G. (1996). Violent vs. nonviolent husbands: Differences in attachment patterns, dependency, and jealousy. *Journal of Family Psychology, 11,* 314–331.

Hudson, S. M., & Ward, T. (1997). Intimacy, loneliness, and attachment style in sexual offenders. *Journal of Interpersonal Violence, 12,* 323–339.

Kaitz, M., Bar-Haim, Y., Lehrer, M., & Grossman, E. (2004). Adult attachment style and interpersonal distance. *Attachment & Human Development, 6,* 285–304.

Kanninen, K., Salo, J., & Punamaki, R. L. (2000). Attachment patterns and working alliance in trauma therapy for victims of political violence. *Psychotherapy Research, 10,* 435–449.

Kazarian, S. S., & Martin, R. A. (2004). Humor styles, personality, and well-being among Lebanese university students. *European Journal of Personality, 18,* 209–219.

Kivlighan, D. M., Jr., Patton, M. J., & Foote, D. (1998). Moderating effects of client attachment on the counselor experience–working alliance relationship. *Journal of Counseling Psychology, 45,* 274–278.

Klein, M. (1940). Mourning and its relationship with manic–depressive states. *International Journal of Psycho-Analysis, 12,* 47–82.

Kobak, R., & Sceery, A. (1988). Attachment in late adolescence: Working models, affect regulation, and representations of self and others. *Child Development, 59,* 135–146.

Lazarus, R. S., & Folkman, S. (1984). *Stress, appraisal, and coping.* New York: Springer.

Ligiero, D. P., & Gelso, C. J. (2002). Countertransference, attachment, and the working alliance: The therapist's contribution. *Psychotherapy, 39,* 3–11.

Lopez, F. G. (2001). Adult attachment orientations, self–other boundary regulation, and splitting tendencies in a college sample. *Journal of Counseling Psychology, 48,* 440–446.

Lopez, F. G., Fuendeling, J., Thomas, K., & Sagula, D. (1997). An attachment-theoretical perspective on the use of splitting defenses. *Counseling Psychology Quarterly, 10,* 461–472.

Lopez, F. G., Melendez, M. C., Sauer, E. M., Berger, E., & Wyssmann, J. (1998). Internal working models, self-reported problems, and help-seeking attitudes among college students. *Journal of Counseling Psychology, 45,* 79–83.

Lyddon, W. J., & Satterfield, W. A. (1994). Relation of client attachment to therapist first- and second-order assessments. *Journal of Cognitive Psychotherapy, 8,* 233–242.

Magai, C., Hunziker, J., Mesias, W., & Culver, L. (2000). Adult attachment styles and emotional biases. *International Journal of Behavioral Development, 24,* 301–309.

Main, M. (1981). Avoidance in the service of attachment: A working paper. In K. Immelmann, G. Barlow, L. Petrinovich, & M. Main (Eds.), *Behavioral development: The Bielefeld interdisciplinary project* (pp. 651–693). New York: Cambridge University Press.

Main, M. (1990). Cross-cultural studies of attachment organization: Recent studies, changing methodologies, and the concept of conditional strategies. *Human Development, 33,* 48–61.

Main, M. (1995). Recent studies in attachment: Overview, with selected implications for clinical work. In S. Goldberg, R. Muir, & J. Kerr (Eds.), *Attachment theory: Social, developmental, and clinical perspectives* (pp. 407–474). Hillsdale, NJ: Analytic Press.

Main, M., & Cassidy, J. (1988). Categories of response to reunion with the parent at age six: Predicted from infant attachment classifications and stable over a one-month period. *Developmental Psychology, 24,* 415–426.

Main, M., & Hesse, E. (1990). Parents' unresolved traumatic experiences are related to infant disorganized attachment status: Is frightened and/or frightening parental behavior the linking mechanism? In M. T. Greenberg, D. Cicchetti, & E. M. Cummings (Eds.), *Attachment in the preschool years: Theory, research, and intervention* (pp. 161–182). Chicago: University of Chicago Press.

Main, M., & Solomon, J. (1990). Procedures for identifying infants as disorganized/disoriented during the Ainsworth Strange Situation. In M. T. Greenberg, D. Cicchetti, & M. Cummings (Eds.), *Attachment in the preschool years: Theory, research, and intervention* (pp. 121–160). Chicago: University of Chicago Press.

Maio, G. R., Fincham, F. D., & Lycett, E. J. (2000). Attitudinal ambivalence toward parents and attachment style. *Personality and Social Psychology Bulletin, 26,* 1451–1464.

Mallinckrodt, B., Coble, H. M., & Gantt, D. L. (1995). Working alliance, attachment memories, and social competencies of women in brief therapy. *Journal of Counseling Psychology, 42,* 79–84.

McWilliams, N. (1994). *Psychoanalytic diagnosis: Understanding personality structure in the clinical process.* New York: Guilford Press.

Mikulincer, M. (1995). Attachment style and the mental representation of the self. *Journal of Personality and Social Psychology, 69,* 1203–1215.

Mikulincer, M. (1998a). Adult attachment style and individual differences in functional versus dysfunctional experiences of anger. *Journal of Personality and Social Psychology, 74,* 513–524.

Mikulincer, M. (1998b). Adult attachment style and affect regulation: Strategic variations in self-appraisals. *Journal of Personality and Social Psychology, 75,* 420–435.

Mikulincer, M., Dolev, T., & Shaver, P. R. (2004). Attachment-related strategies during thought suppression: Ironic rebounds and vulnerable self-representations. *Journal of Personality and Social Psychology, 87,* 940–956.

Mikulincer, M., & Florian, V. (1995). Appraisal of and coping with a real-life stressful situation: The contribution of attachment styles. *Personality and Social Psychology Bulletin, 21,* 406–414.

Mikulincer, M., & Florian, V. (2000). Exploring individual differences in reactions to mortality salience: Does attachment style regulate terror management mechanisms? *Journal of Personality and Social Psychology, 79,* 260–273.

Mikulincer, M., Florian, V., Birnbaum, G., & Malishkevich, S. (2002). The death-anxiety buffering function of close relationships: Exploring the effects of separation reminders on death-thought accessibility. *Personality and Social Psychology Bulletin, 28,* 287–299.

Mikulincer, M., Florian, V., & Tolmacz, R. (1990). Attachment styles and fear of personal death: A case study of affect regulation. *Journal of Personality and Social Psychology, 58,* 273–280.

Mikulincer, M., & Horesh, N. (1999). Adult attachment style and the perception of others: The role of projective mechanisms. *Journal of Personality and Social Psychology, 76,* 1022–1034.

Mikulincer, M., & Nachshon, O. (1991). Attachment styles and patterns of self-disclosure. *Journal of Personality and Social Psychology, 61,* 321–331.

Mikulincer, M., & Orbach, I. (1995). Attachment styles and repressive defensiveness: The accessibility and architecture of affective memories. *Journal of Personality and Social Psychology, 68,* 917–925.

Mikulincer, M., Orbach, I., & Iavnieli, D. (1998). Adult attachment style and affect regulation: Strategic variations in subjective self–other similarity. *Journal of Personality and Social Psychology, 75,* 436–448.

Mikulincer, M., & Shaver, P. R. (2001). Attachment theory and intergroup bias: Evidence that priming the secure base schema attenuates negative reactions to out-groups. *Journal of Personality and Social Psychology, 81,* 97–115.

Mikulincer, M., & Shaver, P. R. (2005). Mental representations of attachment security: Theoretical foundation for a positive social psychology. In M. W. Baldwin (Ed.), *Interpersonal cognition* (pp. 233–266). New York: Guilford Press.

Mikulincer, M., & Shaver, P. R. (2007). *Attachment in adulthood: Structure, dynamics, and change.* New York: Guilford Press.

Mikulincer, M., Shaver, P. R., Gillath, O., & Nitzberg, R. E. (2005). Attachment, caregiving, and altruism: Boosting attachment security increases compassion and helping. *Journal of Personality and Social Psychology, 89,* 817–839.

Mikulincer, M., Shaver, P. R., & Pereg, D. (2003). Attachment theory and affect regulation: The dynamics, development, and cognitive consequences of attachment-related strategies. *Motivation and Emotion, 27,* 77–102.

Murray, H. A. (1971). *Thematic Apperception Test.* Cambridge, MA: Harvard University Press. (Original work published 1936)

Parish, M., & Eagle, M. N. (2003). Attachment to the therapist. *Psychoanalytic Psychology, 20,* 271–286.

Pietromonaco, P. R., & Barrett, L. (1997). Working models of attachment and daily social interactions. *Journal of Personality and Social Psychology, 73,* 1409–1423.

Pyszczynski, T., Greenberg, J., & Solomon, S. (1999). A dual process model of defense against conscious and unconscious death-related thoughts: An extension of terror management theory. *Psychological Review, 106,* 835–845.

Reis, S., & Grenyer, B. F. S. (2004). Fear of intimacy in women: Relationship between attachment styles and depressive symptoms. *Psychopathology, 37,* 299–303.

Riggs, S. A., Jacobvitz, D., & Hazen, N. (2002). Adult attachment and history of psychotherapy in a normative sample. *Psychotherapy: Theory, Research, Practice, Training, 39,* 344–353.

Roisman, G. I., Tsai, J. L., & Chiang, K. H. S. (2004). The emotional integration of childhood experience: Physiological, facial expressions, and self-reported emotional response during the Adult Attachment Interview. *Developmental Psychology, 40,* 776–789.

Rowe, A. C., & Carnelley, K. B. (2005). Preliminary support for the use of a hierarchical mapping technique to examine attachment networks. *Personal Relationships, 12,* 499–519.

Rubino, G., Barker, C., Roth, T., & Fearon, P. (2000). Therapist empathy and depth of interpretation in response to potential alliance ruptures: The role of therapist and patient attachment styles. *Psychotherapy Research, 10,* 408–420.

Satterfield, W. A., & Lyddon, W. J. (1995). Client attachment and perceptions of the working alliance with counselor trainees. *Journal of Counseling Psychology, 42,* 187–189.

Satterfield, W. A., & Lyddon, W. J. (1998). Client attachment and the working alliance. *Counseling Psychology Quarterly, 11,* 407–415.

Sauer, E. M., Lopez, F. G., & Gormley, B. (2003). Respective contributions of therapist and client adult attachment orientations to the development of the early working alliance: A preliminary growth modeling study. *Psychotherapy Research, 13,* 371–382.

Scharf, M., Mayseless, O., & Kivenson-Baron, I. (2004). Adolescents' attachment representations and developmental tasks in emerging adulthood. *Developmental Psychology, 40,* 430–444.

Sharpsteen, D. J., & Kirkpatrick, L. A. (1997). Romantic jealousy and adult romantic attachment. *Journal of Personality and Social Psychology, 72,* 627–640.

Shaver, P. R., & Mikulincer, M. (2007). Adult attachment strategies and the regulation of emotion. In J. J. Gross (Ed.), *Handbook of emotion regulation* (pp. 446–465). New York: Guilford Press.

Shaver, P. R., Mikulincer, M., Lavy, S., & Cassidy, J. (in press). Understanding and altering hurt feelings: An attachment-theoretical perspective on the generation and regulation of emotions. In A. Vangelisti (Ed.), *Feeling hurt in close relationships.* New York: Cambridge University Press.

Solomon, J., & George, C. (Eds.). (1999). *Attachment disorganization.* New York: Guilford Press.

Sonnby-Borgstrom, M., & Jonsson, P. (2003). Models-of-self and models-of-others as related to facial muscle reactions at different levels of cognitive control. *Scandinavian Journal of Psychology, 44,* 141–151.

Spangler, G., & Grossmann, K. E. (1993). Biobehavioral organization in securely and insecurely attached infants. *Child Development, 64,* 1439–1450.

Tasca, G. A., Ritchie, K., Conrad, G., Balfour, L., Gayton, J., Lybanon, V., & Bissada, H. (2006). Attachment scales predict outcome in a randomized controlled trial of two group therapies for binge eating disorder: An aptitude by treatment interaction. *Psychotherapy Research, 16,* 106–121.

Taubman-Ben-Ari, O., Findler, L., & Mikulincer, M. (2002). The effects of mortality salience on relationship strivings and beliefs: The moderating role of attachment style. *British Journal of Social Psychology, 41,* 419–441.

van IJzendoorn, M., & Bakermans-Kranenburg, M. J. (1996). Attachment representations in mothers, fathers, adolescents, and clinical groups: A meta-analytic search of normative data. *Journal of Clinical and Consulting Psychology, 64,* 8–21.

van IJzendoorn, M., Feldbrugge, J., Derks, F., de Ruiter, C., Verhagen, M., Philipse, M., et al. (1997). Attachment representations of personality disordered criminal offenders. *American Journal of Orthopsychiatry, 67,* 449–459.

Wei, M., Heppner, P., & Mallinckrodt, B. (2003). Perceived coping as a mediator between attachment and psychological distress: A structural equation modeling approach. *Journal of Counseling Psychology, 50,* 438–447.

Wood, J. M., Nezworski, M. T., Lilienfeld, S. O., & Garb, H. N. (2003). *What's wrong with the Rorschach?: Science confronts the controversial inkblot test.* San Francisco: Jossey-Bass.

Woodhouse, S. S., Schlosser, L. Z., Crook, R. E., Ligiero, D. P., & Gelso, C. J. (2003). Client attachment to therapist: Relations to transference and client recollections of parental caregiving. *Journal of Counseling Psychology, 50,* 395–408.

Yalom, I. (1980). *Existential psychotherapy.* New York: Basic Books.

Zhang, F., & Hazan, C. (2002). Working models of attachment and person perception processes. *Personal Relationships, 9,* 225–235.

Zimmermann, P., Wulf, K., & Grossmann, K. E. (1997). *Attachment representation: You can see it in the face.* Poster presented at the biennial meeting of the International Society for the Study of Behavioural Development, Québec City, Québec, Canada.

13

An Attachment Perspective on Crying in Psychotherapy

Judith Kay Nelson

Crying occurs frequently in psychotherapy, but it is seldom addressed in clinical literature or in psychotherapy training. The prevailing view, going back to early psychoanalytic affect theory (Breuer & Freud, 1895/1955), has been that crying is discharge behavior designed to relieve negative affect. Although modern affect theory has moved to looking at emotion as interpersonally generated and regulated (Schore, 2003; Vingerhoets & Cornelius, 2001), adult crying, in professional as well as popular psychology, continues to be primarily understood in the context of this earlier quantitative, one-person theory of emotion. By contrast, looking at crying from the standpoint of attachment theory and research shows it to be a two-person, relationship-linked behavior.

Crying, along with smiling, clinging, and sucking, appears on the lists of inborn attachment behaviors (Bowlby, 1969/1982). Of all infant behaviors, crying is the most powerful in terms of establishing and maintaining parent/caregiver proximity (Lester & Boukydis, 1985; Nelson, 2005). Infant crying arouses powerful visceral responses (increased blood pressure, skin conductance, and heart rate)—primarily in parents, but also in anyone who hears an infant cry (Boukydis & Burgess, 1982; Lorberbaum et al., 2002). Infant arousal (crying) creates corresponding caregiver arousal, thereby guaranteeing that there will be a caregiving response, though not necessarily an attuned or regulating one. The caregiving system in adults may be overridden by conscious choice or socialization, or misdirected by early attachment trauma. Optimally, however, the repetition of negative arousal (crying) in the infant, followed by successful affect attunement and regulation (parental caregiving), facilitates the formation of the infant–parent attachment bond (Schore, 2003).

John Bowlby (1969/1982) mentioned that attachment behaviors continue to exist into adulthood, albeit in more complex though functionally similar forms. This chapter looks at the clinical impact of a view of crying as attachment behavior that triggers caregiving behavior throughout life (Nelson, 2000). An attachment–caregiving approach is used to classify different types of crying and inhibited crying, and to describe crying, caregiving, and care-receiving patterns associated with adult attachment styles. Crying is also discussed from the standpoint of the window it provides clinically into the quality of early attachment experiences and current adult bonds, including the therapeutic attachment bond, where they serve as guides for the therapist's responses. The positive and negative effects of crying by the therapist—a neglected aspect of the therapeutic relationship—are also considered from the perspective of the therapeutic attachment bond.

A CLASSIFICATION OF CRYING AND INHIBITED CRYING

The prototypical trigger for infant crying is separation from the caregiver (Bowlby, 1969/1982). But no matter the immediate cause of the crying—separation, fear, hunger, pain—the underlying message to the caregiver is always "Come here; I need you." An infant cannot be cared for without physical contact or physical proximity. The most effective terminators of infant crying are parental presence and physical contact (Bowlby, 1969/1982; Wolff, 1969).

When Bowlby (1960) observed infants separated from their caregivers, he noted a consistent series of reactions, which he labeled *protest, despair,* and *detachment.* In the initial stage of protest, the infant's cry was loud and vigorous, and was accompanied by motor tension and arousal (kicking, flailing, shaking the crib) designed to attract the immediate attention of the caregiver in order to terminate the separation as quickly as possible. If there was no reunion, the physical arousal diminished, and the cry became a low, intermittent wail. This stage, giving up hope of a reunion, Bowlby called despair. Finally, if there was still no reunion and no acceptable substitute caregiver, the child would retreat into a noncrying silence—a life-threatening stage Bowlby called detachment.

The parallel trigger for adult crying is the death of a close loved one (Nelson, 1998, 2005). There is no culture in the world where it is unknown (Habenstein & Lamers, 1963). Even in social groups where crying at a close loved one's death is prohibited, or considered dangerous to the life or health of the bereaved person or to the progress of the departed soul in the next life, there are still individuals who are unable to keep themselves from crying (Kracke, 1981, 1988).

When Bowlby (1961, 1980) observed the reactions of adults following the loss of a close loved one, he noted that they were similar to those of infants separated from their caregivers: protest aimed at undoing or denying the loss, and despair representing abandonment of hope for reunion. Depressed detachment following a permanent loss in adults would only occur in complicated grief reactions. Optimally, in adults, a stage he called *reorganization* would occur, in which the bereaved person would gradually find a way to maintain an inner sense of connection with the departed attachment figure while establishing new attachments or reconfiguring previously existing ones.

If the definition of separation and death is expanded to include the literal, symbolic, threatened, or imagined separations and miniature deaths of everyday life, approximately 95% of childhood or adult crying may be seen as a grief reaction (Nelson, 2005; Vingerhoets, 2001). Even many experiences of crying in happiness or joy include losses that have been averted or overcome (Avery, 1983; Weiss, 1952). The remaining 5% of crying episodes (Nelson, 2005) may be classified as somatic (symptomatic of physiological disorders, such as stroke, multiple sclerosis, seizure disorders, or endocrine disorders) or transcendent (going beyond personal loss to an aesthetic, spiritual, or religious experience of connection, love, or attachment).

Adult crying that is triggered by loss may be classified according to the stage of grief it represents: protest or despair. Inhibited adult crying (here defined as not crying after a major loss), when it is part of withdrawn depression, corresponds to the stage of detachment. Because attachment behavior also triggers caregiving behavior throughout life (Nelson, 2005), each type of crying and inhibited crying may be seen to evoke different types of caregiving responses.

Protest Crying

The aim of protest crying in infancy is to bring about an immediate end to separation. Protest crying over everyday losses throughout life is similarly aimed at undoing or averting a perceived or threatened loss. Corresponding to the motor arousal and piercing cries of infancy, protest crying in adulthood often has a hostile edge and demands caregiving in the form of action rather than soothing. Adult protest crying may also have a physical intensity (clenched fists, squared mouth, or contorted facial expressions) that is more typical of an anger response. Of all adult crying, protest crying is the type most likely to be vocalized. Protest crying is often seen as manipulative, because a caregiver feels induced through guilt or anger, rather than empathy, to redress the crier's loss. Protest crying signals activation of the attachment system and is indicative of hyperactivation when it is particularly persistent and out of keeping with the magnitude of the loss.

A child, for example, may cry because he or she is offered an apple instead of the desired cookie. High-intensity crying, which worked in infancy to terminate a separation, does not have the same desired effect on parental caregivers of a young child, who instead may feel impatient, irritated, or angry with the child's protest tears. Similarly, an adult who cries in frustration over a spouse's refusal to cancel a fishing trip mistakenly scheduled on the day of their wedding anniversary may create resistance, guilt, and irritation in the partner, rather than the desired attuned caregiving response (canceling the trip). The combination of blame and a call for action to avoid or undo the loss is a message that often leaves potential caregivers feeling defensive and irritated rather than wanting to comfort. Even if there is a sympathetic response to protest crying, it is often rejected by the crier, who demands action rather than comfort.

Sad Crying in Despair

Crying in despair or surrender signifies that hope is gone. Infant crying in this stage involves low muscle tone and a quiet, occasional wail. Adult crying in despair is accompanied by the typical slumped posture of sadness, conveying a sense of passivity and resignation. The grief muscles (Darwin, 1872/1965) in the forehead and around the mouth are contracted, though frequently the crier will bury his or her face in a handkerchief or hide behind arms or hands. Unless there is intense sobbing, crying in despair is likely to be silent weeping.

Crying in despair powerfully evokes caregiving in the form of comforting touch or soothing words. A child who is crying because a pet hamster died will encounter sympathetic caregivers willing to soothe and comfort him or her. An adult weeping in despair over a rejection letter from medical school is also likely to receive empathic consolation from friends or loved ones. This is the type of crying that is most helpful in resolving loss and working through grief.

Detached, Inhibited Crying

Detached, inhibited crying in the face of a significant loss distances and frustrates caregivers, who find their comfort resisted, ignored, or attacked. It is, by definition, a deactivating strategy; the detached noncrier handles loss by shutting down the attachment system and moving toward isolation rather than connection. For example, when Brad lost his job, he holed up in the den and played computer games all day. He barked whenever his mother or sister tried to talk or sit with him or to bring him a cup of coffee or a beer.

Not all inhibited crying is of the detached type, however. Noncriers who express their loss and need for comfort in a way that invites responsive caregiving are not deactivating their attachment systems altogether. They may be consciously aware of, and able to verbally acknowledge, their attachment distress with accompanying facial expressions and body language signals of sadness, despair, or concern; they may also reach out to available attachment figures for support or consolation.

Fran, for example, did not shed a tear when Ted abruptly ended their 5-year relationship. However, she shared her pain with several close friends, who touched her shoulder and sometimes hugged her, and she took them up on their offers of movie dates and dinners. She was not crying, but she was expressing her grief verbally and was open to caregiving. Reasons for a reluctance to be openly tearful while still being connected to feeling and amenable to caregiving are discussed in the next section.

ASSESSMENT AND TREATMENT STRATEGIES BASED ON ATTACHMENT STYLE

Crying may occur during a psychotherapy hour or be described to the therapist by the client as part of a narrative. Both the observed and the described crying, along with a person's patterns of crying (or not crying) over time, shed light on attachment style, caregiving history, and the state of current attachment bonds with parents or partners, as well as the therapeutic attachment bond. Together, all of these provide valuable information to the therapist about strategies for treatment.

Secure and *insecure* (*avoidant* or *ambivalent/resistant*) attachment patterns were first identified in infants as part of the Strange Situation research pioneered by Mary Ainsworth (Ainsworth, Blehar, Waters, & Wall, 1978). Subsequently Main and Solomon (1990) added another insecure category, *disorganized/disoriented*.

The Adult Attachment Interview was later developed by Main and her associates (see Hesse, 1999, for a full discussion) to evaluate and categorize parents' attachment experiences in relationship to those of their infants and young children. For adults they used terms parallel, but not identical, to those used for infant attachment styles: *secure/autonomous* for secure, *preoccupied* for ambivalent/resistant, *dismissing* for avoidant, and *unresolved/ disorganized* for disorganized/disoriented. For research into adult romantic relationships, Hazan and Shaver (1987) developed a self-report measure for applying the principles associated with Ainsworth's infant attachment style to three categories of adult attachment styles. In subsequent studies (Bartholomew & Shaver, 1998), adult attachment styles have been reconfigured along two poles representing avoidance and anxiety, resulting in four adult attachment styles: *secure* (low avoidance/low anxiety), *preoccupied* (low avoidance/high anxiety), *dismissing* (high avoidance/low anxiety), and *fearful* (high avoidance/high anxiety). (For in-depth summaries of the development of attachment styles and correlates of each classification, see Shaver & Mikulincer, Chapter 2, and Lopez, Chapter 5, this volume.)

For purposes of clinical assessment, I have expanded the definitions of these four adult attachment styles to include typical crying and caregiving patterns. In addition, I have included the disorganized style of attachment as a fifth residual category for patients who present with unpredictable patterns of attachment. Crying in association with each attachment style is examined from the standpoint of helping the clinician to formulate a clinical impression of attachment style, as well as the attachment wounds to be addressed in the therapy.

Identifying the attachment style and the attachment issues of the client also provides the clinician with guidance as to how to proceed with affect attunement and affect regulation. Attachment styles are described by Schore (1994) as derived from "internalized interactive representations" (p. 449) of early attachment–caregiving experiences, including affect regulation by the caregiver. He points out that in therapy, these "unconscious working models of affect regulation are determined and evaluated as they are expressed in the socioaffective relationship between the patient and therapist, especially during stress" (p. 449). Schore (1994) further states that the therapeutic relationship is the "primary vehicle through which pathological internal object relationships, maladaptive internal working models coding insecure attachment patterns, may be transformed into adaptive models based on more secure attachment programs of affect regulation" (p. 449).

Crying is a clear signal of negative arousal, but therapeutic attunement and regulation vary with the attachment style of the crier and the state of the therapeutic attachment bond. Affect attunement strategies, for example, may range from direct and open compassion to low-key, subtle, and understated sympathy. The types of therapeutic affect regulation also vary according to attachment style and according to whether the affect displayed needs to be regulated in the direction of intensifying or deintensifying painful affect and negative arousal. The felt intersubjective attachment–caregiving connections between therapist and client, along with clinical observations of attachment style, provide valuable information about this complex aspect of therapeutic affect regulation: knowing how and when to intensify affect and when to soothe it. In general, a therapist would think about deintensifying negative affect for clients who:

- Are overwhelmed with grief (protest or despair).
- Overdramatize grief/loss, due to a preoccupied attachment style.
- Have a disorganized attachment style.
- Have an avoidant attachment style and are terrified of crying.
- Have not yet established a solid therapeutic attachment bond.

A therapist would consider intensifying negative affect for clients who:

- Are averse to crying due to an avoidant attachment style, but are on the way to *earned-secure* status (Hesse, 1999) and have a well-established therapeutic attachment bond.
- Suppress or prohibit crying for fear they will be rejected if they display negative affect (e.g., those with fearful attachment styles may do this).

- Are securely attached, but suffer from socially acquired shame about crying.

The most effective techniques for helping a noncrying person to shed tears are indirect. Direct verbal encouragement to cry is seldom appropriate or efficacious. Instead, asking a pointed question about the loss, or gently amplifying caregiving statements and gestures, may help to increase a client's receptivity to shedding tears. As in childhood, the repetition of negative arousal, followed by affect attunement and by interactive affect regulation in the therapeutic relationship (a security-enhancing interaction), leads to the development of the increased ability to tolerate negative arousal, to learn self-regulation, and eventually to acquire a sense of attachment security (Mikulincer & Shaver, 2004). Affect attunement and regulation are discussed below in relationship to each attachment style.

Secure

An adult with a secure style of attachment is confident in the reliability and availability of attachment figures (Mikulincer & Shaver, 2003). Attachment behaviors, such as crying, may be activated when there is separation or loss. Even if there is no overt crying with a significant loss, there is an openly expressed vulnerability. Securely attached adults are comfortable with accepting soothing, caregiving behavior from others, and with giving care to those who cry or show vulnerability in their presence (Feeney & Collins, 2004).

With securely attached patients, crying is experienced as part of a normal grieving process tied to a significant loss. They are open to caregiving comments and show signs of being soothed by the therapist's words, body language, sounds, or tone of voice. This openness is consistent with the observations of secure infants in the Strange Situation studies, who readily turned to and were easily comforted by their mothers (Ainsworth et al., 1978).

Jim, a 38-year-old man, came to therapy because of a relationship crisis with his girlfriend, who had been offered an attractive job in another state. Jim was understandably distressed over the possible separation and cried with anticipatory grief. His expectation, however, was that they would work it out somehow, or else face the possibility that the relationship was perhaps not the right one for the long term. He said he realized that they were in this experience together (she would be separated from him, as well as vice versa), and he felt comforted by that thought. He welcomed my inquiries and ideas as openings for further thought and soothing. Both affect attunement and affect regulation went smoothly. With a securely attached person such as Jim—affect attunement, the sense of being heard and understood— can have a soothing and regulating effect in and of itself.

Social mores that overvalue independence and self-reliance, or that view crying as weak, may impinge upon some crying and caregiving even in securely attached adults. However, their feelings of shame and guilt are more accessible than in a person who resists crying because of insecure attachment. Mild reassurance about crying or "permission" to cry may then be in order, although I rarely if ever directly encourage a person to cry, so as not to confront the defensive structure head on. Instead, I may ask a question or make a caregiving comment designed to intensify the attachment affect. For example, had Jim been a male who felt shamed by his crying, I might have helped him be more expressive of his attachment needs through tears by highlighting (i.e., intensifying) the most painful aspects of his loss. To do so, I might have said something like this: "What a rotten time for this job offer, just when you and Jennifer were starting to talk about moving in together." Or I might have considered relating the grief about this potential loss to early attachment wounds. For example, I might have recalled a cross-country move Jim's family had made for his dad's job when he was a child. As a way to evoke the earlier losses, while at the same time providing affect-regulating caregiving in the present therapeutic attachment relationship, I might have made a caregiving comment such as "And back then there was no one there to say, 'It must be sad and scary leaving all your friends to go so far away to a strange place.'"

Preoccupied

Individuals with a preoccupied attachment style are unable to trust in the availability and reliability of attachment figures (Mikulincer & Shaver, 2003). They demonstrate a desperate desire for connection, along with a strong fear of rejection. They are likely to hyperactivate the attachment system (crying) during times of distress, and to show an anxious, even demanding need for caregiving, coupled with great difficulty in being soothed. They live in constant fear of rejection, and may also be prone to compulsive and intrusive caregiving to others as a way of containing their anxiety and securing the presence and caregiving responses of the attachment figure (Feeney & Collins, 2004).

The preoccupied pattern of behavior is a strategy for coping with inconsistently available parental caregivers in childhood. It is a way of making emotional needs prominent and difficult to ignore. Unfortunately, persistent protest crying often causes attachment figures (especially dismissing ones) to get irritated and to shame the crier, reinforcing the cycle of unpredictability and unavailability, and underscoring the constant threat of rejection.

Although people with a preoccupied style of attachment are often eager to seek therapeutic help, the challenge for the therapist is in dealing with the "difficult-to-soothe" aspect of this attachment style. Persons high in attachment-related anxiety (i.e., preoccupied and fearful styles) are prone to becoming absorbed by, and have difficulty disengaging from, negative affect (Mikulincer & Orbach, 1995). The therapeutic stance must be one of

reliability and availability with consistent affect attunement and attempts
to regulate affect by deintensifying overwhelming and disorganizing emotions. Any crack in the therapist's patience, no matter how slight, will be
sensed immediately and taken as rejection. In that case (and sometimes even
without any obvious precipitant), protest crying may then be aimed at the
therapist with this overt or covert message: "Why don't you do something
to help me?"

Peggy, a young mother of two daughters, was referred for therapy by
her former psychiatrist because of severe anxiety. She described an early
history that fit the prototype of inconsistently available parents, with one
unusual feature: Her mother was consistently rejecting, showing open favor-
itism to a younger sibling, while her father showered Peggy with supportive caregiving in the form of special gifts, attention, and father–daughter
outings. His treatment of Peggy aroused her mother's jealous anger at
him as well as her daughter, which the mother expressed in attacking,
bitter comments that further highlighted her overt rejection of Peggy. The
inconsistency Peggy experienced was the markedly different treatment by
each parent, rather than the more usual experience of one inconsistently
responsive parent.

As an adult, Peggy was not only preoccupied with her adult attachment
relationships; she also remained deeply entangled with her aging parents,
who continued the earlier pattern of maternal rejection and paternal favorit-
ism, leaving her feeling trapped in confusion, anger, anxiety, and self-loathing.
From the beginning of treatment, Peggy cried frequently in protest and anger
as she described her parents' ongoing inconsistencies. My affect attunement
took the form of simple statements, such as "How awful for you," "How
confusing that must have been for you as a child," or "How unfair." She
neutrally accepted my comments, but showed no response or sign of being
soothed. I was low-key in my attempts to soothe her, so as to avoid drawing attention to the fact that she was unable to make use of my caregiving.
I did not want to bring her "difficult-to-soothe" side to the surface, for fear
she would become self-critical for not being a "good patient"—or, worse,
think I was criticizing her and feel rejected. Slowly, the gentle affect attunement began to pay off as the therapeutic attachment bond deepened. She
was gradually able to take in my empathic words as a kind of soothing.
I expanded the attunements over time to include explanations of why she
might have felt a certain way. These explanations served to reassure her and
enabled her to contain and regulate her affect.

Many years into treatment, as Peggy began to cry while recounting a
particularly painful exchange with her mother, I nodded toward the box of
tissues placed near her. She took one, whereas in the past she had pointedly
rummaged in her purse to find one of her own. I saw this small step of using
my tissues as a symbolic acceptance of my caregiving. I might also infer that
she had created an internal working model of me as available and regulating. Over time, interactions such as this one may evolve into more adap-

tive, security-based attachment strategies that overshadow the more typical hyperactivating responses.

Dismissing

Adults with a dismissing style of attachment are also unable to trust in the reliability of attachment figures (Mikulincer & Shaver, 2003). However, they are compulsively self-reliant and defensively rely on deactivating strategies, including inhibition of crying during times of vulnerability and stress. In addition, they tend to be both intolerant of caregiving from others and resistant to giving care to others.

Dismissing individuals, according to insights from infant attachment research, had caregivers who were detached and unavailable, but on a consistent rather than an inconsistent basis. They learned early to deactivate their attachment system and become compulsively self-reliant, and therefore seldom cry. When they do, they often get distressed and angry at themselves for losing control. They are desperate to reclaim their noncrying, self-reliant posture.

Catherine, a long-term client I have written about extensively elsewhere (Nelson, 1998, 2005), said at the beginning of therapy that she was a "noncrier" and described herself as "numb." She came in because she was worried about her inability to separate comfortably from her young son. She was self-reliant and highly functional in her chosen profession, and many people liked and respected her, though she thought of herself as having no close friends.

Because of the threat attachment behavior poses to those with a dismissing style, it does not make sense to encourage them to cry. The caregiving wounds that underlie their crying-averse attachment strategy must first be addressed, and a safe platform for affect attunement and regulation must be established. With the dismissing client, the therapist's job is to attune by respecting the overregulation of affect.

With Catherine, as would be expected with a person having a dismissing attachment style, the therapeutic process was long and painstaking. The early years were spent listening and internally attuning to her narratives. My open affective attunement was mild and understated, allowing her to enter the treacherous terrain of attachment vulnerability and caregiving slowly. For example, when she reported some of her father's sadistic punishments, I would say calmly, "That was so mean," or "Parents have no right to do that." When she talked about her mother's chronic emotional unavailability, I would say something like "How bleak for you and your brother, being left downstairs so much on your own." This is an example of strategic deintensifying, as opposed to, for example, inquiring directly about her feelings or reflecting the depth of what she might have felt. For instance, using "horrible" rather than "bleak" in the statement I made about her mother might have provoked the knee-jerk withdrawal response typical of dismissing persons who are confronted with painful affect. Instead, in the early stage of our relationship, I opted for a more empathically conservative response aimed at maintaining Catherine's engagement and sense of relative safety with me.

Eventually, Catherine began to grieve for her parents' treatment of her through angry protest. During this phase, she began to make some crying sounds that had an infant-like protest quality. Curiously, these sounds frightened her, which lent support to her theory that her father (and perhaps the family's nanny) had punished her for crying even in infancy.

In the next (and, for me, more difficult) phase of treatment, Catherine's protest turned toward me. She angrily challenged my vacation and conference travel schedule, saying that it was "abusive" of me to be so unavailable to her when I knew about her early wounds. My response was to regulate her affect (and my own) by calmly (though sometimes it took great effort not to get irritated) explaining the reasons for a trip and the alternative arrangements made for her care while I was away. It also helped when I would remind her of the many times she had been left for long periods in childhood while her parents traveled, and would label her current reaction a form of "posttraumatic stress disorder." Even though I struggled to deal with my feelings during this phase, I knew that her taking me on directly was a sign that our attachment relationship was deepening (i.e., becoming more secure). She was grieving in real time for the traumatic losses of her past, and becoming open to protest rather than retreating to detachment.

In the later years of treatment, Catherine finally came to be able to shed tears of despair over her many losses in the present as well as the past. As she moved toward a therapeutically earned-secure attachment style, I was able to attune to and regulate her affect in ways that I might do with a securely attached person. Sometimes I would chime in with her to intensify her affect by listing certain related losses she had not mentioned. At other times I would smile and comment humorously on a turn of phrase, as a way of soothing by lightening the grief.

Fearful

A client with a fearful adult attachment style shares high anxiety about rejection with a preoccupied person, but because of this anxiety retreats from closeness and avoids intimacy more like someone with a dismissing style (Mikulincer & Shaver, 2003). In general, activation of attachment behaviors is avoided by maintaining distance from other people. If an attachment relationship does develop, the vulnerability to rejection is extremely high. Attachment behavior (crying) may then be easily activated, but there is acute internal conflict about openly shedding tears, as well as a deep sense of pessimism about the hope of any soothing from a caregiver (even a therapist). If tears do come, the person is at pains to hide them or stop them as quickly as possible.

Because a person with a fearful attachment style is so skittish about closeness and so fearful of rejection, the process of psychotherapy is necessarily a long and often trying one for both client and therapist. For the therapist, this can mean withstanding resistance to and devaluation of therapeutic caregiving for long periods of time when nothing may seem to help or work. In the case of Calvin, a long-term client of mine, it took years of persistent affect attunement before my caregiving was overtly accepted. The entire time, he was questioning the efficacy of therapy; ostensibly his comments were not directly aimed at me, but nonetheless they were devaluing our work and our relationship. In addition, he spoke constantly of expecting criticism and rejection from me.

Like many patients with a fearful style, Calvin's crying was easily activated, but he made conscious and visible efforts to suppress it, his face often contorted with the effort. Beginning therapy had been a last resort in trying to cope with the end of his relationship, though he stayed to become a long-term psychotherapy client. My countertransference feelings in the early years were a mixture of concern, determination, and internally held despair as I did everything possible to make our connection safe. I worked consciously and hard to avoid any semblance of "rejecting" him with direct or implied criticism, confrontation, or impatience. Both affect attunement and affect regulation were extremely important, with little room for error. I had to match his affect almost exactly in order for him to feel understood, and I had to work very hard and consistently in my efforts to soothe him, offering extra sessions and phone calls when our connection was in jeopardy.

With Calvin, a decade-long initial phase culminated in a year of protest over a slight change in scheduling years before. Even though this was an extremely difficult phase of the therapeutic process, I was encouraged by his openly questioning my availability to him, because it gave us an opportunity for him to use me as a secure base to work out in the transference the early wound of inconsistently available caregivers, without fear of criticism or abandonment.

The first sign I saw of a shift in the attachment–caregiving therapeutic bond with Calvin came when he repeated back to me a comment I had made in a previous session—the first time he had ever acknowledged retaining or using any of my words. It was a small sign of our connection and of his being able to use my soothing. To put this another way, Calvin had encoded our security-enhancing interaction and was able to draw upon it at a later date to recapture its soothing quality.

Disorganized

The person with disorganized attachment style has no coherent coping strategy for dealing with loss (Main & Hesse, 1990). He or she has chaotic, confused attachment relationships and shows a mixture of approach and avoidance. Attachment behavior (crying) occurs at unpredictable and often seemingly inappropriate times. Caregiving may be desperately sought and resisted simultaneously. Caregiving attempts from others may evoke hostility or fear, and caregiving needs expressed by others may also be responded to inconsistently—with expansive, even excessive soothing, or alternatively with hostility, fear, or retreat. Narratives about life events are at times nonlinear and difficult to follow. The stories may also be accompanied by inappropriate attachment affect, such as sadistic laughter punctuated by moments of protest crying or angry denial of any feeling. Similarly, the responses to caregiving attempts by the therapist may be "all over the map," from dependent clinging to angry rejection.

This type of person, according to research, has an early attachment history that includes trauma, abuse, severe neglect, or neurologically based developmental disorders (Lyons-Ruth & Jacobvitz, 1999). It may be that some of what appear as chaotic attachment–caregiving strategies are due to the neurological dysfunction and/or defensive dissociation associated with trauma (Schore, 2003).

It is difficult to generalize therapeutic strategies for dealing with the crying of those with disorganized/disoriented attachment styles, because of the erratic and unpredictable behaviors they may show. A man in his early 40s was persuaded to enter therapy by his family after he lost his third job in a year. In the first few sessions, his affect ranged from rage to crying despondency. Occasionally, he would break into a disconnected form of laughter, which was disconcerting to watch and impossible to respond to empathically. The crying, the rage, and the inappropriate laughter functioned to keep me at a distance. I was unable to attune to his affect in this chaotic presentation. When I tried, for example, to translate his tearful despondency into words by saying, "It must have really hurt your feelings when they fired you after such a short time," my comments only served to enrage him further, as he took them to be efforts to minimize his experience or criticize him for taking it so hard.

As with the other forms of insecure attachment, a calm, steady therapeutic presence over time is required before even a modicum of reliable affect attunement or affect regulation is possible. Even with medication, reversals and regressions are to be expected, requiring great patience and tolerance on the part of the therapist. One therapeutic strategy in relation to crying is to ask the client respectfully during a period of calm what kind of response to crying might help him or her, even though the question may trigger hostility or sarcasm. What the question may do therapeutically, however, is to help the client feel safer with a therapist who will not impose or impinge on him or her. If the answer is that the desired response varies with each instance of crying, then signals (nonverbal or verbal) may be devised and agreed upon ahead of time to clue the therapist in to the needs/wishes of the moment.

When there is an early history of trauma, attachment needs and caregiving responses often trigger associations with shame and abuse rather than soothing. (People with certain neurological or psychiatric disorders, such as Asperger disorder, schizophrenia, or bipolar disorders, may also present with a disorganized attachment style.) If the therapist verbalizes this automatic, generally unconscious association between the arousal of attachment needs and caregiving responses with shame and abuse, the interpretation may offer another opportunity for regulating affect and helping to make the therapeutic attachment bond safer. Explaining the natural confusion of a threatened child may also help to create safety and a platform for affect attunement and regulation. As an adjunct to individual therapy, support groups for survivors of childhood abuse may help such survivors learn to regulate affect through the process of attuning to and soothing the negative arousal of other victims.

Providing information about the impact of trauma on brain development may also be helpful in teaching affect regulation. It may be useful to explain that affect regulation may be fitful and difficult when the primitive fear-perceiving parts of the brain are stimulated by trauma, but the cognitive prefrontal cortex is not yet "online" to evaluate the nature and degree of the threat (Schore, 2003). Pointing out the association between early attachment trauma and the defensive use of dissociation may also be effective in attuning to and regulating affect in people with disorganized/disoriented attachment styles (Kalsched, 1996).

CRYING IN THE CLINICAL HOUR

Crying in the clinical hour may be seen from an attachment viewpoint to be an intersubjective, two-person, relationship-linked behavior, mutually generated and mutually regulated. The therapeutic process prototypically involves crying by the client and caregiving by the therapist. At times, however, the process may also include crying by and/or caregiving to the therapist.

Crying by the Client

When a client sheds tears during a therapy hour, it offers invaluable insight into how the intersubjective process of attachment and caregiving is developing between client and therapist, and how the balance between the two is resonating throughout both. These are complex aspects of the therapeutic attachment bond that often defy conscious recognition and verbal articulation. Crying as seen from an attachment–caregiving standpoint offers a way to make these dynamics more available to conscious appraisal by the therapist.

If a client is resistant to soothing by the therapist, for example, it may indicate that there is still substantial insecurity in the therapeutic attachment bond. Resistance to crying itself may signal that the client is fearful of the therapeutic connection, clinging to self-reliance as a defensive posture. Frequent crying may also indicate insecurity in the therapeutic relationship, particularly if the tears leave the therapist feeling ineffective or distanced and the client is difficult to soothe.

For example, Catherine, the woman described above with a dismissing attachment style, entered treatment saying she was "numb." In the early years of treatment, there was no crying, but that pattern changed over the course of the therapy, reflecting progress (or sometimes regression) from insecure to secure in the therapeutic attachment bond. As Catherine moved through her grieving process from detached noncrying to tears of protest and finally to tears of despair, she gradually relinquished her compulsive self-reliance—a sign that she was able to begin trusting in the reliability and availability of my therapeutic caregiving. There were many ups and downs over the course of the years, but her crying and my internal responses to it helped me to clarify the state of the attachment bond and her security with me. Careful observation of her crying also helped me to withstand her withdrawal tendencies and to respond therapeutically as she struggled to trust in this new relationship.

Paying careful attention to the kinds of attachment–caregiving comments that trigger a client's tears, make the therapist feel like crying, or interfere with the client's crying once it has begun also offers a wealth of information about where the therapeutic bond is strong, where it is weak or misdirected, and what is needed by way of affect attunement and regulation. All of these dynamics related to crying enable the therapist to monitor any internal interference or enactments centered around crying that may arise out of the therapist's own discomfort and to understand their source.

For example, I once noticed that I posed a slightly distracting question to a client crying in despair, and wondered if it was because I found her grief and pain intolerable. Upon reflection, however, I saw that she was in fact overwhelmed by despair over her loss and had been so for a long time. My need to distance from it and her need to do so corresponded. My caregiving was aligned with her attachment needs, rather than coming solely from my own sense of discomfort. My intervention served the caregiving function of helping her to feel more secure with me—knowing that I could be with her in her despair, but that I could also help her to regulate it if it became too overwhelming.

Crying by the Therapist

Because crying by the therapist is almost never referred to or discussed in the clinical literature, I did an informal online survey among colleagues on several clinical listserves to which I belong. About two-thirds of the 19 who responded said that they had cried with a client. For most of them it was a rare event, although a few said they cried as often as weekly. Among the one-third who said they had never cried during a session, several noted that they occasionally feel like doing so but suppress their tears.

The most common reason cited by therapists who do cry with patients is empathy. At its best, such crying can represent the strength of the therapeutic attachment bond: The therapist is both sharing the client's pain (caregiving) and underscoring the connection (attachment). I have collected numerous examples where empathic crying by the therapist was an effective and meaningful experience. However, I have an almost equal number of examples where it resulted in a rupture in the treatment.

When crying by the therapist does not go well, the primary disturbing factor is that the client is interpreting the therapist's tears as an appeal for caregiving. This unintended effect appears to be particularly problematic early in a treatment relationship, or when the therapist is unaware of the client's misinterpretation. A middle-aged professional woman made an appointment to see me after having terminated with her therapist of 1 year several years prior. When I asked her about that experience, she reported that she had been talking about a painful argument with her elderly mother when the therapist began to cry. Her first and only thought was that she had to get out of there and never go back, and that was indeed her last session.

This client had grown up with alcoholic parents who were cold and without empathy for her childhood pains, demanding that she learn from an early age to exercise "self-control." In order to get caregiving from her parents, she had to stifle the attachment affect that no doubt upset her parents' equilibrium. On the other hand, when they were drinking, both her mother and father would occasionally exhibit exaggerated, drunken affect, including bouts of tearfulness, which repelled her. The therapeutic attachment bond was still too fragile for her to be able to share her dismay with her therapist's tears or to question their source, leaving her no emotional option except to terminate.

In a well-established treatment relationship with an experienced therapist, however, the therapist's misunderstood tears can be addressed successfully as part of the healing process. For example, one client challenged his empathically crying therapist of 10 years by saying, "I thought this was supposed to be about me!" The therapist explained that the therapy was indeed about the client, but that his story had "touched" the therapist (a connected, attachment–caregiving word in itself), and that this was the reason he had cried. The client accepted this explanation.

In addition to empathy with the client's pain, a number of respondents to my informal survey acknowledged having cried at terminations. Crying at the ending of a mutually meaningful relationship is an understandable human response that underscores the intensity of the attachment bond. However, when terminations are abrupt or conflicted, crying by the therapist may cause difficulties for both parties. In those instances, it makes sense for the therapist to seek consultation so as not to overburden the client's process. Three of the four times that I have cried in my almost 40 years of practice have been at terminations. In two of the instances, the terminations were unexpected, having been triggered by changes in life circumstances: a death and an unplanned pregnancy. My tears (neither client cried) underscored the importance of our connection and enabled the clients to acknowledge their grief. The third sudden termination felt premature and, in my view, represented a repetition of the childhood loss of the client's parent by sudden death. My tears, however, felt to me as though they were interfering with the client's process, and I sought consultation to recover my own more neutral stance; this better enabled us to explore the multiple reasons behind her feeling a need to terminate.

A final category of crying by the therapist that can be either helpful or problematic is when a therapist is personally experiencing an acute grief reaction in his or her own life. For example, one therapist returned to work after losing her husband, and began to cry when a client (who was her son's age) mentioned his father's death. The relationship was solid; the therapist's tears were acknowledged; the reasons for them were briefly discussed; and the outcome was positive. However, in another situation I heard about, a client brought up a difficulty he was having with something his therapist had said and the therapist began to cry, resulting in the client's terminating the therapy. I knew, though the client did not, that the therapist had just lost a close family member 2 weeks before and had returned to work without acknowledging her loss to her clients. Had the therapist felt comfortable sharing the fact of the recent loss, perhaps the awkwardness about the crying could have been overcome. Instead, when the therapist's grief intruded into the treatment, the client was left feeling bewildered and distanced. Because he had no way to process what had happened, he assumed it to be hypersensitivity to the mild criticism he had shared with her.

Attitudes about crying in the presence of patients vary among therapists. Crying is a form of involuntary self-disclosure, and in a traditional one-person psychoanalytic view it would be seen as a countertransferential interference in the treatment. Most of the therapists who responded to my survey said that crying can "sometimes be helpful and sometimes interfere." However, 4 therapists among the 19 respondents said that crying "interferes" with a client's treatment, and that they therefore always suppress their tears.

A therapist does, of course, have a professional responsibility to make the client's attachment needs and the client's grief and loss the focus of the treatment relationship. However, when connection and attachment exist, there is also a mutuality of feeling. One respondent, an experienced therapist, wrote this about the evolution in her attitude: "I've been in practice 28 years. Since I've gotten more confident in being 'relational' I would never suppress a tear, but I think in the old days, when I thought I was supposed to be a blank screen, I probably repressed tears." In addition to theoretical considerations, a high degree of consciousness about the therapist's own attachment and caregiving styles and feelings about crying is required to keep the therapeutic bond in balance.

Crying by the therapist can also evoke caregiving from the client in a positive sense. Although we are well aware of the many pitfalls in looking to a client for caregiving, there are also less obvious pitfalls in rejecting all caregiving directed to us by the client. It is a way for the client to feel a sense of mutuality with the therapist and a sense of his or her own efficacy and agency as part of the therapeutic attachment relationship. As the parent's affirming and accepting reactions to gestures of empathy and caregiving are crucial for the development of the child's attachment–caregiving bond, a client, too, may benefit from being able to care appropriately for the therapist (Bader, 1996).

One of the therapists responding to my survey gave a positive example of crying when a client brought her a latte. She acknowledged her client's generosity and said it had special meaning for her at this time in her own life, without elaborating; they then went comfortably on with the session in the usual way. The therapist, however, said that she took her tears to be a signal that she needed to take some steps to address the massive stress in her life.

CONCLUSIONS

Crying is an integral part of psychotherapy with rich potential for deepening the therapist's understanding of a client's attachment wounds and experiences, both past and present. Crying is also a rich source of information about the therapeutic process and the state of the therapeutic attachment bond. It gives guidance to the therapist in how to respond and intervene— what types of caregiving responses might be most needed and most effective. It also provides insight into what might feel like intuitive therapeutic responses that are, in fact, imbedded in the attachment–caregiving matrix of client and therapist. There are also insights to be gained about interventions that go awry and phases of therapy that seem unproductive or disconnected. Looking at crying from the standpoint of attachment and caregiving may also help the therapist to withstand a protracted or particularly difficult phase of the therapy and the therapeutic relationship.

RECOMMENDATIONS FOR FURTHER READING

Nelson, J. K. (2005). *Seeing through tears: Crying and attachment.* New York: Routledge.—The first part of the book expands on the theory of crying presented briefly here, and includes a thorough exploration of infant and childhood crying useful to professionals or parents. Parts II and III focus on the clinical application of the theory.

Schore, A. S. (2003). *Affect dysregulation and disorders of the self.* New York: Norton.—The entire book provides invaluable background for understanding the neurobiology of attachment. Ch. 3, "Attachment and the Regulation of the Right Brain" (pp. 54–86), is particularly relevant for explaining the role of infant crying and parental caregiving in the early months of life and its impact on affect regulation throughout life.

Wallin, D. J. (2007) *Attachment in psychotherapy.* New York: Guilford Press.— Part IV, "Attachment Patterns in Psychotherapy" (pp. 191–256), provides additional background and suggestions for dealing with the clinical issues in psychotherapy with each of the adult styles of attachment.

REFERENCES

Ainsworth, M. D. S., Blehar, M. C., Waters, E., & Wall, S. (1978). *Patterns of attachment: A psychological study of the Strange Situation.* Hillsdale, NJ: Erlbaum.

Avery, N. (1983). Tears of joy. *Journal of the American Academy of Psychoanalysis, 11,* 251–263.

Bader, M. (1996) Altruistic love in psychoanalysis: Opportunities and resistance. *Psychoanalytic Dialogues, 6,* 741–764.

Bartholomew, K., & Shaver, P. R. (1998). Methods of assessing adult attachment: Do they converge? In J. A. Simpson & W. S. Rholes (Eds.), *Attachment theory and close relationships* (pp. 25–45). New York: Guilford Press.

Boukydis, C. F. Z., & Burgess, R. L. (1982). Adult physiological response to infant cries: Effects of temperament of infant, parental status and gender. *Child Development, 53,* 1291–1298.

Bowlby, J. (1960). Grief and mourning in infancy and early childhood. *Psychoanalytic Study of the Child, 15,* 9–52.

Bowlby, J. (1961). Processes of mourning. *International Journal of Psycho-Analysis, 42,* 317–339.

Bowlby, J. (1980). *Attachment and loss: Vol. 3. Sadness and depression.* New York: Basic Books.

Bowlby, J. (1982). *Attachment and loss: Vol. 1. Attachment* (2nd ed.). New York: Basic Books. (1st ed., 1969)

Breuer, J., & Freud, S. (1955). Studies on hysteria. In J. Strachey (Ed. & Trans.), *The standard edition of the complete psychological works of Sigmund Freud* (Vol. 2, pp. 1–305). London: Hogarth Press. (Original work published 1895)

Darwin, C. (1965). *The expression of the emotions in animals and man.* Chicago: University of Chicago Press. (Original work published 1872)

Feeney, B. C., & Collins, N. L. (2004). Interpersonal safe haven and secure base caregiving processes in adulthood. In W. S. Rholes & J. A. Simpson (Eds.), *Adult attachment: Theory, research, and clinical implications* (pp. 300–338). New York: Guilford Press.

Habenstein, R., & Lamers, W. (1963). *Funeral customs the world over.* Milwaukee: Bulfin.

Hazan, C., & Shaver, P. R. (1987). Romantic love conceptualized as an attachment process. *Journal of Personality and Social Psychology, 52,* 511–524.

Hesse, E. (1999). The Adult Attachment Interview: Historical and current perspectives. In J. Cassidy & P. R. Shaver (Eds.), *Handbook of attachment: Theory, research, and clinical applications* (pp. 395–433). New York: Guilford Press.

Kalsched, D. (1996). *The inner world of trauma: Archetypal defenses of the personal spirit.* New York: Routledge.

Kracke, W. (1981). Kagwahiv mourning. *Ethos, 9,* 258–275.

Kracke, W. (1988). Kagwahiv mourning II. *Ethos, 16,* 209–222.

Lester, B., & Boukydis, C. F. Z. (Eds.). (1985). *Infant crying: Theoretical and research perspectives.* New York: Plenum Press.

Lorberbaum, J., Newman, J. D., Horowitz, A. R., Dubno, J. R., Lydiard, R. B., Hamner, M. B., et al. (2002). A potential role for thalamocingulate circuitry in human maternal behavior. *Biological Psychiatry, 51,* 431–445.

Lyons-Ruth, K., & Jacobvitz, D. (1999). Attachment disorganization. In J. Cassidy & P. R. Shaver (Eds.), *Handbook of attachment: Theory, research, and clinical applications* (pp. 520–554). New York: Guilford Press.

Main, M., & Hesse, E. (1990). Parents' unresolved traumatic experiences are related to infant disorganized attachment status: Is frightened and/or frightening parental behavior the linking mechanism? In M. T. Greenberg, D. Cicchetti, & E. M. Cummings (Eds.), *Attachment in the preschool years: Theory, research, and intervention* (pp. 161–182). Chicago: University of Chicago Press.

Main, M., & Solomon, J. (1990). Procedures for identifying infants as disorganized/ disoriented during the Ainsworth Strange Situation. In M. T. Greenberg, D. Cicchetti, & E. M. Cummings (Eds.), *Attachment in the preschool years* (pp. 121–160). Chicago: University of Chicago Press.

Mikulincer, M., & Orbach, I. (1995). Attachment styles and repressive defensiveness: The accessibility and architecture of affective memories. *Journal of Personality and Social Psychology, 68,* 917–925.

Mikulincer, M., & Shaver, P. R. (2003). The attachment behavioral system in adulthood: Activation, psychodynamics, and interpersonal processes. In M. P. Zanna (Ed.), *Advances in experimental social psychology* (Vol. 36, pp. 53–152). San Diego, CA: Academic Press.

Mikulincer, M., & Shaver, P. R. (2004). Security-based self-representations in adulthood: Contents and processes. In W. S. Rholes & J. A. Simpson (Eds.), *Adult attachment: Theory, research, and clinical implications* (pp. 159–195). New York: Guilford Press.

Nelson, J. K. (1998). The meaning of crying based on attachment theory. *Clinical Social Work Journal, 26,* 9–22.

Nelson, J. K. (2000). Clinical assessment of crying and crying inhibition based on attachment theory. *Bulletin of the Menninger Clinic, 64,* 509–529.

Nelson, J. K. (2005). *Seeing through tears: Crying and attachment.* New York: Routledge.

Schore, A. N. (1994). *Affect regulation and the origin of the self.* Hillsdale, NJ: Erlbaum.

Schore, A. N. (2003). *Affect dysregulation and disorders of the self.* New York: Norton.

Vingerhoets, A. (2001). Appendix. In A. Vingerhoets & R. Cornelius (Eds.), *Adult crying: A biopsychosocial approach* (pp. 303–316). New York: Brunner-Routledge.

Vingerhoets, A., & Cornelius, R. R. (Eds.). (2001). *Adult crying: A biopsychosocial approach.* New York: Brunner-Routledge.

Weiss, J. (1952). Crying at the happy ending. *Psychoanalytic Review, 39,* 338.

Wolff, P. H. (1969). The natural history of crying and other vocalizations in infancy. In B. M. Foss (Ed.), *Determinants of infant behavior IV* (pp. 81–109). London: Methuen.

Part IV

INTEGRATION WITH CLINICAL APPROACHES

14

Adult Psychotherapy from the Perspectives of Attachment Theory and Psychoanalysis

Morris Eagle
David L. Wolitzky

Although attachment research and theory and psychoanalysis developed relatively independently of each other over the course of many years, the original context for attachment theory was psychoanalysis. Bowlby was trained as a psychoanalyst and viewed himself as one throughout his life. Indeed, the point of departure and primary intellectual motivations for the development of attachment theory were Bowlby's dissatisfactions with aspects of Freudian and Kleinian theory, as well as his desire to place psychoanalysis on a more solid scientific footing by grounding it more fully in empirical data and theoretical concepts from other scientific disciplines (such as evolutionary theory, ethology, cognitive psychology, and control systems theory).

During the last number of years, the links between attachment theory and psychoanalysis have been reforged. The psychoanalytic community, especially in the United States, Great Britain, and Italy, has adopted a more favorable stance toward attachment theory and has shown great interest in empirical and theoretical work in the area. Now, as it appears that there is no longer, as Fonagy (2001) has put it, "bad blood" (or less of it) between attachment theory and psychoanalysis, it is time to look at the specific relationship between the two fields. In particular, what can attachment research and theory offer to psychoanalytic approaches to treatment? And conversely, what can psychoanalysis offer to an understanding of attachment phenomena?

Much of the published work relating attachment theory to therapeutic interventions is concerned with problematic parent–child interactions, and

351

in particular with the prevention of insecure attachment and/or the facilitation of secure attachment in the child through work with caregivers (Lieberman & Zeanah, 1999). However, we limit the focus of this chapter to the psychodynamic treatment of adults.

Because attachment theory is now "in," there is somewhat of a bandwagon rush to relate different therapeutic approaches to attachment theory, and to offer workshops and publish articles and books on purported attachment-based approaches to therapy. This enthusiasm is probably due to the significant accumulation of attachment research, in both infancy and adulthood, that has validated central tenets of attachment theory and documented individual differences in attachment as they relate to affect regulation, coping, social confidence, and psychopathology. However, unlike many traditional clinical theories, adult attachment theory has not yet developed its own specific blueprint for carrying out individual adult psychotherapy, though considerable inroads have been made in the infant–parent domain (e.g., Marvin, Cooper, Hoffman, & Powell, 2002) and the couple domain (Johnson, 2004). The absence of a formal approach to adult psychotherapy may have led Slade (1999) to observe "that an understanding of the nature and dynamics of attachment *informs* rather than *defines* intervention and clinical thinking" (p. 577; emphasis in original). We would add that attachment research and theory also offer a potentially useful perspective on conceptualizing the nature of the client–therapist relationship, the nature of therapeutic goals, certain aspects of the therapeutic interaction, and the linking of therapeutic approach to individual differences in attachment style.

Our plan in this chapter is as follows: We begin with a consideration of the client–therapist relationship in attachment theory terms, and focus on the experience of the therapist as a secure base. We then compare an attachment theory and an object relations theory understanding of the client's conflicts. We follow this with a discussion of the nature of therapeutic change from an attachment theory perspective. Next, we take up the issues of different therapeutic approaches for clients with different attachment styles, and of the enhancement of reflective functioning as a central goal of treatment that is informed by both psychoanalysis and attachment theory. We then discuss certain aspects of the relationship between attachment theory and psychoanalysis, including the questions of single versus multiple attachment styles and the role of psychic reality. After summarizing some selected research on attachment and psychotherapy, we end with some comments regarding the ideal relationship between attachment theory and psychoanalysis.

THE CLIENT–THERAPIST RELATIONSHIP

The Therapist as a Secure Base

Perhaps the most obvious implication of attachment theory for psychoanalytic therapy (as well as other forms of therapy) has to do with the central idea that, particularly in long-term treatment, the therapist serves as an attachment figure for the client (Mallinckrodt, Porter, & Kivlighan, 2005; Parish & Eagle, 2003). Of the different functions served by the therapist as an attachment figure, perhaps the most critical is the secure-base function. As Bowlby (1988) noted, one of the main functions of a therapist "is to provide the patient with a secure base from which he can explore the various unhappy and painful aspects of his life, past and present, many of which he finds it difficult or perhaps impossible to think about and reconsider without a trusted companion to provide support, encouragement, sympathy, and, on occasion guidance" (p. 138). In short, for Bowlby, the therapist serves as a secure base from which the client can more safely engage in self-exploration.[1]

The apparent simplicity of the idea of the therapist as a secure base from which to engage in self-exploration is deceptive. According to a careful reading of Bowlby (1988, pp. 140–157), he believed that becoming a secure base is beset with complications and that success requires the use of central psychoanalytic concepts (e.g., *transference* and *countertransference*) in conjunction with attachment ideas (e.g., the role of actual experience, both past and with the therapist). Below we elaborate on some of the more outstanding obstacles to becoming a secure base that are readily understandable from a psychoanalytic viewpoint.

A client with an insecure attachment style (and a corresponding internal working model) is, by definition, someone who has had difficulty in the past and continues to have difficulty in the present experiencing his or her attachment figure as a secure base. There is no reason to expect that the therapist will somehow escape these difficulties and immediately become a secure base. On the contrary, there is every reason to expect that in important respects, the insecurely attached client will experience the therapist in ways similar to the experience of his or her attachment figure; that is, the client will *not* necessarily and automatically have a confident expectation in the availability of the therapist, and indeed will at some level fear and expect rejection, lack of sensitive responsiveness, and lack of empathic understanding on the part of the therapist. In the psychoanalytic context, this is equivalent to recognizing the inevitability of transference in the client's experience of the therapist.[2] An added value of using an attachment frame is that the therapist, via an assessment of attachment style, may be able to foresee (in general terms), the kind of transference a client will engage in (see Tolmacz, Chapter 11, this volume, for a discussion of this topic).

From a psychoanalytic point of view, we can say that much of the therapeutic work, including the analysis of the transference, consists of examining the nature and origins of the client's difficulties in experiencing the therapist as a secure base. Indeed, being capable of experiencing the therapist as a secure base does not constitute a given; rather, it is a central process and outcome *goal* of treatment, and it reflects a relative resolution of the negative transference. The capacity for such an experience would suggest an important positive transformation of the client's internal working model concerning issues of trust and reliability—surely a central therapeutic outcome goal from an attachment theory perspective. This new capacity, in turn, bodes well for the client's ability to experience other potential attachment figures in his or her life as a secure base.

Factors That Contribute to Experiencing the Therapist as a Secure Base

What are the factors that contribute to experiencing the therapist as a secure base? We can answer this question from a number of psychoanalytic perspectives. Consider first the control–mastery theory of Weiss, Sampson, and the Mount Zion Psychotherapy Research Group (1986). According to this theory, a client unconsciously presents *tests* to the therapist (which the latter can pass or fail) in order to determine whether or not the therapist will behave in ways similar to the traumatizing behaviors of early parental figures. In other words, the client presents tests in order to address whether there is a risk of being retraumatized at the therapist's hands (test failure) or whether conditions of safety obtain (test passing). As Weiss et al. (1986) have shown, when the therapist fails the test, the client becomes more defensive; when the therapist passes the test, the client's anxiety is reduced, he or she shows a broadening of interests, and warded-off (repressed) material is more likely to emerge at times even without the therapist's interpretations.[3]

We can understand, in a similar way, one aspect of the therapeutic process described by Kohut (1984). According to Kohut, many clients who come for treatment have experienced early traumatic failures in being empathically mirrored and understood; they hope that the therapist, unlike early parental figures, will empathically understand them. According to Kohut (1984), although certain clients demand perfect mirroring and understanding and may react with rage and despair when this impossible demand is not met, treatment will progress as long as the therapist's failures do not reach traumatic proportions, but rather constitute *optimal failures*. Indeed, the therapist's acknowledgment of his or her optimal failures and other interventions that help the client work them through constitute essential components of treatment, according to Kohut. From an attachment theory perspective, Kohut can be understood as stating that the therapist's repeated "good-enough" empathic understanding, combined with acknowledgment of his or her failures and with the mutual examination of the client's reaction to these failures, contribute importantly to the client's experience of the therapist as a secure base from which the client can, with increasing feelings of safety, explore his or her reactions to empathic failures.

Implied in Kohut's concept of optimal failures is the idea that the client's experience of the therapist as a secure base is not a once-and-for-all accomplishment, but rather an ongoing dynamic process. The inevitable ruptures that occur in treatment, as long as they are followed by repair, can be therapeutically useful (Safran & Muran, 2000)—and, we would add, can serve to enhance the experience of the therapist as a secure base.

Although employing different language, Kohut's (1984) self psychology and Weiss et al.'s (1986) control–mastery theory converge on the conclusion that people who have been traumatized and deprived early in life are the very ones who are most likely to have the greatest difficulty in experiencing the therapist as a secure base. Hence for these clients (and, to a certain extent, for all clients), the critical issues to be explored in treatment are the nature of these difficulties and the processes through which the therapist becomes a secure base—that is, earns his or her status as a secure base. Moreover, Weiss et al.'s and Kohut's ideas extend Bowlby's (1988) belief that in addition to the influence of the client's prior relational experiences, the quality of the therapeutic relationship "is determined no less by the way the therapist treats him [the client]" (p. 141).

In the theories described above as well as in other psychoanalytic approaches, a common factor in the process through which the therapist comes to be experienced as a secure base—or, depending upon one's theoretical language, a *good object,* a *mature self-object,* or a *realistic benevolent figure*—is that the therapist behaves in a way that is presumably different from the behavior of the client's early parental figures. We know from research on infant–mother attachment that the mother's *sensitive responsiveness* (Ainsworth, Blehar, Waters, & Wall, 1978; van IJzendoorn, 1995) contributes to the infant's secure attachment. It is plausible for us to hypothesize that the therapist's sensitive responsiveness to the client will similarly play a major role in the client's experience of the therapist as a secure base—while at the same time recognizing that what constitutes a therapist's sensitive responsiveness to an adult client will undoubtedly be very different from what constitutes a caregiver's sensitive responsiveness to an infant. (Although there are parallels between the two, it is important to avoid facile equations between infant–caregiver and client–therapist attachments. Farber & Metzger elaborate on this issue in Chapter 3, this volume.

What, then, constitutes a therapist's sensitive responsiveness to an adult client? It seems apparent that it will vary with, among other things, the client's developmental level. In the early infant–caregiver context, sensitive responsiveness consists primarily of the caregiver's response to the infant's behavioral and physical signals (e.g., of distress or hunger), and secure attachment may correspondingly consist of the infant's "primitive" expectation that the caregiver be available and will respond to his or her signals. At a later stage in development, sensitive responsiveness may more prominently include representing and understanding the mental states of the other, and secure attachment is, as Fonagy, Steele, Steele, Moran, and Higgitt (1991) have noted, correspondingly likely to include *feeling understood* by the attachment figure. Thus one general answer to the question of what constitutes a therapist's sensitive responsiveness to an adult client is understanding and accurately representing in the therapist's mind the mental states of the client, and then communicating this understanding in such a way that the client feels heard and feels assisted in managing distress. It also includes, of course, the usually emphasized factors of being nonjudgmental, being tactful, and managing one's countertransference.

We would add to the factors noted above *affective presence* as an important component of sensitive responsiveness. Sorce and Emde (1981) have shown that toddlers explore more fully and more comfortably when the attachment figure is emotionally available, as compared with when she is only physically available but engaged in another activity (e.g., reading a newspaper). We suspect that something analogous to this also holds in the therapeutic situation, and in general also characterizes adult attachment. That is, whereas the literal physical availability of the attachment figure may serve a secure-base function and may also be somewhat comforting in times of distress (i.e., may serve a safe-haven function), it is very likely that the emotional availability or affective presence of the attachment figure enhances these functions considerably.

The safe-haven and secure-base functions of the attachment figure can be understood as forming together what Marvin et al. (2002) refer to as a *circle of security*. That is, from a secure base, the child ventures out to explore (play). If the child experiences distress, he or she turns to the attachment figure to be comforted. When the attachment figure is able to provide a safe haven, the child is comforted and returns to exploration. This circle of security implies that repeated experiences of being comforted when distressed are necessary in order for the attachment figure to be experienced as a secure base from which the child can explore. The child learns that the attachment figure can be trusted to be available if the child becomes distressed during exploration. In other words, exploration becomes safe.

We can posit an analogous process in the therapeutic situation. That is, if the therapist can be trusted to be available when the client is distressed and can assist in emotional regulation (i.e., can be a safe haven), self-exploration becomes more possible, particularly given the fact that self-exploration can be painful and distressing. The circle-of-security model makes it clear that the curative factors of the therapeutic relationship on the one hand, and insight and self-knowledge on the other, are inextricably linked. However, it does raise the question of whether repeated experiences of the therapist as a safe haven—quite apart from self-exploration—can be therapeutic itself, probably by implicitly altering the client's internal working model of expectations regarding the attachment figure. It will be noted that we have, in effect, been discussing in attachment theory terms the therapeutic role of *corrective emotional experiences*.

Finally, it should be noted that insecurely attached clients will require repeated experiences of the therapist as a safe haven before any change will occur, whereas securely attached clients are more likely to take this function more or less for granted and can move more readily to self-exploration. What emerges as a general proposition is that in order for the attachment figure to serve as a secure base for exploration, there must be a prior history of experience of the attachment figure as a safe haven in times of distress.

THE NATURE OF THE CLIENT'S CONFLICTS

From the perspective of attachment theory, the client's basic conflict is between the free and appropriate expression and experience of attachment needs on the one hand, and expectations regarding the attachment figure's lack of emotional availability, rejection, abandonment, and so forth, on the other. Thus this is essentially a conflict between expressing one's inner (attachment) needs and expecting psychic pain at the hands of the attachment figure.

However, psychoanalysts are more likely to place greater emphasis on the client's inner conflicts. For example, for an object-relational Fairbairnian therapist, the focus is not so much on the conflict between one's needs and one's expectations from the other, but rather on the conflict between one's needs and one's own rejection of and contempt for those needs. According to Fairbairn (1952), the child internalizes the rejecting parent as an aspect of his or her own personality structure. This means that at the core of the client's difficulties is not simply or primarily that he or she expects rejection or abandonment at the hands of the other, but that the client him- or herself rejects and has contempt for his or her needs. According to this view, the therapeutic goal is centered not so much on altering the client's maladaptive internal working model or representation of the other as on resolving the client's inner conflict and altering the aspect of the self-representation that reflects the early internalization of the rejecting and depriving other as part of oneself. From this perspective, the therapeutic focus is not simply on the client's representation of the current attachment figure as a carryover from early experiences, but on how early negative experiences with the attachment figure have come to be internalized as part of the self.[4]

Many clients are more comfortable talking about the shortcomings, mistreatment, and injustices of external figures (parents, spouses, etc.) than examining their own conflictual feelings. Excessive attention to and support of the former on the part of the therapist may constitute collusion in avoiding dealing with the latter. Although it is obviously important to empathically understand the client's experience of the inadequacies and failures of early and current attachment figures, a therapist working from a psychoanalytic perspective must often help the client also focus inward and recognize that he or she is personally conflicted about and may contemptuously reject the very attachment (and other) needs experienced as not met by external figures.

We are reminded of a client who repeatedly complained about her spouse's and her close friends' unavailability and lack of support, and who always presented convincing evidence to that effect. This is certainly not uncommon in treatment. What the client did not address and was not aware of was the degree to which she herself was conflicted about and rejected the legitimacy of her own needs for closeness, support, and understanding (which probably influenced her experience of others' unavailability, and even her object choice of spouse). She viewed these needs as expressions of dependency and weakness and contemptuously rejected them. Because of these self-attitudes and conflicts, her need and desire for support and caring were expressed as angry demands, in a way that communicated her expectation that her needs would not be met—which, of course, often became a self-fulfilling prophecy. The client showed little recognition of the role that her own projections played in her interactions with others. This pattern was repeatedly explored in the context of the therapeutic relationship.

From the perspective of attachment theory, this brief vignette illustrates how the client's inner conflicts and projections (as well as what they elicit in the therapist) can interfere with his or her experience of the therapist as a safe haven and a secure base—an issue that needs to be addressed in the treatment.

Another factor that played a critical role in this woman's suffering and in the persistence of her maladaptive relationship patterns was what Fairbairn (1952) refers to as *devotion* and *obstinate attachment* to early objects. Such devotion is often motivated by guilt and an unconscious need to protect the attachment figure, often by persisting in self-defeating patterns of behavior. Attachment theory, which of course is concerned with the persistence of internal working models and maladaptive relationship patterns, has relatively little to say about such motivations as loyalty and guilt. It tends to attribute the stability of attachment patterns mainly to the stability of internal working models.

THERAPEUTIC CHANGE

How do we understand the nature of change in successful treatment? And how is that understanding modified when attachment theory and research are brought into the picture? All psychoanalytic perspectives agree that inner *structural* change takes place in successful psychoanalytic treatment. Although the candidates for what constitutes structural change have varied in the history of psychoanalysis—for example, strengthening the observing function of the ego, resolving inner conflict, softening the harshness of the superego, increasing the capacity to delay gratification, increasing the capacity for sublimations, relinquishing infantile wishes, and so on—all of them reflect the basic idea that beyond symptom relief and behavioral change, successful psychoanalytic treatment brings about some change in inner functioning.

Narrative Competence

What is the nature of inner structural change from the perspective of attachment theory and research? According to Holmes (2001), successful treatment increases the client's *narrative competence*. That is, one expects that the client's autobiographical narrative will become more coherent and less fragmented. Holmes's emphasis on narrative competence is partly derived from the role of coherence of discourse in the Adult Attachment Interview (AAI; George, Kaplan, & Main, 1984, 1985, 1996). That is, Holmes's implicit reasoning seems to be that if narrative coherence is a critical criterion for the AAI classification of a secure-autonomous state of mind with respect to attachment, then one should expect increased narrative coherence in successful treatment—a marker of an increase in attachment security. And indeed there is evidence that after 1 year of treatment, some clients with borderline personality disorder shift from a relatively incoherent (insecure attachment style) to a relatively coherent narrative (secure-autonomous attachment style) on the AAI (Levy et al., 2006).

If one defines security of attachment operationally, based on AAI narratives, then indeed one would conclude that these clients have changed from an insecure to a secure-autonomous attachment style. However, this conclusion invites skepticism. Increased narrative coherence on the AAI notwithstanding, it is difficult to believe, given the severity of their pathology, that clients with borderline personality disorder have a secure-autonomous state of mind with respect to attachment after only 1 year of treatment—if, in accord, with the core assumptions of attachment theory, one means by a secure state of mind with respect to attachment such things as a confident expectation in the availability of the attachment figure as a safe haven in times of distress, a secure base for exploration, and a relatively successful internalization of both functions to the point that they become a "natural" and organic part of oneself and of one's self-regulating capacity.

How, then, is one to understand the increased narrative coherence in Levy et al.'s (2006) clients? Is it possible to produce a coherent narrative without necessarily having a state of mind characterized by trust in the availability of the attachment figure, and without having successfully internalized safe-haven and secure-base functions? In order to answer this question empirically, we would need to have independent measures of the latter and then determine their relationship to AAI narrative coherence.

Fonagy and colleagues (Fonagy et al., 1991; Fonagy, Steele, & Target, 1997) have shown that a good deal of the variance in AAI classifications is accounted for by differences in *reflective functioning*. That is, individual differences in narrative coherence on the AAI may well reflect differences in individuals' capacity to reflect on their past attachment experiences, on their own mental states, and on the mental states of others (particularly their attachment figures). Furthermore, this ability to remember and reflect on attachment-related experiences and mental states probably serves to ameliorate the individual's tendency toward an automatic and reflexive repetition of maladaptive responses and patterns. As Santayana noted a long time ago, those who cannot remember (and, one could add, reflect on) the past are doomed to repeat it. Conversely, those who do remember and are able to reflect on the past have at least the opportunity to respond in a different way than they have in the past. In short, we are suggesting that findings such as changes in the narrative coherence of Levy et al.'s (2006) clients after 1 year of treatment (as well as the relationship between a mother's narrative coherence on the AAI and her infant's attachment status) can perhaps be understood as due to increased reflective functioning, which, in turn permits more adaptive responses. Perhaps this may be the first marker that a client is achieving structural personality change. However, more research is needed to show that a change in one domain furthers more coherence in another, and contributes to symptomatic improvement.

First-Order versus Second-Order Change

Implicit in the discussion above is a distinction between, on the one hand, therapeutic changes in reflective functioning (as well as in related areas such as insight, self-awareness, and self-knowledge), and, on the other hand, changes in the very tendencies, states, and affects that one is reflecting on. Consider, for example, in the context of attachment theory, the distinction between, on the one hand, one's implicit and "automatic" expectation (as well as accompanying feelings) of, say, rejection on the part of one's attachment figure and, on the other hand, one's reflection on that implicit and automatic expectation. We are suggesting that at least some positive therapeutic outcomes consist primarily of changes in the latter rather than the former. This is consistent with Crits-Christoph and Luborsky's (1990) findings, based on their use of the Core Conflictual Relationship Theme method, that even in a positive therapeutic outcome, the client's basic wishes do not change; what tend to change are the experienced response of the other and the consequent response of the self. This view is also consistent with Pfeffer's (1993) report that even many years after successful treatment, the client's familiar transference pattern is readily evoked in an interview with a new analyst.

   Thus, even in successful treatment, some individuals may continue to have an automatic expectation of, say, rejection; however, through an increased ability to reflect on and evaluate this automatic expectation, they are better able to modulate the strong negative effects and maladaptive behaviors that in the past have accompanied the implicit and automatic expectation. Such change is very important and can make a great difference in a person's life. However, it is different from change that entails basic modifications in the client's automatic expectations and accompanying affects themselves. In short, we make a general distinction between what we might call *first-order* or fundamental tendencies and structures on the one hand and second-order structures, such as the capacity to reflect on these fundamental tendencies and structures, on the other hand.

   In a previous paper, one of us (Eagle, 2002) described a client who reported that she was always attracted to the "wrong man" (i.e., a man who would not make a commitment, who would reject her, etc.). During the course of treatment, she came to resist her spontaneous desire and temptation to get involved with this kind of man by inserting "Be careful" or "Here I go again" self-warnings, which would serve to keep her from acting on her temptations to get involved in situations that in the past had brought her suffering and distress. However, she continued to be spontaneously attracted to the same kind of "wrong man," despite being aware of the repeated distress that acting on these attractions brought about and despite having some insight into the unconscious basis for this attraction. This client's experience (which is undoubtedly a common one) suggests a distinction between the client's ability to reflect on her spontaneous attraction (i.e., its past consequences, its basis in her history, etc.) and the spontaneous attraction itself. Whereas the former changed in the course of therapy, the latter did not, or at least not appreciably.

Evidence of a deep personality change would be reflected in a notable alteration in the kind of man to whom the client was spontaneously attracted. We are reminded of a statement by Confucius that at a certain point in his life, the dictates of his heart and his sense of right and wrong were one and the same. That is, the spontaneous impulse and the results of self-reflection converged. In the case of the client referred to above, this would mean that her spontaneous desire and her more reflective sense of who was right for her would become one and the same. This would also mean that reflective interventions such as "Be careful" and the like would become less and less necessary.

In the context of attachment theory, we might wonder how often change occurs in a client's attachment style and in his or her underlying internal working model when both are defined not simply in terms of such criteria as narrative competence, but in terms of such factors as an implicit and deeply ingrained level of trust in the availability of the attachment figure as a safe haven and secure base, as well as the degree of internalization of these secure-base and safe-haven functions. This is a question that we believe is worth investigating.

INDIVIDUAL DIFFERENCES IN ATTACHMENT STYLE AND THERAPEUTIC APPROACH

One of the ways in which attachment research and theory can potentially contribute to psychoanalytic treatment and other therapeutic approaches is by sensitizing the therapist to the client's attachment style and encouraging recognition that different attachment styles may require somewhat different therapeutic approaches, particularly when one views insecure attachment styles and their associated use of secondary coping strategies (i.e., hyperactivating and deactivating) partly as defensive maneuvers. Thus individuals with a predominantly dismissing-avoidant attachment style may require a different therapeutic approach than individuals with a preoccupied style may. The former employ *defensive exclusion* (Bowlby, 1980), which deactivates the attachment system (Mikulincer & Shaver, 2003) in relation to attachment experiences. Such clients need to be able to become more in touch with "unexperienced yearning for love and support" (Bowlby, 1977, p. 207) and with "cut-off feelings of loss, sadness, and anger in response to severe disappointments in their relationship with their attachment figure" (Eagle, 1997, p. 226). Hence undoing defensive exclusion in relation to attachment needs would seem to be an appropriate therapeutic aim for clients with an avoidant style.

However, it may not be an appropriate therapeutic approach for preoccupied clients. Whereas dismissing-avoidant individuals defensively deactivate the attachment system, the attachment system is chronically hyperactivated in preoccupied individuals. In working with the latter, one hardly needs to undo defensive exclusion of their attachment needs and experiences. As noted elsewhere, a major problem with these clients is the relative absence of adequate defenses "in the face of intense anxieties, longings, rages, and despair linked to close relationships—the kind of patterns one more likely to see in borderline individuals" (Eagle, 1997, p. 227). If this description is accurate, it would follow that a central therapeutic task for these individuals would not be the undoing of defensive exclusion, but providing help with relinquishing "the fantasy of recovering a lost relationship, a lost relationship that never was, that is itself a fantasy" (Eagle, 1997, p. 227).

ENHANCING REFLECTIVE
FUNCTIONING IN TREATMENT

One area of convergence between attachment theory and psychoanalysis is the importance both assign to the capacity for reflective functioning (for additional discussion of reflective functioning, see Jurist & Meehan, Chapter 4, this volume). The concept of reflective functioning bears a strong family resemblance to the psychoanalytic concept of the observing function of the ego, the strengthening of which was held to be a central goal of psychoanalytic treatment. Similarly, from an attachment theory perspective, there is evidence that reflective functioning in high-risk mothers is a protective factor with regard to their infants' attachment security (e.g., Fonagy et al., 1995). Hence, from an attachment theory perspective as well, enhancing reflective function is an important goal of treatment.

A number of treatment programs attempt to enhance a caregiver's ability to reflect on her behaviors and attributions in relation to her infant with the aim of furthering her infant's security (e.g., Marvin et al., 2002; Toth, Rogosch, & Cicchetti, 2006). For example, Schechter et al. (2006) have a therapist go over videotapes with a mother of her interaction with her infant in the Strange Situation, and try to help her reflect on the infant's mental state and her reactions. In one videotape that we observed, the mother initially interprets her infant's protest in response to her leaving as his attempt to "always control me." Upon examining the videotape with the therapist, she becomes increasingly able to see that her child is upset and distressed rather than controlling. (See also Lieberman, 1999, for a poignant description of working with a mother's fantasies and attributions to her infant.)

It seems to us that a process analogous to what we have described above goes on in adult psychotherapy. Common to work with all clients in psychoanalytic treatment is the therapist's attempt to help the client step back and reflect on his or her implicit assumptions, expectations, fantasies, wishes, and so on in relation to the therapist and other significant figures in the client's life. The therapist's interpretations and reflections can be seen as analogous to the caregiver's and therapist's mutual examination of the videotape in child–mother programs. The therapist models reflective functioning through empathically representing the client's mental states in the therapist's mind. In successful treatment, the client learns to do for him- or herself what the therapist did for the client—that is, "hold" or empathically represent him- or herself in his or her own mind. This can occur either through introjection of the therapist, expressed through invoking the therapist's image and carrying on the dialogue with the therapist, or through internalization of the depersonified therapeutic function (see our later discussion of research on internalization of the therapist).

The barriers to reflective function are likely to vary with individual differences in insecure attachment and, as noted above, may require different therapeutic approaches. The avoidant individual's reliance on defensive exclusion (Bowlby, 1980) is incompatible with being able to reflect on his or her feelings, needs, and so on. Another way to put this is to say that the avoidant individual cannot be expected to become aware of his or her attachment needs and feelings until the person becomes aware of and is able to reflect on the ways in which he or she characteristically excludes these needs and feelings from consciousness. Hence analysis of defense would seem to be an appropriate way of attempting to enhance reflective functioning in these individuals.

For example, during a session with a client who was suffering from an eating disorder, she reported that at the last minute her mother cancelled a date for the two of them to go shopping for new clothes in celebration of the client's job promotion. The client expressed little or no affect in reporting this incident—no hurt, disappointment, or anger. When asked about what happened next, she reported that she binged, not linking it at all to her mother's cancellation. Any feelings having to do, directly or indirectly, with attachment and related needs were defensively excluded on a massive scale. As noted, she had no conscious access at all either to her feelings connected with her mother's cancellation or to a possible link between these unavailable feelings and her bingeing. For this kind of client, it would appear that dealing with her defensive exclusion would be a necessary first step in help-ing her experience her attachment needs and feelings.

The barriers to reflective functioning are somewhat different for the preoccupied individual. They have mainly to do with the individual's inabil-ity to escape long enough from intense affects, such as fear of abandonment, to be able to step back and reflect on the source of these feelings and fears. The therapeutic challenge with such individuals is to effect sufficient regula-tion of intense dysphoric affect that reflective functioning becomes possible. As noted earlier, the therapist's safe-haven function is predominant for long periods of time with these clients. A preoccupied client's dysphoric affects must be sufficiently regulated in order to be able to use the therapist as a secure base for self-exploration and self-reflection.

Work with a client described earlier (see pp. 357–358) illustrates an approach that we believe is likely to be useful with preoccupied clients. This client frequently felt so enraged, self-righteous, and devastated by what she experienced as others' lack of caring that any attempt at interpreta-tion or encouragement of reflection did not work. The negative affect she experienced was too intense for reflective function to operate. Her convic-tion regarding her own righteousness and the uncaring, despicable nature of the others' behavior was absolute, brooking no alternative view. What was required when the client was in this state was an empathic understanding of the depth and intensity of her feelings (see Kohut, 1984). In other words, repeated experiences of the safe-haven function of the therapist (i.e., sooth-ing and comforting in relation to intense negative affect) needed to precede exploration and reflection—activities in which the secure-base function of the therapist is in the forefront.

We have been impressed in our clinical work with the degree to which being able to reflect on one's own and others' mental states can serve affect-regulating functions. An individual who is immersed in a string of negative feelings is hardly able to examine and reflect on the basis of these feelings. The experience of rejection or humiliation or injustice is too strong, too enveloping to permit that. The individual in the grips of these emotions often has a sense of conviction, of certainty, of only one way to construe the situation—the one that utterly justifies the feelings he or she has. This intense psychic state is hardly one that permits reflection. In our experience, when the therapist is able to help the client take even small steps in the direc-tion of reflecting on these intense feelings and of taking the perspective of the other, this can dramatically serve to modulate intense negative feelings. One client described her increased ability to reflect on her feelings and to take the perspective of the other as a new "skill" that kept her from going off into a spiral of increasingly negative feelings.

A subtle interplay between the safe-haven and secure-base functions of the therapist can serve to facilitate the client's ability to engage in reflec-tive functioning. That is, if the therapist can sufficiently soothe the client's intense negative affects, it becomes more possible for the client to use the therapist's secure-base function in order to explore the basis for the intense affects. Repeated experiences of this kind should increase the ability of the client to employ the "skill" of reflective functioning.

From a psychoanalytic perspective, the therapist hopes to facilitate an optimal balance between "experiencing" and "reflecting" on experience. We mention this because the emphasis on reflective functioning needs to be balanced by a consideration of when it may be used excessively, as a defense against experiencing. The client needs to experience the negative affects fully in order for the reflection on them to escape being mere intellectualization. This is especially important for avoidant clients, who may turn the reflective process into an intellectualizing exercise.

SINGLE VERSUS MULTIPLE ATTACHMENT PATTERNS

In the discussion above and throughout this chapter, we have referred to the individual's *attachment style* as if a person is characterized by a singular attachment style—a stable structural trait. This is common practice in the literature and can be quite useful, insofar as it is likely that people do have a predominant attachment style. However, although an individual may show a predominant pattern, we agree with other researchers (e.g., Collins, Guichard, Ford, & Feeney, 2004; Mikulincer & Shaver, 2004) that people have a hierarchy of attachment styles. Each style in the hierarchy is associated with a different threshold for activation, and each pattern is activated by different dynamic factors, as well as by the individual with whom a person is interacting. This idea is partly based on research (e.g., Baldwin, Keelan, Fehr, Enns, & Koh-Rangarajoo, 1996) and partly on the clinical observation that different dynamics can emerge at different points in the treatment. For example, a dismissing style can serve as defense against an underlying preoccupied tendency. One client treated by one of us would go through periods of denying any attachment needs, which was clearly a defense against feelings of abandonment and during that period would present herself as someone with a dismissing style. However, that defense would generally not work, and the predominant preoccupied style would assert itself.

Psychoanalytic clinicians in particular are skeptical about fixed categories, including the fixed category of a single attachment category, because they have observed in their clinical work dynamic fluctuations in behavior and in psychological states as a function of such factors as defense, conflict, object choice, and so on. This observation converges with recent research in attachment assessment (e.g., Fraley & Waller, 1998; Fraley & Spieker, 2003)—which persuasively argues that attachment is best defined by two underlying dimensions, *avoidance* and *anxiety*, rather than by categories of attachment style (see Shaver & Mikulincer, Chapter 2, and Fraley & Phillips, Chapter 7, this volume, for reviews)—as well as with longitudinal research on attachment stability and change (e.g., Cobb & Davila, Chapter 9, this volume; Davila & Cobb, 2003).

ATTACHMENT THEORY, PSYCHOANALYSIS, AND PSYCHIC REALITY

Bowlby objected to what he believed was the overemphasis in psychoanalytic theory, particularly Kleinian theory,[5] on the role of fantasy and the relative neglect of actual events (e.g., loss, separation) in a child's life. In reaction against this state of affairs, Bowlby essentially reversed matters not only by placing virtually exclusive emphasis on the role of actual events, but also by assuming the relative *veridicality* (what he describes as "tolerably accurate reflections"; Bowlby, 1973, p. 202) of the child's representations of early attachment experiences. That is, the child's attachment security and corresponding internal working model are assumed to roughly reflect the attachment figure's actual behavior. For example, an avoidant attachment style is assumed to be the veridical product, so to speak, of the caregiver's actual rejecting behavior. That is, the assumption is that an avoidant attachment style (or an anxious-ambivalent attachment style) is, in large part at least, a response to the caregiver's actual behavior (e.g., rejecting or inconsistent) rather than largely a product of the child's fantasies. And the significant relationship between a caregiver's behavior in the home and a child's attachment style in the Strange Situation found by Ainsworth et al. (1978) supports this assumption. Many analysts, however, have been critical of attachment theory for ignoring the role of fantasy in the representation of events, and generally for minimizing the importance of psychic reality.

Given the reality of temperamental variability among infants, it is unlikely that veridical representation of actual events occurs in any simple sense of the term. As a hypothetical example (Eagle, 1995), imagine two infants, one with a low and with a high threshold for frustration—both waiting, say, 2 minutes to be fed. The infant with low frustration tolerance may encode the experience as a frustrating one, whereas the infant with high frustration tolerance may encode it as a gratifying one. The point here is that the same objective event may be encoded and represented quite differently as a function of an individual's psychic reality. The issue here is not fantasy versus actual events, but the idiosyncratic encoding of actual events. In other words, one can, as Bowlby proposed, give appropriate weight to the role of actual events in the individual's development and life, but nevertheless recognize that there may be variations in how actual events are experienced and represented by different individuals.

There appears to be evidence within attachment research for a defensively driven *nonveridical* representation of actual events—as seen, for example, in the idealization of the attachment figure often found in the AAI narratives of dismissing individuals. One could argue, of course, that the very fact of a dismissing style suggests that, idealization notwithstanding, actual events (e.g., the caregiver's rejecting behaviors) *were* accurately encoded at some level. Why else would the avoidant attachment style have developed? And indeed there is evidence that the idealization is defensively driven, as indicated by the individual's relative inability to instantiate the general idealization through recall of specific episodes. All this suggests that multiple and conflictual representations and internal working models, both veridical and defensively colored, may exist side by side within the same individual (Main, 1995). One could argue that in an important sense, the defensively colored representations and internal working model constitute fantasies, or at least leave the door wide open for unconscious fantasies to operate. Consideration of multiple defensively derived representations of attachment experiences takes one beyond viewing them simply as accurate accounts of events, to an increased recognition of the role of motivational factors in the representations of the attachment figure.

Consider again the idealization of attachment figures in the AAI narratives of avoidant individuals. According to Fairbairn (1952), in the face of rejecting experiences a child views him- or herself as bad, in order to keep the representation of the caregiver good through idealization. Implicit in Fairbairn's formulation is the idea that the rejected child's self-representation as bad and unlovable is not simply a direct product of learning on the basis of repeated rejection, but is also the consequence of a powerful motive to keep a representation of the caregiver as good. If Fairbairn's speculation is valid, it suggests that although the child's representations do reflect the impact of actual events (such as rejection), they do not do so in any simple or direct way. They also reflect the operation of defensive motives, such as the need to keep intact an idealized representation of the caregiver. As Fairbairn (1952) puts it, from the child's perspective, "it is better to be a sinner in a world ruled by God than to live in a world ruled by the devil" (p. 66). By viewing him- or herself as bad and the caregiver as idealized, the child keeps alive the possibility of earning the caregiver's love. That is, if being rejected is due to being bad, one keeps alive the fantasy that one can earn the caregiver's love by being good. In other words, between the extremes of fantasy and accurate representation of events, there is the middle ground of idiosyncratic and defensive encoding of actual events. Whatever the accuracy or inaccuracy of representations, the fact is that as far as treatment is concerned, the focus needs to be on the client's idiosyncratic and often defensive encodings of events—that is, on his or her psychic reality.

ATTACHMENT RESEARCH RELEVANT TO PSYCHOTHERAPY

Some of the potentially fruitful clinical implications of attachment theory as it applies to adults have begun to be studied empirically. Among the relevant research questions one can pose are these: To what extent are different adult attachment styles associated with different forms of psychopathology? What are the implications of different adult attachment styles for the ease or difficulty of forming and sustaining a positive working alliance? Are particular therapeutic modalities differentially suitable for clients with different attachment styles? Within a given modality (e.g., psychoanalytic psychotherapy), which therapeutic techniques need to be adjusted as a function of the client's attachment style? What is the relationship between attachment style and therapy outcome? Are matches and mismatches in attachment style between therapist and client related to outcome? How does the internalization of the therapeutic relationship differ as a function of attachment style? How do we assess changes in the client's internal working models? Other chapters in this volume offer some answers to these questions.

Thus far, the research literature on these kinds of questions shows marked variations across studies in measures of attachment style, level of therapist experience, and degree of client pathology. Many studies rely on self-report scales to measure all variables. The correlations reported, although statistically significant, are generally low or modest. At this early stage of clinically informed research on adult attachment, we do not have a solid body of findings that would generate strong predictions regarding the effectiveness of different types of clinical interventions. Thus Mallinckrodt, Daly, and Wang (Chapter 10, this volume) note that the American Psychological Association's Division 29 (Psychotherapy) Task Force on Psychotherapy Relationships concluded in 2001 that there was insufficient research evidence regarding the role of attachment style on which to base recommendations concerning psychotherapy practice. Mallinckrodt et al. believe that this position is still warranted, and it seems to us that their point is valid.

With this caution in mind, and given our space limitations, we present only a brief, highly selective overview of some of this research; we focus primarily on the key, perhaps overarching issue of which factors impede or facilitate the experience of the therapist as a secure base. Perhaps the first step in a research program directed toward the nature of the client's internalization of the therapist as a secure base would be to show that the therapist indeed has become an attachment figure. Clinically, we assume that the flowering of positive and negative transference indicates that the therapist is becoming an attachment figure—in other words, that he or she is activating internal working models (associative networks) originally formed in relation to the client's initial attachment figures. But there are more direct ways of measuring attachment to the therapist. For example, Parish and Eagle (2003) noted that certain criteria need to be met before we can legitimately say that the therapist has become an attachment figure for the client. Considering multiple components of attachment (e.g., proximity seeking, secure base, safe haven, availability, separation protest, wiser/stronger), they found that all the components were relevant. Secure-base scores (and availability) correlated positively with the strength of a client's working alliance, as measured by the Horvath and Greenberg (1989) scale. Duration of treatment and frequency of sessions correlated with overall degree of attachment to the therapist. As one might expect, dismissing clients reported the lowest intensity of attachment to their therapists.

Dozier and Tyrrell (1998) present a model of therapeutic change in which corrective experiences with the therapist lead to explorations of both current relationships and past relationships with prior attachment figures, which in turn lead to changes in the internal working models of self and other. Their emphasis is on insights that can change the client's internal working model of relationships. However, it also might be that the secure-base experience is healing in its own right, at least for certain clients (Dozier & Bates, 2004). Let us turn to a sampling of empirical research that bears primarily on the internalization of the therapist as a secure base.

Internalization of the Therapist

It has been reported that clients internalize their therapists over the course of psychotherapy (Rosenzweig, Farber, & Geller, 1996; Arnold, Farber, & Geller, 2004). It should be noted that internalization exists on a continuum from *introjection* to *identification* (Schafer, 1968/1990). The process of internalization can take the form of introjection—for example, of an ego-supportive or *holding environment* (Winnicott, 1971) and of the felt availability of a *soothing introject* (Adler & Buie, 1979). It can also take the form of identification, in which there is a change in the client's self-representations in the direction of a greater resemblance to the therapist. Research suggests that clients internalize aspects of their therapists over time (Geller & Farber, 1993), and that their self-representations come to resemble the quality of interpersonal process in sessions (Harrist, Quintana, Strupp, & Henry, 1994). In the case of identification, the depersonalized functions provided by the analyst come to be internalized as part of the client's self; this is what Kohut (1984) meant by *transmuting internalization*.

Shaeffer and Geller (1993) studied clients' representations of their relationship with their therapists. They reported that clients with a secure attachment style, compared with those who were insecurely attached, were more likely to invoke benign and gratifying representations of their therapists. Among their findings were that dismissing subjects, compared with secure subjects, were more apt to show a "failure of benign internalization" and less likely to be involved in "continuing the therapeutic dialogue" outside the session.

It is of interest to know when clients are most apt to invoke representations of their therapists. Geller and Farber (1993) reported that clients were most likely to do so when they were experiencing negative affects. It is reasonable to regard such a tendency toward "out-of-session" silent dialogue with one's therapist as an indication that the therapist is viewed as a safe haven. Invoking the therapist can be regarded as a form of proximity seeking. We should note, however, that current clients who were experiencing negative affect invoked representations of the therapist 53% of the time, while former clients did so 28% of the time. The comparable figures when clients were experiencing conflict were 24% and 19%, respectively. This study did not include a measure of attachment style. It would be of interest to know (1) whether the likelihood of invoking the therapist was related to attachment style, since 47% of current clients did not invoke the therapist between sessions, nor did 72% of former clients; and (2) whether the motivation for and manner of invoking the therapist differed as a function of attachment style.

We might expect that avoidant clients would be less apt to invoke representations of the therapist. Secure and preoccupied clients might invoke the therapist with similar frequency, but one would expect that the preoccupied clients would mainly be looking for soothing and reassurance, while secure clients might be more apt to wonder what their therapist might think about the meanings of their negative affects. As for the marked posttherapy reduction in thinking of the therapist, a client might have progressed from introjection to identification with the therapist and might not need to consciously invoke scenarios of their dialogue. That is, one might suppose that when a client has identified with the therapist's analyzing function and nonjudgmental attitude, the ensuing silent dialogue is a more seamless, automatic, nonconscious event, rather than a conscious (albeit spontaneous) effort to create a sense of connection to the therapist.

Thus, from both an attachment and a psychoanalytic perspective, a significant aspect of what is "curative" is the internalized representation of the therapeutic relationship and the therapist. This internalization can serve as the comforting inner presence of someone who is emotionally available, if only in fantasy, as well as (via an identification with the therapist's analyzing function) a source of enhanced self-understanding (Kantrowitz, Katz, & Paolitto, 1990a, 1990b; Geller & Farber, 1993). In other words, both insight and relationship factors are important components of therapeutic action.

Working Alliance

All writers agree that the promotion and maintenance of a positive therapeutic or working alliance, and the ability to repair inevitable ruptures in it, facilitate therapeutic change (e.g., Safran & Muran, 2000). Insofar as the alliance facilitates exploration leading to insight, as well as being therapeutic in its own right, attachment styles that interfere with an adequate alliance would be inimical to therapeutic progress. It appears that clients with a relatively secure attachment style need little more than an accepting and listening attitude on the part of the therapist in order to collaborate effectively in the therapeutic work. In fact, Kanninen, Salo, and Punamäki (2000), using a paper-and-pencil version of the AAI, reported that clients classified as having a secure state of mind with respect to attachment maintained a stable therapeutic alliance over the course of treatment, whereas clients classified as preoccupied reported a strong alliance only in the later stages of treatment. Those classified as dismissing showed a decline in the alliance near the end of treatment. Consistent with the conception of insecure attachment, issues of trust and a sense of safety would be expected to be more prominent in the internal working models of these clients, and therefore a focus of treatment. Thus the internalization of a benign therapeutic relationship and its reflection in the state of the working alliance should be expected to take time and to depend on experiences with an attachment figure who is more reliable, empathic, and supportive than the original attachment figures. Ordinarily, more secure clients are expected to fare better in therapy. An exception to this general finding is a report by Fonagy et al. (1996) that dismissing-avoidant clients showed the largest gains in treatment. However, a look at the data in that study shows that those clients started at lower levels and had more room to improve.

Client–Therapist Match versus Mismatch in Attachment Style

In addition to attachment style and its associated defensive strategies, we can ask about the relevance of the similarity versus difference in client–therapist attachment styles. In the past, client–therapist match has been studied in relation to personality characteristics, values, demographics, and the like (e.g., Kantrowitz, 1995). Applied to attachment theory, the question is whether client–therapist matches or mismatches in attachment style will make it more or less difficult for clients to internalize a positive, benign therapeutic relationship and to work effectively in the therapy. In a study of case managers working with seriously disturbed clients, Tyrrell, Dozier, Teague, and Fallot (1999) found that cases in which client and therapist were different in attachment style had better outcomes, presumably because the therapist was more likely to challenge the client and less likely to collude with him or her (see also Dozier, Cue, & Barnett, 1994; Dozier, Lomax, Tyrrell, & Lee, 2001).

It is not typically expected that the client will represent an attachment figure for the therapist. Why, therefore, should the therapist's attachment style matter at all in treatment? It would seem that to the extent that the therapist's attachment style is associated with ego-syntonic, trait-like characterological and defensive patterns, it could lead to unrecognized and therefore unmanaged countertransference reactions. For example, a therapist who avoids awareness of emotionally charged issues in his or her own personal functioning may collude with an avoidant client's inclination to avoid focusing on similar emotional issues. A hypothesis to be tested is that the issue of match versus mismatch in attachment style is relevant to the extent that the therapist cannot flexibly adjust his or her style of interaction in relation to clients with different styles of attachment.

Mallinckrodt et al. (Chapter 10, this volume) studied "expert" therapists (i.e., those nominated as skilled in dealing with clients who had problems in close relationships). These therapists were given case vignettes of hypothetical clients who had hyperactivating or deactivating coping strategies. Attachment styles of these therapists were not assessed. However, the therapists showed a strong degree of consensus in their awareness of the importance of monitoring and regulating their behavior, with a view toward maintaining an optimal distance from each client as a function of the client's attachment style as well as phase of treatment. Whether they would indeed act this way, were they actually to treat such clients, is another matter. In the end, it might be that for experienced therapists the time-honored clinical wisdom of optimal timing, tact, and dosage of interpretations, and the flexibility *and relative freedom from unmanaged countertransference* implied in this view, might override the issue of match versus mismatch in therapist–client attachment styles (at least for many, if not all, kinds of clients). It is likely, however, that a therapist's attachment style would be more relevant to behavior in the actual, *more emotionally charged* treatment situation than to the formulation of the case and the planning of treatment strategies. In follow-up studies of Dozier, Tyrrell, and colleagues' findings, it would be useful to examine match and mismatch in attachment styles with less disturbed clients being treated by experienced therapists, such as those in the Mallinckrodt et al. study.

This sampling of research findings suggests a model of therapeutic action that combines in a compatible manner the perspectives of attachment theory and contemporary psychoanalytic theory. A key assumption of both perspectives is that the benign internalization of the therapeutic relationship is healing in its own right, at least for certain clients, and that it also enables clients to explore and modify their internal working models of self, other, and self–other relationships. Insecure attachment (and its associated fear of retraumatization) interferes with the establishment and maintenance of a good working alliance, because the internal working model the patient starts with includes minimal hope that the therapy relationship will be one characterized by the emotional availability, empathic responsiveness, and soothing presence of the therapist. Over time, and with appropriate therapist interventions, these qualities of the therapist lead the insecurely attached client to increased feelings of trust and safety. The strengthening of the alliance allows the client to disclose fears, needs, and negative affects (e.g., shameful impulses) and negative (as well as positive) transference reactions, and to explore their meanings. As discussed earlier, we would hypothesize that therapeutic strategies and tactics would have to be modified, depending on the extent to which the client is inclined toward use of deactivating strategies (i.e., an avoidant attachment style) versus hyperactivating strategies (i.e., an anxious attachment style).

In conclusion, many more empirical studies will be required to test the kinds of hypotheses we have considered in the course of this discussion, and to discover the most fruitful integration of attachment theory with key phenomena addressed by psychoanalytic concepts. The ultimate issue is not just to show that the application of attachment theory to clinical practice enhances our understanding of clients' dynamics and creates new options for therapeutic intervention, but to develop a body of findings about whether (and, if so, to what extent) a solid grounding in attachment theory and in the clinical research it generates actually improves our clinical effectiveness.

CONCLUSIONS

One of the potentially fruitful interactions between psychoanalysis and attachment theory and research is the psychoanalytic exploration of the individual meanings of trends and patterns identified by attachment research and theory. Although it can be very useful information, it is unlikely—and rightly so—that an analyst will be content with viewing a client as, say, avoidant or preoccupied. This is partly so because having an avoidant, a preoccupied, or any other attachment style will always be idiosyncratic and embedded in a complex individual life in which conflicts, defenses, wishes, and fantasies are present.

Although certain dynamics may be associated with a particular attachment style, they are not equivalent to each other. Thus, for example, although the dynamic underlying an agoraphobic client's relationship with her mother—"If I separate, I will be harming or destroying my mother"— may be associated with a preoccupied attachment style, it is not equivalent to it. It needs to be described in its own terms. There is little to be gained by attempting to "squeeze" or reduce idiosyncratic clinical patterns into one or another "standard" attachment category when there is not a good fit. Given the current popularity of attachment theory, this is a real danger. This misuse of attachment ideas will not do justice to the complexity of the clinical phenomena. It is also likely that in the course of trying to squeeze everything into the framework of attachment theory, the central concepts, ideas, and hypotheses of that theory will become so diluted as to lose any precision of meaning and any possibility of empirical test. It must be acknowledged that although attachment is a vital area of human functioning and experience, it does not constitute all of personality development and functioning.

We believe that the ideal relationship between attachment theory and psychoanalysis is one in which the findings and concepts emerging from attachment research and theory serve to sensitize analysts (and other therapists) to certain issues and phenomena and to provide a new perspective; conversely, it is one in which phenomena emerging from the clinical situation serve to challenge and refine the formulations of attachment theory. At present, we believe there are not sufficient empirical or conceptual grounds for proposing a specific kind of attachment-based treatment for individual adults. Therapists should be skeptical regarding the current bandwagon. However, as outlined in this chapter, attachment theory and psychoanalysis have much to offer each other. For the present, we reiterate our agreement with Slade (1999, p. 577) "that an understanding of the nature and dynamics of attachment *informs* rather than *defines* intervention and clinical thinking."

NOTES

1. Although not stated in attachment theory terms, the idea of the therapist as a secure base from which the patient can more safely engage in self-exploration finds expression in a number of different theoretical psychoanalytic contexts—a similarity Bowlby (1988, p. 140) readily acknowledged. Some examples include Sandler's (1960/1987) concept of *background of safety*; Weiss, Sampson, and the Mount Zion Psychotherapy Research Group's (1986) central idea that *conditions of safety* facilitate the emergence of warded-off material; and Fairbairn's (1952) recognition that the analyst needs to be experienced as a *good object* by the patient in order for the latter to be capable of confronting the painful *bad object* situation of the past.
2. Given the history of rejection and lack of empathy that many clients have experienced prior to therapy, it would be foolhardy, given such clients' fear of retraumatization at the hands of the therapist, for them simply to assume that the therapist will be sensitively responsive and serve reliably as a safe haven and a secure base.
3. Insofar as a broadening of interests can be seen as an increase in exploratory behavior, the finding that test passing leads to such a broadening especially supports the idea that presentation of tests is related to the status of the therapist as a secure base.
4. As Fairbairn (1952) has noted, the model for the internalized *bad object* is Freud's concept of the *superego*. Although the superego's origins lie in the reactions of parental figure, these reactions have become part of the self. Therefore, the issue is not simply a matter of expecting harsh and condemning judgments from others, but of experiencing harsh and condemning judgments from oneself. It is the latter that, according to Fairbairn, needs to be "exorcised" in treatment.
5. The objection could be equally directed to Freudian theory, once Freud shifted from an emphasis on actual seduction to seduction fantasies.

RECOMMENDATIONS FOR FURTHER READING

Dozier, M., & Tyrrell, C. (1998). The role of attachment in therapeutic relationships. In J. A. Simpson & W. S. Rholes (Eds.), *Attachment theory and close relationships* (pp. 221–248). New York: Guilford Press—This chapter provides a useful overview of the significance of attachment in the context of psychotherapy.
Fonagy, P. (2001). *Attachment theory and psychoanalysis.* New York: Other Press—Fonagy's book offers a broad overview of the relationship between attachment theory and various schools of psychoanalytic thought.

REFERENCES

Adler, G., & Buie, D. H. (1979). Aloneness and borderline psychopathology: The possible relevance of child developmental issues. *International Journal of Psycho-Analysis, 60,* 83–96.

Ainsworth, M. D. S., Blehar, M., Waters, E., & Wall, S. (1978). *Patterns of attachment: A psychological study of the Strange Situation.* Hillsdale, NJ: Erlbaum.

Arnold, E. G., Farber, B., & Geller, J. (2004). Termination, posttermination, and internalization of the therapy and the therapist: Internalization and psychotherapy outcome. In D. P. Charman (Ed.), *Core processes in brief psychodynamic psychotherapy: Advancing effective practice* (pp. 289–308). Mahwah, NJ: Erlbaum.

Baldwin, M. W., Keelan, J. P. R., Fehr, B., Enns, V., & Koh-Rangarajoo, E. (1996). Social-cognitive conceptualization of attachment working models: Availability and accessibility effects. *Journal of Personality and Social Psychology, 71,* 94–109.

Bowlby, J. (1973). *Attachment and loss: Vol. 2. Separation: Anxiety and anger.* New York: Basic Books.

Bowlby, J. (1977). The making and breaking of affectional bonds: Aetiology and psychopathology in the light of attachment theory. *British Journal of Psychiatry, 130,* 201–210.

Bowlby, J. (1980). *Attachment and loss: Vol. 3. Loss: Sadness and depression.* New York: Basic Books.

Bowlby, J. (1988). *A secure base.* London: Routledge.

Collins, N. L., Guichard, A. C., Ford, M. B., & Feeney, B. C. (2004). Working models of attachment: New developments and emerging themes. In W. S. Rholes & J. A. Simpson (Eds.), *Adult attachment: Theory, research, and clinical implications* (pp. 196–239). New York: Guilford Press.

Crits-Christoph, P., & Luborsky, L. (1990). Changes in CCRT pervasiveness during psychotherapy. In L. Luborsky & P. Crits-Christoph (Eds.), *Understanding transference* (pp. 133–146). New York: Basic Books.

Davila, J., & Cobb, R. J. (2003). Predicting change in self-reported and interview-assessed adult attachment: Tests of the individual differences and life stress models of attachment change. *Personality and Social Psychology Bulletin, 29,* 1383–1395.

Dozier, M., & Bates, B. C. (2004). Attachment state of mind and the treatment relationship. In L. Atkinson & S. Goldberg (Eds.), *Attachment issues in psychopathology and intervention* (pp. 167–180). Mahwah, NJ: Erlbaum.

Dozier, M., Cue, K. L., & Barnett, L. (1994). Clinicians as caregivers: Role of attachment organization in treatment. *Journal of Consulting and Clinical Psychology, 62,* 793–800.

Dozier, M., Lomax, L., Tyrrell, C. L., & Lee, S. W. (2001). The challenge of treatment for clients with dismissing states of mind. *Attachment & Human Development, 3,* 62–76.

Dozier, M., & Tyrrell, C. L. (1998). The role of attachment in therapeutic relationships. In J. A. Simpson & W. S. Rholes (Eds.), *Attachment theory and close relationships* (pp. 221–248). New York: Guilford Press.

Eagle, M. (1995). The developmental perspectives of attachment and psychoanalytic theory. In S. Goldberg, R. Muir, & J. Kerr (Eds.), *Attachment theory: Social, developmental, and clinical perspectives* (pp. 123–150). Hillsdale, NJ: Analytic Press.

Eagle, M. (1997). Attachment and psychoanalysis. *British Journal of Medical Psychology, 70,* 217–229.

Eagle, M. (2002). Some clinical issues in the light of attachment research and theory. *Journal of Infant, Child, and Adolescent Psychotherapy, 2,* 11–17.

Fairbairn, W. R .D. (1952). *Psychoanalytic studies of the personality.* London: Tavistock.

Fonagy, P. (2001). *Attachment theory and psychoanalysis.* New York: Other Press.

Fonagy, P., Leigh, T., Steele, M., Steele, H., Kennedy, R., Mattoon, G., et al. (1996). The relation of attachment status, psychiatric classification, and response to psychotherapy. *Journal of Consulting and Clinical Psychology, 64,* 22–31.

Fonagy, P., Steele, M., Steele, H., Moran, G., & Higgitt, A. (1991). The capacity for understanding mental states: The reflective self in parent and child and its significance for security of attachment. *Infant Mental Health Journal, 12,* 201–218.

Fonagy, P., Steele, M., Steele, H., Leigh, T., Kennedy, R., Mattoon, G., et al. (1995). Attachment, the reflective self, and borderline states. In S. Goldberg, R. Muir, & J. Kerr (Eds.), *Attachment theory: Social development and clinical perspectives* (pp. 233–278). Hillsdale, NJ: Analytic Press.

Fonagy, P., Steele, M., & Target, M. (1997). *Reflective-functioning manual, version 4.1, for application to Adult Attachment Interviews.* London: University College London.

Fraley, R. C., & Spieker, S. J. (2003). What are the differences between dimensional and categorical models of individual differences in attachment?: Reply to Cassidy (2003), Sroufe (2003), Waters (2003), and Beauchaine (2003). *Developmental Psychology, 39,* 423–429.

Fraley, R. C., & Waller, N. G. (1998). Adult attachment patterns: A test of the typological model. In J. A. Simpson & W. S. Rholes (Eds.), *Attachment theory and close relationships* (pp. 77–144). New York: Guilford Press.

Freud, S. (1958). Remembering, repeating, and working through. In J. Strachey (Ed. & Trans.), *The standard edition of the complete psychological works of Sigmund Freud* (Vol. 12, pp. 145–156). London: Hogarth Press. (Original work published 1913)

Geller, J. D., & Farber, B. A. (1993). Factors influencing the process of internalization in psychotherapy. *Psychotherapy Research, 3,* 166–180.

George, C., Kaplan, N., & Main, M. (1984). *Adult Attachment Interview protocol.* Unpublished manuscript, University of California, Berkeley.

George, C., Kaplan, N., & Main, M. (1985). *Adult Attachment Interview protocol* (2nd ed.). Unpublished manuscript, University of California, Berkeley.

George, C., Kaplan, N., & Main, M. (1996). *Adult Attachment Interview protocol* (3rd ed.). Unpublished manuscript, University of California, Berkeley.

Harrist, R. S., Quintana, S. M., Strupp, H. H., & Henry, W. P. (1994). Internalization of interpersonal process in time limited dynamic psychotherapy. *Psychotherapy, 31,* 49–57.

Holmes, J. (2001). *The search for the secure base.* New York: Brunner/Mazel.

Horvath, A., & Greenberg, L. S. (1989). Development and validation of the Working Alliance Inventory. *Journal of Counseling Psychology, 36,* 223–233.

Johnson, S. M. (2004). Attachment theory: A guide for healing couple relationships.

In W. S. Rholes & J. A. Simpson (Eds.), *Adult attachment: Theory, research, and clinical implications* (pp. 367–387). New York: Guilford Press.

Kanninen, K., Salo, J., & Punamäki, R. (2000). Attachment patterns and working alliance in trauma therapy for victims of political violence. *Psychotherapy Research, 10,* 435–449.

Kantrowitz, J. L. (1995). The beneficial aspects of the patient–analyst match. *International Journal of Psychoanalysis, 76*(2), 299–313.

Kantrowitz, J. L., Katz, A. L., & Paolitto, F. (1990a). Follow-up of psychoanalysis five to ten years after termination: II. Development of the self-analytic function. *Journal of the American Psychoanalytic Association, 38,* 637–654.

Kantrowitz, J. L., Katz, A. L., & Paolitto, F. (1990b). Follow-up of psychoanalysis five to ten years after termination: III. The relation between the resolution of the transference and the patient–analyst match. *Journal of the American Psychoanalytic Association, 38,* 655–678.

Kohut, H. (1984). *How does analysis cure?* Chicago: University of Chicago Press.

Levy, K. N., Meehan, K. B., Kelly, K. M., Reynoso, J. S., Weber, M., Clarkin, J. F., et al. (2006). Change in attachment patterns and reflective function in a randomized control trial of transference-focused psychotherapy for borderline personality disorder. *Journal of Consulting and Clinical Psychology, 74,* 1027–1040.

Lieberman, A. F. (1999). Negative maternal attributions: Effects on toddlers' sense of self. *Psychoanalytic Inquiry, 19,* 737–756.

Lieberman, A. F., & Zeanah, C. H. (1999). Contributions of attachment theory to infant–parent psychotherapy and other interventions with infants and young children. In J. Cassidy & P. R. Shaver (Eds.), *Handbook of attachment: Theory, research, and clinical applications* (pp. 555–574). New York: Guilford Press.

Main, M. (1995). Recent studies in attachment: Overview, with selected implications for clinical work. In S. Goldberg, R. Muir, & J. Kerr (Eds.), *Attachment theory: Social, developmental, and clinical perspectives* (pp. 407–474). Hillsdale, NJ: Analytic Press.

Mallinckrodt, B., Porter, M., & Kivlighan, D. (2005). Client attachment to therapist, depth of in-session exploration and object relations in brief psychotherapy. *Psychotherapy: Theory, Research, Practice, Training, 42,* 85–100.

Marvin, R., Cooper, G., Hoffman, K., & Powell, B. (2002). The Circle of Security project: Attachment-based intervention with caregiver–preschool child dyads. *Attachment & Human Development, 4,* 107–124.

Mikulincer, M., & Shaver, P. R. (2003). The attachment behavioral system in adulthood: Activation, psychodynamics, and interpersonal processes. In M. P. Zanna (Ed.), *Advances in experimental social psychology* (Vol. 35, pp. 53–152). San Diego, CA: Academic Press.

Mikulincer, M., & Shaver, P. R. (2004). Security-based self-representations in adulthood: Contents and processes. In W. S. Rholes & J. A. Simpson (Ed.), *Adult attachment: Theory, research, and clinical implications* (pp. 159–195). New York: Guilford Press.

Parish, M., & Eagle, M. (2003). The therapist as an attachment figure. *Psychoanalytic Psychology, 20,* 271–286.

Pfeffer, A. Z. (1993). After the analysis: Analyst as both old and new object. *Journal of the American Psychoanalytic Association, 141,* 323–337.

Rosenzweig, D., Farber, B., & Geller, J. D. (1996). Clients' representations of their therapists over the course of psychotherapy. *Journal of Clinical Psychology, 52,* 197–207.

Safran, J., & Muran, J. C. (2000). *Negotiating the therapeutic alliance: A relational treatment guide.* New York: Guilford Press.

Sandler, J. (1987). The background of safety. In J. Sandler (Ed.), *From safety to superego: Selected papers of Joseph Sandler* (pp. 1–8). London: Karnac. (Original work published 1960)

Schafer, R. (1990). *Aspects of internalization.* Madison, CT: International Universities Press. (Original work published 1968)

Schechter, D., Meyers, M., Brunelli, S., Coates, S., Zeanah, C., Davies, M., et al. (2006). Traumatized mothers can change their minds about their toddlers: Understanding how a novel use of video feedback supports positive maternal attributions. *Infant Mental Health Journal, 27,* 429–447.

Shaeffer, C., & Geller, J. D. (1993). *Attachment, affect regulation, alexithymia, and patients' representations of the psychotherapy relationship.* Paper presented at a meeting of the Society for Psychotherapy Research, Pittsburgh, PA.

Slade, A. (1999). Attachment theory and research: Implications for the theory and practice of individual psychotherapy with adults. In J. Cassidy & P. R. Shaver (Eds.), *Handbook of attachment: Theory, research, and clinical applications* (pp. 575–594). New York: Guilford Press.

Sorce, J. F., & Emde, R. N. (1981). Mother's presence is not enough: Effect of emotional availability on infant exploration. *Developmental Psychology, 17,* 737–745.

Toth, S. L., Rogosch, F. A., & Cicchetti, D. (2006). The efficacy of toddler–parent psychotherapy to reorganize attachment in the young offspring of mothers with major depressive disorder. *Journal of Consulting and Clinical Psychology.*

Tyrrell, C. L., Dozier, M., Teague, G. B., & Fallot, R. D. (1999). Effective treatment relationships for persons with serious psychiatric disorders: The importance of attachment states of mind. *Journal of Consulting and Clinical Psychology. 67,* 725–733.

van IJzendoorn, M. H. (1995). Adult attachment representations, parental responsiveness, and infant attachment: A metaanalysis of the predictive validity of the Adult Attachment Interview. *Psychological Bulletin, 117,* 387–403.

Weiss, J., Sampson, H., & the Mount Zion Psychotherapy Research Group. (1986). *The psychoanalytic process: Theory, clinical observation, and empirical research.* New York: Guilford Press.

Winnicott, D. W. (1971). *Playing and reality.* New York: Basic Books.

15

An Interpersonal Approach to Attachment and Change

Paul Florsheim
Laura McArthur

This chapter integrates attachment theory and interpersonal theories of psychotherapy, with an emphasis on the nature of therapeutic action. We have two primary objectives. The first is to articulate how attachment theory can clarify the goals of interpersonally oriented treatment. From an attachment perspective, the goal of therapy, like the goal of development, is to enhance attachment security—that is, "a sense that one can rely on close relationship partners for protection and support, can safely and effectively explore the environment, and can engage effectively with other people" (p. 159). (Mikulincer & Shaver, 2004). Although clients often enter therapy with a specific, tangible goal in mind (to diminish symptoms, resolve interpersonal disputes, etc.), it is useful to consider symptoms and interpersonal problems within the context of attachment theory. Having an attachment-informed focus helps the therapist guide the client through the process of symptom reduction to a more complete, gratifying, and (ideally) enduring resolution.

Our second objective is to describe interpersonal models for revising maladaptive patterns of interpersonal behavior that stem from attachment insecurity. It is a well-established research finding that the quality of the therapist–client relationship accounts for a respectable proportion of the variance in psychotherapeutic change across treatment models (Lambert & Barley, 2001; Martin, Garske, & Davis, 2000; Norcross, 2002). This research underscores the important role of interpersonal techniques in facilitating positive change in attachment security. Whereas attachment theory helps clarify overarching therapeutic goals, interpersonal theory helps the therapist understand and define the processes involved in reaching those goals (Henry & Strupp, 1994; Henry, Schacht, & Strupp, 1986).

We present the case of a young couple—Ana and Juan—to illustrate the integration of attachment and interpersonal theories. Following the initial case presentation, we discuss several points of theoretical convergence and complementarity. We then describe several existing models of interpersonal therapy and illustrate how each uniquely addresses attachment insecurity. Throughout this chapter, we argue that attachment theory's emphasis on the interplay between attachment and exploration can help interpersonal therapists integrate the goal and process of therapy. According to Bowlby and Ainsworth, attachment and exploration are mutually supportive systems, in that secure attachment sets the stage for competent exploration, and exploration in the context of a supportive and caring atmosphere further enhances security (Ainsworth, 1991; Bowlby 1969/1982; Grossmann, Grossmann, & Zimmerman, 1999).

Interpersonal exploration (i.e., behavior that extends the realm and depth of close relationships) is the primary means through which security is expressed, negotiated, and developed. Attachment researchers have demonstrated that through the process of interpersonal exploration and experimentation, the parent–infant bond develops and the self evolves (Thompson, Easterbrooks, & Padilla-Walker, 2003; Volling, McElwain, & Notaro, 2002). In part, it is through this process of exploration that internal working models are elaborated and attachment strategies forged. Thinking about the therapy process as an interplay between security seeking and exploration can enhance our understanding of how therapeutic change occurs (Bateman & Fonagy, 2004; Slade, 2004; Stern, 2004).

CASE STUDY: ANA AND JUAN

Ana, an 18-year-old pregnant woman, and Juan, her 20-year-old boyfriend, were recruited into co-parenting counseling as part of a research study for high-risk expectant parents. The goal of the program was to help young expectant couples communicate more effectively, so as to provide their child with a more secure interpersonal environment.

Juan and Ana had met through mutual gang affiliations and had dated on and off since Juan was released from prison 8 months earlier. Consistent with their history of reckless behavior, Ana and Juan rarely used birth control, and soon Ana became pregnant. Ana was not happy about the prospect of becoming a mother, but felt pressured by Juan and her mother to keep the baby.

Ana had been raised in a violent, chaotic family with a rich criminal history. She had a strained and distant relationship with her mother, who was alternately controlling and neglectful. Her mother had been an adolescent mother herself and had a long history of substance use problems, which contributed to the family's chronic instability. Ana reported a more positive relationship with her father, who had been sent to prison when she was 10 and then deported to Mexico. Although she was not able to say much about this relationship, she seemed to regard her father as warmly watching over her from a great distance. Just prior to entering our intervention research study, Ana was released from a drug treatment center after a 2-month stay. The staff at this center were pessimistic about Ana's prognosis; although she was no longer using substances, she had been consistently resistant to therapy.

Juan's parents were traditional Mexican immigrants who spoke little English and worked long hours. According to Juan, it was a mystery why he and his brothers, also gang-involved, ended up in so much trouble. If there were family troubles beneath the surface, Juan kept them to himself. He was open about the fact that he had always struggled with overwhelming feelings of jealousy and anger, and said he would like to change his habit of overreacting to small slights. As a child, his jealousy was directed toward his brothers, but currently he felt jealous of Ana's family and friends. Fortunately, Juan was reflective enough to recognize that his jealousy was negatively affecting his relationship with Ana.

When Ana and Juan were recruited into the Young Parenthood Program, their relationship was "on again, off again." The director, who is a senior clinician (Paul Florsheim), took the case because during the initial assessment, it became clear that Ana and Juan presented a number of interpersonal challenges associated with a history of attachment problems, drug use, gang affiliation, and criminal behavior. The first clinical contact was preceded by a series of phone calls in which the therapist played go-between. Ana and Juan had recently broken up and were no longer speaking. Ana's mother disliked Juan and had talked her into dumping him. For reasons that never became clear, a friend of Ana's had threatened Juan by putting a gun to his head. Despite this drama and conflict, Juan and Ana independently told the therapist that each was willing to meet *if* the other one wanted to meet. The therapist negotiated a first session.

This pattern of reluctant engagement with each other continued throughout the program. When they were on speaking terms, Ana and Juan would make plans to be together, and then one or the other would often fail to show up. When Juan failed to show, Ana would become more removed. When Ana failed to show, Juan would lose his temper, yell at Ana, and disengage for days. After cooling down, he would try to make up.

Initially, Ana seemed profoundly detached, as if she had constructed a brick wall around herself. Although she attended her appointments, she was unwilling to open up in Juan's presence, except to say that she was depressed about becoming a mother. She was monosyllabic and sometimes spoke no more than a dozen or so words during an entire session. The therapist considered a number of explanations for this behavior, including the possibility that Ana was intellectually impaired and did not understand what was happening around her. This hypothesis was eventually rejected, as Ana revealed that she was a sharp observer with a quick, biting wit. Eventually the therapist began to work from the assumption that Ana's silence reflected a fear of investing in others, whom she regarded as undependable and transient. We feel confident that Ana would be classified as dismissing, according to the most common attachment classification systems (e.g., Brennan, Clark, & Shaver, 1998; Hesse, 1999): Her parental relationships were characterized by inconsistent availability and hostility; her interpersonal demeanor was cool and distant; and her narrative style was brief and nondisclosing.

Although Juan was somewhat more open than Ana and invested in having a relationship with her, he felt confused, insulted, and dismissed by her "silent treatment." Just before beginning therapy, Juan quit the job his parole officer had helped him find and began hanging out with his gang buddies. When asked about this, Juan said that going back to prison did not bother him. He was angry at his parole officer, who was breathing down his neck, and angry at Ana for her detachment. Juan may have been trying to get some declaration of investment from Ana. If this was the case, the plan backfired: Ana only became more disdainful and distant. She seemed to regard Juan's behavior as confirmation that it was wise to expect nothing from him.

Both Ana and Juan were more willing to open up when speaking privately to the therapist, and each seemed to anticipate that he would help relay information to the other that could not be expressed directly. The therapist accepted this somewhat unusual role, with the goal of helping them learn to express themselves more directly. That a middle-aged, European American university professor would find himself playing go-between for a couple of angry young Mexican Americans with gang affiliations and serious attachment problems seems like the premise for a bad movie; that Ana and Juan would open themselves to a therapist who represented a world both foreign and inaccessible seems implausible. Yet the interpersonal problem presented by Ana and Juan, and the sociocultural divide between this couple and their therapist, are common clinical experiences and provide an opportunity to consider the nature and limits of therapeutic action.

The case of Ana and Juan raises a number of theoretical and practical challenges that provide a context for integrating attachment and interpersonal theories of intervention. What could be done to support Ana and Juan's sense of attachment security, both as individuals and as co-parents? Should the therapist attempt to facilitate the security of this couple's attachment? Should he assist them in exploring the quality of their parental attachments, in an effort to increase their capacity to nurture their child's security? Or should treatment focus on the quality of the attachment to the therapist, as a way to engender attachment security?

INTEGRATION OF ATTACHMENT
AND INTERPERSONAL THEORIES

Harry Stack Sullivan is regarded as the father of interpersonal psychotherapy (Greenberg & Mitchell, 1983). Influenced by the leading social and cultural theorists of his day (Cooley, 1902; Mead, 1934), Sullivan (1938, 1953) proposed that we all experience ourselves through our relationships with others. Sullivan's peers adhered to the traditional psychoanalytic perspective that we are driven by libidinal and aggressive instincts, and that we operate in response to intrapsychic structures (Freud, 1940/1964). By contrast, Sullivan regarded human behavior as motivated by relationships, which seemed more variable, subtle, and flexible.

There are striking points of convergence between interpersonal and attachment theories. Both Sullivan and Bowlby challenged classical psychoanalytic theory by redefining *instincts* in relational terms. Both believed that human beings are primarily motivated to seek security through interpersonal relations, and both recognized that the fundamental human goal of maintaining contact with significant others has significant clinical implications. If human beings are *driven* to become attached, then psychotherapy is primarily about the development and elaboration of relationships and relational capacities.

Like Bowlby, Sullivan believed that throughout the lifespan, and particularly during infancy and childhood, we internalize *interpersonal schemas*. These "me–you" schemas set the stage for interpersonal expectations. We focus our attention and interpret cues on the basis of previous interpersonal experiences; we forecast how interpersonal situations are likely to transpire; and we regulate our behaviors accordingly in both adaptive and maladaptive ways (Scarvalone, Fox, & Safran, 2005). Sullivan's schemas or *personifications* are very similar to Bowlby's *internal working models*, and it is not difficult to integrate these two perspectives (Florsheim, Henry, & Benjamin, 1996). Working models of self and other derive from early attachment experiences; shape beliefs, attitudes, and expectations in intimate encounters; and influence interpersonal strategies used to achieve attachment needs. In addition, internalized representations of attachment figures can be *identified with* (i.e., copied as models for self-action), *internalized* (i.e., reacted to as expectations), and/or *introjected* (i.e., used in treatment of the self that mirrors the treatment of the self by others).

Whether children of abusive parents become aggressive or depressed depends on whether the children identify with or introject the behavior of attachment figures. Children who identify with the attachment figures learn to treat others as they have been treated. Children who internalize early experiences regard themselves as the products of how they were treated by others. When such children are confronted with interpersonal events that are inconsistent with their internalized models of self and others, they tend to shut them out in ways that were originally self-preserving but that can become profoundly maladaptive. Ana's restricted capacity for expression and her staunch independence were probably based on the internalization of a parent–child dynamic in which her feelings and needs were not reflected, or even tolerated.

Sullivan and Bowlby regarded the avoidance of interpersonal anxiety as a primary motivating factor in the developmental process, closely related to the basic human drive to seek relationships and form attachments; we are all personally shaped by our earliest efforts to reduce anxiety in our interpersonal worlds (Bowlby, 1969/1982; Sullivan, 1953). Anticipating Bowlby, Sullivan believed that anxiety is generated when relationships are threatened. As such, anxiety motivates us to maintain contact with significant others, but also to protect ourselves from interpersonal threats. This may result in seemingly contradictory behaviors. If a mother wants to be left alone, then the need to leave others alone may become part of how her child defines him- or herself and relates to others. Ironically, the interpersonal strategy of leaving significant others alone is an effort to maintain primary connections.

As defined by interpersonal and attachment theories, psychopathology is characterized by overriding feelings of distrust, jealousy, hostility, neglect, fear, and/or detachment. These traits are particularly prominent under stressful circumstances, but are also likely to become apparent in most psychotherapeutic contexts. From an integrated interpersonal–attachment perspective, psychopathology is always profoundly relational (Florsheim et al., 1996). Even in the bleakest of interpersonal situations, the primary drive to maintain connections with significant others is never fully suppressed, but often distorted or derailed. Both Bowlby and Sullivan suggested that insecure or anxiety-ridden relationships (and associated interpersonal deficits) undermine constructive developmental processes. In many cases, the effort to reduce anxiety and maintain connections does not necessarily lead to increased security. Avoidant persons (such as Ana) seek a connection with others (such as Juan and her mother), but maintain distance. This ambivalent stance allowed the avoidantly attached Ana to manage her interpersonal anxieties of rejection and abandon, but it did little to facilitate her development of healthier relationships.

Attachment and interpersonal theories also complement one another in important ways. According to attachment theory, security tends to beget security, in the sense that securely attached individuals engage with others in ways that foster confidence, intimacy, and mutual trust. Accumulating research suggests that securely attached parents are more likely to have securely attached children, who are in turn more likely to develop close, trusting relationships with friends, romantic partners, and others. (Benoit & Parker, 1994; Sroufe, 2005; van IJzendoorn, Goldberg, & Kroonenberg, 1992). It is also the case that insecurity tends to be self-perpetuating and developmentally limiting.

Following Bowlby's emphasis on intrapsychic structures, a generation of attachment researchers successfully demonstrated that working models tend to endure over time and are resistant, but not impervious, to change (Fraley, 2002). For example, Ana had a history of selecting friends and boyfriends who tended to be aggressive, aloof, and undependable, which confirmed her expectation that others would alternately control, dismiss, or abandon her. Moreover, she was reluctant to explore the possibility that other interpersonal options were available—either that there might be "other fish in the sea," or that Juan could be experienced as less controlling and more reliable. She also refused to explore her own feelings or demonstrate any interest in the feelings of others, including Juan.

Because Sullivan was fundamentally suspicious of a psychology built upon unobservable internal structures, he focused on interpersonal process and the repetition of those processes over time. Sullivan introduced the idea that our behaviors and personalities are continually shaped by interpersonal processes which become internalized, forming the substance of our intrapersonal lives. In the introductory issue of the journal *Psychiatry,* which he founded in 1938, Sullivan wrote, "Personality is made manifest in interpersonal relations and not otherwise" (p. 32). In this sense, Sullivan's interpersonal theory is more fully a theory of relationships than attachment theory. Sullivan believed that we are dynamically related to the social contexts in which we live.

Related to his interest in a process-oriented approach to diagnosis and intervention, Sullivan defined the role of the psychiatrist (he wrote to an audience of psychiatrists) as that of a participant-observer: someone who cannot be regarded as entirely separate from the subject he or she is studying (or treating). Though this is hardly a radical reformulation of the therapist's role by today's standards, Sullivan was among the first to question Freud's notion of the psychoanalyst as the detached scientist. To a large degree, Sullivan's fluid, egalitarian, and intersubjective notion of human development and therapeutic exchange is the essence of what he meant by *interpersonal.* His cautiousness about what can be known or determined to be true introduced the notions of uncertainty and subjectivity to the predominantly positivist world of psychological science and practice. This aspect of Sullivan's clinical theory relates to subsequent theoretical developments on the intersubjective nature of knowledge and the constructivist understanding of therapy (Greenberg & Mitchell, 1983; Hoffman, 1998; Stolorow, 2000).

Sullivan's explicit emphasis on the interpersonal, and his skepticism about unobserved psychological certainties, were misunderstood by some as a form of behavioralism (Greenberg & Mitchell, 1983). Rather, Sullivan's interest in observed interpersonal events allowed for a more careful and intricate understanding of how human exchanges, including therapist–client exchanges, shape experience and meaning. As the therapist forgoes presumptions about the unobserved meaning of interpersonal events, he or she is required to focus more carefully on the quality of the interpersonal exchange. From the interpersonal perspective, deriving meaning is a highly interactive process; as such, interpersonal theorists hone in on the concrete details of the therapeutic process (Teyber, 2006; Wachtel, 1993). Whereas Bowlby emphasized the development of internal psychic structures, Sullivan emphasized interpersonal developmental processes. These points of contrast are not absolute or mutually exclusive; when considered in tandem, interpersonal and attachment theories provide a comprehensive understanding of the process and structural elements of psychopathology and psychotherapy.

In their classic text on psychoanalysis, Greenberg and Mitchell (1983) underscore the contributions of Sullivan to our understanding of human development and therapeutic process, but also point out Sullivan's greatest theoretical flaw: his failure to articulate a theory of psychological health. Sullivan revolutionized psychoanalysis by highlighting the role of the interpersonal in psychological processes, but his perspective on interpersonal anxiety suggests that if we could only find a way to live in an anxiety-free world, development would proceed without impediment. Without a definition of *psychological health,* it is difficult to articulate a compelling set of therapeutic goals or expectations regarding outcome. The reduction of interpersonal anxiety as the ultimate outcome of development (and therapy) seems an inadequate aspiration. However, attachment theory's emphasis on the link between security and exploration helps define psychological health as fundamentally characterized by (1) an open, trusting interpersonal style; (2) an appreciation of the psychological needs of self and others; and (3) the capacity to express and receive care.

ATTACHMENT THEORY AND PSYCHOTHERAPY

Although attachment researchers were initially interested in documenting the stability of attachment security (Fraley, 2002), more recent researchers have turned their attention to change in working models and associated shifts in security (Bakermans-Kranenburg, van IJzendoorn, & Juffer, 2003; Davila, Burge, & Hammen, 1997; Fraley, 2002; Grossmann, Grossmann, & Waters, 2005). Attachment theory suggests that if the insecurely attached client is able to revise his or her internal working models and develop new security-based attachment strategies, substantial, sustainable therapeutic change is likely to occur (Harris, 2004; Holmes, 2001; Slade, 2004; Travis, Bliwise, Binder, & Horne-Mayer, 2001). For example, Holmes (2001) has described the therapy process as a rewriting of the client's personal narrative in ways that open him or her up to new ways of experience the self and others.

Bowlby was more of a developmentalist than a clinical theorist, but in *A Secure Base,* Bowlby (1988) described five therapeutic tasks related to facilitating attachment capacities. The first task of the therapist is to provide a secure base for exploring painful affect and experience (support, encouragement, sympathy, guidance). Bowlby wrote the following description of the therapeutic relationship:

> In providing his patient with a secure base from which to explore and express his thoughts and feelings the therapist's role is analogous to that of a mother who provides her child with a secure base from which to explore the world. The therapist strives to be reliable, attentive, and sympathetically responsive to his patient's exploration, and so far as he can, to

see and feel the world through his patient's eyes, namely to be empathic. (1988, p. 152)

By drawing an analogy between therapist and mother, Bowlby suggests that the *relationship* between therapist and client plays a critical role in the therapeutic process. As straightforward as this point may seem, it raises some difficult questions about how this relationship can facilitate the development of secure attachments and psychological well-being. Technically and practically speaking, what does a therapist do to help an adult client replace his or her insecure attachment system with something more interpersonally adaptive? Theoretically speaking, what does it mean for the therapist to take on the role of an attachment figure (Farber, Lippert, & Nevas, 1995)?

Bowlby's explanation of the four other therapeutic tasks clarifies his perspective on the ultimate goal of therapy and are remarkably similar to tasks outlined by Sullivan (1953, pp. 376–377). The second task of the therapist is to assist the client in exploring how he or she engages in current interpersonal relationships. The third task—closely related to the first and second—is to encourage the client to examine his or her relationship with the therapist in regard to how internal working models manifest themselves. The fourth task is to encourage the client to consider how his or her current perceptions and expectations, feelings, and actions relate to childhood experience and relations with primary attachment figures. Finally, the therapist should help the client to recognize his or her models of self and other, to determine the experiences from which these models derive, and to see how these models may no longer be functional in current relationships. The second through fifth tasks suggest that once a secure base has been established, the primary therapeutic goal is to understand the link between past and current relationships and the potentially dysfunctional influence of internal models of self and others. Security within the therapeutic relationship is a necessary precondition for therapeutic progress, but the second through fifth tasks underscore the role of insight in the process of reworking internal structures. A core theme of Bowlby's version of attachment-oriented intervention, therefore, involves individuation and differentiation from earlier, less adaptive attachment patterns.

Bowlby's emphasis on individual insight in psychotherapy may seem ironic, given that he championed the importance of the relational processes in development. However, Bowlby did not regard attachment and insight as opposing forces (Mitchell, 2000). Attachment theory proposes that security does not just beget more security; it also leads to and allows for exploration. A securely attached individual is more willing to explore the world and to embrace new developmental challenges. Such a person is also more able to create new relationships, expanding his or her domain of security (Grossmann et al., 1999). Sullivan (1950), who proposed that individuation cannot be conceived outside the context of a relationship, compels us to consider the notion of exploration from an interpersonal perspective; just as we explore the physical world, we also explore the relational world, including the interior of our relationships. The securely attached individual is more open to the feelings and thoughts of others, *and* more open to his or her own feelings and thoughts about others.

We can infer from Bowlby's writings that exploration facilitates the development of security via insight and individuation. Attachment theorists and researchers describe healthy attachment relations as supporting the interplay between safe-haven behaviors (i.e., seeking reassurance, support, dependability, and attunement) and exploratory behaviors. Providing the client with a safe, stable, and secure therapeutic context will support the client's interest in the thoughts and feelings of self and others. Attachment theory proposes that security leads to exploration, but the relationship between security and exploration can be more reciprocal. Exploratory behavior—including the exploration of feelings and other perspectives—supports the development of secure attachments. In child–parent dyads, romantic partnerships, and therapy relationships, gently delivered challenges can help widen the sphere of security and deepen intimate bonds. By helping the client observe current relations and recognize that old attachment behaviors are no longer adaptive in current interpersonal circumstances, the therapist encourages the development of new, more adaptive strategies (Slade, 2004; Travis et al., 2001).

In the case of Ana, the therapist used statements that conveyed the message "Here is what I think might be going on with you." In this way, the therapist indicated that he had been thinking about her and was trying, cautiously but sympathetically, to make sense of why she shut others out. By reframing her dismissive behavior in terms of her fears about commitment and intimacy, and by casting these fears in the light of past disappointments (e.g., her father's desertion), the therapist demonstrated an interest in what lay behind her ambiguous behavior. Accurate or not, the effort to make empathic interpretations is akin to using (exploratory) insight to create a holding environment (Winnicott, 1971). It also conveyed that the therapist would not be put off by her apparent nonchalance. This was reassuring to Ana, and it helped Juan to avoid personalizing Ana's aloofness.

According to Bowlby (1969/1982), when infants feel secure, they will begin to explore their environment and engage with what is unfamiliar. They explore to expand their sphere of security and to become progressively more adapted to their environment. When they are feeling less secure or in need of emotional refueling, exploration is likely to stop, and the infants will return to what is comfortable and reassuring. This constant switching back and forth between attachment and exploration persists throughout development. Bretherton (1996) describes the relationship between the attachment and exploration systems in the following way:

> The complementarity of attachment and exploration is central to Bowlby's thinking. He regarded the two tendencies, though antithetical on the surface, as co-evolved behavioral systems. Thus self reliance is not viewed as

opposed to attachment, but as co-developing with it from the beginning. … Bowlby contended that optimal functioning depends on the appropriate interplay between familiarity preserving, stress reducing behavioral systems and novelty or information seeking systems. (pp. 34–35)

Exploration is not necessarily about the past. Under many therapeutic circumstances—such as those in the case of Ana—exploration of the past would be unlikely to engender change. As we discuss later, change is most likely to occur when the client feels more fully engaged with others (including the therapist) in a way that feels creative and new. Freud saw the work of psychotherapy as akin to archaeology, with the analyst leading the client down into the bug-infested crypt of past experience. We believe it is more fitting to use the analogy of an explorer venturing *with* the client into uncharted territories.

INTERPERSONAL PSYCHOTHERAPY: CONNECTION AND EXPLORATION

The idea that therapy ought to facilitate a sense of attachment security helps to anchor and direct the work of psychotherapy. It is not difficult to justify a primary focus on relationships as a means to achieve security; there is ample evidence that relationship problems have devastating effects on psychological well-being, mediated through conflict-ridden marriages, divorce, child maltreatment and dysfunctional parenting, deviant peer relations, and so forth (Grant et al., 2006; van IJzendoorn, Schuengel, & Bakermans-Kranenburg, 1999). Bowlby's five therapeutic tasks notwithstanding, the question of *how* to change attachment system in adults is theoretically complex and raises difficult technical questions about the nature of the therapist–client relationship (Farber et al., 1995). How do we as therapists engage with different types of attachment-related problems? How do we address the limitations of time on our psychotherapeutic endeavors? How do we balance providing security with encouraging exploration? In this section, we discuss several theories of interpersonal psychotherapy, each of which provides a different perspective on how to increase a sense of attachment security. We begin with the idea of the *corrective emotional experience* in therapy, which marked a shift in thinking about the mechanisms of change relevant to contemporary interpersonal theories.

Relationship-Focused Therapy and the Corrective Emotional Experience

In 1946, Franz Alexander and Thomas French introduced the idea of the *corrective emotional experience*. This concept created controversy, because it suggested a very different sort of therapeutic activity from that espoused by psychoanalysis. Psychoanalysts focused on insight and interpretation as the primary mechanisms of therapeutic change. Alexander and French explicitly questioned the value of insight and described a more relationship-focused alternative.

There are two primary components of the corrective emotional experience. The first component is to disconfirm the client's expectations. The typical client expects people to respond in particular ways to his or her behavior, feelings, and thoughts. These expectations derive from relations with significant others and are based on years of experience. When the therapist does not respond as expected, the client is able to see (this often requires some work) that new sorts of experiences might be possible (Teyber, 2006). But the therapist's interpersonal restraint (his or her effort to avoid interpersonal traps) is not enough to enact therapeutic change. The second component of the corrective emotional experience involves providing something new that the client presumably failed to receive from his or her original caregivers. Moreover, this new interpersonal experience must address unmet developmental needs, which vary from client to client, even among those with the same diagnosis. Deemphasizing the role of insight in the process of reconciling the client with his or her past relational experiences, Alexander and French (1946) highlighted the interpersonal role of the therapist:

> Because the therapist's attitude is different from that of the authoritative person of the past, he gives the patient an opportunity to face again and again, under more favorable circumstances, those emotional situations which were formerly unbearable and to deal with them in a manner different from the old. This can be accomplished only through actual experience in the patient's relationship to the therapist; intellectual insight alone is not sufficient. A completely neutral psychoanalyst does not exist in reality, nor would he be desirable. While it is necessary that the therapist maintain an objective, helpful attitude at all times, within this attitude lies the possibility of a great variety of responses to the patient. (pp. 67–68)

This idea of the corrective emotional experience is related to a wide range of clinical theories, including attachment theory. Rogers (1957) emphasized unconditional positive regard; Winnicott (1971) introduced the idea of the holding environment; Kohut (1995) trumpeted the value of mirroring and empathy. Working from different perspectives, each of these clinical theorists has articulated how different components of the therapeutic process support the development of what attachment theorists would call a *secure base* (Bowlby, 1988). The secure-base behaviors of the therapist serve the primary functions of soothing distress and helping the client to become more open, flexible, and adaptively engaged with the environment (Mallinckrodt, Porter, & Kivlighan, 2005). Theoretically, these interpersonal experiences become internalized over the course of psychotherapy, enabling the client to develop a more secure attachment orientation toward others and to regulate emotions more adaptively (Harris, 2004).

The idea that therapy can undo past developmental lapses is compelling but controversial for two reasons (Blatt & Behrends, 1987; Gill, 1990). First, even though it may be possible for a therapist to function as an attachment figure for his or her clients, under many circumstances it is impractical. Few therapists can provide a relational experience that truly makes up for what their clients missed at an earlier phase of their development. Many clients have experienced profound deprivation and trauma, and it is unlikely that therapists can provide the sorts of nurturance, sustained attunement, and reflective encouragement that were lacking in their lives. Correcting the past is a tall order, particularly in settings where clients and therapists are expected to wrap things up in 20 sessions or less.

It has also been suggested that when the corrective emotional experience becomes the central focus of treatment, we are implicitly assuming that the presenting problem is due to past failures in the client's environment (Levenson, 2003). This assumption may be correct, but many clients play some role in maintaining the problem. The most astute and empathic therapist cannot "correct" the past without also attending to (and challenging) the client's contribution to current difficulties.

Despite these practical and theoretical concerns, it is hardly controversial to suggest that the therapist–client relationship is critical to the therapeutic process and the enactment of meaningful change (Kiesler, 1996; Lambert & Barley, 2001; Levenson, 2003; Teyber, 2006). The therapeutic impact of the *relationship* between therapist and client has been well documented in the research literature (Barber, Connolly, Crits-Christoph, Gladis, & Siqueland, 2000; Beutler, Machado, & Neufeldt, 1994; Norcross, 2002). When therapists demonstrate consistently high levels of empathy, attentiveness, and appreciation, clients are more likely to have positive treatment outcomes (Henry et al., 1986; Horvath & Luborsky, 1993; Norcross, 2002). According to Lambert and colleagues, therapist (i.e., relational) effects outweigh the effects of specific techniques and placebos (Lambert & Barley, 2001; Lambert & Okiishi, 1997). Consistent with the principles of interpersonal theory, therapist warmth facilitates positive treatment outcome because clients internalize their representations of the therapist–client relationship (Harrist, Quintana, Strupp, & Henry, 1994). When the therapeutic process is warm, the internalized representation is more likely to be positive (Henry et al., 1986). Conversely, an empirically supported model of psychotherapy is unlikely to be effective when delivered by a diligent but interpersonally unskilled therapist (Holtforth & Castonguay, 2005; Henry et al., 1986). Recent clinical theorists have suggested that *relationship* and *technique* are not so easily differentiated (Goldfried & Davila, 2005; Norcross, 2002). From the perspective of some interpersonal theorists, the relationship *is* the primary technique of psychotherapy.

In the most recent edition of his classic text on interpersonal process in psychotherapy, Teyber (2006) illustrates how providing understanding and promoting intimacy invite clients to explore their internal experiences, including their experience of the therapy relationship. Like Alexander and French (1946), Teyber focuses primarily on avoiding old, dysfunctional interpersonal traps and meeting the client's developmental needs through interpersonal engagement. Teyber emphasizes that positive and negative moments in therapy are mediated by the therapist's word choice, phrasing, and tone. He concretely describes how some therapist responses are likely to be more effective than others, with respect to helping the client (1) feel understood and appreciated, (2) develop an internal focus for changing interpersonal problems, and (3) address personal obstacles to developmental progress. Teyber also underscores the importance of response specificity: Clients experience others in different ways, which challenges the therapist to find an approach that is respectful of the client's interpersonal defenses (and underlying fears), but that actively invites, entices, and lures the client into a healthier, more adaptive *interpersonal space*. In the next section, we discuss how some interpersonal theorists define this idea of interpersonal space, locate the various types of attachment within that space, and conceptualize the process of moving clients toward a greater sense of attachment security.

Interpersonal Diagnosis and Treatment Planning

Attachment researchers have developed well-validated, developmentally based systems for identifying attachment styles in adolescents and adults (see Levy & Kelly, Chapter 6, and Fraley & Phillips, Chapter 7, this volume). However, from a clinical perspective, identifying attachment style is only a first step. The next step is to delineate an interpersonally oriented treatment plan for facilitating change in attachment (Florsheim et al., 1996).

How can we nurture clients' sense of attachment security, induce them to experiment with security-based strategies, and enhance their ability to provide an atmosphere of security for partners and offspring? It may seem obvious that Ana would benefit from becoming more open and engaged, but knowing how to approach her and draw her into a more secure interpersonal space is not so obvious. Knowing how to dislodge insecurity depends on a number of interrelated factors including (1) the therapist's understanding of the client's working models of self and other; (2) the client's receptivity to the interpersonal behaviors of significant others, including the therapist; and (3) a clear idea of the client's interpersonal goals. A strength of the interpersonal approach is its ability to systematically identify each of these.

Sullivan was neither an empirical scientist nor a psychometrician, but his followers developed his ideas into well-defined systems for measuring interpersonal processes. Leary (1957) used Sullivan's theory of interpersonal psychiatry to develop the *interpersonal circumplex*, which has had an enduring impact on the study of personality, psychopathology, and therapeutic process (Benjamin, 1996; Horowitz, Rosenberg, & Bartholomew, 1993; Kiesler, 1996; Leary & Coffey, 1955). The interpersonal circumplex is a tool for systematically describing interpersonal behavior and linking behavior to underlying personality characteristics and intrapsychic processes. Circumplex models are based on two orthogonal dimensions: warmth–hostility and enmeshment–autonomy. The different versions of the interpersonal circumplex offer different perspectives on the organization of interpersonal processes.

For example, the Structural Analysis of Social Behavior (SASB; Benjamin, 1974) is a circumplex model that describes interpersonal behavior and associated intrapsychic processes as more or less affiliative (warm or hostile), more or less autonomous (assertive or submissive), and more or less controlling (managing or letting go). As illustrated in Figure 15.1, the SASB operationalizes interpersonal and intrapsychic process across three circumplex surfaces. The first surface (descriptors are written in bold) describes interpersonal behavior that focuses on the other; the second surface (descriptors are underlined) describes interpersonal behavior that focuses on the self; and the third surface (in italics) describes intrapsychic behaviors.

The SASB model proposes that individual differences in psychopathology are based on the specific quality of internalized interpersonal processes. Like attachment theory, the SASB defines normality in terms of a balance between warm enmeshment and friendly differentiation. Psychological well-being and healthy interpersonal process are represented by a balance of behaviors in Clusters Two, Three, and Four (Figure 15.1; Benjamin, 1996). Conversely, relationships marked by Clusters Six, Seven, and Eight are manifestations of insecurity; these clusters undermine the interpersonal conditions through which secure attachments and normative differentiation are achieved.

Florsheim et al. (1996) described how the SASB model can help delineate interpersonal and introjected processes associated with different attachment styles. In the broadest terms, insecure attachments are described as overly hostile, excessively enmeshed, or excessively differentiated (or alternating between these extremes). For example, individuals categorized as preoccupied are likely to engage in highly enmeshed relationships; individuals classified as dismissing-avoidant or fearful-avoidant would consistently behave in a highly differentiated manner. In SASB language, Ana's behavior toward Juan and her therapist could be easily described in terms of the upper left-hand quadrant of Figure 15.1 (e.g., ignoring). Presumably, this behavior was a learned response to her introjected mother, who undermined Ana's sense of security by ignoring and dismissing her fundamental needs.

Some circumplex models, including the SASB, are also prescriptive. Once the interpersonal problem has been described, the model can be used to (1) identify targets for change and (2) clarify the sort of therapeutic maneuvers likely to engender such change. Most often the SASB prescribes

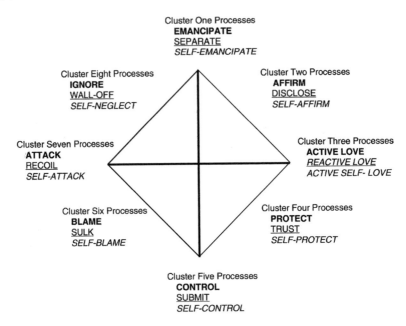

FIGURE 15.1. The simplified SASB cluster model. **Focus on other in bold.** <u>Focus on self underlined.</u> *Focus on intrapsychic italicized.* Adapted from Benjamin (1996). Copyright 1996 by The Guilford Press. Adapted by permission.

interventions that are antithetical to the identified problem (i.e., behaviors on the opposite side of the circumplex). When the problems are extreme or rigid, however, a gradual approach toward the prescribed solution is necessary (Benjamin, 2003). For example, an automatic or typical response to Ana's dismissing attachment style would be to disengage. This was what happened at the residential treatment center, where Ana's aloofness was seen as untenable resistance. A different, more generous approach would be to provide Ana with the nurturance and structure she missed as a child (i.e., the antithesis to ignoring). However, such an approach would probably be perceived by Ana as too controlling; an immediate emphasis on nurturance could backfire because of her need for autonomy. Alternatively, the therapist could steer a more acceptable course that would involve avoiding the natural tendency to control or dismiss Ana and encouraging her to move toward greater connection by gently challenging her to be more disclosing. Modeling warm, autonomous behavior, the therapist would look for opportunities to express his positive impressions of Ana's interpersonal style and his curiosity about what might be going on inside her head. Such an approach in the context of couple counseling would also help Juan learn to be more affirming and open with Ana.

To illustrate further, a highly anxious-preoccupied client is prone to interpret autonomy-giving or autonomy-taking behavior (expressed by a partner or therapist) as potentially abandoning, uncaring, and dismissive. Thus, in the interest of gently moving this client toward an increased capacity for engaging with others in a more autonomous fashion, the therapist might temper any movement toward openness (warm autonomy) with a dose of reassurance (warm control). Conversely, when working with a client who is dismissing-avoidant, the therapist might temper nurturance with a dose of autonomy-granting behavior.

These complex communications can often be delivered sequentially and straightforwardly. For example, a client who is avoiding a connection with a therapist by missing appointments will benefit from an approach that increases his or her capacity for sustained engagement and intimacy. The therapist might say, "I realize that my wanting to keep regular appointments might feel controlling and too involved, but I want to emphasize that the ball is in your court; you are the expert on what is best for you and are in the best position to decide the right level of involvement." In this case, the value of a therapeutic relationship is underscored, but the threat of becoming entangled and the need for autonomy are acknowledged and appreciated.

Developing Security-Based Attachment Strategies

Most readers are likely to associate the term *interpersonal psychotherapy* with the model developed by Klerman and Weissman and commonly referred to as IPT (Klerman & Weissman, 1993; Weissman, Markowitz, & Klerman, 2000). Drawing inspiration from Sullivan and Bowlby, IPT is a short-term, empirically supported approach for treating depression among adults. Since its inception, IPT has been expanded to include the treatment of depression in adolescents and a range of other disorders (Bleiberg & Markowitz, 2005; Cyranowski et al., 2002; Rosselló & Bernal, 1999). In keeping with Sullivan's proposition that there is a dynamic interplay among relationships, symptoms, and underlying psychopathology, the IPT therapist addresses symptom reduction and work to improve the client's interpersonal relations with significant others.

In IPT, attachment insecurity is addressed by focusing on present influential relationships; IPT therapists are instructed to avoid engaging in transference-based treatment approaches, processing past relations, or focusing on intrapsychic processes. Instead, the role of the therapist is to support and advise the client throughout the process of trying new interpersonal strategies intended to foster a sense of security. This is accomplished by using a combination of supportive and interpersonally oriented cognitive-behavioral techniques, including restructuring cognitions about self and others and engaging in interpersonal experiments with significant others. For example, Weissman et al. (2000) describe the case of a man with severe interpersonal deficits consistent with an avoidant attachment style, who benefited from some relatively simple, straightforward instructions about how to negotiate interpersonally challenging situations with his boss, girlfriend, and peers.

The IPT model focuses on helping a client develop supports outside the therapeutic relationship, assuming that people (coworkers, family, friends, and romantic partners) will respond to positive changes in the client's interpersonal behavior. Indeed, there is evidence that altering the quality of the client's interpersonal behavior predicts symptom reduction and positive outcomes (de Mello, de Jesus Mari, Bacaltchuk, Verdeli, & Neugebauer, 2005). Moreover, research from a variety of theoretical camps suggests that helping the client to alter the quality of his or her support system will improve both the client's individual and interpersonal functioning (Davidson, Shahar, Stayner, Chinman, & Tebes, 2004; Lutgendorf et al., 1998).

IPT is designed to focus on the individual client, but obviously relates to couple and family therapy. If the goal of therapy is to help the client develop improved (secure) interpersonal relations, then it makes sense to work with viable attachment figures in the client's interpersonal world. In the case of Ana and Juan, the goal of therapy was to help them build a sense of security with each other. The interpersonal solution proposed by Weissman and Klerman makes sense, given recent research on how attachments formed in adolescence and adulthood can help reconfigure working models of self and others (Moretti & Holland, 2003). There is some evidence that clients who have participated in IPT report higher levels of relationship satisfaction and decreased symptoms across a broad range of conditions (Markowitz, 2003).

Individuation from Insecure Attachments

Another interpersonal approach to addressing attachment problems involves helping the client individuate from insecure attachments. Theoretically, this process supports the development of more secure working models of self and others, freeing the client to find new, healthier attachments. Therapeutic action focuses on modifying the link between intrapsychic processes and interpersonal patterns of behavior (Horowitz et al., 1993). Unlike traditional psychoanalytic therapy, this type of insight-oriented therapy is "attachment-oriented" in its emphasis on the need to address old loyalties and is "interpersonal" in its focus on altering relationship dynamics. Therapist and client work together to identify how internal working models of self and other (derived from past attachments) shape current interpersonal behaviors in both positive and negative ways. Once these intrapersonal processes are identified, the goal of therapy is to differentiate the self from dysfunctional internalized representations.

For example, interpersonal reconstructive therapy (IRT; Benjamin, 2003) is based on the premise that interpersonal change will occur when the client is able to loosen automatic links between old but potent attachment relations and current interpersonal processes. IRT emphasizes the role of dysfunctional loyalties to attachment figures in the development and maintenance of psychopathology. Benjamin (2003) describes the collaboration between therapist and client as a *circumscribed attachment* that provides a secure base for identifying and exploring new, more adaptive patterns.

Insight is a central component of the IRT model. Learning about the origin and function of relationship patterns is the essence of insight in IRT. Referring explicitly to Bowlby, Benjamin (2003) writes that dysfunctional attachment relationships perpetuate problem patterns and are therefore a main focus of treatment. Using the term *gift of love*, Benjamin describes how we repeat early patterns of behavior, no matter how dysfunctional, as a way to remain emotionally connected to attachment figures. From this perspective, Ana's rejection of Juan and her reckless, nihilistic history could be construed as a gift of love to her mother and her father.

Benjamin (2003) addresses how to move from understanding the interpersonal problem to finding an interpersonal solution, and she proposes that change occurs through three primary channels. First, the therapist uses the SASB model to differentiate between maladaptive and adaptive interpersonal and intrapsychic processes. Once this distinction is made explicit in treatment, the therapist actively blocks maladaptive behavior by reminding the client when old dysfunctional loyalties are interfering with the development of more adaptive interpersonal solutions. In this sense, the therapist is supporting both intrapsychic and interpersonal exploration through reflection and confrontation (see Bateman & Fonagy, 2004).

Second, as a counterbalance to maladaptive interpersonal patterns, the therapist uses positive feedback to actively support the development of adaptive solutions to old interpersonal problems. Practically, the therapist may encourage the client to spend time with nurturing and caring friends. If there is a lack of nurturing relationships in the client's life, then cultivating healthy relationships becomes a priority. If all goes well, the client will begin to experience him- or herself (and others) as occupying a different, more adaptive, and more satisfying interpersonal space.

The success of IRT depends on the client's *will* to change. If the client is no longer the passive victim of unconscious, unfulfilled longings and dysfunctional loyalties, then she can become master of her own fate. In Ana's case, her unacknowledged loyalty to her mother reinforced her disdain for Juan. Acknowledging that she felt torn between these two opposing forces helped her feel that she could choose for herself or refuse to be forced into making such a choice. The client's will to change is reinforced by the therapist's encouragement to give up unrealistic hopes regarding past attachment figures.

IRT contributes to the integration of attachment and interpersonal theories in several respects. First, Benjamin (2003) embraces the idea that attachment dysfunction underlies a great deal of personality-based psychopathology. Second, IRT demonstrates how the interpersonal circumplex can help the therapist formulate and enact interpersonal antidotes that specifically address client's more problematic tendencies. Third, the IRT therapist is expected to play an active role in blocking maladaptive behaviors and encouraging adaptive solutions. Despite a strong learning focus, Benjamin suggests that the IRT therapist—insofar as he or she is meant to engender will—does more than provide support and insight. The therapist challenges the client to reflect upon and revise interpersonal patterns. If the IRT process is successful, the client will begin to engage in healthy forms of exploratory behavior (developing new relationships, new interests, etc.). In this sense, the change process begins with an exploration of intrapsychic processes, but moves to a more outwardly focused exploratory endeavor.

Interpersonal Exploration and Fostering Attachment Security

There are several schools of interpersonal psychoanalysis that build upon Sullivan's theoretical innovations and are relevant to the therapeutic implications of attachment theory (Hoffman, 1998; Levenson, 1991; Mitchell, 1988; Safran, 2002). Interpersonal (or relational) psychoanalysts emphasize the role of transference and countertransference as the crux of therapeutic action. In this section, we discuss how the interpersonal psychoanalytic model helps clarify how the therapist–client relationship can be used to revise old patterns of attachment.

From the interpersonal psychoanalytic perspective, therapist and client will inevitably engage in ways that are consistent with each person's attachment history. For the client, interactions will involve dysfunctional interpersonal patterns directly related to his or her reasons for seeking therapy. For the therapist, the patterns may not be dysfunctional, but they will be consistent with his or her interpersonal history and in keeping with his or her interpersonal repertoire. Ideally, the therapist's interpersonal repertoire will be greater than the client's capacity to determine the direction of the relationship. The job of the therapist is to work with the client to find a way out of the old dysfunctional patterns and create a new (i.e., more secure) sort of relationship with new possibilities. This process is highly transactional. What happens between therapist and client is not simply a replication of the client's past or something the client imagines. The client pulls for certain behaviors in the therapist, and the therapist responds in ways that highlight certain aspects of his or her character. The therapist plays an active, personal role in the relationship.

Whereas traditional psychoanalysts (and cognitively oriented therapists) regard insight as the primary mechanism of change, interpersonal psychoanalysts use insight to "grease the wheels" of a more relationship-focused approach to change (Mitchell, 1988). The emphasis on relational processes over self-discovery is particularly important in working with clients with attachment problems, because the process of developing increased attachment security requires experience-based learning within the context of a close relationship (i.e., with the therapist). Drawing upon Sullivan's more participatory, process-oriented approach to therapy, interpersonal psychoanalysts focus on helping clients experience themselves more fully in current relations, particularly the therapeutic relationship (Mitchell, 1988).

Several interpersonally oriented psychoanalysts (Gill, 1990; Hoffman, 1998; Mitchell, 1988) suggest that the therapist must become personally engaged in the client's interpersonal reality by allowing him- or herself to fall into the client's relational traps. However, unlike the more traditional psychoanalysts, these theorists acknowledge that therapists are prone to fall into clients' traps in idiosyncratic ways. When the therapist's role in the making of these traps is acknowledged, the process of engagement becomes more ambiguous and dynamic. Neither therapist nor client is the arbiter of what's *really* happening between them (Hoffman, 1987). Acknowledging the ambiguity and uncertainty inherent in the therapeutic process is important, because it sends a message of openness to new experiences—a willingness to explore.

The structure of the therapeutic relationship, and the separate role the therapist occupies in the life of the client, allow the therapist to say things that would otherwise seem intrusive and perhaps frightening. It also allows the client to divulge information and feelings that are often omitted from his or her other relationships. The unusual nature of the therapist–client relationship (what some clients might perceive as its artificial quality) increases its potential for change, because it creates a context of safety in which intrapersonal and interpersonal exploration is possible. Therapist and client are continually (and implicitly) engaged in addressing questions about the nature of reality, the relationship between past and present, and the quality and relevance of their relationship. Clients often will pose questions (to themselves or out loud) about whether their therapists really care, or whether the relationship is real or relevant to the world out there. Therapists will often gauge whether the clients are being honest, whether they are ready to change, and so on. From the interpersonal psychoanalytic perspective, these questions are part and parcel of the exploratory and transformational process, and there are no clearly correct answers.

This willingness of the therapist to fall into the relationship reflects the "participant" part of Sullivan's participant-observer therapist. It is essential for this to happen, because it helps the therapist to understand the client experientially, and helps the client to experience the genuine presence of the therapist. Mitchell (1988) suggests that the collaborative effort of therapist and client to discover new channels to engage one another is the crucible of therapeutic change. By focusing on those aspects of the relationship that seem overly constrained or underdeveloped, the therapist gains insight into how he or she might move the process forward more quickly. If the therapist feels critical, bored, timid, or unsympathetic in ways that seem somewhat atypical or overdrawn, these experiences offer important clues about what is missing from the relationship.

The "observer" part of Sullivan's participant-observer therapist avoids becoming destructively entwined with the client by attending to how each exchange offers the opportunity for interpersonal growth. This emphasis on reciprocity and spontaneity does not diminish the importance of structure in the therapeutic process. Hoffman (1998) has suggested that the somewhat rigid structure of the therapeutic frame helps to set the stage for something new and exciting to happen. There is a dialectical tension between the highly regulated domain of the psychotherapy session and the spontaneity of intimate interpersonal engagement (Hoffman, 1998). Ironically, it is within this highly ritualized setting that the client feels freer to experience something interpersonally new and to discover underdeveloped aspects of the self.

Over the course of several sessions, Juan began to open up about how difficult it was to find work. He did not have a high school diploma; he lacked the interpersonal skills to schmooze; he had a prison record; he looked like the gang member he had been … what were his chances of finding work? He had applied for several jobs in the neighborhood, but received no call-backs. Juan's parole officer was threatening to send him back to prison for parole violation, and Ana was rolling her eyes. The therapist felt a mix of compassion and frustration in response to Juan's helplessness. Was Juan up against an unforgiving social structure, was he developmentally incapable of venturing out into the world on his own, or was he being defiant? Believing that all these factors might be involved, the therapist took a step outside the therapeutic frame in an effort to become more fully engaged with this interpersonal obstacle. He told Juan that next week, during their regular meeting time, he (the therapist) would walk the neighborhood with him (Juan) and help him put in job applications. There were dozens of businesses within a stone's throw of the therapist's office. A look of shock, appreciation, and fear seemed to flitter across Juan's face. By the following week he had found a job on his own. Later, as they processed this exchange, Juan confirmed that the idea of looking for a job with his therapist in tow had shaken him up, but it had also meant a great deal that the therapist was willing to do that for him. Ana seemed intrigued and relieved that some movement had occurred.

Some readers might (correctly) point out that this intervention was a countertransference enactment; the therapist seems to have reacted to his own upper-middle-class guilt, to Juan's helpless passivity, or to some combination of both. It turned out all right in this instance, but it could have gone sour. Juan could have felt intruded upon, or the therapist might have tried to help Juan find a job and failed miserably. But such enactments often occur without becoming countertherapeutic if the therapist remains watchfully open to the impact of this form of participation. This is not to say that "anything goes"; going with Juan to scout for jobs might have been paternalistic, intrusive, or pathetic, but even the worst outcome could have been dealt with in a potentially useful, interesting way. On the other hand, the therapist's hiring Juan as an employee would have been an ethical violation. If we stay within the boundaries of our ethics code, countertransference enactments can bring underlying dynamics to the surface and offer opportunities for change.

A client is not simply struggling with (or against) past attachments projected onto the current therapist. From Mitchell's and Hoffman's perspectives, therapy is far more personal. The client is using old, automatic, and idiosyncratic strategies to connect with a *particular* therapist. From this interpersonal psychoanalytic perspective, the therapeutic process involves two people, each of whom takes up his or her fair share of interpersonal space and requires some sort of accommodation from the other; the interpersonal process is truly *interpersonal*. Rather than engage in a process that is either formulaically neutral/objective or nurturing/empathic, the therapist strives to offer the client something less scripted, more unique to the particular dynamics of *their* relationship, and ultimately more "real" or genuine. The genuineness of the process provides the active ingredient of change. The therapist focuses on how development might occur, rather than where development didn't occur.

How does this happen? With highly educated, professional adults, the process of therapeutic exchange often involves detailed examination of the therapist–client relationship, but this intense focus on transference–countertransference exchange is not a necessity. For many adolescents and adults who are less educated and articulate, the process of interpersonal exchange and discovery is often implicit, as it was in the case of Ana. The therapist working with Ana gently teased her about her unwillingness to speak in session by pretending to read the slightest change in her facial expression as important clues about her thoughts and feelings. In response, Ana became visibly looser and seemed to enjoy the idea that her therapist (and Juan) were attempting to understand what might be going on beneath her mask. In addition to getting her to laugh at herself, the therapist hoped *she* would consider what she was feeling and wanted to communicate. To prevent her from feeling he was making fun of her, the therapist prefaced the teasing by acknowledging that it was difficult for her to express feelings directly or even recognize how she felt.

When we see clients becoming more reflective and *making use* of their insights in relationships, it usually indicates that therapeutic progress has occurred. Without denying the value of reflection in the development of secure attachments, we believe that it is important to distinguish between reflection as process and product (see Jurist & Meehan, Chapter 4, this volume, for a discussion of reflective functioning). When therapists engage their clients in ways that warmly challenge, cajole, or tease them into considering other perspectives, they are doing more than increasing their capacity for insight or reflection. As Mitchell (1988) and Hoffman (1998) indicate, the therapist is inviting the client to share in a new type of relationship, unbounded by old rules. The therapist is carving out interpersonal space for him- or herself and inviting the client to share that space. We believe that the creation of this space—often achieved through reflection—is what allows interpersonal changes to occur.

CONCLUSIONS

Clinical theorists from most psychotherapy camps tend to emphasize safety and security as prerequisites for effective intervention. But security in the context of most therapeutic relationships is fundamentally different from the sort of security provided by a primary attachment relationship. The therapist cannot offer some of the essential ingredients of primary security, such as proximity and availability, or the sort of comfort and soothing that mothers (and fathers) should provide. Nonetheless, the therapeutic relationship is set up to provide something akin to a secure base. Like the "good-enough" mother, the therapist is focused on and attuned to the client (Winnicott, 1971); the therapist's presence is predictable, and he or she behaves in ways designed to help the client to establish a greater sense of coherence and internal integrity.

The client is expected to act *as if* he or she is in the presence of an attachment figure: to open his or her mind and heart to the therapist and absorb what that therapist has to offer. Indeed, the effectiveness of the therapeutic encounter partly depends on the client's capacity to suspend belief with respect to the actual security provided by the therapist. Remarkably, this often happens with little prodding—partly due to the ritualized, structured nature of the encounter, and partly due to the attitude of the therapist. The therapist is equally engaging in this "as if" attachment experience, insofar as he or she holds the client in mind, attends to the client's developmental needs, and provides stability and containment. Although the goal of providing an actual secure base is often unrealistic and potentially misguided, anchoring therapy in these tangible attachment-like experiences provides the client with a new version of the self in relation to others. The "as if" quality of therapy helps the therapist and client cope with the limitations and boundaries of their relationship while engaging in a highly intimate, personal level of exchange. It allows attachment processes to occur without requiring that the therapist step fully into the role of an attachment figure. When clients protest that therapy is not a real relationship, they are correct, but are missing the point. It may be useful to acknowledge, "Yes, there are limits to what the therapist can provide," but then to add that because the relationship is set apart from "reality," the client is permitted more interpersonal freedom to take risks and grow.

Writing from an object relations perspective, Winnicott (1971) regarded the capacity for play as important to living a full life. In a classic paper, he remarked that if a client (child or adult) is not able to be playful, then play should become a major focus of the therapeutic process:

> Psychotherapy takes place in the overlap of two areas of playing, that of the patient and that of the therapist. Psychotherapy has to do with two people playing together. The corollary of this is when playing is not possible, then the work done by the therapist is directed towards bringing the patient from a state of not being able to play into a state of being able to play. (p. 38)

Winnicott defined play as an activity that occurs along the boundary between the individual's private self and the world outside that self. In therapy, play involves a form of engagement with the therapist that allows the client to step outside the rigid internal structure he or she has spent a lifetime constructing. The precarious nature of play—one never knows where it is going—is fundamentally healthy and growth-promoting.

On two occasions, Ana met with the therapist alone. During these meetings, she confessed to not wanting a baby and feeling worried that she lacked maternal instincts. She was thinking about giving the child up for adoption, but she felt pressured by others (particularly Juan and her mother) to keep the baby. She also had serious doubts about whether she and Juan could make it work as a couple, because she did not trust him and was afraid to depend on him for anything. The therapist let her know that if she chose to give the baby up (it was too late for an abortion) or break off her relationship with Juan, he would support her and help her figure out how to live with the decision. He also said that he knew her well enough to say with some conviction that getting close to others, including any baby or any boyfriend, would be a struggle for her. Then he pointed out that despite this basic sense of distrust, she was opening up to him in ways that probably surprised her as much as they surprised him, and that this seemed like a pretty good start.

After this session, Ana began to be more open with Juan about her feelings and more demanding, which the therapist regarded as a greater investment in the relationship. Eventually Ana moved in with Juan and his family, and Juan managed to stay on the right side of the law. After the program ended, Ana stayed in phone contact with the therapist. She let him know that things were okay but not perfect; that the baby was sick but getting better; and that now that Juan was working so much, she missed him.

Much of what we have discussed in this chapter draws from the vast literature on clinical theory. We have made reference to a diverse body of relevant research, ranging from maternal influences on infant development to the role of the working alliance in treatment outcome, but we acknowledge that there is limited research on attachment processes within the context of psychotherapy (Harris, 2004). We believe that interpersonal process research, focusing on therapist–client interactions, could greatly contribute to our understanding of how secure-base behavior might relate to positive, adaptive changes in the client's internal working models of self and other and the quality of his or her own attachment-related behaviors (security seeking, exploration).

For example, it would be possible to use the SASB (Benjamin, 1974) to measure therapist behaviors that challenge the client's current construal of self and others, and that are conveyed empathically in the service of supporting exploration. As indicated earlier, we could reasonably predict that some strategies would be more effective than others, depending on a client's particular attachment style (i.e., dismissing clients might respond better to autonomy-supporting interventions than to nurturing interventions). If we could demonstrate that particular therapeutic strategies led to short-term positive changes in the client's experience of felt security, it seems reasonable to suggest that such changes would represent "as if" attachment processes. Such processes could be assessed in a variety of ways, including daily diaries in which clients report thoughts about the therapist, self-report measures of emotion regulation, or experimental techniques designed to detect subtle changes in felt security (e.g., Shaver & Mikulincer, 2005)

In this chapter, we have presented several interpersonal models of psychotherapy, underscoring the diversity of therapeutic approaches generated by Sullivan's original theory. Each approach stands on its own and contributes something unique to the goal of facilitating attachment security. As such, we have highlighted the differences between them and the strengths of each. Using the case of Ana and Juan as a point of reference, we have illustrated how these various approaches can be used in combination with each other to enact the specific components of the therapeutic process, and to meet the formidable challenge of helping our clients develop an increased sense of attachment security and use it to build more satisfying relationships.

NOTE

1. The authors' clinical work was supported by National Institute of Mental Health grant 5R21MH67652.

RECOMMENDATIONS FOR FURTHER READING

Greenberg, J., & Mitchell, S. (1983). *Object relations in psychoanalytic theory*. Cambridge, MA: Harvard University Press.—A sophisticated integration of object relations with psychoanalytic theory. Excellent sections on Harry Stack Sullivan provide a solid description of his theory and impact on the field.

Hoffman, I. (1998). *Ritual and spontaneity in the psychoanalytic process: A dialectical constructivist view*. Hillsdale, NJ: Analytic Press.—A theoretically complex approach to understanding dialectical processes; it includes excellent case examples.

Teyber, E. (2006). *Interpersonal process in therapy: An integrative model (5th ed.).* Belmont, CA: Thomson Brooks/Cole.—A modern classic that provides a practical introduction to interpersonal theory and technique. It offers plenty of concrete examples that bring the theoretical material alive. A "must-read" for graduate students.

REFERENCES

Ainsworth, M. D. S. (1991). Attachments and other affectional bonds across the life cycle. In C. M. Parkes, J. Stevenson-Hinde, & P. Marris (Eds.), *Attachment across the life cycle* (pp. 33–51). New York: Routledge.

Alexander, F., & French, T. M. (1946). *Psychoanalytic therapy: Principles and application.* New York: Ronald Press.

Bakermans-Kranenburg, M. J., van IJzendoorn, M. H., & Juffer, F. (2003). Less is more: Meta-analyses of sensitivity and attachment interventions in early childhood. *Psychological Bulletin, 129,* 195–215.

Barber, J. P., Connolly, M. B., Crits-Christoph, P., Gladis, L., & Siqueland, L. (2000). Alliance predicts patients' outcomes beyond in-treatment change in symptoms. *Journal of Consulting and Clinical Psychology, 68,* 1027–1032.

Bateman, A. W., & Fonagy, P. (2004). Mentalization-based treatment of BPD. *Journal of Personality Disorders, 18,* 36–51.

Benjamin, L. S. (1974). The Structural Analysis of Social Behavior. *Psychological Review, 81,* 392–425.

Benjamin, L. S. (1996). *Interpersonal diagnosis and treatment of personality disorders* (2nd ed.). New York: Guilford Press.

Benjamin, L. S. (2003). *Interpersonal reconstructive therapy: Promoting change in nonresponders.* New York: Guilford Press.

Benoit, D., & Parker, K. C. H. (1994). Stability and transmission of attachment across three generations. *Child Development, 65,* 1444–1456.

Beutler, L. E., Machado, P. P. P., & Neufeldt, S. A. (1994). Therapist variables. In A. E. Bergin & S. L. Garfield (Eds.), *Handbook of psychotherapy and behavior change* (4th ed., pp. 229–269). New York: Wiley

Blatt, S. J., & Behrends, R. S. (1987). Internalization, separation–individuation, and the nature of therapeutic action. *International Journal of Psycho-Analysis, 68,* 279–297.

Bleiberg, K. L., & Markowitz, J. C. (2005). A pilot study of interpersonal psychotherapy for posttraumatic stress disorder. *American Journal of Psychiatry, 162,* 181–183.

Bowlby, J. (1982) *Attachment and loss: Vol. 1. Attachment* (2nd ed.). New York: Basic Books. (1st ed., 1969)

Bowlby, J. (1988). *A secure base: Clinical applications of attachment theory.* London: Routledge.

Brennan, K. A., Clark, C. L., & Shaver, P. R. (1998). Self-report measurement of adult attachment: An integrative overview. In J. A. Simpson & W. S. Rholes

(Eds.), *Attachment theory and close relationships* (pp. 46–76). New York: Guilford Press.

Bretherton, I. (1996). Bowlby's legacy to developmental psychology. *Child Psychiatry and Human Development, 28,* 33–43.

Cooley, C. H. (1902). *Human nature and the social order.* New York: Scribner's.

Cyranowski, J. M., Bookwala, J., Feske, U., Houck, P., Pilkonis, P., Kostelnik, B., et al. (2002). Adult attachment profiles, interpersonal difficulties, and response to interpersonal psychotherapy in women with recurrent major depression. *Journal of Social and Clinical Psychology, 21,* 191–217.

Davidson, L., Shahar, G., Stayner, D. A., Chinman, M. J., & Tebes, J. K. (2004). Supported socialization for people with psychiatric disabilities: Lessons from a randomized controlled trial. *Journal of Community Psychology, 32,* 453–477.

Davila, J., Burge, D., & Hammen, C. (1997). Why does attachment style change? *Journal of Personality and Social Psychology, 73,* 826–838.

de Mello, M. F., de Jesus Mari, J., Bacaltchuk, J., Verdeli, H., & Neugebauer, R. (2005). A systematic review of research findings on the efficacy of interpersonal therapy for depressive disorders. *European Archives of Psychiatry and Clinical Neuroscience, 255,* 75–82.

Farber, B. A., Lippert, R. A., & Nevas, D. B. (1995). The therapist as attachment figure. *Psychotherapy: Theory, Research, Practice, Training, 32,* 204–212.

Florsheim, P., Henry, W., & Benjamin, L. S. (1996). Integrating individual and interpersonal approaches to diagnosis: The structural analysis of social behavior and attachment theory. In F. W. Kaslow (Ed.), *Handbook of relational diagnosis and dysfunctional family patterns* (pp. 81–101). New York: Wiley.

Fraley, R. C. (2002). Attachment stability from infancy to adulthood: Meta-analysis and dynamic modeling of developmental mechanisms. *Personality and Social Psychology Review, 6,* 123–151.

Freud, S. (1964). An outline of psycho-analysis. In J. Strachey (Ed. & Trans), *The standard edition of the complete psychological works of Sigmund Freud* (Vol. 23, pp. 139–207). London: Hogarth Press. (Original work published 1940)

Gill, M. M. (1990). The analysis of transference. In A. H. Esman (Ed.), *Essential papers on transference* (pp. 362–381). New York: New York University Press.

Goldfried, M. R., & Davila, J. (2005). The role of relationship and technique in therapeutic change. *Psychotherapy: Theory, Research, Practice, Training, 42,* 421–430.

Grant, K. E., Compas, B. E., Thurm, A. E., McMahon, S. D., Gipson, P. Y., Campbell, A. J., et al. (2006). Stressors and child and adolescent psychopathology: Evidence of moderating and mediating effects. *Clinical Psychology Review, 26,* 257–283.

Greenberg, J., & Mitchell, S. (1983). *Object relations in psychoanalytic theory.* Cambridge, MA: Harvard University Press.

Grossmann, K. E., Grossmann, K., & Waters, E. (Eds.). (2005). *Attachment from infancy to adulthood: The major longitudinal studies.* New York: Guilford Press.

Grossmann, K. E., Grossmann, K., & Zimmermann, P. (1999). A wider view of attachment and exploration: Stability and change during the years of immaturity. In J. Cassidy & P. R. Shaver (Eds.), *Handbook of attachment: Theory, research, and clinical applications* (pp. 760–786). New York: Guilford Press.

Harris, T. (2004). Discussion of the special issue: Chef or chemist? Practicing psychotherapy within the attachment paradigm. *Attachment & Human Development, 6,* 191–207.

Harrist, R. S., Quintana, S. M., Strupp, H. H., & Henry, W. P. (1994). Internalization of interpersonal process in time-limited dynamic psychotherapy. *Psychotherapy: Theory, Research, Practice, Training, 31,* 49–57.

Henry, W. P., Schacht, T. E., & Strupp, H. H. (1986). Structural Analysis of Social Behavior: Application to a study of interpersonal process in differential psychotherapeutic outcome. *Journal of Consulting and Clinical Psychology, 54,* 27–31.

Henry, W. P., & Strupp, H. H. (1994). The therapeutic alliance as interpersonal process. In A. O. Horvath & L. S. Greenberg (Eds.), *The working alliance: Theory, research, and practice* (pp. 51–84). New York: Wiley.

Hesse, E. (1999). The Adult Attachment Interview: Historical and current perspectives. In J. Cassidy & P. R. Shaver (Eds.), *Handbook of attachment: Theory, research, and clinical applications* (pp. 395–433). New York: Guilford Press.

Hoffman, I. (1987). The value of uncertainty in psychoanalytic practice: An ambivalent challenge. *Contemporary Psychoanalysis, 23,* 205–214.

Hoffman, I. (1998). *Ritual and spontaneity in the psychoanalytic process: A dialectical-constructivist view.* Hillsdale, NJ: Analytic Press.

Holmes, J. (2001). *The search for the secure base: Attachment theory and psychotherapy.* Hove, UK: Brunner-Routledge.

Holtforth, M. G., & Castonguay, L. G. (2005). Relationship and techniques in cognitive-behavioral therapy: A motivational approach. *Psychotherapy: Theory, Research, Practice, Training, 42,* 443–455.

Horowitz, L. M., Rosenberg, S. E., & Bartholomew, K. (1993). Interpersonal problems, attachment styles, and outcome in brief dynamic psychotherapy. *Journal of Consulting and Clinical Psychology, 61,* 549–560.

Horvath, A. O., & Luborsky, L. (1993). The role of the therapeutic alliance in psychotherapy. *Journal of Consulting and Clinical Psychology, 61,* 561–573.

Kiesler, D. J. (1996). *Contemporary interpersonal theory and research: Personality, psychopathology, and psychotherapy.* New York: Wiley.

Klerman, G. L., & Weissman, M. M. (1993). Interpersonal psychotherapy for depression: Background and concepts. In G. L. Klerman & M. M. Weissman (Eds.), *New applications of interpersonal psychotherapy* (pp. 3–26). Washington, DC: American Psychiatric Association.

Kohut, H. (1995). Introspection, empathy, and psychoanalysis: An examination of the relationship between mode of observation and theory. *Journal of Psychotherapy Practice and Research, 4,* 163–177.

Lambert, M. J., & Barley, D. E. (2001). Research summary on the therapeutic relationship and psychotherapy outcome. *Psychotherapy: Theory, Research, Practice, Training, 38,* 357–361.

Lambert, M. J., & Okiishi, J. C. (1997). The effects of the individual psychotherapist and implications for future research. *Clinical Psychology: Science and Practice, 4,* 66–75.

Leary, T. (1957). *Interpersonal diagnosis of personality.* New York: Ronald Press.

Leary, T., & Coffey, H. S. (1955). Interpersonal diagnosis: Some problems of methodology and validation. *Journal of Abnormal and Social Psychology, 50,* 110–124.

Levenson, E. A. (1991). *The purloined self: Interpersonal perspectives in psycho-analysis.* New York: Contemporary Psychoanalysis Books.

Levenson, H. (2003). Time-limited dynamic psychotherapy: An integrationist per-spective. *Journal of Psychotherapy Integration, 13,* 300–333.

Lutgendorf, S., Antoni, M., Ironson, G., Starr, K., Costello, N., Zuckerman, M., et al. (1998). Changes in cognitive coping skills and social support during cogni-tive behavioral stress management intervention and distress outcomes in symp-tomatic HIV seropositive gay men. *Psychosomatic Medicine, 60,* 204–214.

Mallinckrodt, B., Porter, M. J., & Kivlighan, D. M., Jr. (2005). Client attachment to therapist, depth of in-session exploration, and object relations in brief psycho-therapy. *Psychotherapy: Theory, Research, Practice, Training, 42,* 85–100.

Markowitz, J. C. (2003). Interpersonal psychotherapy. In R. E. Hales & S. C. Yudof-sky (Eds.), *The American Psychiatric Publishing textbook of clinical psychiatry* (4th ed., pp. 1207–1223). Washington: American Psychiatric Publishing.

Martin, D. J., Garske, J. P., & Davis, M. K. (2000). Relation of the therapeutic alliance with outcome and other variables: A meta-analytic review. *Journal of Consulting and Clinical Psychology, 68,* 438–450.

Mead, G. H. (1934). *Mind, self, and society from the standpoint of a social behav-iorist.* Chicago: University of Chicago Press.

Mikulincer, M., & Shaver, P. R. (2004). Security-based self-representations in adult-hood: Contents and processes. In W. S. Rholes & J. A. Simpson (Eds.), *Adult attachment: Theory, research, and clinical implications* (pp. 159–195). New York: Guilford Press.

Mitchell, S. A. (1988). *Relational concepts in psychoanalysis: An integration.* Cam-bridge, MA; Harvard University Press.

Mitchell, S. A. (2000). *Relationality: From attachment to intersubjectivity.* Hillsdale, NJ: Analytic Press.

Moretti, M. M., & Holland, R. (2003). The journey of adolescence: Transitions in self within the context of attachment relationships. In S. M. Johnson & V. E. Whiffen (Eds.), *Attachment processes in couple and family therapy* (pp. 234–257). New York: Guilford Press.

Norcross, J. C. (Ed.). (2002). *Psychotherapy relationships that work: Therapist con-tributions and responsiveness to patient needs.* New York: Oxford University Press.

Rogers, C. R. (1957). The necessary and sufficient conditions of therapeutic person-ality change. *Journal of Consulting Psychology, 22,* 95–103.

Rosselló, J., & Bernal, G. (1999). The efficacy of cognitive-behavioral and interper-sonal treatments for depression in Puerto Rican adolescents. *Journal of Con-sulting and Clinical Psychology, 67,* 734–745.

Safran, J. D. (2002). Brief relational psychoanalytic treatment. *Psychoanalytic Dia-logues, 12,* 171–195.

Scarvalone, P., Fox, M., & Safran, J. D. (2005). Interpersonal schemas: Clinical theory, research, and implications. In M. W. Baldwin (Ed.), *Interpersonal cog-nition* (pp. 359–387). New York: Guilford Press.

Shaver, P. R., & Mikulincer, M. (2005). Attachment theory and research: Resur-rection of the psychodynamic approach to personality. *Journal of Research in Personality, 39,* 22–45.

Slade, A. (2004). Two therapies: Attachment organization and the clinical process.

In L. Atkinson & S. Goldberg (Eds.), *Attachment issues in psychopathology and intervention* (pp. 181–206). Mahwah, NJ: Erlbaum.

Sroufe, L. A. (2005). Attachment and development: A prospective, longitudinal study from birth to adulthood. *Attachment & Human Development, 7,* 349–367.

Stern, D. N. (2004). The motherhood constellation: Therapeutic approaches to early relational problems. In A. J. Sameroff, S. C. McDonough, & K. L. Rosenblum (Eds.), *Treating parent–infant relationship problems: Strategies for intervention* (pp. 29–42). New York: Guilford Press.

Stolorow, R. D. (2000). From isolated minds to experiential worlds: An intersubjective space odyssey. *American Journal of Psychotherapy, 54,* 149–151.

Sullivan, H. S. (1938). Psychiatry: Introduction to the study of interpersonal relations. *Psychiatry: Journal for the Study of Interpersonal Processes, 1,* 121–134.

Sullivan, H. S. (1950). The illusion of personal individuality. *Psychiatry: Journal for the Study of Interpersonal Processes, 13,* 317–332.

Sullivan, H. S. (1953). *The interpersonal theory of psychiatry.* New York: Norton.

Teyber, E. (2006). *Interpersonal process in therapy: An integrative model* (5th ed.). Belmont, CA: Thomson Brooks/Cole.

Thompson, R. A., Easterbrooks, M. A., & Padilla-Walker, L. M. (2003). Social and emotional development in infancy. In I. B. Weiner (Series Ed.) & R. M. Lerner, M. A. Easterbrooks, & J. Mistry (Vol. Eds.), *Handbook of psychology: Vol. 6. Developmental psychology* (pp. 91–112). New York: Wiley.

Travis, L, A., Bliwise, N. G., Binder, J. L., & Horne-Moyer, H. L. (2001). Changes in clients' attachment styles over the course of time-limited dynamic psychotherapy. *Psychotherapy: Theory, Research, Practice, Training, 38,* 149–159.

van IJzendoorn, M. H., Goldberg, S., & Kroonenberg, P. M. (1992). The relative effects of maternal and child problems on the quality of attachment: A meta-analysis of attachment in clinical samples. *Child Development, 63,* 840–858.

van IJzendoorn, M. H., Schuengel, C., & Bakermans-Kranenburg, M. J. (1999). Disorganized attachment in early childhood: Meta-analysis of precursors, concomitants, and sequelae. *Development and Psychopathology, 11,* 225–249.

Volling, B. L., McElwain, N. L., & Notaro, P. C. (2002). Parents' emotional availability and infant emotional competence: Predictors of parent–infant attachment and emerging self-regulation. *Journal of Family Psychology, 16,* 447–465.

Wachtel, P. L. (1993). *Therapeutic communication: Principles and effective practice.* New York: Guilford Press.

Weissman, M. M., Markowitz, J. C., & Klerman, G. L. (2000). *Comprehensive guide to interpersonal psychotherapy.* New York: Basic Books.

Winnicott, D. W. (1971). *Playing and reality.* London: Tavistock.

16

Attachment Theory and Emotionally Focused Therapy for Individuals and Couples

Perfect Partners

Susan M. Johnson

Experiential therapies, such as emotionally focused therapy (EFT; Greenberg, Rice, & Elliott, 1993; Johnson, 2004), share with John Bowlby's (1969/1982, 1988) attachment theory a focus on the way we deal with basic emotions, engage with others on the basis of these emotions, and continually construct a sense of self from the drama of repeated emotionally laden interactions with attachment figures. The relevance of attachment theory to understanding change in adult psychotherapy, whether individual or couple therapy, has become clearer because of the enormous amount of research applying attachment theory to adults in the last two decades (Cassidy & Shaver, 2008). Attachment theory is now used explicitly to inform interventions in individual therapy (Fosha, 2000; Holmes, 1996), and it forms the basis of one of the best-validated and most effective couple interventions—EFT for couples (Johnson, 2004; Johnson, Hunsley, Greenberg, & Schindler, 1999). This chapter considers how the attachment perspective helps the humanistic experiential therapist address individual problems such as anxiety and depression, as well as the relationship distress that accompanies and maintains these problems. The current humanistic experiential model of individual psychotherapy is perhaps best represented by the systematic and evidence-based interventions of the EFT school (Greenberg et al., 1993). This approach has received considerable empirical validation both for anxiety/trauma-related problems and for depression in individuals (Elliott, Greenberg, & Lietaer, 2004).

POINTS OF CONTACT

The theoretical points of contact between experiential therapies such as EFT and attachment theory are many. Both take a transactional view of personality: Internal aspects of a person, such as affect regulation abilities, interact with the quality and nature of present close relationships in a dynamic and reciprocal manner. Both link dancer and dance, self and system, in a holistic evolving process (Johnson & Best, 2002). More specifically, in both models the responsiveness and acceptance offered by key others are crucial in facilitating the effective processing and ordering of experience into coherent meaning frames. These frames then guide adaptive action. For the individual to be emotionally accessible and flexibly responsive to self and others is the hallmark of health in both approaches.

In general, the concepts of health and dysfunction seem very consistent across the two perspectives. Attachment research (Mikulincer, 1995) and theory predict that securely attached adults will have a more organized, coherent or articulated, and positive sense of self. Others are seen as basically trustworthy, and the self is viewed as lovable and competent. Rogers (1961), the founding father of the humanistic experiential model of therapy, also focused on how safe emotional connection with others builds a positive and empowered sense of self. This connection not only maximizes flexibility and adaptability, but promotes resilience in the face of stress and trauma. A secure orientation (and the coherent positive sense of self associated with it), seems to promote cognitive exploration and flexibility, helps people stay open to new information, and helps them deal with ambiguity (Mikulincer, 1997; Mikulincer & Shaver, 2003). In brief, it promotes the ability to learn and adapt. As Rogers (1961) pointed out, the presence of an attuned empathic other who offers acceptance enhances exploration and self-actualization. A secure orientation also allows an adult to consider alternative perspectives and engage in metacognition (Kobak & Cole, 1991; see also Jurist & Meehan, Chapter 4, this volume). The ability to reflect on, discuss, and so revise realities is enhanced. The experience of felt security with another is associated with more open, direct communication styles, as well as with more ability to self-disclose and assert one's needs. In general, a secure attachment style allows for the continued expansion of a positive sense of self and the ability to respond to one's environment, whereas insecurity is associated with constriction of experience and a lack of responsiveness.

In EFT, health is described as the ability to fully listen to and engage inner experience (particularly emotional experience), to trust this experience, and to create meanings that can then direct behavioral responses. As

Greenberg et al. (1993, p. 28) state, when this therapy works, clients learn to "trust their own experience and to accept their own feelings. They learn that they are able to be themselves in relation to one another. They are confirmed in their existence as worthwhile people." Rogers (1961) believed that the growth tendency propelling people toward health is innate, as did Bowlby (1988, p. 152), who stated that "the human psyche, like human bones, is strongly inclined towards self-healing." Rogers saw this tendency as a genetic blueprint; however, a safe, validating environment enables this tendency. Greenberg (1996) also points out that although Rogers spoke of dysfunction in terms of the conflict between experience and one's self-concept, this formulation has waned in importance, whereas blocks to listening to emotions and fully processing key experiences have become key to understanding dysfunction. Health, then, is being able to fully engage in current moment-to-moment experience and use this experience to make active choices in how to define the self and relate to others. Key experiences are explored, integrated, and used to expand the range of an individual's responses, rather than being denied or distorted. The value of being authentic—trusting one's experience and being true to oneself—is implicit in this model and intricately linked to intimate connection to others. Humanistic therapists view themselves as helping people make active choices, understand how they actively construct their experience of self and of others, and listen to their emotional experiences and needs. Therefore, the views of health set out both in attachment theory and in experiential writings seem to me to be complementary and to share a common view of people's basic needs—for acceptance, connection, and the safety that leads to exploration and growth. Both look within and between individuals, and at how intra- and interindividual realities reflect and create each other. Both perspectives suggest that when these needs are not met, the processing of experience and engagement with others becomes distorted or constricted. John Bowlby would surely have agreed with Rogers's comment that therapy should lead someone from "defensiveness and rigidity" to "openness to experience" (1961, p. 115).

In terms of how clients are seen, both attachment and experiential perspectives are inherently nonpathologizing. Bowlby stressed that if we understand the relational environment in which a person learned to relate and adapt, then we would appreciate that the person's behavior is a "tolerably accurate reflection" of what actually happened to him or her. This parallels the emphasis experiential therapy places on the therapist's unconditional acceptance of a client's experience and empathic understanding of the client. In both perspectives, strategies or ways of dealing with emotions that land people in trouble are seen as having originated as defensive maneuvers to maintain connections with loved ones or ward off a sense of the self as unlovable and helpless. Both models speak of coherence, or the ability to integrate different experiences or parts of self, as being an ongoing process aimed at health. The integration of implicit, overlooked, or silenced aspects of self, spoken of in the experiential literature (Elliott, Watson, Goldman, & Greenberg, 2004) parallels the focus in attachment theory on the secure person's ability to create coherent integrative narratives of key attachment experiences and tell these stories congruently (Hesse, 1999; Main, Kaplan, & Cassidy, 1985).

Both attachment and experiential viewpoints privilege emotion. Bowlby (1991) noted that the main function of emotion is to communicate one's needs, motives, and priorities to both oneself and others. I believe he would have endorsed the EFT concept that being tuned out of emotional experience is like navigating through life without an internal compass. Both perspectives see emotion as essentially adaptive and compelling—as organizing core cognitions and responses to others. Both perspectives also include the view that affect regulation is the core issue underlying the constricted responses that bring people into therapy. Bowlby stated, "The psychology and psychopathology of emotion is ... in large part the psychology and pathology of affectional bonds" (1979, p. 130). The processing of emotional experience is viewed as the vital organizing element in how the self and others are experienced and how models of self are constructed (Bowlby, 1988; Elliott, Watson, et al., 2004). Both experiential therapists and attachment theorists view emotion as the vital element in guiding perception, cueing internal models of self and other and interactional responses. Indeed, research suggests that affect may function as the "glue" that binds information within mental representations (Niedenthal, Halberstadt, & Setterlund, 1999).

The concept of emotion has become more differentiated, and its role in therapy more clearly articulated, than was the case when attachment theory was originally formulated. It is perhaps easier to use emotion in therapy when, for example, we understand clearly that there are six or seven main universal emotional responses (Frijda, 1986; Izard, 1991; Tomkins, 1962–1992). Attachment theorists talk mostly of insight into emotion as a primary change mechanism in therapy, whereas experiential therapists attempt to create new corrective emotional experiences rather than insight per se.

The focus on moment-to-moment emotional processing—which is so fundamental to experiential therapies such as EFT, where the therapist literally tracks and aids in the moment-to-moment construction of an individual's experience—has a parallel in the basic observational technique used in developing attachment theory: the coding of emotional responses and behavior in the Strange Situation (Ainsworth, Blehar, Waters, & Wall, 1978). Both an experiential therapist and an attachment theorist focus on bottom-up processing. Just as an experiential therapist focuses on what happens in a key emotional situation, so Bowlby and Ainsworth focused on what happens in key moments when a vulnerable child is left by an attachment figure in a strange context. Both the attachment theorist-researcher and the experiential therapist in a therapy session note how emotion arises and is dealt with in key situations when vulnerability is present and compelling. Both then focus on how an individual responds and either protects the self (perhaps by shutting down or becoming overemotional) or reaches out into the environment to get needs met. Both will examine the consequences of that choice for the sense of self and for interactions with others. Both note how an individual pulls others close or drives them away and sends out congruent or conflictual signals. Both ask this question: Can people integrate emotions and move confidently into the world trusting themselves and their own realities, or not? The focus on emotional processing and how it creates patterns of interpersonal responses and models of self is the same. This concern with process is also reflected in the work of Mary Main and colleagues (e.g., Main et al., 1985), who interview people about their past and present attachments. The focus in this work is not on the content of these memories, but on how they are formulated—specifically, on the openness and coherence with which they are retrieved and articulated.

The goals of therapy also seem to be similar. Both the attachment theorist and the EFT therapist expect a client at the end of a therapy process to be more open to his or her experience, more able to engage with strong emotion, and more able to create a coherent and meaningful frame and narrative about the self and key relationships. EFT therapists want to help clients create change in emotional reactions that define key relationships. They want to help clients regulate their emotions and not become stuck in strategies such as avoidance that lead to disorientation and incongruence (Greenberg & Paivio, 1997). They want to help clients connect with, reflect on, and integrate traumatic experience and create positive meaning frames that promote resilience. Attachment-oriented therapists such as Fosha (2000) and Holmes (1996) would endorse all of these goals.

Since both perspectives stress attunement, responsiveness, and emotional engagement—that is, since both contend that genuine connection is the key to growth and adaptation—many of the general conditions of therapy will then be similar. Both models suggest, using slightly different language, that the therapy session should be a safe haven. Empathy and emotional connection have to be key parts of the therapeutic alliance and necessary conditions for change. The need for validation, support, and caring from the therapist is stressed in both perspectives. To depend on others is seen as part of the human condition—not as an immature or dysfunctional response to be ameliorated. In general, the therapist in EFT sounds very much like the security-promoting attachment figure of attachment theory. The therapist is emotionally present and genuine, attuned, accepting, and responsive. The therapist responds to the client's pain and helps the client struggle with that pain; what is sharable becomes bearable (Siegel, 1999). The EFT therapist is a process consultant who stands with clients as they encounter and organize their experience. This role parallels that of the loving parent who provides safety and a secure base as a child reaches out to life. The therapist's validation and presence provide a safe haven, and the therapist's responsiveness creates a secure base from which the client can explore the edges and depth of his or her experience and make sense of it.

Although attachment theory has become well integrated into EFT for couples (Johnson, 2003, 2008), it has not been explicitly used in EFT for individuals, at least as described in the literature. How then does attachment theory hone and refine the experiential approach to change in individual EFT?

ATTACHMENT-INFORMED EFT

Although Bowlby did not focus a great deal on the implications of his theory for the practice of psychotherapy, he sometimes described cases in ways that very closely parallel experiential interventions. For example, he described a case where a therapist offered suggestions as to how a young mother at risk for abusing her baby felt frightened, angry, and helpless as a child and longed for secure connection. The young mother was then able to express these emotions herself and so to make progress in therapy (Bowlby, 1988, p. 155). However, most of the time Bowlby and other attachment theorists, while noting the primacy of affect, seemed to suggest a more analytic, insight-oriented approach to change (Holmes, 1996). The humanistic perspective that forms the basis of EFT is essentially a theory of intervention, whereas attachment theory is a theory of personality and development. How can EFT therapists use current attachment theory and research to hone and refine their work with individual clients?

First, the attachment perspective emphasizes the crucial part played by the therapeutic alliance in the change process. EFT has always stressed the importance of accurate empathy, attunement to the client, and genuine engagement. The focus in therapy is on the person rather than the problem. The therapist strives to be authentic with the client, honoring and processing the client's ongoing experience as a collaborative consultant. The existentialists, who were part of the development of humanistic models, stressed that authentic dialogue and genuine encounter allow for the emergence of the client's authentic self (Cain, 2002). The attachment perspective stresses the need for the alliance also to provide a safe haven and a secure base— that is, an explicit source of comfort, reassurance, and validation. Bowlby (1979, p. 94) spoke of a therapist's sympathizing with a grieving widow's "unrealism and unfairness" in such a way that the therapist became her champion and supporter, rather than telling her to be more realistic. Acceptance, validation, and the offering of comfort at times of great pain become vital parts of the therapy process. For example, when a client cries, ashamed of her "pathetic weakness" and vulnerability, and says that she prefers to "numb out" (something that actually happened in the case of Alexis and Keith, described in more detail later), I would make my voice softer and slower and reflect her pain. I think of my response as holding her with my voice and also letting her know that her pain is seen and respected. "Feeling felt" and attuned to by another is a vital element in the creation of safe connection in attachment theory. It enables the ability to distill, trust, and "own" one's emerging experience. I also provide validation—saying in this case, for example, that of course Alexis would choose to "shut down," since for her in her family it would have been dangerous to allow these feelings to emerge. The ability to numb out had, in effect, saved her life, allowing her to stay connected with those she depended upon. In the safety of the interaction with me, she could then allow herself to weep for all the times she dared not connect with that vulnerability. The creation of a safe haven in therapy allows for new levels of engagement with key emotional experiences—the experiences that define the self.

In cases of extreme trauma or lack of any kind of secure attachment, the therapist may become a surrogate attachment figure; this gives the client a glimpse of another world where others are responsive and accessible, and where safe engagement with inner experience and with others is possible. The therapist also helps contain overwhelming affect at certain times, as a supportive attachment figure does in normal life. The EFT therapist may use grounding techniques during a traumatic flashback (see the example in Johnson & Williams-Keeler, 1998), or may directly use engagement with the therapist as an active experiment in connection. The therapist might say, for example, "What is it like to say these things right now with me here? How is it for you that I am here—seeing your vulnerability? You say you are sure that I must be feeling contempt for you listening to this; can you look at my face and see if that is what you see?" The alliance then becomes a safe platform for exploration, and is also used in and of itself as a tool to explore the client's habitual sensitivities and ways of engaging others. However, in EFT the focus is not so much on using the therapist as a surrogate attachment figure per se and working on forms of transference from the client; it is on using the alliance as a platform for the tasks of distilling primary or core emotions and processing these emotions, so that they move the client toward new responses to self and other.

Attachment theory also offers a guide to primary emotional experience. Attachment theorists (e.g., Fosha, 2000; Siegel, 1999) and experiential writers (Greenberg & Paivio, 1997; Johnson, 2004) both stress that emotion involves an initial orientation ("Pay attention—this is important. It is good or bad, threatening or safe"), a body response, a process of meaning creation, and an action tendency. The word *emotion* comes from the Latin *emovere* to move—"to motivate." When an emotion is reprocessed and expanded (e.g., when reactive irritation melts into sorrow), the action tendency and the meanings associated with the emotional experience change. Emotions communicate to the self and others what a person needs and is motivated to move toward (Bowlby, 1991). It organizes experience and interaction. Emotion theorists tell us that six emotions are universal across all cultures: joy, anger, surprise, shame, sadness/anguish, and fear (e.g., Ekman, 1992). Attachment theory gives us an encompassing metaframework in which to place these emotions.

In the context of attachment, our most basic human need is for safe emotional engagement with precious others on whom we can depend and to whom we matter. In the deeper, more primary emotional experiences that emerge in a therapy session, there are a number of primary attachment themes. Fear of isolation and abandonment, or the inability to deal with the threat of disconnection from others, and the longing for a safe-haven relationship form the underlying "music" of many problems that bring people into therapy. Themes of deprivation and violation by attachment figures—which result in either the deactivation or hyperactivation of the attachment system (Mikulincer & Shaver, 2003) and the emotions that go with either of these, especially anxiety and anger—are common. Bowlby saw these themes as key sources of problems in adult life. Studies of the phenomenology of emotional hurt stress the power of abandonment or rejection and the lack of self-valuing implicit in most problematic issues (Feeney, 2004). Problems of depression, if placed in an attachment frame, are seen in terms of loss of connection with and trust in others, or loss of the sense of self as worthy of love and connection. The working models of self outlined in attachment theory focus the therapist on the client's need to experience others as trustworthy and as a source of safety, and to view the self as competent and lovable. Attachment theory offers a map to key needs and to key emotional responses and the meanings associated with them. It explains and clarifies the power of emotion to shape cognitive models, to bring out our most compelling needs and fears, and to define our interactions with others. It supports the EFT therapist's stance that emotion has *control precedence* and so is the most powerful route to change.

Attachment theory also offers a guide to new, transforming emotional experiences. In EFT for couples, these key change events involve partners' taking new risks with each other in order for each to give clear attachment signals that move the other to become responsive and engaged (Johnson, 2004). In individual EFT, the overall task is the reprocessing of primary emotional experience, but the therapist can engage the client in many task experiments that lead to corrective emotional experiences. These experiences always involve a deepening engagement with primary emotions, and these most often concern (i.e., are paths into) attachment issues. This engagement also then creates a new awareness of needs and so a new readiness for action. For example, one task outlined in the EFT literature involves integration of conflicting elements in emotional experience by helping the client give voice to and engage with two opposing parts of the self ("I want to take risks, but I am afraid, so I hide out"). Another task is to confront blocks in experiencing or contacting emotions, which prevent movement into adaptive action and therefore keep the client frozen or paralyzed. These tasks help to uncover the client's internal working models of self and the affect regulation strategies learned in attachment contexts. They also promote the construction of a coherent narrative that offers a framework for dealing with emotions, as set out in the work of Main and colleagues (summarized by Hesse, 1999).

Some of the tasks of individual EFT are more clearly interpersonal and involve new ways of engaging others or dealing with inner representations of others. The therapist will help a client deal with painful unfinished issues with an attachment figure by having the client imagine that the person is sitting in an empty chair in the therapy room and engage in an imaginary dialogue with that person. In my experience, it is also extremely useful to evoke attachment figures to help a client confront a block in experiencing emotions. For example, a depressed client who came to me for therapy could not empathize with his own pain, and so could not stand up to his wife and ask for a separation even after decades of an extremely disengaged relationship. In a key change event, I asked him to connect with the attachment figure who most loved him and might understand his pain. I then asked that he express his pain to this figure (his mother) while visualizing her with his eyes closed. I encouraged him to "hear" and articulate his mother's loving empathic response. He was able, in his mother's voice, to reassure himself that he had been a good partner and must now listen to his own pain. He then gave himself permission to move into an assertive stance with his wife. This significantly affected his depression. Attachment research also supports the benefits of purposely evoking secure representations; this often leads to increased empathy and positive affect (Mikulincer, Gillath, et al., 2001; Mikulincer, Hirschberger, Nachmias, & Gillath. 2001).

From an attachment standpoint, transforming change events in therapy include the discovery, distillation, and disclosing of core emotions, which allow for better regulation of these emotions and enhanced emotional intelligence (Salovey & Mayer, 1990). These events also modify core models of self and others. New appraisals of behavior arise, and old constricting expectations are challenged. New behaviors can then be explored, and new risks can be taken in relation to basic needs for connection with others and a valued sense of self. Clients can then achieve a *working distance* (Gendlin, 1996) from emotion and so use it as a compass to guide their adaptive responses.

In summary, attachment theory offers a compelling rationale for many aspects of EFT practice:

- Attachment theory supports and validates the concern for a safe, collaborative validating alliance with the therapist as a prerequisite for engagement in the change process. Each therapy session becomes a safe haven and a secure base from which to explore and move into new experiences.
- Attachment theory offers deeper understanding and support for the phenomenology of hurts, fears, and longings that EFT therapists focus on and explore. The themes of abandonment, traumatic isolation, rejection, helplessness, and anxiety, and the ways these are dealt

with (by shutting down and restricting experience, or becoming reactive and so creating more of the same), are placed in an existential context and clarified by the attachment perspective. The EFT therapist then has a clearer map of common human misery and human motivation.

• Attachment theory supports the primacy of emotional experience and the necessity of engaging emotion in the change process. Emotion organizes inner and outer realities. Corrective emotional experiences are able to change representational models of self and others and to cue new responses.

• Attachment research also promotes a focus on the moment-to-moment processing of present experience and how it is constructed, rather than a coaching or "let's get somewhere else" model. As Main (1991) stresses, the coherence and congruence of experience and its integration into coherent narratives and meanings are the keys to adaptive, flexible coping, rather than the nature or content of that experience.

• Lastly, the change events of EFT—where a client more deeply engages in his or her inner world, with the therapist acting as an emotionally present process consultant and support—are inherent in attachment theory, even if Bowlby did not stipulate specific change processes (such as how to explore and expand working models).

TYPES OF INTERVENTIONS

How does an EFT therapist who explicitly uses an attachment frame intervene? Given the creation of a safe-haven/secure-base alliance in couple or in individual therapy, the two main foci of therapy are the accessing and reprocessing of emotion and the use of new emotional experiences to restructure behavioral responses to self and others. The main types of interventions can be described as follows:

1. Empathetically attuning to the client, the therapist tracks and reflects the client's experience, with a clear focus on emotions and key emotional responses to attachment figures. Reflection serves many purposes. It structures the session by slowing dialogue down and focusing it on emotional responses. It invites a deeper engagement with the key issues and emotions. It also creates safety and a positive alliance, affirming the client's sense of self. A good reflection organizes and distills experience, letting the superfluous aspects drop away and bringing the central aspects into the light. Reflection, when repeated, also allows the client to savor, revisit, and so further integrate complex emotional experience.

2. The EFT therapist validates emotion and the defenses we all use against overwhelming emotion or feared responses from key others. Attach-

ment theory helps with this validation by giving the "reasons" behind many responses. For example, the fearful clinging and hostile defensiveness of many clients labeled as having borderline personality disorder is easier to connect with if it is seen as fearful-avoidant attachment, based on experiences in which key others have been both a source of safety and a source of violation. Such a client has experienced being left in an impossible, paradoxical position and is still caught in the mode of "Come here, I so need you—but go away, I can't trust you." However, in EFT the focus is not primarily on using the therapist as a surrogate attachment figure per se and working on forms of transference. It is on using the alliance as a platform for the tasks of distilling primary or core emotions and processing these emotions so that they move the client toward new responses to self and other.

3. The therapist evokes deeper engagement in the session by tracking, reflecting, and replaying moment-by-moment interpersonal process—whether between client and therapist, between partners, or within the emotional and representational world of an individual. Evocative questions are the main tools here, as well as replays of key moments. So the therapist might offer the following questions:

> "What happens to you when you speak of this? How does it feel—in your body—when you say this to me? You seem very agitated as we speak of this. What do you want to do right now? What do you say to yourself when these emotions come up? Do you say, 'I shouldn't feel this way—it's pathetic'? What happens to you when I say you have a right to feel this way—can you tell me? What happens when you hear your father's voice in your head saying you must grow up? What is it like to tell Peter, who has just told you he loves you right here in this session, that you are afraid? How do you 'numb out' as you say it and then shut Peter out?"

With such questions the therapist will validate secondary reactive emotions, such as anger at an attachment figure, and evoke the more primary underlying emotions, such as fear of abandonment and rejection.

4. The EFT therapist follows the attachment model by addressing deactivating and hyperactivating strategies. To contain the emotional extremes of each strategy, he or she will reflect and help to better organize expressed emotions, placing them in a specific context, or will use grounding, externalization, or the therapeutic alliance to soothe the client. As an example of grounding, a therapist might say,

> "Can you just slow down a little and listen to your breath? We are talking about something very difficult here. Can you feel your feet on the ground? You are here with me, and we are working this out. This fear comes up precisely when ... and that makes sense. We can hold it for a

little bit and look at it—then we will put it away and deal with it some more when you are ready."

However, most of the time, the EFT therapist will heighten emotion. This is achieved through repetition, through the use of images, and through a focus on somatic responses. Key emotional events or moments are identified and replayed, and the elements of emotion, cues, initial responses, body reactions, meaning appraisals, and action tendencies are reviewed. The interpersonal context and attachment significance are evoked. The therapist uses nonverbal cues and slow, simple speech (Johnson, 2004) to make the implicit explicit, the vague specific, and the muted vivid. So the therapist might say,

> "Can we go back a moment? You just said that your partner's anger 'swept you away.' What happens to you as you say that? That is a very powerful image—to feel swept away. That is like 'overwhelmed,' and it sounds dangerous—yes?"

5. The therapist uses interpretation or conjecture in EFT. This is not the cognitive, insight-oriented intervention usually associated with the word *interpretation*. As the therapist discovers the client's experience with him or her and goes to the leading edge of that experience, where it is unformulated or difficult to access, the therapist may go one step beyond the client's words and offer a conjecture. For example, an EFT therapist working with a couple might say,

> "So you're getting very 'uncomfortable' right now as we are discussing what happens when you reach for Harry and he does not respond. I wonder—this uncomfortable feeling—is that the scary part? For most of us, it is very hard to take the risk of asking our lover for a response and our partner possibly being unable to respond. We often feel even more alone then. But maybe that does not fit for you?"

Within the explanatory framework of attachment theory, emotions do not appear haphazard or difficult to understand. As a result, conjectures become easier to make, and when made they are more relevant to the client.

6. The therapist reframes certain emotions and responses in ways that lead to positive possibilities. Attachment theory is a rich source of such reframes. For example, trauma symptoms can be externalized and framed as a dragon that comes for the client and pushes the client against a wall of helplessness, rather than as an inner set of symptoms the client should be able to cope with. The angry protest that is part of distress in unhappy couples can be reframed as a sign of love and the importance of the other partner, rather than as hostility and contempt.

7. The therapist sets up enactment experiments. *Enactments* are struc-

tured experiences that can occur between two opposing parts of the self or two conflicting attachment strategies (e.g., the avoidant part of self that does not wish to risk depending on others, and the part that longs for connection); between self and the representation of an attachment figure (e.g., a depressed woman who obsesses about her distant, unresponsive mother but cannot confront her); or between partners in couple therapy. Before such an enactment, relevant emotional experience is heightened and distilled. The enactment is then set up, as in "Can you talk to that numb part of you—that little girl part of you—and tell her ... " or "So, Mary, can you please tell Jim directly: 'It is too hard for me to reach out for you, to tell you how much I need you.' " The therapist helps the person(s) stay focused and move through the enactment, dealing with the emotions as they arise. Next, the therapist helps the client or the couple process what happened in the enactment and make sense of it. In couple therapy, this last step most often involves placing the event in an attachment frame and integrating the attachment meanings that arise.

Let us now look at two moments of change—one in an individual and one in a couple EFT session—that demonstrate different types of interventions.

BURNED OR ALONE:
NOTES FROM AN INDIVIDUAL SESSION

Leslie was a factory worker in her early 40s, referred by her family doctor. She had many symptoms of posttraumatic stress, which had developed following an extremely violent marriage where she was repeatedly assaulted and raped. When she left the marriage, she was then stalked by her ex-husband for 4 years, but in her words, "no one cared." Her family, especially her mother, did not support or protect her. She deliberately chose night shift work in a large factory so that she would not have to be with people, and she lived with a small cat that she idolized. Chris, the only man she had allowed to come close to her in recent years, had become depressed, felt rejected by her, and left the country 2 years earlier. In addition, Leslie had recently discovered she could no longer work in the factory, due to serious somatic complaints brought on by the factory environment. Her only family relationships (with her mother and sister) were very tenuous, and her few friendships were distant. She came to see me because she could not sleep, had massive headaches, could not make the decisions necessary for this life transition, and was obsessed with the fear that something might happen to her cat. If her cat died, then life was "not worth the trouble." The following is a transcript from the 10th session. My goal in this session was to help Leslie begin to step past her bitterness and defensive hostility, and access her vulnerabilities and needs. Seeing Leslie as a person with a fearful-avoidant attachment style and as a trauma survivor helped me attune to her.

LESLIE: I'm calling the factory and going back on shift. What difference does it make, anyway? It was my birthday yesterday, and no one bothered to call—why bother? At least when I am running that huge machine, I am somebody. That is the biggest machine in the place. Even the men would look at me and say I could handle it well.

THERAPIST: I'm hearing a lot here. Part of you wants to go back—back to the sense of running the huge machine—that gave you a sense of being someone being special, especially since the alternative seems to be feeling vulnerable. All these headaches, and your family isn't there for you even when you are not working nights and more available. You are still alone and you feel like nobody. They didn't recognize your birthday. So part of you says, "Why struggle? What is it all for? Is that it?"

LESLIE: Right. With my mum, it's always my brother—(*sarcastic simpering voice*) "Oh, poor Terry. We must help him." I'm mad at the whole world. And you said last time that my cat was not all there was. Well, aren't we the clever therapist!

THERAPIST: Hm. Your cat never lets you down.

LESLIE: (*Nods.*)

THERAPIST: I guess I am included in the world you are mad at.

LESLIE: (*Smiles affirmatively.*)

THERAPIST: Okay. I think I did ask if your cat was enough for you last time. Maybe that wasn't so clever, because I know that you count on your cat—she anchors and comforts you—

LESLIE: (*Nods.*)

THERAPIST: —especially when you feel you have lost the one thing that made you feel like somebody—gave you a sense of control, and you feel nobody sees you—is there for you, remembers your birthday. It's like you came out of the factory and no one was waiting for you. That is hard.

LESLIE: (*Looks down and away from me.*)

THERAPIST: So you get mad—at all of us?

LESLIE: (*Nods.*)

THERAPIST: But you don't look mad right now. How are you feeling at this minute?

LESLIE: Like telling everyone to screw off. I had to go for a test—the medical test I told you about—didn't want to go by myself, but everyone was busy. So screw off.

THERAPIST: So no one was there on your birthday, and no one would come with you for the test? So you say "Screw off" to all of us, but your face tells me that it's hard to not have someone say "Happy birthday" or come to a test with you. That is so hard.

LESLIE: (*Becomes tearful.*)

THERAPIST: What happens for you as I say this?

LESLIE: I guess it's hard. (*Looks away out the window.*)

THERAPIST: Hard to not be able to count on someone to come to the test with you, hard to have people miss your birthday, hard to have lost the sense of running that huge machine. That was important to you, wasn't it? You felt in control there. And your body is hurting. This is such a struggle.

LESLIE: I was good at running that machine. And at night in that place, it was me that was running it. I knew how to run it. It was my kingdom, and no one else was there.

THERAPIST: Yes. You mattered. You knew how to run the big machine well. You felt strong, confident, and safe there. But you made the choice. You knew that that aloneness and that life was killing you. It was safe but deadly, no?

LESLIE: My cat is the only good thing in my life, No one loves me like her, so I get scared if she looks sick. I just don't trust people.

THERAPIST: Yes. And you have good reasons for that. It's amazing that you have the courage to come here and risk talking about all these things with me.

LESLIE: You challenge me sometimes, but you don't scare me.

THERAPIST: But other people do, don't they, Leslie? They really scare you. There isn't much room for trust, or even giving people a chance. Did you tell people it was your birthday?

LESLIE: (*Looks away.*)

THERAPIST: What is happening as I ask this?

LESLIE: Nothing. Well, I did tell Mary, my neighbor down the road. And, well, she asked me to come over. She invited me for supper, but I didn't go. What was the point?

THERAPIST: Could you help me? How do you feel as you say that? You refused her offer. She is the one you like, yes?

LESLIE: (*Nods.*)

THERAPIST: And she reached and you refused. You were important enough for her to ask you to come to be with her, but you pushed her away, kept the door shut tight. How do you feel right now?

LESLIE: (*Very quietly*) I feel angry. (*Looks at me, and I raise my eyebrows and smile.*). All right. I don't know. I feel sad, I guess (*Tearfully*). It's a bit like Chris.

THERAPIST: Yes. It's like you said last time. You decide it's safer to be alone, but the longing is still there, isn't it?

LESLIE: (*Sheds tears.*)

THERAPIST: You wanted your mom to remember your birthday—and part of you wanted to go to your neighbor's supper—and wanted to let Chris in. It's sad to want that and not be able to risk it?

LESLIE: If you let people in, you get burned. My mum says to me, "You are better off alone."

THERAPIST: Other people are too scary. They burn you. And you feel so vulnerable, and you have been so burned. You were burned by your dad—we talked of that. You so wanted his approval, but he just gave orders and demands. And then you trusted your husband, and he burned you. So now you tell yourself, and your mother tells you, "It's better—the only way to stay safe, Leslie—to be closed off." Your tears tell me that being closed off and shutting everyone out isn't such a safe place, either. You would like to have been able to let Chris in a little, to take your neighbor up on her offer, but . . .

LESLIE: I cry all the time. If I let them in, I'll be a doormat.

THERAPIST: If you listen to the sadness and the longing and how much the aloneness hurts and risk, you will be burned, helpless again.

LESLIE: (*Weeps.*)

THERAPIST: And you promised yourself "Never again." You fought for your life in that abusive relationship. You took control. But now, with leaving the factory, you have lost that. You feel more alone, but too scared to let anyone in?

LESLIE: (*Nods.*)

THERAPIST: All this fear and sadness. And if someone sees that, you would be so easily burned. A doormat?

LESLIE: No one knows how sad I am, but I don't need love, don't let people see me. I don't want love. It's shit.

THERAPIST: So when I see you right now? How is it for you? You do let me in?

LESLIE: It's scary. But I can walk away from here. My mother says she loves me. That is shit.

THERAPIST: (*In a soft, slow voice.*) So can you see your mum if you close your eyes? Can you see her telling you, "I love you, Leslie"?

LESLIE: (*Closes eyes and weeps.*)

THERAPIST: That brings up sadness, hurt in you? Yes? 'Cause she isn't there when you need her, and you are so alone and vulnerable. She even tells you it's better to be alone, but it hurts.

LESLIE: (*Nods.*)

THERAPIST: Can you tell her?

LESLIE: It's not better. It's not better. (*Long pause*) But it's too scary. Can't open the door. (*Weeps.*) I couldn't even go to the neighbors. They are nice. They like me.

THERAPIST: So you're telling your mother, "It's not better to be alone with no one to count on, to feel you matter, to trust. But it's so hard to risk letting anyone in." Can you tell her?

LESLIE: How can you tell me it's better to be alone? I never had the choice. I was alone or I was burned, and you were never there, and I can't live like this any more.

THERAPIST: Can you say that again, Leslie?

LESLIE: I can't live like this. It's too hard. You let me down. But I can't be angry all the time and not letting anyone in.

THERAPIST: What is that like to say that? "I got hurt, abandoned, let down, but it's too hard to live with all the doors closed." To never risk is to be closed in behind those doors, maybe? But it was your way of fighting to survive.

LESLIE: Yes. I could never trust you, and then so much hurt. So I closed the door. Had to do it to stay alive. But now I wanted to go to the dinner. I wanted to let Chris in. I'd give anything to have him back. With him, I felt I was good for something. I mattered, but then he let me down, so I cut him off.

THERAPIST: So can you tell her, "You are wrong. I got mad and shut everyone out to stay alive. But it's cost me and I am so sad and scared and alone. It's too hard just to have Smiley [her cat]. I can cut everyone off, but then I am so sad. I cry all the time."

LESLIE: Yes. Like she said. (*Points to me and laughs.*) It's stupid, but it feels good to say this.

THERAPIST: It makes sense to me. You are a fighter. You fought in one way that got you out of a furnace, but then it got you stuck, and it's hard to turn around and start to risk and trust. But you are in here taking risks with me. What did you say last week? Maybe you didn't want to live all encased in barbed wire, feeling like you were good for nothing.

LESLIE: (*Relaxes and smiles.*) Yes, that's right. But I trust you a little 'cause you are just a silly therapist. (*We both laugh.*)

I then summarized the process above with Leslie, and we agreed that she would write it down in a journal when she got home. Journaling enabled her to make a more coherent narrative out of the intense emotions she had experienced. Being able to impose order on experience and still be engaged with it is part of functional living and secure attachment. Leslie also volunteered that she was going to go see her neighbor and tell her that it had been too hard to accept her invitation for the birthday supper. The huge number of issues—loss, deprivation, trauma, a model of self as "nothing" and of others as "dangerous," and a major life transition that confronted Leslie with all her vulnerabilities (difficult life adjustments and health problems)—complicated the therapy process. However, staying with the thread of primary emotions and attachment themes helped me stay focused and present with Leslie. In this session, she had already come a long way from her initial statements of "I hate people" and "I want to change my life—but without being with people."

No Touch: Notes from a Couple Session

Alexis and Keith were a highly intellectual professional couple; they had been married for 15 years, and had two children ages 8 and 6. Ten years ago, they had emigrated to Canada and left all their family and friends in another country. They were extremely easy to create a positive alliance with. They arrived for the first session displaying a dance of mutual withdrawal after a recent fight. During the fight, Keith had insisted that Alexis change her hair before they left for a party together, but she refused. He then told her that if she did not change her hair, she did not love him, and they should separate. The tiff made them realize how alienated from each other they had become, and this scared them.

Among couples, the content of fights is typically irrelevant; the strong emotions embedded in attachment themes are the heart of the matter. Such was the case with Keith. Keith reported that he had lost his wife when the first child was born. He withdrew into his work, felt more and more rejected by Alexis, and as a result asked for less and less connection. Similarly, Alexis had felt rebuffed and isolated by Keith's "irritability." To cope, she "built a wall" around herself, dealing with every issue by staying "in control" and analyzing everything in her head. The couple had not made love in 2 years and described their lives as "empty routine." After seven sessions, during which their negative cycle of angry withdrawal by Keith followed by numbing and distancing by Alexis had been articulated and framed as the enemy that kept each partner isolated and anguished, Keith began to open up and express his "loss" of Alexis to motherhood. He was able to express his hurt, his fear of asking for connection, and his "automatic shutdown" that occurred whenever he felt shut out by her. He experienced his wife as "behind glass," and expressed his "loneliness" and his need for reassurance. Alexis was quite responsive to Keith's frankness, and soon after, the partners resumed their sexual relationship and began to confide in each other. Keith shared that he felt "abandoned" by her in favor of the children, and that this paralleled his experience with his distant parents. He also felt "judged" by her. As a result of these disclosures, he became more accessible and responsive and was able to share his needs with Alexis.

The goal was now to help Alexis experience and be moved by her attachment emotions, and to engage more intimately with her partner. She articulated that she had had an unpredictable and verbally abusive home life as a child and wanted harmony at whatever price. She found negative emotions very disturbing, and to cope she habitually "numbed them out." As in many other couples, her habitual way of dealing with key emotions in childhood specifically shaped the way she engaged with her spouse, especially in the context of closeness and vulnerability. Let us take a small segment of her key responses and examine how I attempted to work with them to produce a *softening* change event in EFT. In a softening event, a previously distant or critical spouse risks engaging with his or her newly responsive partner (who has already reengaged) from a position of vulnerability, and asking for his or her attachment needs to be met in a way that elicits a positive response from the partner. This event results in mutual accessibility and responsiveness, and in moments of secure bonding that transform the relationship.

Again and again Alexis returned to the incident of the fight about how she wore her hair to the party, so we stayed there and mined the moment. As I helped her focus on her feelings, the process flowed as follows:

ALEXIS: I am numb, barren as a desert. I have just put my feelings aside. Under control. I was the pillar in my family. I kept everyone together. But that night it felt awful. I felt so vulnerable. There was no sense of being desired. He didn't think I was beautiful. He could just turn away. (*Weeps.*)

THERAPIST: In that moment you could not numb out. You were so vulnerable, and what you heard was that he did not want you, need you. He turned away.

ALEXIS: (*Nods.*)

THERAPIST: You were not desired—have not felt desired—but rejected—alone.

ALEXIS: I am so lonely, and I am inhibited. It is hard for me to show myself.

THERAPIST: Ah-ha. Hard to show that soft side. That vulnerability, that longing to be desired. Can you ask, Alexis? Can you ever ask Keith for reassurance, attention, touch? Can you ask for a hug?

ALEXIS: (*Recoils in chair, shakes head, and cries.*)

THERAPIST: I see the answer is no—no? That would be too hard, too risky?

ALEXIS: (*Nods.*)

THERAPIST: It's too scary to reach out and ask?

ALEXIS: I have built a wall. It is scary. I can't touch him. We didn't touch for months and months.

THERAPIST: It is too hard to feel all that longing to be desired, to feel so lonely, so vulnerable. And to reach, to ask, to show him you and your need?

ALEXIS: Yes. I can't do it. (*Puts face in hands.*) So I just numb out. Go in my head and try to stay calm.

THERAPIST: Yes. It's overwhelming to feel this vulnerable, so you shut down, and Keith then feels shut out.

KEITH: (*Nods in agreement.*)

THERAPIST: And he gets angrier and more distant. And you feel more rejected and put up more of a wall. This is the dance that took over your relationship and has left you both alone. Keith, how do you feel as your wife talks about this? How scary it is for her to even protest your distance, to call out for you, to reach for you?

KEITH: It is so sad. It's sad. We got so caught in that. I want her to be able to reach for me.

ALEXIS: But you are so silent. And we do not touch. I cannot.

THERAPIST: What does the silence say to you, Alexis?

ALEXIS: That he does not even like me. And the only safety is in me—to stay in my head so I have ... silence is so awful. (*Turns to Keith.*) You shut me out too.

KEITH: I did shut you out. In those fights we had years ago, I heard that you despised me. Like we talked about here. I heard that I had failed, felt I had lost you to the kids, felt left out. But we are here now.

THERAPIST: What you are saying, Keith, is that you both went behind walls, and now you want to reach out and get Alexis to risk, to trust, to let you in, to ask for the love she needs?

KEITH: (*Stares at Alexis intently, leans forward.*) Yes, yes.

THERAPIST: Can you tell her, please? (*Here I am setting up an enactment where the attuned and responsive partner reaches out and encourages the more fragile partner to risk connecting with attachment needs and sending clear attachment signals.*)

KEITH: I want you to risk with me. I don't want you to be lonely. I don't want to be lonely. I want you to trust me, to support you. I don't want to lose you. I want you to be able to ask. I will be there. So you can ask for a hug, maybe?

ALEXIS: That is terrifying. To ask for a hug, to ask to be held. I can't do that. Being that open in my family ... well ... (*Throws up her arms.*)

THERAPIST: That was suicide in your family, yes? The only safety was in shutting down. It would be like being naked to ask—exposed. What happens to you when Keith asks you to risk? Can you look at him?

ALEXIS: (*Looks at Keith.*)

THERAPIST: What happens when he says, "Risk with me, trust me, ask me"?

ALEXIS: (*Long silence*) I hear it a long way off. (*Cries.*) I do need him. (*Turns to Keith.*) I want to let you in, but it's so scary. We have to go slow. It's sad that I just can't ask.

THERAPIST: Yes. All those lonely years—in your family and with Keith. What was the word you used a few weeks ago? All that "lonely anguish." Maybe even doubting that you were entitled, deserved, had a right to ask for his touch, his love? (*Alexis weeps and nods.*) So can you tell him, "I want to let you in, but it is so scary"?

ALEXIS: Yes. (*Turns to Keith and says in a very soft voice:*) I do need you, but it's so hard to say it.

KEITH: (*Stands up and holds her.*)

I then replayed and helped the couple process this event, distilling meanings and validating attachment needs.

The responsiveness in this kind of softening event offers an antidote to negative cycles of interaction that foster insecurity and alienation. As emotions—the music of the attachment dance—change, so do the dance and the dances. Individual and interpersonal change occurs in such events, and the events themselves are associated with positive outcomes and recovery from distress in EFT. They are so powerful that they appear to revise models of self and other and to create new ways of dealing with attachment needs. Understood this way, softening events may explain the low rates of relapse in EFT even among at-risk couples (Clothier, Manion, Gordon-Walker, & Johnson, 2002). The therapist uses the attachment figure, attachment emotions, and needs as they arise to help each person reach past his or her habitual ways of dealing with emotion and engaging others. Perhaps couple therapy can be so powerful precisely because the main attachment figure is present in the room; the dramas of attachment and self-definition are immediate. This is in contrast to more analytic or even psychodynamic interventions, where much time must be spent in engaging emotions and eliciting key habitual responses.

CONCLUSIONS

Integrating an attachment perspective with EFT interventions seems to be a powerful combination for change. John Bowlby developed a brilliant theory of human functioning and development. It seems to me that the attachment perspective streamlines and extends the experiential perspective on change, and that EFT, as a specific model of change, shares much common conceptual ground with attachment theory. EFT also involves a systematic set of interventions that extends attachment theory into the realm of clinical practice. Bowlby always made it clear that emotion and emotion regulation are the primary issues in health and dysfunction, but interventions based on attachment have focused mostly on therapeutic techniques that depend on cognitive insight to create change. Even when attachment theorists expressly embrace a focus on emotion as a change agent—for example, when Holmes (1996, p. 33) states that the royal route to change is when "previously warded off or repressed affect is evoked, focused on, turned into narrative, experimented with and finally mastered"—the systematic techniques, process maps, and interventions to work with emotion are missing. The stated goal of attachment-informed therapy has often been to change internal working models. EFT assumes that the fastest way to change such models is through new corrective emotional experiences that are placed in the context of and used to transform attachment responses. I believe and hope that Bowlby would have shared my view that EFT is a model of change easily bonded to attachment theory, and that it is almost tailor-made to be attachment theory's clinical arm.

RECOMMENDATIONS FOR FURTHER READING

Ekman, P. (2003). *Emotions revealed: Recognizing faces and feelings to improve communication and emotional life.* New York: Times Books.—A book that summarizes some of the most fascinating research on emotion.

Goleman, D. (2006). *Social intelligence: The new science of human relationships.* New York: Bantam Books.—A book that presents and integrates a mosaic of the new threads of this science.

Karen, R. (1994). *Becoming attached: First relationships and how they shape our capacity to love.* New York: Oxford University Press.—The fascinating story of attachment theory.

Johnson, S. (2008). *Hold me tight: Seven conversations for a lifetime of love.* New York: Little, Brown.—An easy-to-read version of attachment theory and how it revolutionizes our view of couple relationships.

Mikulincer, M., & Shaver, P. R. (2007). *Attachment in adulthood: Structure, dynamics, and change.* New York: Guilford Press.—A fine synthesis of the last 15 years of thinking and research on adult attachment.

REFERENCES

Ainsworth, M. D. S., Blehar, M. C., Waters, E., Wall, S. (1978). *Patterns of attachment: A psychological study of the Strange Situation.* Hillsdale, NJ: Erlbaum.

Bowlby, J. (1979). *The making and breaking of affectional bonds.* London: Routledge.

Bowlby, J. (1982). *Attachment and loss: Vol. 1. Attachment* (2nd ed.). New York: Basic Books. (1st ed., 1969)

Bowlby, J. (1988). *A secure base.* New York: Basic Books.

Bowlby, J. (1991). Postscript. In C. M. Parkes, J. Stevenson-Hinde, & P. Marris (Eds.), *Attachment across the life cycle* (pp. 293–297). London: Routledge.

Cain, D. J. (2002). Defining characteristics, history and evolution of humanistic psychotherapies. In D. J. Cain & J. Seeman (Eds.), *Humanistic psychotherapies: Handbook of research and practice* (pp. 3–54). Washington, DC: American Psychological Association.

Cassidy, J., & Shaver, P. R. (Eds.). (2008). *Handbook of attachment: Theory, research, and clinical applications* (2nd ed.). New York: Guilford Press.

Clothier, P., Manion, I., Gordon-Walker, J., & Johnson, S. M. (2002). Emotionally focused interventions for couples with chronically ill children: A 2 year follow-up. *Journal of Marital and Family Therapy, 28,* 391–398.

Ekman, P. (1992). Facial expressions of emotion: New findings, new questions. *Psychological Science, 3,* 34–38.

Elliott, R., Greenberg, L. S., & Lietaer, G. (2004). Research on experiential psychotherapies. In M. Lambert (Ed.), *Bergin and Garfield's handbook of psychotherapy and behavior change* (5th ed., pp. 493–540). New York: Wiley.

Elliott, R., Watson, J. C., Goldman, R. N., & Greenberg, L. S. (2004). *Learning emotion-focused therapy: The process-experiential approach to change.* Washington, DC: American Psychological Association.

Feeney, J. A. (2004). Hurt feelings in couple relationships: Towards integrative models of the negative effects of hurtful events. *Journal of Social and Personal Relationships, 21,* 487–508.

Fosha, D. (2000). *The transforming power of affect: A model for accelerated change.* New York: Basic Books.

Frijda, N. H. (1986). *The emotions.* Cambridge, UK: Cambridge University Press.

Gendlin, E. (1996). *Focusing-oriented psychotherapy: A manual of the experiential method.* New York: Guilford Press.

Greenberg, L. S. (1996). The power of empathic exploration. In B. Farber, D. Brink, & P. Raskin (Eds.), *The psychotherapy of Carl Rogers: Cases and commentary* (pp. 251–260). New York: Guilford Press.

Greenberg, L. S., & Paivio, S. (1997). *Working with emotions in psychotherapy.* New York: Guilford Press.

Greenberg, L. S., Rice, L., & Elliott, R. (1993). *Facilitating emotional change.* New York: Guilford Press.

Hesse, E. (1999). The Adult Attachment Interview: Historical and current perspectives. In J. Cassidy & P. R. Shaver (Eds.), *Handbook of attachment: Theory, research, and clinical applications* (pp. 395–433). New York: Guilford Press.

Holmes, J (1996). *Attachment, intimacy and autonomy: Using attachment theory in adult psychotherapy.* Northvale, NJ: Aronson.

Izard, C. E. (1991). *The psychology of emotions.* New York: Plenum Press.

Johnson, S. M. (2003). Attachment theory: A guide for couple therapy. In S. M. Johnson & V. Whiffen (Eds.), *Attachment processes in couple and family therapy* (pp. 103–123). New York: Guilford Press.

Johnson, S. M. (2004). *The practice of emotionally focused couple therapy: Creating connection* (2nd ed.). New York: Brunner-Routledge.

Johnson, S. M. (2008). *Hold me tight: Seven conversations for a lifetime of love.* New York: Little Brown.

Johnson, S. M., Hunsley, J., Greenberg, L., & Schindler, D. (1999). Emotionally focused couples therapy: Status and challenges. *Clinical Psychology: Science and Practice, 6,* 67–79.

Johnson, S. M., & Best, M. (2002). A systemic approach to restructuring attachment: The EFT model of couple therapy. In P. Erdman & T. Caffery (Eds.), *Attachment and family systems: Conceptual, empirical and therapeutic relatedness* (pp. 165–192). New York: Springer.

Johnson, S. M., & Williams-Keeler, L. (1998). Creating healing relationships for couples dealing with trauma: The use of emotionally focused marital therapy. *Journal of Marital and Family Therapy, 24,* 25–40.

Kobak, R., & Cole, C. (1991). Attachment and meta-monitoring: Implications for adolescent autonomy and psychopathology. In D. Cicchetti (Ed.), *Rochester Symposium on development and psychopathology: Vol. 5. Disorders of the self* (pp. 267–297). Rochester, NY: University of Rochester Press.

Main, M. (1991). Metacognitive knowledge, metacognitive monitoring and singular (coherent) vs. multiple (incoherent) model of attachment: Findings and directions for future research. In C. M. Parkes, J. Stevenson-Hinde, & P. Marris (Eds.), *Attachment across the life cycle* (pp. 127–159). London: Routledge.

Main, M., Kaplan, N., & Cassidy, J. (1985). Security in infancy, childhood, and adulthood: A move to the level of representation. In I. Bretherton & E. Waters (Eds.), Growing points of attachment theory and research. *Monographs of the Society for Research in Child Development, 50*(1–2, Serial No. 209), 66–104.

Mikulincer, M. (1995). Attachment style and the mental representation of the self. *Journal of Personality and Social Psychology, 69,* 1203–1215.

Mikulincer, M. (1997). Adult attachment style and information processing: Individual differences in curiosity and cognitive closure. *Journal of Personality and Social Psychology, 72,* 1217–1230.

Mikulincer, M., Gillath, O., Halevy, V., Avihou, N., Avidan, S., & Eshkoli, N. (2001). Attachment theory and reactions to others' needs: Evidence that activation of the sense of attachment security promotes empathic responses. *Journal of Personality and Social Psychology, 81,* 1205–1224.

Mikulincer, M., Hirschberger, G., Nachmias, O., & Gillath, O. (2001). The affective component of the secure base schema: Affective priming with representations of attachment security. *Journal of Personality and Social Psychology, 81,* 305–321.

Mikulincer, M., & Shaver, P. R. (2003). The attachment behavioral system in adulthood: Activation, psychodynamics, and interpersonal processes. In M. Zanna (Ed.), *Advances in experimental social psychology* (Vol. 35, pp. 53–152). San Diego, CA: Academic Press.

Niedenthal, P., Halberstadt, J. B., & Setterlund, M. B. (1999). Emotional response categorization. *Psychological Review, 106,* 337–361.

Rogers, C. (1961). *On becoming a person.* Boston: Houghton Mifflin.

Salovey, P., & Mayer, J. D. (1990). Emotional intelligence. *Imagination, Cognition, and Personality, 9,* 185–211.

Siegel, D. J. (1999). *The developing mind: How relationships and the brain interact to shape who we are.* New York: Guilford Press.

Tomkins, S. (1962–1992). *Affect, imagery, consciousness* (4 vols.). New York: Springer.

17

Attachment Theory and Cognitive-Behavioral Therapy

Carolina McBride
Leslie Atkinson

Since John Bowlby presented his first theoretical paper to the British Psychoanalytic Society in 1957, attachment theory has been largely airbrushed out of not only psychoanalytic thinking, but other clinical approaches as well. Recently, however, attachment theory has increasingly attracted the attention of psychodynamic clinicians and clinically oriented researchers. By comparison, attachment theory is largely still a stranger to cognitively oriented clinicians and researchers—despite, as we will show, the many points of contact between it and the cognitive theory (CT) that underlies cognitive-behavioral therapy (CBT). We also explore how attachment theory can inform the practice of CBT. We are not proposing a new adaptation of CBT, but instead outline how attachment theory and research can supplement the theoretical and applied aspects of CBT. We use case examples to illustrate key points. The chapter is divided into three main sections. In the first section, we present general tenets of CT and summarize its points of contact with attachment theory. In the second section, we discuss how attachment theory can inform and enrich cognitive conceptualizations and interventions used in clinical practice, using the five key therapeutic tasks outlined by Bowlby as a framework for our discussion. Finally, in the third section, the clinical application of attachment theory in CBT is illustrated with a clinical case study.

POINTS OF CONTACT
BETWEEN CT AND ATTACHMENT THEORY

Overview of CT

CT (Beck, 1967, 1976, 1987) is one of the most influential theories about the nature and cause of psychological disorders. Though the gist of CT is

widely known—that what we think influences how we feel and behave—
CT consists of a coherent set of propositions (Alford & Beck, 1997). First
and foremost among these is that people create cognitive representations
of their experience called *schemas*, a construct now central to all cognitive
accounts of personality and psychopathology. Introduced by Aaron T. Beck
(1967), schemas are meaning-making tools that consist of beliefs, attitudes,
and rules about oneself, others, and the world. They are constructed during
early childhood experiences with significant others, and their purpose is to
adapt the then current environmental circumstances in order to facilitate
survival.

In CT, schemas constitute the cognitive equivalent of personality. Interactions with the environment are interpreted through the lens of schemas,
and the resulting meanings coordinate the action of affective and behavioral
systems. For example, some individuals will respond to failures with dejec-
tion and withdrawal, whereas others will approach them with curiosity and
renewed effort. The idiosyncratic meanings that schemas assign, and the
feelings and actions to which they lead, are the result of the learning history
each person develops in a unique array of circumstances, people, pressures,
and culture. This characteristic of schemas is called *cognitive content specificity*.

Schemas play a crucial role in assigning meaning and do this via what
Beck (2002) calls the *cognitive continuum*—the processes of perception,
attention, working memory, knowledge storage, and recall. Beck proposed
that schemas influence each phase of information processing in a top-down
manner. Schemas sift through the bewildering barrage of daily stimuli and
extract the essential elements, usually those consistent with the content of the
schemas themselves (Taylor & Crocker, 1981). Processing that is directed by
schemas is necessarily biased; it often yields cognitive errors or distortions
and, in extreme instances, psychopathology (Beck, 1967; Beck, Rush, Shaw,
& Emery, 1979; Segal & Shaw, 1986; Young, 1994; Young & Gluhoski,
1996). For instance, if a schema containing the belief "I am unlovable" is
activated and conducts information processing, a relatively neutral event
(e.g., a friend not returning a phone call) may be interpreted and personal-
ized as rejection, and may thus reinforce both a negative mood state and the
belief. Numerous cognitive errors, such as minimizing and selective abstrac-
tion, have been observed (for a complete listing of errors, see J. S. Beck,
1995). Some schemas predispose people to make specific errors, a tendency
called *cognitive vulnerability*.

Dysfunctional or maladaptive schemas, the origin of psychopathology
in CT (e.g., Abramson, Metalsky, & Alloy, 1989; Abramson, Seligman, &
Teasdale, 1978; Beck, 1967; Young, 1990), result in such a degree of bias
and distortion that negative affects predominate and optimal functioning is
undermined. Because schemas were originally developed to foster adaptation to an early childhood that was punctuated by negative events, they tend
to block new and creative solutions to the challenges of present-day living

(Alford & Beck, 1997). The rigidity of dysfunctional schemas guarantees that the actions of psychological systems (e.g., affective and behavioral) will remain restricted, and that resulting environmental contingencies are likely to reinforce existing beliefs and attitudes. Thus schemas, at least dysfunctional ones, are relatively stable structures.

Schemas lie dormant until activated by events. Once activated, schemas assign meaning, foment automatic thoughts, lead to errors in processing, and trigger affective and behavioral systems (Beck, 1996). For example, the dysfunctional schema "Others are unlovable" may be triggered by a breakup. The schema stirs up such thoughts as *I'll always be alone,* may result in personalizing others' schedule changes, and may lead to depression and withdrawal. The functioning of schemas is not always conscious. CT recognizes that cognition has preconscious (i.e., automatic), conscious, and metacognitive levels (i.e., decentering and distancing; Alford & Beck, 1997).

Theoretical Similarities between CT and Attachment Theory

Beck and Bowlby independently formulated their ideas in response to their dissatisfaction with psychoanalytic theory and technique. Beck (1967) reacted to the underestimation of reasoning to solve problems and the view of people as helpless in the face of unconscious impulses, whereas Bowlby (1969/1982) took issue with the neglect of real-life experiences, with feeding or oral gratification as the origins of mother love, and with psychoanalysts' lack of interest in empirical data. However, both men were influenced by the cognitive revolution in psychology—a fact that creates several points of contact between CT and attachment theory.

Mental Representations

Bowlby's *internal working model* (IWM) is analogous to Beck's cognitive schema. (For an in-depth review of IWMs, see Cobb & Davila, Chapter 9, this volume.) Both constructs describe mental representations or cognitive structures, the content of which includes beliefs, attitudes, and memories. Both also describe models of oneself, others, and the world. However, several characteristics are unique to IWMs but complement Beck's ideas. First, although cognitive theory clearly states that schemas evolve from childhood experiences with significant others (e.g., Beck, 1987), attachment theory specifies the kinds of experiences that are most influential in the construction of IWMs—namely, repeated interactions with primary caregivers (attachment figures) during which needs for safety, comfort, and exploration are negotiated (Bowlby, 1973). In other words, motivational goals (e.g., the need for security) and emotion regulation processes are embedded in IWMs. Second, whereas schemas can be general in nature, IWMs are explicitly set in interpersonal terms; they are designed to inform a person's perceptions, forecasts, and actions in encounters with intimate partners. Third, encoded in IWMs are plans and strategies (e.g., behaviors, defense mechanisms) for relieving the sense of insecurity caused by distress and the unavailability of attachment figures. (For further discussion of the differences between schemas and IWMs, see Shaver, Collins, & Clark, 1996.)

Activation, Processing, and Appraisal

Similar to schemas, IWMs can be activated by internal (thoughts) or external (events) stimuli, although the language used to describe this activation is slightly different. In CT, dysfunctional schemas are seen as latent until triggered by events that rouse cognitive vulnerabilities (e.g., when the belief "I am unlovable" is coupled with rejection; Beck, 2002). The use of schemas is so well practiced that their implementation is automatic and just outside the sphere of consciousness. These ideas are highly compatible with those in attachment theory. IWMs are considered chronically accessible structures; that is, idiosyncratic beliefs and expectations are readily brought to mind in response to stimuli (Collins, Guichard, Ford, & Feeney, 2004). IWMs also operate largely out of awareness (Bowlby, 1973). For example, in a study by Mikulincer, Gillath, and Shaver (2002), participants subliminally exposed to threat words (e.g., *failure, separation*) brought to mind representations of attachment figures more quickly than representations of other known persons.

Just as schemas are thought to conduct information processing, IWMs are regarded as containing "a set of rules for obtaining or limiting access to … information" (Main, Kaplan, & Cassidy, 1985, p. 67). Like Beck (1967, 1976, 1987), Bowlby (1980) argued that people have a limited ability to attend to and process information. Therefore, sensory inflow is appraised out of awareness before conscious processing occurs. Experience renders some environmental features more subjectively salient than others. On this basis, Bowlby (1980) argued that an individual's attachment history influences what is and what is not processed consciously.

Furthermore, just as Beck (1967, 1976, 1987) has done, Bowlby (1980) suggested that unfamiliar stimuli are interpreted through the lens of existing mental representations. He argued that humans process perceptions in two directions simultaneously. On the one hand, a sensory stimulus triggers an automatic series of analyses that starts at the sense organs and continues up the chain of processing stages. On the other hand and simultaneously, the stimulus triggers experience-based processing that conceptually drives interpretation of the stimulus. Thus, the perception of a stimulus is based not only on the stimulus itself, but also on individual differences in people's IWMs. These predictions have been borne out in numerous studies (e.g., Baldwin, Fehr, Keedian, Seidel, & Thompson, 1993; Mikulincer, Hirschberger, Nachmias, & Gillath, 2001; for a review, see Mikulincer & Shaver, 2007).

Individual Differences in Mental Representations

Not only do CT and attachment theory suppose that mental representations underlie personality, but there is some overlap in how the two theories conceive individual differences in personality. The *sociotropic* and *autonomous* personalities in CT share features with the *anxious* and *avoidant* attachment styles.

Beck (1987) proposed that personality differences are associated with distinctive presentations of psychopathology (e.g., depression) and precipitating factors. Two specific personality types, *sociotropic* and *autonomous,* may render an individual more vulnerable to psychopathology (Beck, Epstein, & Harrison, 1983; Sacco & Beck, 1995). Highly sociotropic individuals are excessively concerned about and sensitive to the disapproval of others; their sense of worth is based on receiving love and acceptance from others and on maintaining close relationships. A common core belief of sociotropic individuals is "I must be loved in order to be happy." In contrast, autonomous individuals strive for independence and goal achievement, and their self-worth is based on productivity, achievement, and control. Autonomous individuals often believe that "I must be a success in order to be worthwhile." According to Beck (1987), when negative life events provoke the emotional vulnerabilities of the sociotropic or autonomous personality, the respective dysfunctional schemas are activated and precipitate psychopathology (a diathesis–stress model). For example, a relationship breakup would lead to emotional distress for a sociotropic individual, whereas being fired would result in emotional distress for an autonomous individual.

Attachment theory is also a model of personality differences, some of which make individuals susceptible to mental health difficulties (Bowlby, 1988; Mikulincer & Shaver, 2007). CT's sociotropy resembles attachment-related anxiety. Anxiously attached adults are highly dependent on the affection and approval of others, are inordinately sensitive to the possibility of rejection by others, and engage in clinging and controlling behaviors to garner attention and support. Such adults experienced early attachment figures as inconsistently available and responsive; the lack of emotional support has often left them overwhelmed by worries and unsure of their self-worth. The dimension of attachment closest to CT's autonomous personality is attachment-related avoidance. Avoidantly attached persons value emotional self-sufficiency, control, and interpersonal distance (Mikulincer & Shaver, 2007). Avoidant adults are motivated to suppress feelings or needs that might activate the attachment system, because in the past their expression has been met with aloofness, outright rejection, or punishment. As such, avoidant adults are inclined to block awareness of personal vulnerability, defensively enhance their self-worth, and devalue others and relationships (Mikulincer & Shaver, 2007).

Interpersonal Schemas

Theorists have long emphasized the vital importance of social environment and functioning to the etiology of psychopathology. One of the main criticisms of cognitive accounts has been that little attention is paid to these developmental issues and to the role of social environment in the development and maintenance of psychopathology (Coyne & Gotlib, 1983, 1986; Gilbert, 1992; Gotlib & Hammen, 1992). In response to the accumulating evidence of the association between interpersonal and social factors and emotional disorders (Joiner & Coyne, 1999), a more recent development in the cognitive field has been the cognitive–interpersonal approach (Gotlib & Hammen, 1992; Safran & Greenberg, 1991; Safran & Segal, 1990/1996; Schmidt, Schmidt, & Young, 1999). This approach directly incorporates aspects of attachment theory into cognitive principles. Cognitive–interpersonal approaches place a critical emphasis on attachment relationships in understanding vulnerability to psychopathology and the way in which attachment patterns become internalized as cognitive schemas (e.g., Gotlib & Hammen, 1992; Safran, Segal, Hill, & Whiffen, 1990).

To characterize the interpersonal nature of the self, Safran (Safran, Vallis, Segal, & Shaw, 1986; Safran, 1990) has introduced the notion of the *interpersonal schema*. Interpersonal schemas are generalized cognitive representations of interactions with others that initially develop from patterns of interactions with attachment figures, and that allow an individual to predict interactions with significant others and maximize the probability of maintaining relatedness (Hill & Safran, 1994). This depiction of interpersonal schemas also precisely describes mental representations with respect to attachment. Interpersonal schemas and mental representations contain information of the form "If I do X, others will do Y" (e.g., "If I assert myself, others will put me down"). Psychologically healthy individuals are presumed to have interpersonal schemas that predict interpersonal relatedness to be accessible, regardless of how they act or feel ("If I am sad, I will be comforted"). This profile is akin to a secure IWM.

Confidence in the support of others allows them to act and feel in a wide range of ways without risk of jeopardizing the attachment relationship (in attachment terms, they can explore their environment freely because they have a secure base). In contrast, individuals prone to psychopathology have interpersonal schemas predicting that interpersonal relatedness is unattainable and that a wide range of feelings and behaviors can threaten close relationships (e.g., "If I am sad, I will be rejected"). As a result, such individuals have a highly constricted sense of how they must act and feel to retain relationships (Safran & Segal, 1990/1996). This pattern is similar to insecure attachment.

In the cognitive–interpersonal approach, interpersonal schemas are believed to be maintained according to Kiesler's (1983, 1996) principle of *complementarity* (Safran, 1990; Safran & Segal, 1990/1996), which states that two people's behaviors, emotions, and thoughts are mutually and causally interconnected, with specific interpersonal behaviors from one individual predictably pulling for specific interpersonal behaviors from another individual in an interaction. Complementarity can be operationalized by using Kiesler's (1983) *interpersonal circle,* which represents interpersonal behaviors as a combination of two basic motivations: *control* and *affiliation.* Control (dominance vs. submissiveness) is placed on the vertical axis, and affiliation (friendliness vs. hostility) is placed on the horizontal axis. Complementary behaviors on the control axis are thought to be on opposite poles (submission pulls for dominance; dominance pulls for submission), whereas complementary behaviors on the affiliation axis are thought be on the same pole (friendliness pulls for friendliness; hostility pulls for hostility). As an example of how dysfunctional cognitive–interpersonal cycles can maintain, say, depression, imagine an individual with an interpersonal schema that anticipates rejection from others (e.g., "If I express myself, others will reject me"). This individual will selectively interpret neutral behavior as rejecting and antagonistic, and will respond accordingly with anger or withdrawal (dominant or submissive behavior). Either behavior may distance the other, confirming and strengthening the individual's interpersonal schema that expressing oneself leads to rejection from others. Thus, according to cognitive–interpersonal approaches, schemas are not only responsible for erroneously *construing* the environment, but they are also involved in the *construction* of an individual's environment through these dysfunctional cognitive–interpersonal cycles (Safran & Segal, 1990/1996).

Very similar points have been made within the attachment framework. Attachment theory also predicts a self-fulfilling prophecy, whereby IWMs lead an individual to behave in ways that are consistent with how he or she expects to be treated by others (Hazan, 2003). In turn, these behaviors elicit reactions from others that are consistent with the individual's expectations. Attachment-related IWMs, therefore, are reinforced and internalized as cognitive representations of self and others that drive how an individual perceives, interprets, and responds to his or her environment (Shorey & Snyder, 2006).

Overall, CT and attachment theory appear extraordinarily complementary. It is not difficult to ascertain how each might inform the other, and how both in combination might lead to new insights in the practice of psychotherapy.

CLINICAL APPLICATIONS OF ATTACHMENT THEORY IN CBT

In this section, we explore the clinical applications of attachment theory in CBT. We discuss the implications of attachment theory and research for determining the client's suitability to CBT and conceptualizing cases and interventions. We also examine CBT in the light of the five suggestions Bowlby made for using attachment theory in psychotherapy.

Suitability for CBT

Research suggests that insecure attachment style adversely affects clients' approach to psychotherapy (for reviews, see Farber & Metzger, Chapter 3, and Mikulincer, Shaver, Cassidy, & Berant, Chapter 12, this volume). Adults classified as having dismissing states of mind with respect to attachment are less likely to report a history of psychotherapy (Riggs, Jacobvitz, & Hazen, 2002) and are less willing to seek psychotherapy than either preoccupied or secure adults are (Lopez, Melendez, Sauer, Berger, & Wyssmann, 1998). Once in therapy, dismissing adults are evaluated by their therapists as less disclosing about personal issues, more rejecting of treatment, less able to assist their therapists in constructing a joint coherent narrative to aid in comprehending early and painful attachment experiences, and less cooperative (Dozier, 1990; Dozier & Tyrrell, 1998; Dozier, Lomax, Tyrrell, & Lee, 2001; Hardy et al., 1999). Preoccupied adults are thought to be demanding of and dependent on their therapists, to present as needy in therapy (Slade, 1999), and to experience more tension in the therapeutic alliance (Eames & Roth, 2000). In working with preoccupied adults, therapists tend to avoid interpretation, work to contain the clients' emotion and to help them reflect on their experience, and support (rather than challenge) the clients' interpretation of experience (Hardy et al., 1999).

Research also shows that adult attachment style may interact with treatment type to influence treatment outcome. In a study examining the effects of brief dynamic therapy, Horowitz, Rosenberg, and Bartholomew (1993) found that clients reporting problems consistent with avoidant attachment (e.g., being domineering and cold) showed less improvement. In a more stringent test of the interaction between attachment style and treatment, Tasca et al. (2006) examined the role of attachment in predicting outcome in two group treatments for binge-eating disorder, one CBT and one psychodynamic–interpersonal. Attachment-related anxiety was positively associated with improvement in CBT but not in the psychodynamic treatment. Attachment-related avoidance was not related to improvement in either treatment, but was associated with dropping out of CBT.

We have detected somewhat similar patterns in our own research. We (McBride, Atkinson, Quilty, & Bagby, 2006) conducted a randomized controlled trial in which we investigated whether attachment-related anxiety and avoidance moderated treatment outcomes for depressed individuals undergoing a course of either CBT or interpersonal psychotherapy (IPT; Weissman, Markowitz, & Klerman, 2000). The results showed that avoidant clients enrolled in CBT showed a greater reduction in depression than avoidant adults enrolled in IPT did. One possible reason for this finding is that CBT's focus on logic may have been congruent with avoidant clients' valuing of cognition over emotion. IPT's focus on relationships and communication may have been too threatening for avoidant clients because of their propensity to regulate affect by deactivating thoughts and feelings related to attachment. Anxiously attached clients appeared to do equally well in either manualized treatment. Together, these early studies show that having an understanding of attachment theory and research can inform clinical thinking by encouraging therapists to take clients' attachment style into consideration when selecting a clinical approach.

Safran and Segal (1990/1996) developed a CBT suitability rating scale that aids clinicians in deciding whether or not a client is likely to respond to CBT. Examples of items on the scale include accessibility to automatic thoughts, differentiation of emotions, and compatibility with the cognitive rationale. Although the McBride et al. (2006) results need to be replicated, and research examining the relationship between attachment security and treatment outcome is needed, clinical information about attachment security could also be used to determine suitability for CBT. It would be expected that CBT would be most suitable for clients who are low on both attachment-related avoidance and attachment-related anxiety (i.e., secure), followed by clients who are high on avoidance and low on anxiety (i.e., dismissing), followed by clients who are low on avoidance and high on anxiety (i.e., preoccupied). CBT might be least suitable for clients who are high on both avoidance and anxiety (i.e., fearful), although this group would likely present the most challenges to any psychotherapeutic approach.

Cognitive Assessment and Case Formulation

Conducting effective CBT requires ongoing cognitive assessment to aid in the development of a specific case formulation. The key aspect of the case formulation is that it ties together all of a client's problems and provides a guide for understanding and treating the client's current difficulties (Persons, 1989). Because CT sees dysfunctional schemas as constituting a root cause of the client's presenting problems, clearly describing them is fundamental to a strong CBT-based case formulation. A good working hypothesis of the relationship between a client's overt difficulties and the underlying schemas helps the therapist understand the association among problems endorsed by the client, predict the client's behavior, decide on a treatment plan, and choose appropriate interventions.

The process of developing hypotheses about underlying schemas is challenging, partly because schemas are not readily accessible to conscious thought. Having information about a client's attachment style is an extremely useful tool in case formulation; it provides important clues about the underlying schemas that precipitated and are maintaining the psychopathology. According to Liotti (2002), those with avoidant attachment construct schemas in which the self is portrayed as bound to loneliness and self-reliance, and others are portrayed as unwilling to provide comfort. Anxiously attached individuals, in contrast, construct working models wherein the self is viewed as helpless, and others are viewed as unpredictable and intrusive. Finally, the schemas of those with a disorganized or disoriented pattern of attachment portrays both self and others as unavailable in times of distress.

In psychotherapy it is not always possible to conduct a lengthy assessment of adult attachment, such as the Adult Attachment Interview (George, Kaplan, & Main, 1984, 1985, 1996). Self-report measures that focus on close relationships are also useful tools that help the therapist understand the underlying schemas. Having assessed a client's attachment style as preoccupied, for example, the therapist could hypothesize from the outset that schemas of the self would be in the realm "I'm unlovable," schemas of others would be in the realm "Others are unavailable," and interpersonal schemas would be in the realm "If I express my needs, others will reject me." By examining early experiences with parents and patterns in peer relationships, the therapist can draw more specific conclusions about these hypothesized schemas that are based on a client's attachment style. To illustrate these ideas, consider the following vignette:

Kate, a 30-year-old woman, was referred for CBT by her family doctor. She presents with anxiety and depression symptoms. Her symptoms began after the breakup of a long-term relationship. She often cries for no apparent reason, and she has lost weight in the last month. She has also had a few panic attacks when ruminating on her sense of loneliness. Kate is feeling responsible for the dissolution of the relationship, noting that she "drove him away." She describes herself in relationships as initially very assertive and confident, but over time as needy and dependent. As an example, she reported being extremely anxious if she was unable to get hold of her partner. She tended to "fear the worst" and to call him repeatedly until she reached him. Kate admitted that she was similar as a child and would have "separation anxiety" if away from her mother. Kate described her upbringing as "turbulent." Her parents bitterly divorced when she was 5 or 6, and she remembered being involved in a lengthy custody battle. She was raised by her mother, whom she described as "overprotective" and "anxious." Kate noted that her mother was afraid for her safety and health and would seldom allow Kate to "do normal kid things" (e.g., have sleepovers, climb trees). Although her mother was strict in some ways, she was, in Kate's words, "emotionally dependent" on her, and Kate noted that her mother treated her "more as a friend than a daughter." Her mother would often disclose her loneliness to Kate. She eventually remarried, but Kate did not get along well with her stepfather.
When Kate was 16 years old, her older brother unexpectedly died. She was very close to him, and his death greatly affected her. Since his death, Kate has become hypervigilant and highly anxious about her own health and the health of those close to her. She often misinterprets physical sensations as evidence that she has some form of cancer, even

though extensive medical tests have always come back negative. In terms of romantic relationships, Kate noted that she tends to be attracted to "dominating and self-confident" men. An examination of her relationship history revealed that her first serious boyfriend was unfaithful to her on numerous occasions. Therefore, her anxiety increases if she perceives romantic partners as emotionally unavailable, often fearing that they will be unfaithful to her or break up with her. Kate reacts to these fears by putting others' needs before her own and with reassurance-seeking behavior—qualities that she does not like about herself.

Having knowledge of Kate's attachment pattern in close relationships, coupled with information about her upbringing and relationship history, helps the therapist develop a good working hypothesis of the underlying schemas. A self-report inventory reveals that Kate has a preoccupied attachment style. Kate's description of her mother as overinvolved and role-reversing suggests that the mother was herself preoccupied—a possibility consistent with the high degree of intergenerational transmission that characterizes IWMs of attachment (van IJzendoorn, 1995). Preoccupied mothers tend to place their own emotional needs before those of their children and respond inconsistently to their infants' bids for comfort and reassurance (Ainsworth, Blehar, Waters, & Wall, 1978). Kate probably developed both the view that she had to be strong for others (i.e., bear the weight of her mother's loneliness) in order to receive love, and the view that she was vulnerable in a world not forthcoming in stable support. Her first experience in a romantic relationship was (coincidentally) negative, and thus reinforced her insecure attachment style. The therapist can theorize that Kate's childhood and early romantic relationship experiences led to the development of schemas of instability and abandonment in relationships, and to schemas of the self as unlovable and helpless. Furthermore, her mother's own anxiety and overprotection regarding Kate's health and safety, together with her brother's untimely death, probably resulted in the schemas "I'm vulnerable" and "The world is an unsafe place." Finally, her interpersonal schemas are probably in the realm of "If I let my guard down, others will abandon, leave, or reject me." The treatment plan can be to help revise her core beliefs of self and others within relationships, and to reduce her sense of vulnerability and anxiety about her own and other's health and safety. Additional goals can include helping Kate reduce her insecure attachment-related behaviors (e.g., intense reassurance seeking) directly linked to her underlying mental representations of self, others, and the interaction of the two.

CBT Interventions

Once maladaptive schemas have been identified and an initial case conceptualization has been developed, CBT interventions can be used for cognitive restructuring and behavioural change. In CBT, various interventions are useful in accomplishing these goals, including *automatic thought records* (ATRs), behavioral experiments, and action plans, as well as various schema change interventions (e.g., the *positive data log*, continuum methods, historical tests of schemas). Knowledge of a client's attachment style can inform these clinical interventions by providing the therapist with a framework of the mental representations that are negatively influencing cognitions and behaviors.

ATRs are used in CBT to help clients identify, evaluate, and challenge errors in thinking. To continue with the example of Kate, having knowledge of her preoccupied attachment style will help the therapist anticipate that in interpersonal situations, she is susceptible to particular instantiations of *personalization* (seeing negative events as indicative of a personal characteristic) and *mind reading* (concluding that others are negatively reacting to you) cognitive errors. Given her anxiety about the loss of attachment relationships, she is probably also prone to *catastrophizing* errors, particularly related to the misinterpretation of the whereabouts of others as well as her own physical health. The therapist can customize and tailor CBT interventions by giving her a specific rationale for why these thoughts are emerging, given her attachment style and attachment history, so that she can learn to anticipate and readily challenge predictable patterns of cognitive errors by using ATRs.

Knowledge of the client's attachment style can also assist the therapist in appreciating the adaptive value and historical significance of clients' current and past approaches to coping their presenting problems and how their selections serve to maintain problematic cognitive–interpersonal patterns. For example, having a childhood experience of attachment figures as distant and cold can result in a working model of self as unlovable and incompetent, and a working model of others as unreliable and distant. As adults, these individuals are prone to reacting to interpersonal problems by devaluing the importance of relationships and maintaining interpersonal distance (i.e., avoidance). Avoidant behavior, however, decreases communication with others and interferes with the ability to assert needs. The end result is that others are either unaware of what these individuals' needs are, or react negatively to their avoidance, reinforcing a view of the self as unlovable/incompetent and of others as unreliable/distant. Behavioral experiments and action plans can be used to help break avoidance behavior, and test the negative interpretation that "others will not respond" if one asserts needs and increases communication.

Knowledge of a client's attachment style can also usefully inform interventions aimed at schema change. The positive data log, for example, is an intervention that is used to help strengthen new adaptive schemas by correcting information-processing errors (Padesky, 1994). The positive data log is set up as a task to encourage the client to actively look for information to support the new and more adaptive schema; the client is encouraged to observe and record on a daily basis information that is consistent with the new schema, no matter how small or insignificant it might seem. As noted by Padesky (1994), a therapist can assume that a client will discount, distort, and resist information that is not consistent with the old schema, and the challenge for the therapist is to support and encourage clients to perceive and record data they do not believe exist. Knowledge that a client's attachment style is preoccupied will allow the therapist to hypothesize that maladaptive IWMs of self may include "I'm unlovable" and IWMs of others may include "Others will abandon me," whereas knowing that a client has an avoidant attachment style will allow the therapist to hypothesize that IWMs of self may include "I'm incompetent" and IWMs of others may include "Others will reject me." The therapist can also anticipate the type of information that will be discounted by the client. A preoccupied client, for example, will have a tendency to minimize experiences where others are encouraging and supportive, whereas an avoidant client will discount experiences where others respond to his or her needs.

CBT and Bowlby's Five Therapeutic Tasks

As discussed earlier, Bowlby argued that attachment theory plays a key role in the psychotherapeutic process and suggested five key tasks through which psychotherapy could accomplish the goals of restructuring representational models of self and attachment figures. Although attachment theory and principles are not explicit components of CBT, CBT can be readily framed in terms of Bowlby's tasks.

According to Bowlby, the first task of the therapist is to provide clients with a secure base from which to explore painful and previously unexamined aspects of life. As in all psychotherapies, the therapeutic relationship is of utmost importance in CBT, though it has not traditionally been given a central role. The therapeutic relationship is a nonspecific factor common to all psychotherapies and is known to be a powerful predictor of outcomes (Zuroff & Blatt, 2006; Wampold, 2001). The CBT therapist works to establish a safe, trusting, nonjudgmental environment (i.e., a secure base) in which the client feels free to explore thoughts and feelings. Although CBT is a here-and-now therapy, and therefore painful aspects of a client's current life are the focus of treatment, past experiences are examined when a present focus has not provided sufficient relief (J. S. Beck, 1995) or when personality change is the explicit goal of treatment (e.g., in schema-focused therapy; Young, 1990).

Bowlby's second suggestion was that therapists should explore patterns in relationships (expectations, feelings, and behaviors). In CBT, patterns in relationships are explored in the context of schemas. Schemas of self, others, and self and others in interaction are examined, and thoughts, emotions, and behaviors that are congruent with these schemas are identified. Interventions are aimed to change the underlying schemas, and therefore the enduring, constricted, and predictable patterns of thoughts, emotions, and behaviors.

The third suggestion was that psychotherapy should include an exploration of how attachment patterns influence the therapeutic relationship. Although use of the therapeutic relationship is not an explicit intervention used in CBT, information gathered from the therapeutic relationship can inform the therapist of underlying schemas driving information processing. Recent advances in CBT, however (e.g., the cognitive–interpersonal approach; Safran & Segal, 1990/1996), make explicit recommendations for how the therapeutic relationship can be used to facilitate schema change.

Bowlby's fourth suggestion was that therapists should explore how attachment patterns influence current relationships. In CBT, an exploration of how attachment patterns influence current relationships can be done in the context of ATRs and behavioral experiments, if the focus of these interventions is an interpersonal situation. Examining the cognitive–interpersonal cycles, wherein the exploration is on how underlying schemas influence how a client interacts with and elicits responses from significant others, also accomplishes this goal.

Finally, Bowlby suggested that therapists should help their clients recognize and alter maladaptive models of self and other derived either from past experiences or from parent–child interactions. This suggestion is an implicit goal in CBT. In particular, the aim in CBT is to help the clients identify and change maladaptive schemas that are driving information processing and influencing thoughts, emotions, and behaviors. In essence, CBT is helping the clients recognize and alter models of self and others that developed as a result of early life experiences (including parent–child interactions).

THE INTEGRATION OF CBT AND ATTACHMENT: A CLINICAL CASE STUDY

In this section, we present a clinical case to illustrate in detail how attachment theory and research can inform a 16-week CBT protocol. The client, Laura (her name has been changed to protect confidentiality), is currently being treated for recurrent major depression and social phobia by one of us (Carolina McBride), using a CBT approach. Laura has completed 9 sessions of a 16-week treatment protocol. She has consented to disclosure of her information, but her identifying data have been altered.

Background Information

Laura is a 47-year-old woman who presently lives with her common-law partner of 15 years. They do not have any children, and Laura noted at intake that this was her explicit decision, as she never wanted any. Laura has a bachelor of arts and a law degree, and is currently employed as a partner in a law firm. Her family doctor referred her for treatment of depression and requested either IPT or CBT.

History of Presenting Problem

Laura presented with a history of chronic feelings of dissatisfaction with her life, marked by recurrent periods of major depression. She reported that her most recent episode of depression, which began approximately 8 months prior to the intake appointment, was precipitated by a number of stressors, including the departure of several coworkers (which resulted in an increase in her workload). She felt that she did not have a good balance between personal life and work; she often skipped lunches and worked until 8:00 P.M. In addition, Laura reported that she was saddened this summer when her family doctor advised her that she is currently in menopause. She indicated that although she never wanted to have children, the fact that this chapter of her life has closed has been difficult for her to accept. Finally, Laura indicated that since the death of her father 5 years ago, she has been increasingly involved in her 86-year-old mother's care. She has always found her mother to be a difficult woman and has been having increasing conflict with her, which leaves her feeling both resentful that the responsibility has fallen on her shoulders and guilty for having these negative feelings and thoughts.

At intake, the results from the Structured Clinical Interview for DSM-IV Axis I Disorders (First, Spitzer, Gibbon, & Williams, 1997) were consistent with a diagnosis of major depressive disorder, recurrent, moderate, as defined by the most recent version of the *Diagnostic and Statistical Manual of Mental Disorders,* fourth edition, text revision (DSM-IV-TR; American Psychiatric Association, 2000). Her symptoms of depression included sad mood, loss of interest, difficulties sleeping (e.g., middle insomnia), fatigue, difficulties concentrating, and self-criticism. Laura also reported symptoms that would meet DSM-IV-TR criteria for social phobia, generalized. She reported experiencing anxiety in a number of different social situations (e.g., parties, meetings, speaking to people in authority, being assertive, formally speaking to peers, and maintaining conversations). She reported fears that she will not have anything to say; that she will appear "boring," "socially inept," or foolish; or that others might become upset, grow defensive, and reject her. Laura indicated that she invariably experiences anxiety in these situations and recognized that her fear is excessive. She believed that her anxiety was interfering with work (e.g., being less able to network, turning down speaking engagements), and that she might have more friends if it were not for her anxiety.

Family History

Laura grew up with both parents and two younger brothers. Her mother was formally trained as a nurse, but stayed home to raise her children on the insistence of her father, a pharmacist. She indicated that her mother was the matriarch of the household. Laura recalled that her parents frequently fought in front of the children, with her mother typically becoming angry and screaming at her father while he ignored her and read the newspaper. She suspected that her mother was unhappy in their marriage and felt very isolated. Both parents would often physically punish the children, hitting them very hard with boards. She remembered several instances of abuse where her mother or father would walk her down to a cold room in the basement or the back shed and repeatedly hit her with a board (40 or 50 blows)—enough to leave her "black and blue for weeks." This abuse stopped when she was about 14 years old. She also noted that her mother often made her feel as if she was "a sneaky, bad child," whose natural tendency would be toward dishonesty and malevolent behavior were it not for strict discipline. As a result, Laura would often overcompensate and be "extra good" to prove to her mother that she was not devious and troublesome. She also had memories of her father as an emotionally distant and cold person. She did not remember receiving any physical affection from him and noted that he would become visibly uncomfortable if she gave him a hug (which she rarely did). She found that she could only connect with him when talking about work, and was terribly saddened after his death because she felt she had lost the opportunity to "really get to know him." Regarding her upbringing, Laura wrote in her diary, "I never got the message [that] someone would love me—that I was loveable. I NEVER got that latter message."

Laura suspects that her mother might have suffered from depression, but is unsure because her mother has always been reluctant to discuss these emotional difficulties, preferring to show a "stiff upper lip." She reported that a distant relative committed suicide during the Great Depression. She also reported that both of her grandfathers were "alcoholics."

Relationship History

In terms of friendships, Laura felt she had let many friendships slip away over the years due to increased job stress, especially over the past 4–5 years. She rarely disclosed personal issues or troubles to friends, including her romantic partner, for fear of upsetting others or being seen as a complainer.

Laura described a good relationship with her partner, but she admitted to "keeping her distance" and being uncomfortable opening up and sharing her private thoughts and feelings with him. Laura had not had many boyfriends before him, commenting, "I wasn't ever much into relationships." It was her decision never to marry or have any children. She noted that she never saw herself as being "maternal" and was never interested in being a mother. As a result, she was confused as to why she is so saddened by menopause and the knowledge that she can never have children, but she did note that menopause "underscores my feeling that I don't really love anyone."

Psychological Assessment

Test results were obtained for the following self-report instruments:

1. Beck Depression Inventory–II (BDI-II; Beck, Steer, & Brown, 1996)
2. Beck Anxiety Inventory (BAI; Beck & Steer, 1990)
3. Experiences in Close Relationships (ECR; Brennan, Clark, & Shaver, 1998)
4. Dysfunctional Attitudes Scale (DAS; Weissman & Beck, 1979)

Laura's depression was moderate (BDI-II), and she endorsed a higher-than-average number of depression-related attitudes (DAS), which suggested a perfectionistic streak and strong needs for approval. On the ECR, Laura reported feelings and behaviors consistent with a dismissing attachment style; she described herself as content and comfortable without close relationships, and emphasized her preference for self-sufficiency and her discomfort with either depending on others or being depended on.

Mental Status

Laura arrived on time for her intake appointment. She was very well groomed and formally dressed. Her affect appeared depressed, which was congruent with her reported mood. She cried at several points during the interview, but appeared uncomfortable with the tears and apologized for becoming emotional. There was nothing remarkable about her speech, and no motor or perceptual abnormalities were noted. Laura was friendly and cooperative throughout the assessment, and her alliance potential was judged to be good. There was no evidence of active suicidal ideation or intent.

Recommendations

Laura was deemed to be an appropriate candidate for psychotherapy. Although the IPT approach might seem suitable, as several interpersonal events were linked to the onset of her depression (menopause, increased work demands, conflict with her mother, grief over her father's death), the therapist decided to use a CBT approach for several reasons. Laura admitted to being more "cerebral" than "emotional," and noted that she is goal-oriented and focused. She endorsed a CBT rationale for her depression: "I need to change the way I think about things." Her ability to access automatic thoughts and differentiate emotions was deemed to be good, and she appeared motivated for treatment. Results from her responses to the ECR also played an important role in the decision. In particular, her dismissing style in close relationships indicated that CBT would probably be a better choice of treatment than IPT.

Case Conceptualization

At the second appointment, Laura was provided with feedback on the self-report questionnaires she completed, including her romantic attachment style. Laura agreed that in romantic relationships she tends to be distant and avoidant and is uncomfortable opening up and being close to her partner. The therapist linked her attachment style to Laura's early life experiences, and together they created a working hypothesis of the underlying schemas that were influencing her thoughts and mood. In particular, it was hypothesized that her mother's authoritarian discipline and cold, distant interpersonal style, coupled with the modeling of her parents' unhappy marriage, resulted in core beliefs about the self as "bad" and beliefs about others as "unavailable." It was also hypothesized that Laura had a core belief that others think she is "malicious," "stupid," and "incompetent." Given that both her mother and her father were punitive and would use physical means of disciplining, she learned early that it was better to inhibit her emotions and not irritate her parents, thereby decreasing the probability that they would negatively respond to her. Given her attachment style, interpersonal schemas that were formulated included "If I assert my needs, I will be punished" and "If I express emotion, others will not respond."

These core beliefs were hypothesized to be negatively influencing Laura's current thoughts and behavior, leading to depression and social anxiety. In particular, her view of self as bad and her perception that others view her negatively have led to personalization and mind-reading cognitive errors that maintain her anxiety in social situations. In particular, she is continually fearful that others will judge her harshly and negatively, increasing her anxiety around and avoidance of others. Furthermore, in order to compensate for what she believes others think of her, Laura admitted to working twice as hard as her colleagues and never saying "no" to extra work demands. This unassertiveness at work has resulted in an increased workload, which ultimately precipitated her most recent depressive episode. Furthermore, she is unable to stand up to her mother for fear of repercussions, and therefore has agreed to be her primary caregiver without complaint.

Based on this cognitive conceptualization, treatment goals included helping Laura reduce the amount of time she spent at work, assisting her in asking for help regarding the care of her mother, and increasing her social support system. The therapist and Laura also agreed to target her grief about her father's death and her difficulty in accepting menopause. The therapist explained to Laura the CBT interventions that would be used to accomplish these goals, including an activity schedule, ATRs, and exposure work.

CBT Interventions

Given that Laura identified one of her strengths as being a goal-oriented and driven individual, the first task of therapy was to help her reduce the amount of time she spent at work and to increase her pleasurable activities. An activity schedule was initially used in order for the therapist to get a clear understanding of how much time she was spending at work. A review of the activity schedule, in which Laura recorded her daily activities and her associated mood, indicated that she was staying at work until 8 or 9 P.M. on most nights and that this was having a substantial negative impact on her mood. The therapist and Laura then tackled her work schedule, using a graduated approach. Her first homework assignment was to leave work every day at 7 P.M. (Laura came up with a time she thought would be attainable and realistic). She stated that her ultimate goal would be to leave work by 6 P.M. Monday through Thursday and by 5 P.M. on Fridays. Because of her dismissing attachment style and her social anxiety, the therapist suggested that if Laura did not leave work by 7 P.M., she would need to call or e-mail the therapist. More specifically, her dismissing attachment style would suggest that Laura values self-reliance and would rather avoid reaching out for help. Laura agreed readily to the plan and admitted that she would be more likely to leave work in time if this were the consequence, as it would be easier than approaching the therapist and admitting "failure." After Laura successfully completed the first homework assignment, the time she had to leave work was gradually changed in 10-minute increments (6:50 P.M., 6:40 P.M., etc). By session 8, Laura was leaving work by 6:30 P.M. Monday through Thursday and by 5:30 P.M. on Friday. ATRs were used concurrently in order to address her negative beliefs about how others would view her if she left work earlier than her usual standard. The automatic thoughts within these records were identified and linked to her underlying schemas of self and others, as well as to her early attachment experiences with her mother and father. Once the thoughts were identified, Laura learned effective ways to challenge them. The activity and ATRs markedly improved her mood. By session 4, her depression scores on the BDI-II had improved from the moderate to the mild range.

In order to revise her underlying core beliefs, a positive data log was introduced in session 4 to help Laura gather evidence for a new core belief that she is competent and well regarded by peers. Initially, Laura had difficulty with this task. As is common with dismissing persons, she tended to discount information consistent with the new adaptive schema, despite its abundance. To dislodge this self-confirming habit, she and the therapist tackled her discounting through the use of ATRs.

Exposure work was used to tackle Laura's high level of attachment-related avoidance, both in her romantic relationship and with friends. The therapist and Laura developed an anxiety and avoidance hierarchy in session 5, in which her ultimate goals included being assertive with coworkers, inviting friends over for dinner, asking her brothers to become more involved in the care of their mother, and confiding more in her partner. Initial exposure exercises included situations that provoked moderate levels of anxiety or avoidance. These situations included calling friends during the week, disclosing her feelings to her partner, and saying "no" when coworkers asked her for extra work. Laura's dismissing attachment style helped maximize her homework compliance, which is known to be a positive predictor of treatment outcome in CBT (Addis & Jacobson, 2000). Dismissing adults are overly concerned about the possibility of failure and base their sense of self-worth on productivity, achievement, and control; therefore, Laura approached all homework tasks with diligence and attentiveness. Because interpersonal closeness was tackled in a hierarchical, graduated manner, Laura was able to regulate and minimize her anxiety about approaching others.

The next few sessions continued with graduated exposure to interpersonal connection, ATRs, positive data log, and reducing the amount of time spent at work. Laura's BDI-II was in the normal, nondepressed range by session 8. She reported that her sleep, concentration, and interest levels were markedly improved. She also noted that she was more aware of her self-critical thoughts and of how her views of self and others had developed. Although her old schemas were still active, Laura admitted that through the positive data log she was slowly improving her self-concept.

In session 8, the therapist and Laura began targeting the grief of her father's death. They explored how her relationship with him (and, in particular, the abuse she had endured) contributed to her construction of negative IWMs of self and other. Underlying schemas of self as "unlovable" and of others as "unavailable" that developed from her early attachment experiences were linked to her overt problems with depression and social anxiety, including negative automatic thoughts (e.g., "Others will judge me") and avoidant behaviors (e.g., having difficulty confiding in her partner, not asserting her needs at work). These early life experiences were also linked to her tendency to react to current interpersonal problems with her mother and partner by deactivating the importance of these relationships and maintaining interpersonal distance.

Laura also identified strong feelings of shame regarding the abuse, and ATRs were used to explore and challenge thoughts associated with these feelings. The links between these feelings of shame and her avoidant and nonassertive behavior were also highlighted, and behavioral experiments were used to help Laura increase interpersonal connection and assertion. Laura expressed regret about not knowing her father and not feeling connected to him. Knowledge of her attachment relationship with her father helped the therapist provide a context for reasons why interpersonal closeness was not possible with him. It is likely that her father also had a dismissing attachment style, as evidenced by his reaction to the few times she had tried to increase communication and connection. Laura, however, was able to write down her feelings toward her father and express what she would have liked to communicate to him. She found this intervention quite helpful, and was encouraged to think of ways in which she could increase communication and connection with the remaining members of her family, as well as with her partner and friends.

In summary, Laura has responded well to treatment thus far. Scores on the BDI-II indicate that her depressive symptoms are still in remission. Knowledge of her attachment style has helped to enrich the CBT case conceptualization and interventions and to improve outcome.

CONCLUSIONS

In this chapter we have illustrated how attachment theory can be easily integrated into the CBT approach. Attachment theory and CT are complementary—a fact that facilitates their integration in the psychotherapeutic context. As we have seen, knowledge of a client's attachment style is extremely useful for a therapist using the CBT approach, as it can inform the cognitive conceptualization and enrich the interventions used in clinical practice. We know that attachment theory provides a useful framework for understanding the development and maintenance of psychopathology. In addition, however, the importance of the social environment and attachment can provide the therapist with a greater understanding of the developmental and interpersonal issues driving schema formation and maintenance. Attachment theory and research provide the therapist with a solid framework of the mental representations that are negatively influencing a client's cognitions and behaviors. CBT is already a powerful treatment with proven efficacy for several different disorders. Our hope is that what we have presented here can be used to supplement this therapeutic approach, and to assist the CBT therapist in preparing a case formulation and treatment plan informed by theory and research in close relationships.

RECOMMENDATIONS FOR FURTHER READING

Baldwin, M. W. (Ed.). (2005). *Interpersonal cognition.* New York: Guilford Press.— This volume examines the processes by which people understand past and present interpersonal experiences, and how interpersonal cognition affects current interactions and sense of self.

Riso, L. P., du Toit, P. L., Stein, D. J., & Young, J. E. (Eds.). (2007). *Cognitive schemas and core beliefs in psychological problems: A scientist-practitioner guide.* Washington, DC: American Psychological Association.—This volume provides up-to-date information on the evaluation and utility of the schema concept as it applies to the research and treatment of a variety of clinical problems. The emphasis on cognitive schemas reflects several trends in CBT, including an increased focus on the developmental antecedents of psychopathology.

REFERENCES

Abramson, L. Y., Metalsky, G. I., & Alloy, L. B. (1989). Hopelessness depression: A theory-based subtype of depression. *Psychological Review, 96,* 358–372.

Abramson, L. Y., Seligman, M. E., & Teasdale, J. (1978). Learned helplessness in humans: Critique and reformulation. *Journal of Abnormal Psychology, 87,* 49–74.

Addis, M. E., & Jacobson, N. S. (2000). A closer look at treatment rationale and homework compliance in cognitive–behavioral therapy for depression. *Cognitive Therapy and Research, 24,* 313–324.

Ainsworth, M. D. S., Blehar, M. C., Waters, E., & Wall, S. (1978). *Patterns of attachment: A psychological study of the Strange Situation.* Hillsdale, NJ: Erlbaum.

Alford, B. A., & Beck, A. T. (1997). *The integrative power of cognitive therapy.* New York: Guilford Press.

American Psychiatric Association. (2000). *Diagnostic and statistical manual of mental disorders* (4th ed., text rev.). Washington, DC: Author.

Baldwin, M. W., Fehr, B., Keedian, E., Seidel, M., & Thompson, D. W. (1993). An exploration of the relational schemata underlying attachment styles: Self-report and lexical decision approaches. *Personality and Social Psychology Bulletin, 19,* 746–754.

Beck, A. T. (1967). *Depression: Clinical, experimental and theoretical aspects.* New York: Harper & Row.

Beck, A. T. (1976). *Cognitive therapy and the emotional disorders.* New York: International Universities Press.

Beck, A. T. (1987). Cognitive models of depression. *Journal of Cognitive Psychotherapy, 1,* 2–27.

Beck, A. T. (1996). Beyond belief: A theory of modes, personality, and psychopathology. In P. Salkovskis (Ed.), *Frontiers of cognitive therapy* (pp. 1–25). New York: Guilford Press.

Beck, A. T. (2002). Cognitive models of depression. In R. L. Leahy & E. T. Dowd (Eds.), *Clinical advances in cognitive psychotherapy: Theory and application* (pp. 29–61). New York: Springer.

Beck, A. T., Epstein, N., & Harrison, R. (1983). Cognitions, attitudes and personality dimensions in depression. *British Journal of Cognitive Psychotherapy, 1,* 1–16.

Beck, A. T., Rush, J., Shaw, B. F., & Emery, G. (1979). *Cognitive therapy of depression.* New York: Guilford Press.

Beck, A. T., & Steer, R. A. (1990). *Manual for the Beck Anxiety Inventory.* San Antonio, TX: Psychological Corporation.

Beck, A. T., Steer, R. A., & Brown, G. K., (1996). *Manual for the Beck Depression Inventory–II.* San Antonio, TX: Psychological Corporation.

Beck, J. S. (1995). *Cognitive therapy: Basics and beyond.* New York: Guilford Press.

Bowlby, J. (1973). *Attachment and loss: Vol. 2. Separation: anxiety and anger.* New York: Basic Books.

Bowlby, J. (1980). *Attachment and loss: Vol. 3. Loss: Sadness and depression.* New York: Basic Books.

Bowlby, J. (1982). *Attachment and loss: Vol. 1. Attachment* (2nd ed.). New York: Basic Books. (1st ed., 1969)

Bowlby, J. (1988). *A secure base.* New York: Basic Books.

Brennan, K. A., Clark, C. L., & Shaver, P. R. (1998). Self-report measurement of adult attachment: An integrative overview. In J. A. Simpson & W. S. Rholes (Eds.), *Attachment theory and close relationships* (pp. 46–76). New York: Guilford Press.

Collins, N. L., Guichard, A. C., Ford, M. B., & Feeney, B. C. (2004). Working models of attachment: New developments and emerging themes. In W. S. Rholes & J. A. Simpson (Eds.), *Adult attachment: Theory, research, and clinical implications* (pp. 196–239). New York: Guilford Press.

Coyne, J. C., & Gotlib, I. H. (1983). The role of cognition in depression: A critical appraisal. *Psychological Bulletin, 9,* 4472–4505.

Coyne, J. C., & Gotlib, I. H. (1986). Studying the role of cognition in depression: Well-trodden paths and cul-de-sacs. *Cognitive Therapy and Research, 10,* 794–812.

Dozier, M. (1990). Attachment organization and treatment use for adults with serious psychopathological disorders. *Development and Psychopathology, 2,* 47–60.

Dozier, M., Lomax, L., Tyrrell, C. L., & Lee, S. W. (2001). The challenge of treatment for clients with dismissing states of mind. *Attachment & Human Development, 3,* 62–76.

Dozier, M., & Tyrrell, C. (1998). The role of attachment in therapeutic relationships. In J. A. Simpson & W. S. Rholes (Eds.), *Attachment theory and close relationships* (pp. 221–248). New York: Guilford Press.

Eames, V., & Roth, A. (2000). Patient attachment orientation and the early working alliance: A study of patient and therapist reports of alliance quality and ruptures. *Psychotherapy Research, 10,* 421–434.

First, M. B., Spitzer, R. L., Gibbon, M., & Williams, J. B. W. (1997). *User's Guide for the Structured Clinical Interview for DSM-IV Axis I Disorders (SCID-I).* Washington, DC: American Psychiatric Press.

George, C., Kaplan, N., & Main, M. (1984). *Adult Attachment Interview protocol.* Unpublished manuscript, University of California, Berkeley.

George, C., Kaplan, N., & Main, M. (1985). *Adult Attachment Interview protocol* (2nd ed.). Unpublished manuscript, University of California, Berkeley.

George, C., Kaplan, N., & Main, M. (1996). *Adult Attachment Interview protocol* (3rd ed.). Unpublished manuscript, University of California, Berkeley.

Gilbert, D. T. (1992). "How mental systems believe": Reply. *American Psychologist, 4,* 670–671.

Gotlib, I. H., & Hammen, C. L. (1992). *Psychological aspects of depression: Toward a cognitive–interpersonal integration.* New York: Wiley.

Hardy, G. E., Aldredge, J., Davidson, C., Rowe, C., Reilly, S., & Shapiro, D. A. (1999). Therapist responsiveness to client attachment styles and issues observed in client-identified significant events in psychodynamic–interpersonal psychotherapy. *Psychotherapy Research, 9,* 36–53.

Hazan, C. (2003). The essential nature of couple relationships. In S. M. Johnson & V. E. Whiffen (Eds.), *Attachment processes in couple and family therapy* (pp. 43–63). New York: Guilford Press.

Hill, C. R., & Safran, J. D. (1994). Assessing interpersonal schemas: Anticipated responses of significant others. *Journal of Social and Clinical Psychology, 13,* 366–379.

Horowitz, L. M., Rosenberg, S. E., & Bartholomew, K. (1993). Interpersonal problems, attachment styles, and outcome in brief dynamic psychotherapy. *Journal of Consulting and Clinical Psychology, 61,* 549–560.

Joiner, T., & Coyne, J. C. (1999). *The interactional nature of depression: Advances in interpersonal approaches.* Washington, DC: American Psychological Association.

Kiesler, D. J. (1983). The 1982 interpersonal circle: A taxonomy for complementarity in human transactions. *Psychological Review, 90*, 185–214.

Kiesler, D. J. (1996). *Contemporary interpersonal theory and research: Personality, psychopathology, and psychotherapy.* New York: Wiley.

Liotti, G. (2002). Patterns of attachment and the assessment of interpersonal schemata: Understanding and changing difficult patient–therapist relationships in cognitive psychotherapy. In R. L. Leahy & T. E. Dowd (Eds.), *Clinical advances in cognitive psychotherapy: Theory and application.* New York: Springer.

Lopez, F. G., Melendez, M. C., Sauer, E. M., Berger, E., & Wyssmann, J. (1998). Internal working models, self-reported problems, and help-seeking attitudes among college students. *Journal of Counseling Psychology, 45*, 79–83.

Main, M., Kaplan, N., & Cassidy, J. (1985). Security in infancy, childhood, and adulthood: A move to the level of representation. In I. Bretherton & E. Waters (Eds.), Growing points of attachment theory and research. *Monographs of the Society for Research in Child Development, 50*(1–2, Serial No. 209), 66–104.

McBride, C., Atkinson, L., Quilty, L. C., & Bagby, R. M. (2006). Attachment as moderator of treatment outcome in major depression: A randomized control trial of interpersonal psychotherapy versus cognitive behavior therapy. *Journal of Consulting and Clinical Psychology, 74*, 1041–1054.

Mikulincer, M., Gillath, O., & Shaver, P. R. (2002). Activation of the attachment system in adulthood: Threat related primes increase the accessibility of mental representations of attachment figures. *Journal of Personality and Social Psychology, 83*, 881–895.

Mikulincer, M., Hirschberger, Nachmias, O., & Gillath, O. (2001). The affective component of the secure base schema: Affective priming with representations of attachment security. *Journal of Personality and Social Psychology, 81*, 305–321.

Mikulincer, M., & Shaver, P. R. (2007). *Attachment in adulthood: Structure, dynamics, and change.* New York: Guilford Press.

Padesky, C. (1994). Schema change processes in cognitive therapy. *Clinical Psychology and Psychotherapy, 1*, 267–278.

Persons, J. B. (1989). *Cognitive therapy in practice: A case formulation approach.* New York: Norton.

Riggs, A., Jacobvitz, D., & Hazen, N. (2002). Adult attachment and history of psychotherapy in a normative sample. *Psychotherapy: Theory, Research, Practice, Training, 39*, 344–353.

Sacco, W. P., & Beck, A. T. (1995). Cognitive theory and therapy. In E. E. Beckham & W. R. Leber (Eds.), *Handbook of depression* (2nd ed., pp. 329–351). New York: Guilford Press.

Safran, J. D. (1990). Towards a refinement of cognitive therapy in light of interpersonal theory: Interpersonal theory. *Clinical Psychology Review, 10*, 87–105.

Safran, J. D., & Greenberg, L. S. (Eds.). (1991). *Emotion, psychotherapy, and change.* New York: Guilford Press.

Safran, J., & Segal, Z. V. (1996). *Interpersonal process in cognitive therapy.* Northvale, NJ: Aronson. (Original work published 1990)

Safran, J. D., Segal, Z. V., Hill, C., & Whiffen, V. (1990). Refining strategies for research on self-representations in emotional disorders. *Cognitive Therapy and Research, 14*, 143–160.

Safran, J. D., Vallis, T. M., Segal, Z. V., & Shaw, B. F. (1986). Assessment of core cognitive processes in cognitive therapy. *Cognitive Therapy and Research, 10,* 509–526.

Schmidt, N. B., Schmidt, K. L., & Young, J. E. (1999). Schematic and interpersonal conceptualizations of depression: An integration. In T. Joiner & J. C. Coyne (Eds.), *The interactional nature of depression: Advances in interpersonal approaches* (pp. 127–148). Washington, DC: American Psychological Association.

Segal, Z. V., & Shaw, B. F. (1986). Cognition in depression: A reappraisal of Coyne and Gotlib's critique. *Cognitive Therapy and Research, 10,* 671–693.

Shaver, P. R., Collins, N. L., & Clark, C. L. (1996). Attachment styles and internal working models of self and relationship partners. In G. J. O. Fletcher & J. Fitness (Eds.), *Knowledge structure in close relationships: A social psychological approach* (pp. 25–61). Mahwah, NJ: Erlbaum.

Shorey, H. S., & Snyder, C. R. (2006). The role of adult attachment styles in psychopathology and psychotherapy outcomes. *Review of General Psychology, 10,* 1–20.

Slade, A. (1999). Attachment theory and research: Implications for the theory and practice of individual psychotherapy with adults. In J. Cassidy & P. R. Shaver (Eds.), *Handbook of attachment: Theory, research, and clinical applications* (pp. 575–594). New York: Guilford Press.

Tasca, G. A., Ritchie, K., Conrad, G., Balfour, L., Gayton, J., Lybanon, V., et al. (2006). Attachment scales predict outcome in a randomized controlled trial of two group therapies for binge eating disorder: An aptitude by treatment interaction. *Psychotherapy Research, 16,* 106–121.

Taylor, S. E., & Crocker, J. (1981). Schematic bases of social information processing. In E. T. Higgins, P. Herman, & M. Zanna (Eds.), *The Ontario Symposium: Vol. 1. Social cognition* (pp. 89–134). Hillsdale, NJ: Erlbaum.

van IJzendoorn, M. H. (1995). Adult attachment representation, parental responsiveness, and infant attachment: A meta-analysis on the predictive validity of the Adult Attachment Interview. *Psychological Bulletin, 117,* 387–403.

Wampold, B. E. (2001). *The great psychotherapy debate: Models, methods, findings.* Mahwah, NJ: Erlbaum.

Weissman, A. N., & Beck, A. T. (1978). *Development and validation of the Dysfunctional Attitude Scale: A preliminary investigation.* Paper presented at the annual meeting of the Association for Advancement of Behavior Therapy, Chicago.

Weissman, M. M., Markowitz, J. C., & Klerman, G. L. (2000). *Comprehensive guide to interpersonal psychotherapy.* New York: Basic Books.

Young, J. E. (1990). *Cognitive therapy for personality disorders: A schema-focused approach* (rev. ed.). Sarasota, FL: Professional Resource Exchange.

Young, J. E. (1994). *Cognitive therapy for personality disorders: A schema-focused approach* (rev. ed.). Sarasota, FL: Professional Resource Press.

Young, J. E., & Gluhoski, V. L. (1996). Schema-focused diagnosis for personality disorders. In F. W. Kaslow (Ed.), *Handbook of relational diagnosis and dysfunctional family patterns* (pp. 300–321). New York: Wiley.

Zuroff, D. C., & Blatt, S. J. (2006). The therapeutic relationship in the brief treatment of depression: Contributions to clinical improvement and enhanced adaptive capacities. *Journal of Consulting and Clinical Psychology, 74,* 130–140.

Part V

FUTURE DIRECTIONS

18

Attachment-Informed
Psychotherapy Research with Adults

Ety Berant
Joseph H. Obegi

Two enduring strengths of an attachment perspective are that it is anchored by a cohesive theory with considerable explanatory power and that it is paired with a tradition of empirical rigor. The contributors to this volume have capitalized on both strengths. Although attachment theory is viewed by some as an oversimplification of the human experience, our chapter authors use the theory to give rich descriptions of complex clinical phenomena, such as therapeutic relationship, therapeutic process, transference, and defensive functioning, while simultaneously grounding their observations in empirical research from both the clinical and nonclinical literatures. In addition, many contributors point out where more research is needed. Although research-oriented readers can sift chapters for suggestions, we hope to make this somewhat easier by collecting them here and adding our own observations.

Our primary task, however, is to provide a qualitative review of attachment-informed clinical studies produced to date. We attend only to studies that included clinical samples of adults, samples of mental health professionals or trainees, and nonclinical samples of adults in which clinical process variables were examined (e.g., interest in psychotherapy). We collected studies from the chapters of this volume, other recent comprehensive reviews (e.g., Daniel, 2006; Mikulincer & Shaver, 2007), and our own search of the PsycINFO and PubMed databases. Our review is organized into two broad areas: attachment security as it relates to therapeutic process and to outcome. Along the way, we note unresolved theoretical issues and emerging themes in attachment-informed psychotherapy. Before beginning, we wish to note that in the current atmosphere of empirically supported treatments, it is somewhat less common for researchers to study how personality influences psychotherapy process and outcome. However, as Norcross (2002) persuasively argues, manualized treatments tend to reduce clients to a set of symptoms and to ignore what is readily apparent to all clinicians—that is, "different types of clients respond better to different types of treatments and relationships" (p. 6). In this regard, attachment theory and research are poised to deepen our understanding of how personality differences influence clinical presentation, the therapeutic relationship, in-session behavior of clinicians, and the interaction of all these variables in shaping outcome.

ATTACHMENT STYLE AND PROCESS VARIABLES

Perhaps the largest gap between research findings on adult attachment and the practice of adult psychotherapy is between what we know about the intra- and interpersonal correlates of attachment security as they appear in nonclinical samples, and whether and how these correlates manifest themselves in psychotherapy. Indeed, the clinical descriptions of attachment styles offered throughout this volume often rely on an amalgam of inferences based on studies of nonclinical samples and clinical experience. As one example, Farber and Metzger (Chapter 3) note that although disclosure has been well studied by psychotherapy and attachment researchers, no studies have examined whether, for instance, dismissing *clients* are as reluctant to disclose private information as their nonclinical counterparts. Studies of the interactions between attachment security and process variables are sorely needed. (Researchers interested in this topic will find ample inspiration in Orlinsky, Rønnestad, & Willutzki's [2004], expert review of the psychotherapy process literature.) However, because attachment researchers have studied constructs that, in one way or another, overlap with process variables, there is a substantial literature on which to base new hypotheses. In the sections that follow, we summarize findings of process-oriented research to date.

Treatment Seeking, Engagement, and Alliance

Theoretically, avoidant adults place such a high value on independent problem solving and are so reluctant to admit distress that seeking psychotherapy would be a last resort. Conversely, anxious adults might readily enter treatment; they lack confidence in their coping abilities and suspect that handling problems independently will alienate supportive others. Three studies to date, using nonclinical samples, support these hypotheses (Table 18.1). Avoidant adults express less interest in psychological treatment even when they are distressed (Lopez, Melendez, Sauer, Berger, & Wyssmann, 1998; Vogel & Wei, 2005), and they are less likely to have a history of treat-

TABLE 18.1. Published Attachment-Informed Studies of Treatment Seeking, Engagement, and Alliance

Study	Outcome variable	Attachment scale	Main finding
Seeking psychotherapy			
Lopez et al. (1998)***	Interest in tx	RQ	Anxiety (ns), avoidance (–)
Riggs et al. (2002)***	Hx of tx	AAI	Secure > preoccupied > dismissing
Vogel & Wei (2005)***	ISCI	ECR	Anxiety (+), avoidance (–)
Therapeutic engagement			
Dozier (1990)	Engagement	AAI	Anxiety (–), avoidance (–)
Korfmacher et al. (1997)	Commitment	AAI	Secure > dismissing, disorganized
Goldman & Anderson (2007)	Dropout	AAS	Insecurity (ns)
Client attachment style and alliance			
Mallinckrodt et al. (1995)	WAI-C	CATS	Secure (+), preoccupied (+), avoidant-fearful (–)
Satterfield & Lyddon (1995)	WAI-C	AAS	Anxiety (ns), avoidance (–)
Hardy et al. (1998)	ARM	IIP	Anxiety (ns), avoidance (ns)
Satterfield & Lyddon (1998)	WAI-C	RQ	Secure (+), fearful (–)
Hardy et al. (2001)	TUI	IIP	Anxiety (ns), avoidance (–)
Tyrrell et al. (1999)**	WAI-C	AAI	Deactivating strategies (ns)
Kivlighan et al. (1998)	WAI-C	AAS	Anxiety (ns), avoidance (–)
Eames & Roth (2000)	WAI-C	RSQ	Fearful (–)
	WAI-T	RSQ	Secure (+)
	Ruptures-T	RSQ	Preoccupied (+)
Kanninen et al. (2000)	WAI-C	AAI*	(ns) at session 1, pattern differences
Parish & Eagle (2003)	CAQ	RQ	Secure (+), dismissing (–)
Sauer et al. (2003)	WAI-C	AAQ	Anxiety (ns), avoidance (ns)
Reis & Grenyer (2004)	WAI-C	RQ	Secure (+), dismissing (–)
Mallinckrodt et al. (2005)	WAI-C	ECR	Anxiety (–), avoidance (ns)
Hietanen & Punamaki (2006)	WAI-C	RQ	Secure > dismissing, fearful for W
			Secure, fearful > dismissing, preoccupied for M
	WAI-T		Secure, fearful > dismissing for M
Fuertes et al. (2007)	WAI-C	CATS	Secure (ns), preoccupied (ns), avoidant-fearful (–)
	WAI-T	CATS	Secure (ns), preoccupied (ns), avoidant-fearful (ns)
Goldman & Anderson (2007)	WAI-C	AAS	Security (+)
Therapist attachment style and alliance			
Dunkle & Friedlander (1996)	WAI-C	AAS	Anxiety (ns), avoidance (–)
Tyrrell et al. (1999)	WAI-C	AAI	Deactivating strategies (ns)
Ligiéro & Gelso (2002)	WAI-T	RQ	(ns)

(continued)

TABLE 18.1. (*continued*)

Sauer et al. (2003)	WAI-C	AAQ	Anxiety (+) at session 1, (–) over time; avoidance (ns)
Black et al. (2005)	ARM	ASQ	Anxiety (–), avoidance (–)
Client–therapist matching on attachment style and alliance			
Tyrrell et al. (1999)**	WAI-C	AAI	Client deactivation × therapist deactivation

Note. (+), positive association; (–), negative association; (ns), nonsignificant effects; *, adaptation of instrument; **, sample of nontherapists; ***, nonclinical sample; Hx of tx, history of mental health treatment; AAI, Adult Attachment Interview; AAQ, Adult Attachment Questionnaire; AAS, Adult Attachment Scale; ARM, Agnew Relationship Measure; ASQ, Attachment Style Questionnaire; CAQ-T, Components of Attachment Questionnaire targeting therapists; CATS, Client Attachment to Therapist Scale; ECR, Experiences in Close Relationships questionnaire; IIP, Inventory of Interpersonal Problems; ISCI, Intentions to Seek Counseling Inventory; M, men; RQ, Relationship Questionnaire; RSQ, Relationship Style Questionnaire; Ruptures-T, therapist report of therapeutic ruptures; TUI, Therapist Understanding and Involvement Scale (from the California Psychotherapy Alliance Scales); W, women; WAI-C, Working Alliance Inventory–Client version; WAI-T, Working Alliance Inventory–Therapist version.

ment (Riggs, Jacobvitz, & Hazen, 2002), whereas anxious adults exhibit the opposite patterns. Because avoidant adults have misgivings about professional support, particular care must be taken to ensure positive experiences early in psychotherapy. Unfortunately, we know little about the specific kinds of intervention that either avoidant or anxious adults perceive as welcoming, encouraging of continued engagement, or therapeutically helpful.

Several contributors to this volume (Farber & Metzger, Chapter 3; Nelson, Chapter 13; Florsheim & McArthur, Chapter 15), echoing other writers (e.g., Dozier & Tyrrell, 1998), point out the strong resemblance between many client behaviors and attachment behaviors in both their form (e.g., seeking proximity to therapists, crying) and their function (regulating distress). As such, secure-base dynamics (exploring versus seeking comfort) should be evident in interactions with therapists, and attachment insecurity should mold these in theoretically consistent ways. Only two studies have examined the impact of insecurity on therapeutic engagement (Table 18.1). Once in treatment, avoidant adults appear less engaged and appeal for help less often than other adults, but anxious adults also seem to struggle with getting the most out of treatment (Dozier, 1990; Korfmacher, Adam, Ogawa, & Egeland, 1997).

We currently know little about how attachment security predicts premature termination. Theoretically, both avoidance and anxiety may be related to termination, though for different reasons. Avoidant clients may be more inclined to exit treatment when the early focus of therapy challenges their attachment-related goals (i.e., self-sufficiency, controlling distress). Pursuing interventions such as a strong focus on emotional intimacy (e.g., pressures to disclose, intense focus on affect or interpersonal process) or examining personal weakness (e.g., focus on deficiencies) early in treatment is likely to trigger deactivating strategies—an extreme form of which is to abort an emotionally challenging relationship. In contrast, anxious clients enter treatment with a high subjective sense of distress. When they are not able to elicit some degree of comfort or sympathy from therapists (i.e., therapists do not appear to be viable attachment figures), their distress may be amplified to such an extent that they disengage from treatment in order to find a different, more responsive figure. Only one published study, with nonsignificant results, has examined these hypotheses (Goldman & Anderson, 2007). In an unpublished study by Berant, Mikulincer, and Loebel (2008), clients high in either avoidance or anxiety, as measured at intake, were more likely to leave a psychodynamic therapy (of up to 1 year) before reaching the 10th session.

We need to learn considerably more about how insecure clients behave in treatment and why they find treatment frustrating or satisfying. As an example of the former, when avoidant adults do enroll in treatment, they are (theoretically) inclined to discuss problems in an impersonal and intellectual way, externalize them, and minimize the importance of their therapists. Indeed, some of these qualities are plainly evident in transcripts of avoidant individuals' responses to the Adult Attachment Interview (AAI; George, Kaplan, & Main, 1984, 1985, 1996). However, although the AAI's questions somewhat resemble those asked by clinicians, they do not include a central focus of treatment: discussing and exploring presenting problems. Attachment-informed research using, for example, Hill's (1986) scheme for coding client utterances could enhance our knowledge in this area, as could work on the relationship between forms of insecurity and particular errors in mentalizing. Regarding dyadic interactions, McCluskey, Hooper, and Miller (1999) have taken an initial theoretical step by describing client–therapist communications in secure-base terms, though empirical studies of their ideas are needed.

The most frequently studied process variable in the clinical literature on adult attachment is the therapeutic alliance (Table 18.1). The alliance is a natural focus because of the numerous similarities between the client–therapist relationship and an attachment, between negotiating intimate issues in session and negotiating attachment needs with significant others, and between the dialectic of ambivalence and change in therapy and that of proximity seeking and exploration in secure-base dynamics. As contributors to this volume note (e.g., Farber & Metzger, Chapter 3; Mallinckrodt, Daly, & Wang, Chapter 10), insecurity—and the evidence appears particularly strong for avoidant clients—undermines alliance strength. How insecurity exerts its effect is, empirically, less clear. For anxious clients, one study suggests that the frequency of ruptures may play a role (Eames & Roth, 2000), though we know little about the kinds of ruptures either anxious or avoidant clients are prone to experience (e.g., empathic failures vs. perceptions of insufficient support from the therapist) or whether they exhibit different *rupture markers* (Samstag, Muran, & Safran, 2004). A combination of qualitative and quantitative approaches to studying alliance ruptures may be particularly helpful.

A current trend in alliance research is to examine patterns of alliance strength over the course of treatment, although this approach has met with mixed results so far (Horvath & Bedi, 2002). Taking insecurity into account in future studies could be fruitful. For example, Kanninen, Salo, and Puna-maki (2000) found that, compared to secure clients, insecure clients exhib-ited less optimal trajectories of alliance strength over 10–12 months of treat-ment. If replicated, this finding suggests that it is imperative for therapists to adapt their approach to the attachment style of their clients—a conclusion enthusiastically endorsed by the expert therapists consulted by Mallinck-rodt et al. (Chapter 10). Ignoring individual differences in attachment secu-rity could result in a mismatch of interpersonal styles that jeopardizes the quality of the alliance—perhaps the most important tool therapists have in their arsenal for promoting change (Martin, Garske, & Davis, 2000).

Of course, therapists are not neutral in their contribution to the alliance. Abundant evidence suggests that various personal qualities of therapists are related to strong or weak alliances (Ackerman & Hilsenroth, 2001, 2003). Theoretically, secure therapists are likely to possess alliance-enhancing char-acteristics (e.g., warmth, sensitivity), and therefore better able to create the atmosphere of security (i.e., to become a secure base) that Bowlby (1988) viewed as a prerequisite for productive therapeutic work. In general, find-ings from five studies examining this issue are supportive (Table 18.1). In addition to replicating these findings, researchers might consider examining the kinds of attitudes, pacing, and techniques secure therapists employ, as well as the flexibility of their responding to client communications. As Eagle and Wolitzky (Chapter 14) suggest, operationalizing Ainsworth's concept of sensitive responding (Ainsworth, Blehar, Waters, & Wall, 1978) in terms of clinicians' behavior is a potential starting point. More complex research questions include how the attachment styles of clients and therapists jointly influence the degree to which clients feel secure in the therapeutic alliance, and how this client–therapist matching influences therapeutic process and outcome. We discuss these questions further in the next section.

We suspect that attachment theory and research are poised to make important contributions to the alliance concept and to its role in therapeutic change. First, as we have already discussed, attachment theory can revital-ize the study of personality as it relates to the development and patterning of the therapeutic alliance. In creating a pan-theoretical vision of the alli-ance, Bordin (1979, p. 257) essentially disconnected alliance from theories of personality, despite his belief that how well clients can forge a bond to therapists hinges on their attitudes about intimacy.

Second, because attachment theory is in part a theory of how people idiosyncratically form, maintain, and dissolve emotional bonds, it is a natu-ral tool for studying how differences in attachment security influence the unfolding bond between clients and therapists. For example, one could ask:

How does attachment security promote treatment retention? How do insecure ways of relating interfere with the development of a strong alliance?

Third, although the concept of the therapeutic alliance has been the "flagship" of the scientist-practitioner model (Constantino, Castonguay, & Schut, 2002), it has several shortcomings. Specifically, alliance theory lacks a sophisticated view of how an emotional bond unfolds between client and therapist (Horvath, 2005; Obegi, in press). An attachment-informed view suggests that the alliance consists of two components: attachment security, the rough equivalent of *confident collaboration* as discussed in the alliance literature (Hatcher, 1999); and the attachment bond itself, the equivalent of the relatively underelaborated concept of the *therapeutic bond* in pan-theoretical formulations of the alliance. Translating the alliance in this way leads to a bounty of important questions: What factors contribute to an anxious versus an avoidant client's feeling of security in the therapeutic relationship? Is the stage model of attachment development, as framed by Bowlby (1969/1982) and Ainsworth (Ainsworth et al., 1978), applicable to the formation of attachment to the therapist? If so, how does attachment style impinge on or facilitate the client's development of an attachment to the therapist? And, finally, how is security in therapeutic relationships related to change, and to what extent is a clear-cut attachment required for change?

Attachment Style, Intervention, and Client–Therapist Matching

Three preliminary studies—one qualitative (Hardy et al., 1999) and two quantitative (Hardy, Stiles, Barkham, & Startup, 1998; Rubino, Barker, Roth, & Fearon, 2000)—have examined the relationship between the kinds of interventions therapists use and clients' attachment styles (Table 18.2). Together, the findings suggest that therapists are drawn to use more empathic reflections with anxiously attached clients. We suspect that this is because the narratives of anxious clients are laden with intense distress and desperate requests for support and validation. The findings regarding the use of interpretation are less clear. Whereas Hardy et al. (1999) found that therapists responded to client utterances indicative of a dismissing style with interpretation, Rubino et al. (2000) found that fearful clients elicited the most depthful interpretations. Clearly, more research in this area is desirable.

Three studies have examined clients' perceptions of their sessions (Table 18.2). Mallinckrodt, Porter, and Kivlighan (2005) found that as of sessions 3–7, clients' ratings of session depth and smoothness—the combination of which the researchers called *exploration*—were associated with feelings of security with respect to their therapists, but not to their more global sense of security in relationships. However, Mohr, Gelso, and Hill (2005) found that clients reporting a fearful style in relationships rated their sessions as less valuable and pleasant (security–insecurity with respect to the therapist was not measured). In contrast to these studies, Hardy et al. (1998)

TABLE 18.2. Published Attachment-Informed Studies of Therapeutic Intervention

Study	Outcome variable	Attachment scale	Main finding
Client attachment style and intervention			
Hardy et al. (1998)	Affective interventions	IIP	Anxiety (+)
	Cognitive interventions		Avoidance × treatment condition
	Depth		Anxiety × treatment condition
			Avoidance × treatment condition
	Smoothness		Anxiety (ns), avoidance (ns)
Hardy et al. (1999)†	Reflection	AAI*	Preoccupied (+)
	Interpretation		Dismissing (+)
Rubino et al. (2000)***	Empathic responding	Vignette	Fearful > secure, dismissing
	Interpretive depth		Fearful > secure, dismissing
Mallinckrodt et al. (2005)	Depth, smoothness	CATS	Secure (+), preoccupied (ns), avoidant-fearful (−)
		ECR	Anxiety (ns), avoidance (ns)
Mohr et al. (2005)***	Depth, smoothness	ECR	Fearful (−)
Therapist attachment style and intervention			
Dozier et al. (1994)**	Intervention depth	AAI	(ns)
	Dependency needs		Preoccupied > dismissing
Rubino et al. (2000)	Empathic responding	RSQ	Anxiety (−), avoidance (ns)
	Interpretive depth		Anxiety (ns), avoidance (ns)
Client–therapist match based on attachment style and intervention			
Dozier et al. (1994)**	Intervention depth	AAI	Client preoccupied × therapist secure
	Dependency needs		Client preoccupied × therapist secure
Rubino et al. (2000)***	Empathic responding	RSQ	Client fearful, secure × therapist anxiety
	Interpretive depth		(ns)
Mohr et al. (2005)***	Depth, smoothness	ECR	(ns)

Note. †, a qualitative study. Other symbols and abbreviations as in Table 18.1.

examined clients' ratings of *depth* (i.e., their perception of a session's value and power) in two kinds of psychotherapy. They found a modest tendency for avoidant clients in a 16-week cognitive-behavioral treatment to report greater depth than avoidant clients in either a shorter (8-week) cognitive-behavioral treatment or in a psychodynamic–interpersonal therapy (of 8 or 16 weeks). Anxious clients, on the other hand, reported greater depth in an

8-week psychodynamic–interpersonal therapy than did anxious clients in any of the other treatment conditions. To state the findings another way, there was a trend for clients to perceive more value in a treatment that resonated with their attachment-related goals.

These studies also highlight an important measurement issue: Which type of attachment scale—one focused on the therapy dyad, or one focused on relationships generally—is the "right" tool for the job? In work with non-clinical samples, adult attachment researchers have found that the strength of associations decreases when the domain tapped by an attachment scale is increasingly removed from the domain of relationships tapped by the independent variable under study (Crowell, Fraley, & Shaver, 1999). We suspect that a similar phenomenon will appear in the clinical literature on attachment. In addition, we wonder whether the predictive power of global assessments of security will decline as therapy advances. Theoretically, the influence of insecure and global internal working models should wane as a client develops a model specific to a therapist (and, ideally, one that is more secure; Obegi, in press). As the model of the therapist becomes elaborated and more accessible, it should have a stronger influence on thoughts, feelings, and behavior than global models.

Regarding therapists, it is not yet clear how their attachment styles are related to the frequency of particular kinds of interventions, or how they adapt their interventions to the attachment styles of their clients. Only two studies have examined this issue. Dozier, Cue, and Barnett (1994) found that less securely attached case managers were more likely to take dependency needs into account when intervening with clients, whereas Rubino et al. (2000) found that anxiously attached graduate-level therapists were less empathic overall than less anxious ones. Neither study found a relationship between a therapist's attachment style and the overall tendency to use "deeper" interventions (e.g., exploring emotions, depthful interpretations).

The picture becomes somewhat clearer when the interaction between clients' and therapists' attachment styles is considered (Table 18.2). In the Dozier et al. (1994) study, insecure case managers were especially likely to attend to dependency needs and intervene at greater depth when their clients were anxiously attached. In the Rubino et al. (2000) study, more anxious clinical graduate students responded less empathically to vignettes of fearful and secure clients. Taken together, these results might suggest that insecure case managers more readily perceive and respond to the emotional needs of their clients, but that this ability may not always result in more empathic interventions. More research is necessary to sort out how complementary and noncomplementary attachment styles affect the frequency of various therapeutic interventions. To borrow a commonly used mantra in discussions of empirically supported treatments, we need to know, in terms of attachment security, what kinds of therapists say and do what kinds of things with what kinds of clients.

A related question concerns how client–therapist matching on attachment style is related to the resolution of alliance ruptures. Initial research suggests that resolving ruptures improves therapeutic outcomes (Safran, Muran, Samstag, & Stevens, 2002). From an attachment-informed viewpoint, alliance ruptures can be understood as existing on a continuum ranging from mild disruptions in a client's sense of security in psychotherapy or in secure-base dynamics to full-blown attachment injuries[1] that seriously threaten the viability of therapeutic relationships. Farber and Metzger (Chapter 3) speculate that insecure therapists may be less well equipped to handle ruptures, especially with insecure clients. In the only study we are aware of that has examined this issue, Rubino et al. (2000) found that anxious therapists were rated as less empathic in response to therapeutic ruptures expressed by client actors in videotaped vignettes, especially when an actor portrayed a fearfully attached client. Examination of the relationship between attachment security and rupture repairs with actual therapy dyads is an exciting next step.

In closing this section, we wish to note that some studies relied on "homegrown" scales that were vaguely defined or lack demonstrated validity, thus making the interpretation of positive or null findings problematic. When possible, we encourage researchers to use field-tested rating scales and coding systems for analyzing and describing therapist interventions. For example, researchers interested in psychodynamic interpretation might consider the scales used by Hoglend (e.g., Hoglend, Johansson, Marble, Bogwald, & Amlo, 2007) in his excellent studies of the benefit of psychodynamic interpretation. Researchers interested in a more comprehensive analysis of therapist verbalizations might consider one of the many coding systems designed for this purpose (e.g., Hill, 1986).

Transference and Countertransference

The negative associations between insecurity and process variables discussed so far suggest that therapy-interfering transferences may be in play. However, only a few clinical studies have directly examined the relationship between attachment style and transference (Table 18.3). In a way, this is surprising in light of (1) the numerous studies that have documented the role of transference in close relationships (for a review, see Andersen & Saribay, 2005); (2) the overwhelming evidence that attachment style shapes how people think, feel, and behave in close relationships (for reviews, see Cobb & Davila, Chapter 9, this volume; Mikulincer & Shaver, 2007); (3) growing evidence that attachment style influences transference (Brumbaugh & Fraley, 2006, 2007); and (4) Bowlby's (1988) belief that resolving problematic transferences is essential to positive therapeutic outcome. Yet capturing transference in action is challenging; it currently requires complex experimental designs, time-consuming coding of narratives, or reliance on clinical judges.

As Tolmacz (Chapter 11, this volume) notes, anxiously attached clients are expected to exhibit a pattern of positive and negative transferences,

TABLE 18.3. Published Attachment-Informed Studies of Transference and Countertransference

Study	Outcome variable	Attachment scale	Main funding
Client attachment style and transference			
Diamond et al. (2003)	Transference	AAI, PT-AAI	AAI, PT-AAI concordance
Waldinger et al. (2003)	Autonomy wishes Closeness wishes	AAI	Dismissing > preoccupied (ns)
Woodhouse et al. (2003)	Neg. transf.	CATS	Secure (+), preoccupied (–), avoidant-fearful (ns)
Client attachment style and countertransference			
Martin et al. (2007)***	Pos. countertr.	Vignette	Secure, preoccupied > dismissing
	Well-being		Secure > dismissing, preoccupied
	Friendliness		Secure > dismissing, preoccupied
	Hostility		Dismissing > secure, preoccupied
Mohr et al. (2005)***	Neg. count. ratings	ECR	(ns)
Therapist attachment style and countertransference			
Ligiéro & Gelso (2002)	Neg. count. ratings	RQ	Secure (–)
Marmarosh et al. (2006)	Neg. expectations	SGAP	Anxiety (+), avoidance (ns)
Martin et al. (2007)	Pos. countertr.	RQ	(ns)
	Well-being		(ns)
	Friendliness		(ns)
	Hostility		(ns)
Mohr et al. (2005)	Neg. count. ratings	ECR	Dismissing (+)
Client–therapist match based on attachment style and countertransference			
Mohr et al. (2005)	Neg. count. ratings	ECR	Anxiety × Avoidance
Martin et al. (2007)	Pos. countertr.	RQ	(ns)

Note. Neg. count. ratings, supervisor ratings of therapists' countertransference behaviors; Neg. expectations, therapists' negative expectations of clients; Pos. countertr., therapists' ratings of positive countertransference; PT-AAI, Patient–Therapist Adult Attachment Interview; SGAP, Social Group Attachment Scale. Other symbols and abbreviations as in Table 18.1.

whereas dismissing clients should exhibit primarily negative transferences. Only one study has examined these predictions in a clinical sample. In a study of clients in ongoing psychotherapy, high scores on the Preoccupied/Merger scale of the Client Attachment to Therapist Scale (CATS; Mallinckrodt, Gantt, & Coble, 1995) and, unexpectedly, on the Secure scale were positively associated with ratings of negative transference by therapists (Woodhouse, Schlosser, Crook, Ligiero, & Gelso, 2003). Surprisingly, the Preoccupied/Merger scale was not associated with positive transference. The researchers speculated that preoccupied clients engaged in negative transference due to an unmet need for closeness, whereas secure clients did so because they felt more comfortable exploring difficulties relating to their therapists. Replication and extension of these findings are necessary.

The role of transference is implicated by clients' narratives of their parental relationships. In a small sample of persons with and without a history of psychiatric hospitalizations in adolescence, Waldinger et al. (2003) used the Core Conflictual Relationship Theme (CCRT) method (Luborsky & Crits-Christoph, 1998) and found that participants classified as dismissing included wishes for autonomy in their narratives of relationships more often than did secure or preoccupied participants. Contrary to theoretical predictions, wishes for closeness were not related to preoccupied states of mind. Berant et al. (2008) also used the CCRT method, though with somewhat different results. In a sample of clients receiving 1 year of psychodynamic psychotherapy, they found that among avoidant clients who completed treatment, avoidance was negatively associated with wishes for independence but positively associated with wishes to be able to trust parental figures. Avoidance was also associated with the perception of parental figures as less controlling. (These associations may in part explain why avoidant clients remained in treatment, despite their distancing orientation to relationships.) In contrast, avoidant clients who dropped out of treatment tended to perceive parental figures as not understanding or accepting.

An interesting hypothesis put forward by Tolmacz (Chapter 11, this volume) is that transference is a failure to fully mentalize, rather than a simple misapplication of internal working models. Diamond, Stovall-McClough, Clarkin, and Levy (2003) provide indirect evidence for this idea. In a sample of 10 clients diagnosed with borderline personality disorder, they found that clients' state of mind with respect to the therapist, on a tailored version of the AAI, tended to match their insecure state of mind on the AAI. In other words, clients tended to represent therapists in their minds in much the same terms as they did their parents, suggesting that insecure clients tend to assimilate therapists into what they already believe about attachment figures, rather than to consider that the therapists may have unique feelings and motivations (i.e., such clients fail to mentalize). Indeed, there is strong evidence that insecurity is associated with less capable mentalizing (e.g., Fonagy, Steele, Steele, Moran, & Higgitt, 1991). Clearly, the intriguing relationship among attachment insecurity, mentalizing, and transference warrants more research with larger samples, both clinical and nonclinical.

Another important focus of future research is the potential for a mismatch of attachment styles to produce therapy-damaging transferences. For example, we imagine that the tendency of highly anxious clients to exhibit negative transference will be exacerbated when they are working with therapists who are uncomfortable with unmet needs for closeness and comfort (i.e., avoidant). Future research in this area should also explore whether or not the antecedents of transference (i.e., the therapist's behavior) differ among insecure clients. Theoretically, anxious clients should be more sensitive to boundary setting and encouragements to examine the evidence for their beliefs, whereas avoidant clients may be triggered by persistent emphatic comments or encouragements to examine the feelings underlying their behavior.

Like transference, countertransference has received modest empirical attention, but in general the findings highlight insecurity as a risk factor developing destructive feelings toward clients (Table 18.3). Insecure clients tend to evoke a wide range of countertransferential feelings, and the potential for these to become damaging countertransference enactments may be especially strong when insecure clients are paired with insecure therapists. For example, Mohr et al. (2005) found that when clients were paired with therapists who had opposing attachment strategies (e.g., highly anxious clients saw highly avoidant therapists), hostile or distancing countertransferences were more likely. They speculated that this phenomenon occurs because insecure pairings involve contradictory attachment-related goals—a virtual clash of cultures. Avoidant therapists, who value emotional coolness and self-sufficiency, may feel overwhelmed by anxious clients' pressing needs for intimacy and soothing, and so reflexively resort to rejecting behaviors. Conversely, anxious clients may judge themselves as ineffective when avoidant clients consistently meet their interventions with aloofness and surface disclosures, and as a result become impatient and critical. A mismatch of attachment styles poses significant therapeutic challenges, so there is considerable value in studying the joint contribution of clients' and therapists' attachment style in creating the potential for therapy-interfering feelings and behaviors.

ATTACHMENT STYLE AND OUTCOME

Studies of attachment style and outcome fall into two groups: studies of how attachment style moderates treatment progress, and, less frequently, how treatment affects insecure attachment (Table 18.4). Thirteen studies have examined the former, and a relatively clear pattern of findings has emerged: Consistent with predictions of attachment theory, secure clients appear to fare better than insecure clients in psychotherapy. At the end of treatment, secure clients tend to function better overall, and their symptoms are less severe (Meyer, Pilkonis, Proietti, Heape, & Egan, 2001; Strauss et al., 2006; Travis, Bliwise, Binder, & Horne-Moyer, 2001), though they may enter treatment less disturbed than their insecure counterparts (Travis et al., 2001). Two studies have found that fearful clients may require longer treatments before their symptoms remit (Cyranowski et al., 2002; Reis & Grenyer, 2004).

Of course, the pressing question is how treatment can be modified to optimize outcomes for insecure clients. That is, given a particular form of insecurity, what combination of treatment approaches and therapist quali-

TABLE 18.4. Published Attachment-Informed Studies of Therapeutic Outcome

Study	Outcome variable	Attachment scale	Main finding
Outcome as treatment progress			
Fonagy et al. (1996)	GAF	AAI	Dismissing > preoccupied > secure
Hardy et al. (1998)	BDI, SCL-90-R	IIP	Anxiety (ns), avoidance (ns)
Tyrrell et al. (1999)**	GAF	AAI	Client deactivation × therapist deactivation
Hardy et al. (2001)	BDI	IIP	Anxiety (+), avoidance (+)
Meyer et al. (2001)	GAF	AP	Secure (+)
Travis et al. (2001)	GAS	HAI*	Secure (+)
	SCL-90-R		Secure (−)
Cyranowski et al. (2002)	Time to remission	RQ	Fearful (+)
Reis & Grenyer (2004)	Remission	RQ	Fearful (−)
Stalker et al. (2005)	PTSD sx, SCL-90-R	RAQ	Feared loss of attachment figure (+)
McBride et al. (2006)	HRSD, remission	RSQ	Avoidance × treatment condition
Strauss et al. (2006)	SCL-90-R	AAPR	Secure (−)
Tasca et al. (2006)	Dropout	ASQ	Avoidance × treatment condition
	Days binged		Anxiety × treatment condition
Fuertes et al. (2007)	COM	CATS	Secure (+), preoccupied (ns), avoidant-fearful (ns)
Goldman & Anderson (2007)		AAS	Insecurity (ns)
Diamond et al. (1999)†	AAI, RF	AAI, RF	↑ proportion of secures, RF (+)
Travis et al. (2001)	RQ	RQ	↑ proportion of secures
Stovall-McClough & Cloitre (2003)	AAI	AAI	↓ proportion of unresolved
Levy et al. (2006)	AAI, RF	AAI, RF	Secure (+), coherence (+), RF (+)
McBride et al. (2006)	RSQ	RSQ	Anxiety ↓, avoidance (ns)

Note. (+), positive outcomes; (−), negative outcomes; ↑, increase in; ↓, decrease in; AAPR, Adult Attachment Prototype Rating; AP, Attachment Prototype; BDI, Beck Depression Inventory; COM, Counseling Outcome Measure; GAF, Global Assessment of Functioning scale; GAS, Global Assessment Scale; HAI, History of Attachment Interview; HRSD, Hamilton Rating Scale for Depression; PTSD sx, posttraumatic stress disorder symptoms; RAQ, Reciprocal Attachment Questionnaire; RF, reflective functioning; SCL-90-R, Symptom Checklist 90—Revised. Other symbols and abbreviations as in Tables 18.1 and 18.2.

ties will be the best match? In a review of the literature on client–therapist matching, Bernier and Dozier (2002) concluded that there was modest support for complementary and noncomplementary matching. Specifically, they concluded that early in treatment complementarity (i.e., responding in a manner consistent with clients' expectations) seemed to be essential for the formation of a strong alliance, but that over the course of treatment a mismatch of global interpersonal (attachment) styles seemed to yield better outcomes.

Bernier and Dozier's (2002) conclusions are in line with Bowlby's (1988) implicit endorsement of a flexible therapeutic stance. His first treatment goal, establishing a secure base, suggests that complementary responding should dominate early; persistently confronting clients' insecure attachment strategies too early may leave clients feeling criticized and invalidated to such an extent that they may consider withdrawing from psychotherapy. Later in treatment, Bowlby advocated a more active, challenging stance to assist clients in reexamining their characteristic ways of relating and eventually changing them. Here the research is nascent. The findings of Tyrrell, Dozier, Teague, and Fallot (1999), the only attachment researchers to have studied the issue, supported Bowlby's approach: They did not find that more secure case managers had better overall outcomes. Rather, clients who had case managers with attachment strategies opposite to their own were more likely to improve.

A modern interpretation of Bowlby's recommendation to gently confront a client's typical way of perceiving and relating might be to use the therapeutic approach that leverages the client's attachment strategy to promote change. For example, reasoning that avoidant adults prefer emotional restraint, McBride, Atkinson, Quilty, and Bagby (2006) hypothesized, and found, that avoidant clients presenting with depression did better in cognitive-behavioral treatment than in interpersonal short-term treatment. (This finding remained even after the researchers controlled for avoidant and obsessive–compulsive personality styles.) Interestingly, McBride et al.'s results converge with those of Bakermans-Kranenburg, Juffer, and van IJzendoorn (1998). In a study of interventions directed at maternal sensitivity, these researchers found that avoidant mothers did better in a video feedback condition than in a condition in which video feedback was paired with exploration of childhood experiences. Contrary to these two studies, Tasca et al. (2006) showed that avoidant clients tended to drop out of group cognitive-behavioral treatment for binge-eating disorders, though anxious clients had better outcomes in a group psychodynamic–interpersonal psychotherapy.

Five studies have investigated whether treatment mitigates attachment insecurity. The paucity of studies examining changes in security is perhaps not surprising, given the focus of empirically supported treatments on symptom reduction rather than on how personality differences influence those reductions (but see Blatt, Shahar, & Zuroff, 2002). On the other hand, a long-term goal of psychodynamic therapies generally, and therapies for personality disorders more specifically, is structural change. An increase in security is potentially a global indicator that improvement has occurred in some area of psychological functioning, be it interpersonal adaptation, emotion regulation skills, or cognitive representations of self and others. Travis et al. (2001) found that at intake no clients described themselves as secure on a self-report measure of attachment, whereas after approximately 21 sessions of time-limited dynamic therapy (Strupp & Binder, 1984), 7 of 29 insecure clients (24%) did so. In a randomized clinical trial of clients reliably diagnosed with borderline personality disorder (Levy et al., 2006), clients enrolled in transference-focused psychotherapy were more likely to be classified as secure and to show increases in reflective functioning at the end of 1 year of treatment than were clients receiving either dialectical behavior therapy (Linehan, 1993) or supportive psychotherapy (Appelbaum, 2005). Diamond et al. (1999) gave a detailed report of two clients, each receiving 1 year of transference-focused psychotherapy, who progressed from insecure to secure states of mind. In a small sample ($N = 18$) of female clients diagnosed with posttraumatic stress disorder (PTSD), Stovall-McClough and Cloitre (2003) found that the proportion of clients with the unresolved AAI classification decreased following a 16-session treatment (72% vs. 28%). Finally, in McBride et al.'s (2006) study, clients' self-reported anxiety, but not avoidance, decreased by the end of 16–20 sessions, regardless of treatment approach (cognitive-behavioral treatment or interpersonal psychotherapy); this finding suggests that attachment-related anxiety may be more amenable than avoidance to treatment. The nonsignificant change in avoidance mirrors results in two nonclinical samples. In a large cross-sectional study, Mickelson, Kessler, and Shaver (1997) found that avoidant attachment was stable across age groups, whereas secure attachment was more common and anxious attachment less common in the older age groups. Similarly, Klohnen and Bera (1998) observed that avoidance showed substantial stability in a sample of women over a period of 25 years.

In summary, early research into the relationship between attachment style and outcome is promising, but hypotheses about client–therapist matching or client–treatment matching based on attachment style need further investigation. Moreover, though treatment can enhance attachment security, we know little about how this occurs or whether such changes moderate treatment progress. More sophisticated studies of outcome should include wait-list controls, should control for other explanatory variables (personality disorders, neuroticism, initial severity of psychopathology), and should include practicing psychotherapists.

ADDITIONAL RESEARCH ISSUES

Measurement Issues

As can be seen in our four tables, many different attachment measures have been used, with self-report versions being by far the most common. A drawback of this heterogeneity is that it makes comparing findings and judging the reliability of findings difficult. With respect to self-report measures, we recommend that clinical researchers use multi-item measures of adult attachment that yield scores for anxiety and avoidance, two dimensions found to underlie the construct of attachment (Fraley & Spieker, 2003; Fraley & Waller, 1998). At the moment, the Experiences in Close Relationships (ECR) questionnaire (Brennan, Clark, & Shaver, 1998) and its revision (Fraley, Waller, & Brennan, 2000) are among the strongest psychometric choices. Shorter and more flexible versions are also under development (Fraley, 2007). In addition, we urge researchers to create norms for community and clinical populations. Norms will help clinicians judge the severity of insecurity and promote wider use of self-report measures of attachment in clinical settings. (For an initial attempt to create outpatient norms for the ECR-R, see Obegi et al., 2008.) More research into the validity of measures that tap clients' sense of security with their therapists—for instance, the CATS (Mallinckrodt et al., 1995) and the Components of Attachment Questionnaire (CAQ; Parish & Eagle, 2003)—is also needed. Finally, some have raised concerns that self-report measures of attachment are susceptible to conscious and unconscious distortions (due to lack of insight, symptomatology, or low reading ability, e.g., Bifulco, 2002). These concerns especially apply to clinical populations. Clients mandated to treatment have a reputation for manipulating their self-reports, and in our own experience with using the ECR clinically, we have occasionally witnessed marked differences between what clients with low insight report and our own clinical impressions of their attachment styles (for an empirical test of this point, see Gjerde, Onishi, & Carlson, 2004). Traditional means of assessing reliability of reporting (e.g., checks for random patterns of responses, similar to the VRIN scale of the Minnesota Multiphasic Personality Inventory) may be a useful addition to future versions of self-report measures of attachment.

Regarding interview-based assessment of attachment, a small number of researchers have adapted existing interviews or their scoring systems, presumably in an effort to more easily integrate attachment assessment into clinical settings and to overcome the considerable training, cost, and effort required to score the AAI and its sister interviews (e.g., Meyer et al., 2001; Travis et al., 2001; Strauss et al., 2006). Although we do not wish to discourage the creation of new attachment measures that may be more suitable for clinical populations, issues of validity should not be overlooked: Does a new measure produce a network of correlates consistent with predictions of attachment theory? How does the new measure compare to existing, well-studied attachment measures?

We are aware of two instruments in development that were designed expressly for clinical settings and that sidestep at least some of the limitations of measures used by adult attachment researchers. The first is the Attachment Questionnaire (AQ) designed by Westen, Nakash, Thomas, and Bradley (2006). This clinician-rated questionnaire is unique in that it includes items that tap narrative markers *and* items that tap current interpersonal behavior, thus combining the hallmark features of the interview and self-report traditions of attachment assessment. An initial study of the AQ's validity and factor structure is promising, and further validity work is under way. The second measure is Bifulco's Attachment Style Interview (ASI; Bifulco, Lillie, Ball, & Moran, 1998). Compared to the AAI, the ASI is a more easily coded interview that focuses on current attitudes and behavior in attachment relationships, rather than on coherence in describing childhood experiences with parents. The results of two initial validity studies, using epidemiological samples of women (Bifulco, Moran, Ball, & Bernazzani, 2002; Bifulco, Moran, Ball, & Lillie, 2002), are encouraging.

In selecting a measure, researchers should attend to the domain of attachment most relevant to their investigation. Considerable research suggests that interview and self-report measures are not readily interchangeable, and that each seems better suited to measuring different classes of correlates (Roisman et al., 2007). When the effect of a target's global sense of security in relationships is of interest, self-report measures, such as the ECR, are more appropriate. When the effect of a client's sense of security with his or her therapist is of greater interest, the CATS or the CAQ is more appropriate. The AAI, with its emphasis on the quality of discourse about early attachment experiences, is well suited to assesses reflective functioning and the specifics of internal working models of parental attachments; it was not designed to assess overall security in relationships or models of current intimate partners or therapists (although see Levy & Kelly, Chapter 6, this volume, for a discussion of several alternative AAI-inspired interviews that tap these variables).

Attachment-Based Interventions

One conclusion that can be drawn from the chapters of Part IV is that the respective techniques of dominant clinical approaches (e.g., interpretation in psychodynamic work, thought records in cognitive-behavioral therapy) can be applied to mitigate attachment insecurity.

In Chapter 2, Shaver and Mikulincer hypothesize that the principal techniques of psychotherapy (e.g., establishing a therapeutic alliance), implicitly or otherwise, mitigate attachment insecurity by contributing to what they call a *broaden-and-build* cycle of attachment security. This cycle consists of events that "augment a person's resources for maintaining emotional stability in times of stress, encourage intimate and deeply interdependent bonds with others, maximize personal adjustment, and expand the person's perspectives and capacities" (p. 32, this volume). Indeed, a remarkable and reliable finding is that experimentally enhancing attachment security via conscious or preconscious priming boosts several clinically relevant variables, such as the positivity of self-views, mood (Carnelley & Rowe, 2007; Rowe & Carnelley, 2003), empathy, and compassion (Mikulincer & Shaver, 2005). An interesting approach will be to adapt these priming techniques to the clinical setting (perhaps in the form of well-known clinical methods, such as guided imagery, meditation, or journaling) and empirically examine their effects on symptom severity, coping, in-session exploration, and accuracy of self- and other-perceptions. In a clinical vignette, Johnson (Chapter 6, this volume) describes one convincing implementation of security priming.

The Neuroscience of Attachment Security and Therapeutic Change

The neural correlates of attachment security and insecurity constitute an exciting and mostly unexplored frontier in adult attachment research. Although there are several neuroimaging studies of adult love (e.g., Bartels & Zeki, 2004; Fisher, Aron, & Brown, 2005), as well as several theoretical papers and research summaries on the neurobiology of attachment more generally (e.g., Carter et al., 2005; Insel, 2000; Schore, 1994), to our knowledge only three studies have investigated individual differences in adult security as it relates to neurological functioning (Cohen & Shaver, 2004; Gillath, Bunge, Shaver, Wendelken, & Mikulincer, 2005; Zhang, Li, & Zhou, 2008). From the standpoint of psychotherapy, intriguing questions include how priming security influences brain activity and how the pre- and postpriming levels of brain activity compare (if at all) to measures of brain activity taken before and after an initial session, or an entire course, of psychotherapy. Researchers have just begun to document the neurological impact of psychotherapy (for reviews, see Beitman & Viamontes, 2006; Etkin, Pittenger, Polan, & Kandel, 2005), and doing so within a framework of personality differences is an exciting prospect.

Cultural Differences

It goes without saying that being mindful of cultural issues is good psychotherapeutic practice. In fact, a recent meta-analysis suggests that culturally adapted interventions yield substantial benefits (Griner & Smith, 2006). Unfortunately, we know little about what attachment security means in the context of different cultures and how insecurity varies in adults from culture to culture (for an initial investigation of the latter, see Wei, Russell, Mallinckrodt, & Zakalik, 2004). In the context of infant attachment, some have argued that we need to be conscious of the Western biases in current articulations of attachment concepts (Rothbaum, Weisz, Pott, Miyake, & Morelli, 2000, 2001). Wang and Mallinckrodt (2006) provide a good illustration of these issues in a sample of Taiwanese and U.S. college students. Using a self-report measure of attachment, these researchers found that Taiwanese students described the ideal adult as moderately more anxious and avoidant than did a predominantly European American sample of U.S. students. (Excellent illustrations using the AAI are also available as well; see, for example, Onishi & Gjerde, 2002.) The implication is clear: If we are to properly assess and promote security in our clients, we must understand the culture-specific meanings of security in order to optimally adapt the therapeutic relationship and design interventions consonant with those meanings. Further inspiration for research in this area can be found in the groundbreaking work of Harwood, Miller, and Irizarry (1995). Using a combination of qualitative and quantitative approaches, these research- ers found that Puerto Rican and European American mothers understood security in different terms, and that these differences were realized in their respective methods of child rearing.

Psychopathology and Attachment Styles

Although the literature on attachment and psychopathology falls outside the focus of this chapter and this volume, several points are worth noting. Attachment measures such as the AAI or ECR are not diagnostic tools, and the assessment of attachment styles is not a substitute for a *Diagnostic and Statistical Manual of Mental Disorders* (DSM)-based diagnosis, on either Axis I or Axis II. Attachment styles are nonpathological ways of describ- ing personality functioning, and no style is unconditionally associated with mental illness or any one disorder (Mikulincer & Shaver, 2007). Similarly, attachment styles cannot be inferred from diagnostic schemes derived from the DSM or Kernberg's structural diagnosis. Rather, as several researchers have pointed out (Egeland & Carlson, 2004; Dozier, Stovall-McClough, & Albus, 2008; Mikulincer & Shaver, 2007), insecure attachment is a general risk factor for mental health and adjustment problems that are realized only when combinations of other factors are present (e.g., genetic loadings, lack of social support). That said, an assessment of attachment style can assist a clinician in arriving at a person-specific formulation of how the atheoretical DSM-based diagnosis may have developed, how it is being maintained, and why a specific subset of symptoms is being manifested. Based on all of these things, an attachment-informed view may assist the clinician in creating a person-centered treatment plan that takes into account the idiosyncrasies of attachment style.

CONCLUSIONS

In the preface to his 1988 collection of lectures, Bowlby expressed dis- appointment with the rate at which clinicians, and presumably clinical researchers, had adopted attachment theory and tested its postulates. As evidenced by the number of studies cited in this chapter (44) and the count- less theoretical articles on attachment and adult psychotherapy published since Bowlby's death in 1990, the climate of interest has clearly changed. We are aware of only four empirical articles examining the intersection of adult attachment, clinical process, and therapeutic outcomes that were published from 1990 to 1995; this number jumped to 17 by 2000 and to 35 by 2005.

We suspect that this growth has much to do with the advent of reliable tools for assessing adult attachment, and with the upswell of basic research that followed and continues unabated today. That said, attachment-informed clinical research is still in its infancy, and many unanswered questions and theoretical hurdles remain. Every area reviewed in this chapter requires further empirical attention, be it in the form of replications, extensions, or controlled clinical trials. Nevertheless, Bowlby's and Ainsworth's lucid theoretical formulations appear to be holding up well in clinical adult samples. It is our fervent hope that their ideas will continue to inspire innovative clinical studies, spawn new treatments, and fortify our understanding of factors that promote positive therapeutic outcomes.

Although we are both clinical psychologists and researchers who were already interested in the clinical value of adult attachment theory, collaborating on this volume has engaged us more deeply in applying it to our own work with clients, critically evaluating its utility, and studying the supporting data more closely. We have come away with a greater appreciation of where we need to learn more, but also more optimistic about the promise of attachment theory as a clinical frame of reference for working with adult clients.

NOTE

1. The term *attachment injury,* coined by Johnson, Makinen, and Millikin (2001), was originally used to describe a serious incident of abandonment or violation of trust that occurs between couples. However, to us, the term is equally applicable to any in-progress or clear-cut attachment, including the attachment a client may form with a therapist.

REFERENCES

Note. References marked by an asterisk denote studies cited in this chapter's tables.

Ackerman, S. J., & Hilsenroth, M. J. (2001). A review of therapist characteristics and techniques negatively impacting the therapeutic alliance. *Psychotherapy: Theory, Research, Practice, Training, 38,* 171–185.

Ackerman, S. J., & Hilsenroth, M. J. (2003). A review of therapist characteristics and techniques positively impacting the therapeutic alliance. *Clinical Psychology Review, 23,* 1–33.

Ainsworth, M. S., Blehar, M. C., Waters, E., & Wall, S. (1978). *Patterns of attachment: A psychological study of the Strange Situation.* Hillsdale, NJ: Erlbaum.

Andersen, S. M., & Saribay, S. A. (2005). The relational self and transference: Evoking motives, self-regulation, and emotions through activation of mental representations of significant others. In M. W. Baldwin (Ed.), *Interpersonal cognition* (pp. 1–32). New York: Guilford Press.

Appelbaum, A. H. (2005). Supportive psychotherapy. In J. M. Oldham, A. E. Skodol, & D. S. Bender (Eds.), *The American Psychiatric Publishing textbook of personality disorders* (pp. 335–346). Washington DC: American Psychiatric Publishing.

Bakermans-Kranenburg, M. J., Juffer, F., & van IJzendoorn, M. H. (1998). Interventions with video feedback and attachment discussions: Does type of maternal internal insecurity make a difference? *Infant Mental Health Journal, 19,* 202–219.

Bartels, A., & Zeki, S. (2004). The neural correlates of maternal and romantic love. *NeuroImage, 21,* 1155–1166.

Beitman, B. D., & Viamontes, G. I. (2006). The neurobiology of psychotherapy. *Psychiatry Annals, 36,* 214–220.

Berant, E., Mikulincer, M., & Loebel, S. J. (2008). *The contribution of clients' attachment orientation and representations of relationships to early dropout from time-limited dynamic therapy.* Unpublished manuscript.

Bernier, A., & Dozier, M. (2002). The client–counselor match and the corrective emotional experience: Evidence from interpersonal and attachment research. *Psychotherapy: Theory, Research, Practice, Training, 39,* 32–43.

Bifulco, A. (2002). Attachment style measurement: A clinical and epidemiological perspective. *Attachment & Human Development, 4,* 180–188.

Bifulco, A., Lillie, A., Ball, B., & Moran, P. (1998). *Attachment Style Interview (ASI) training manual.* Unpublished manuscript, Royal Holloway, University of London.

Bifulco, A., Moran, P. M., Ball, C., & Bernazzani, O. (2002). Adult attachment style: I. Its relationship to clinical depression. *Social Psychiatry and Psychiatric Epidemiology, 37,* 50–59.

Bifulco, A., Moran, P. M., Ball, C., & Lillie, A. (2002). Adult attachment style: II. Its relationship to psychosocial depressive-vulnerability. *Social Psychiatry and Psychiatric Epidemiology, 37,* 60–67.

Black, S., Hardy, G., Turpin, G., & Parry, G. (2005). Self-reported attachment styles and therapeutic orientation of therapists and their relationship with reported general alliance quality and problems in therapy. *Psychology and Psychotherapy: Theory, Research and Practice, 78,* 363–377.*

Blatt, S. J., Shahar, G., & Zuroff, D. C. (2002). Anaclitic/sociotropic and introjective/autonomous dimensions. In J. C. Norcross (Ed.), *Psychotherapy relationships that work: Therapist contributions and responsiveness to patients* (pp. 315–333). New York: Oxford University Press.

Bordin, E. S. (1979). The generalizability of the psychoanalytic concept of the working alliance. *Psychotherapy: Theory, Research, and Practice, 16,* 252–260.

Bowlby, J. (1982). *Attachment and loss: Vol. 1. Attachment* (2nd ed.). New York: Basic Books. (1st ed., 1969)

Bowlby, J. (1988). *A secure base: Parent–child attachment and healthy human development.* New York: Basic Books.

Bradley, R., Heim, A. K., & Westen, D. (2005). Transference patterns in the psychotherapy of personality disorders: Empirical investigation. *British Journal of Psychiatry, 186,* 342–349.

Brennan, K. A., Clark, C. L., & Shaver, P. R. (1998). Self-report measurement of adult attachment: An integrative overview. In J. A. Simpson & W. S. Rholes

(Eds.), *Attachment theory and close relationships* (pp. 46–76). New York: Guilford Press.

Brumbaugh, C. C., & Fraley, R. C. (2006). Transference and attachment: How do attachment patterns get carried forward from one relationship to the next. *Personality and Social Psychology Bulletin, 32,* 552–560.

Brumbaugh, C. C., & Fraley, R. C. (2007). Transference of attachment patterns: How important relationships influence feelings toward novel people. *Personal Relationships, 14,* 513–530.

Carnelley, K. B., & Rowe, A. C. (2007). Repeated priming of attachment security influences later views of self and relationships. *Personal Relationships, 14,* 307–320.

Carter, C. S., Ahnert, L., Grossmann, K. E., Hrdy, S. B., Lamb, M. E., Perges, S. W., et al. (2005). *Attachment and bonding: A new synthesis.* Cambridge, MA: MIT Press.

Cohen, M. X., & Shaver, P. R. (2004). Avoidant attachment and hemispheric lateralization of the processing of attachment- and emotion-related words. *Cognition and Emotion, 13,* 799–813.

Constantino, M. J., Castonguay, L. G., & Schut, A. J. (2002). The working alliance: A flagship for the "scientist-practitioner" model in psychotherapy. In G. S. Tryon (Ed.), *Counseling based on process research: Applying what we know* (pp. 81–131). Boston: MA: Allyn & Bacon.

Crowell, J. A., Fraley, R. C., & Shaver, P. R. (1999). Measurement of individual differences in adolescent and adult attachment. In J. Cassidy & P. R. Shaver (Eds.), *Handbook of attachment: Theory, research, and clinical applications* (pp. 434–465). New York: Guilford Press.

Cyranowski, J. M., Bookwala, J., Feske, U., Houck, P., Pilkonis, P., Kostelnik, B., et al. (2002). Adult attachment profiles, interpersonal difficulties, and response to interpersonal psychotherapy in women with recurrent major depression. *Journal of Social and Clinical Psychology, 21,* 191–217.*

Daniel, S. I. F. (2006). Adult attachment patterns and individual psychotherapy: A review. *Clinical Psychology Review, 26,* 968–984.

Diamond, D., Clarkin, J., Levine, H., Levy, K., Foelsch, P., & Yeomans, F. (1999). Borderline conditions and attachment: A preliminary report. *Psychoanalytic Inquiry, 9,* 831–884.*

Diamond, D., Stovall-McClough, K. C., Clarkin, J. F., & Levy, K. N. (2003). Patient–therapist attachment in the treatment of borderline personality disorder. *Bulletin of the Menninger Clinic, 67,* 227–259.*

Dozier, M. (1990). Attachment organization and treatment use for adults with serious psychopathological disorders. *Development and Psychopathology, 7,* 47–60.*

Dozier, M., Cue, K. L., & Barnett, L. (1994). Clinicians as caregivers: Role of attachment organization in treatment. *Journal of Consulting and Clinical Psychology, 62,* 793–800.*

Dozier, M., Stovall-McClough, K. C., & Albus, K. E. (2008). Attachment and psychopathology in adulthood. In J. Cassidy & P. R. Shaver (Eds.), *Handbook of attachment: Theory, research, and clinical applications* (2nd ed., pp. 718–744). New York: Guilford Press.

Dozier, M., & Tyrrell, C. (1998). The role of attachment in therapeutic relationships. In J. A. Simpson & W. S. Rholes (Eds.), *Attachment theory and close relationships* (pp. 221–248). New York: Guilford Press.

Dunkle, J. H., & Friedlander, M., L. (1996). Contribution of therapist experience and personal characteristics to the working alliance. *Journal of Counseling Psychology, 43,* 456–460.*

Eames, V., & Roth, A. (2000). Patient attachment orientation and the early working alliance: A study of patient and therapist reports of alliance quality and ruptures. *Psychotherapy Research, 10,* 421–434.*

Egeland, B., & Carlson, E. A. (2004). Attachment and psychopathology. In L. Atkinson & S. Goldberg (Eds.), *Attachment issues in psychopathology and intervention* (pp. 27–48). Mahwah, NJ: Erlbaum.

Etkin, A., Pittenger, C., Polan, H. J., & Kandel, E. R. (2005). Toward a neurobiology of psychotherapy: Basic science and clinical applications. *Journal of Neuropsychiatry and Clinical Neurosciences, 17,* 145–158.

Fisher, H., Aron, A., & Brown, L. L. (2005). Romantic love: An fMRI study of a neural mechanism for mate choice. *Journal of Comparative Neurology, 493,* 58–62.

Fonagy, P., Leigh, T., Steele, M., Steele, H., Kennedy, R., Mattoon, G., et al. (1996). The relation of attachment status, psychiatric classification, and response to psychotherapy. *Journal of Consulting and Clinical Psychology, 64,* 22–31.*

Fonagy, P., Steele, M., Steele, H., Moran, G. S., & Higgitt, A. C. (1991). The capacity for understanding mental states: The reflective self in parent and child and its significance for security of attachment. *Infant Mental Health Journal, 12,* 201–218.

Fraley, R. C. (2007). *Relationship Structures (RS) Questionnaire.* Retrieved from *www.psych.uiuc.edu/~rcfraley/measures/relstructures.htm*

Fraley, R. C., & Spieker, S. J. (2003). Are infant attachment patterns continuously or categorically distributed?: A taxometric analysis of Strange Situation behavior. *Developmental Psychology, 39,* 387–404.

Fraley, R. C., & Waller, N. G. (1998). Adult attachment patterns: A test of the typological model. In J. A. Simpson & W. S. Rholes (Eds.), *Attachment theory and close relationships* (pp. 77–114). New York: Guilford Press.

Fraley, R. C., Waller, N. G., & Brennan, K. A. (2000). An item response theory analysis of self-report measures of adult attachment. *Journal of Personality and Social Psychology, 78,* 350–365.

Fuertes, J. N., Mislowack, A., Brown, S., Gur-Arie, S., Wilkinson, S., & Gelso, C. J. (2007). Correlates of the real relationship in psychotherapy: A study of dyads. *Psychotherapy Research, 17,* 423–430.*

Gillath, O., Bunge, S. A., Shaver, P. R., Wendelken, C., & Mikulincer, M. (2005). Attachment style differences in the ability to suppress negative thoughts: Exploring the neural correlates. *NeuroImage, 28,* 835–847.

George, C., Kaplan, N., & Main, M. (1984). *Adult Attachment Interview protocol.* Unpublished manuscript, University of California, Berkeley.

George, C., Kaplan, N., & Main, M. (1985). *Adult Attachment Interview protocol* (2nd ed.). Unpublished manuscript, University of California, Berkeley.

George, C., Kaplan, N., & Main, M. (1996). *Adult Attachment Interview protocol* (3rd ed.). Unpublished manuscript, University of California, Berkeley.

Gjerde, P. F., Onishi, M., & Carlson, K. S. (2004). Personality characteristics associated with romantic attachment: A comparison of interview and self-report methodologies. *Personality and Social Psychology Bulletin, 30,* 1402–1415.

Goldman, G. A., & Anderson, T. (2007). Quality of object relations and security of attachment as predictors of early therapeutic alliance. *Journal of Counseling Psychology, 54,* 111–117.*

Griner, D., & Smith, T. B. (2006). Culturally adapted mental health intervention: A meta-analytic review. *Psychotherapy: Theory, Research, Practice, Training, 43,* 531–548.

Hardy, G. E., Aldridge, J., Davidson, C., Rowe, C., Reilly, S., & Shapiro, D. A. (1999). Therapist responsiveness to client attachment styles and issues observed in client-identified significant events in psychodynamic–interpersonal psychotherapy. *Psychotherapy Research, 9,* 36–53.*

Hardy, G. E., Cahill, J., Shapiro, D. A., Barkham, M., Rees, A., & Macaskill, N. (2001). Client interpersonal and cognitive styles as predictors of response to time-limited cognitive therapy for depression. *Journal of Consulting and Clinical Psychology, 69,* 841–845.*

Hardy, G. E., Stiles, W. B., Barkham, M., & Startup, M. (1998). Therapist responsiveness to client interpersonal styles during time-limited treatments for depression. *Journal of Consulting and Clinical Psychology, 66,* 304–312.*

Harwood, R. L., Miller, J. G., & Irizarry, N. L. (1995). *Culture and attachment: Perceptions of the child in context.* New York: Guilford Press.

Hatcher, R. L. (1999). Therapists' views of treatment alliance and collaboration in therapy. *Psychotherapy Research, 9,* 405–423.

Hietanen, O. M., & Punamaki, R.-L. (2006). Attachment and early working alliance in adult psychiatric inpatients. *Journal of Mental Health, 15,* 423–435.*

Hill, C. E. (1986). An overview of the Hill counselor and client verbal response modes category systems. In L. S. Greenberg & W. M. Pinsof (Eds.), *The psychotherapeutic process: A research handbook* (pp. 131–159). New York: Guilford Press.

Hoglend, P., Johansson, P., Marble, A., Bogwald, K.-P., & Amlo, S. (2007). Moderators of the effects of transference interpretations in brief dynamic psychotherapy. *Psychotherapy Research, 17,* 160–171.

Horvath, A. O. (2005). The therapeutic relationship. Research and theory: An introduction to the special issue. *Psychotherapy Research, 15,* 3–7.

Horvath, A. O., & Bedi, R. P. (2002). The alliance. In J. C. Norcross (Ed.), *Psychotherapy relationships that work: Therapist contributions and responsiveness to patients* (pp. 37–69). New York: Oxford University Press.

Insel, T. R. (2000). Toward a neurobiology of attachment. *Review of General Psychology, 4,* 176–185.

Johnson, S. M., Makinen, J. A., & Millikin, J. W. (2001). Attachment injuries in couple relationships: A new perspective on impasses in couples therapy. *Journal of Marital and Family Therapy, 27,* 145–155.

Kanninen, K., Salo, J., & Punamaki, R. (2000). Attachment patterns and working alliance in trauma therapy for victims of political violence. *Psychotherapy Research, 10,* 435–449.*

Kivlighan, D. M. J., Patton, M. J., & Foote, D. (1998). Moderating effects of client attachment on the counselor experience–working alliance relationship. *Journal of Counseling Psychology, 45,* 274–278.*

Klohnen, E. C., & Bera, S. (1998). Behavioral and experiential patterns of avoidantly and securely attached women across adulthood: A 31-year longitudinal perspective. *Journal of Personality and Social Psychology, 74,* 211–223.

Klohnen, E. C., & John, O. P. (1998). Working models of attachment: A theory-based prototype approach. In J. A. Simpson & W. S. Rholes (Eds.), *Attachment theory and close relationships* (pp. 115–140). New York: Guilford Press.

Korfmacher, J., Adam, E., Ogawa, J., & Egeland, B. (1997). Adult attachment: Implications for the therapeutic process in a home visitation intervention. *Applied Developmental Science, 1,* 43–52.*

Levy, K. N., Meehan, K. B., Kelly, K. M., Reynoso, J. S., Weber, M., Clarkin, J. F., et al. (2006). Change in attachment patterns and reflective function in a randomized control trial of transference-focused psychotherapy for borderline personality disorder. *Journal of Consulting and Clinical Psychology, 74,* 1027–1040.*

Ligiéro, D. P., & Gelso, C. J. (2002). Countertransference, attachment, and the working alliance: The therapist's contribution. *Psychotherapy: Theory, Research, Practice, Training, 39,* 3–11.*

Linehan, M. (1993). *Cognitive-behavioral treatment of borderline personality disorder.* New York: Guilford Press.

Lopez, F. G., Melendez, M. C., Sauer, E. M., Berger, E., & Wyssmann, J. (1998). Internal working models, self-reported problems, and help-seeking attitudes among college students. *Journal of Counseling Psychology, 45,* 79–83.*

Luborsky, L., & Crits-Christoph, P. (1998). *Understanding transference: The Core Conflictual Relationship Theme Method.* Washington, DC: APA Books.

Mallinckrodt, B., Gantt, D. L., & Coble, H. M. (1995). Attachment patterns in the psychotherapy relationship: Development of the Client Attachment to Therapist Scale. *Journal of Counseling Psychology, 42,* 307–317.*

Mallinckrodt, B., Porter, M. J., & Kivlighan, D. M. J. (2005). Client attachment to therapist, depth of in-session exploration, and object relations in brief psychotherapy. *Psychotherapy: Theory, Research, Practice, Training, 42,* 85–100.*

Marmarosh, C. L., Franz, V. A., Koloi, M., Majors, R. C., Rahimi, A. M., Ronquillo, J. G., et al. (2006). Therapists' group attachments and their expectations of patients' attitudes about group therapy. *International Journal of Group Psychotherapy, 56,* 325–338.*

Martin, A., Buchheim, A., Berger, U., & Strauss, B. (2007). The impact of attachment organization on potential countertransference reactions. *Psychotherapy Research, 17,* 46–58.*

Martin, D. J., Garske, J. P., & Davis, M. K. (2000). Relation of the therapeutic alliance with outcome and other variables: A meta-analytic review. *Journal of Consulting and Clinical Psychology, 68,* 438–450.

McBride, C., Atkinson, L., Quilty, L. C., & Bagby, R. M. (2006). Attachment as moderator of treatment outcome in major depression: A randomized control trial of interpersonal psychotherapy versus cognitive behavior therapy. *Journal of Consulting and Clinical Psychology, 74,* 1041–1054.*

McCluskey, U., Hooper, C.-A., & Miller, L. B. (1999). Goal-corrected empathic attunement: Developing and rating the concept within an attachment perspective. *Psychotherapy: Theory, Research, Practice, Training, 36,* 80–90.

Meyer, B., Pilkonis, P. A., Proietti, J. M., Heape, C. L., & Egan, M. (2001). Attachment styles and personality disorders as predictors of symptom course. *Journal of Personality Disorders, 15,* 371–389.

Mickelson, K. D., Kessler, R. C., & Shaver, P. R. (1997). Adult attachment in a nationally representative sample. *Journal of Personality and Social Psychology, 73*, 1092–1106.

Mikulincer, M., & Shaver, P. R. (2005). Attachment security, compassion, and altruism. *Current Directions in Psychological Science,* 34–38.

Mikulincer, M., & Shaver, P. R. (2007). *Attachment in adulthood: Structure, dynamics, and change.* New York: Guilford Press.

Mohr, J. J., Gelso, C. J., & Hill, C. E. (2005). Client and counselor trainee attachment as predictors of session evaluation and countertransference behavior in first counseling sessions. *Journal of Counseling Psychology, 52*, 298–309.*

Norcross, J. C. (2002). Empirically supported therapy relationships. In J. C. Norcross (Ed.), *Psychotherapy relationships that work: Therapist contributions and responsiveness to patients* (pp. 3–16). New York: Oxford University Press.

Obegi, J. H. (in press). The development of the client–therapist bond through the lens of attachment theory. *Psychotherapy: Theory, Research, Practice, Training.*

Obegi, J. H., Bousman, C. A., Norman, S. B., Twamley, E. W., Heaton, R. K., Thibeault, M. A., et al. (2008). Validity of the ECR–R in an outpatient psychiatric sample. Manuscript submitted for publication.

Onishi, M., & Gjerde, P. F. (2002). Attachment strategies in Japanese urban middle-class couples: A cultural theme analysis of asymmetry in marital relationships. *Personal Relationships, 9*, 435–455.

Orlinsky, D. E., Rønnestad, M. H., & Willutzki, U. (2004). Fifty years of psychotherapy process–outcome research: Continuity and change. In M. J. Lambert (Ed.), *Bergin and Garfield's handbook of psychotherapy and behavior change* (5th ed., pp. 307–389). New York: Wiley.

Parish, M., & Eagle, M. N. (2003). Attachment to the therapist. *Psychoanalytic Psychology, 20*, 271–286.*

Reis, S., & Grenyer, B. F. S. (2004). Fearful attachment, working alliance and treatment response for individuals with major depression. *Clinical Psychology and Psychotherapy, 11*, 414–424.*

Riggs, S. A., Jacobvitz, D., & Hazen, N. (2002). Adult attachment and history of psychotherapy in a normative sample. *Psychotherapy: Theory, Research, Practice, Training, 39*, 344–353.*

Roisman, G. I., Holland, A., Fortuna, K., Fraley, R. C., Clausell, E., & Clarke, A. (2007). The adult attachment interview and self-reports of attachment style: An empirical rapprochement. *Journal of Personality and Social Psychology, 92*, 678–697.

Rothbaum, F., Weisz, J., Pott, M., Miyake, K., & Morelli, G. (2000). Attachment and culture: Security in the United States and Japan. *American Psychologist, 55*, 1093–1104.

Rothbaum, F., Weisz, J., Pott, M., Miyake, K., & Morelli, G. (2001). Deeper into attachment and culture. *American Psychologist, 56*, 827–829.

Rowe, A., & Carnelley, K. B. (2003). Attachment style differences in the processing of attachment-relevant information: Primed-style effects on recall, interpersonal expectations, and affect. *Personal Relationships, 10*, 59–75.

Rubino, G., Barker, C., Roth, T., & Fearon, P. (2000). Therapist empathy and depth of interpretation in response to potential alliance ruptures: The role of therapist and patient attachment styles. *Psychotherapy Research, 10*, 408–420.*

Safran, J. D., Muran, J. C., Samstag, L. W., & Stevens, C. (2002). Repairing alliance ruptures. In J. C. Norcross (Ed.), *Psychotherapy relationships that work: Therapist contributions and responsiveness to patients* (pp. 235–254). New York: Oxford University Press.

Samstag, L. W., Muran, J. C., & Safran, J. D. (2004). Defining and identifying alliance ruptures. In D. P. Charman (Ed.), *Core processes in brief psychodynamic psychotherapy: Advancing effective practice* (pp. 187–214). Mahwah, NJ: Erlbaum.

Satterfield, W. A., & Lyddon, W. J. (1995). Client attachment and perceptions of the working alliance with counselor trainees. *Journal of Counseling Psychology, 42*, 187–189.*

Satterfield, W. A., & Lyddon, W. J. (1998). Client attachment and the working alliance. *Counselling Psychology Quarterly, 11*, 407–415.*

Sauer, E. M., Lopez, F. G., & Gormley, B. (2003). Respective contributions of therapist and client adult attachment orientations to the development of the early working alliance: A preliminary growth modeling study. *Psychotherapy Research, 13*, 371–382.*

Schore, A. N. (1994). *Affect regulation and the origin of the self: The neurobiology of emotional development.* Hillsdale, NJ: Erlbaum.

Stalker, C. A., Gebotys, R., & Harper, K. (2005). Insecure attachment as a predictor of outcome following inpatient trauma treatment for women survivors of childhood abuse. *Bulletin of the Menninger Clinic, 69*, 137–156.*

Stovall-McClough, K. C., & Cloitre, M. (2003). Reorganization of unresolved childhood traumatic memories following exposure therapy. *Annals of the New York Academy of Sciences, 1008*, 297–299.

Strauss, B., Kirchmann, H., Eckert, J., Lobo-Drost, A., Marquet, A., Papenhausen, R., et al. (2006). Attachment characteristics and treatment outcome following inpatient psychotherapy: Results of a multisite study. *Psychotherapy Research, 16*, 573–586.*

Strupp, H. H., & Binder, J. L. (1984). *Psychotherapy in a new key: A guide to time-limited dynamic psychotherapy.* New York: Basic Books.

Tasca, G. A., Ritchie, K., Conrad, G., Balfour, L., Gayton, J., Lybanon, V., et al. (2006). Attachment scales predict outcome in a randomized controlled trial of two group therapies for binge eating disorder: An aptitude by treatment interaction. *Psychotherapy Research, 16*, 106–121.*

Travis, L. A., Bliwise, N. G., Binder, J. L., & Horne-Moyer, H. L. (2001). Changes in clients' attachment styles over the course of time-limited dynamic psychotherapy. *Psychotherapy: Theory, Research, Practice, Training, 38*, 149–159.*

Tyrrell, C. L., Dozier, M., Teague, G. B., & Fallot, R. D. (1999). Effective treatment relationships for persons with serious psychiatric disorders: The importance of attachment states of mind. *Journal of Consulting and Clinical Psychology, 67*, 725–733.*

Vogel, D. L., & Wei, M. (2005). Adult attachment and help-seeking intent: The mediating roles of psychological distress and perceived social support. *Journal of Counseling Psychology, 52*, 347–357.*

Waldinger, R. J., Seidman, E. L., Gerber, A. J., Liem, J. H., Allen, J. P., & Hauser, S. T. (2003). Attachment and core relationship themes: Wishes for autonomy and closeness in the narratives of securely and insecurely attached adults. *Psychotherapy Research, 13*, 77–98.*

Wang, C.-C. D. C., & Mallinckrodt, B. S. (2006). Differences between Taiwanese and U.S. cultural beliefs about ideal adult attachment. *Journal of Counseling Psychology, 53,* 192–204.

Wei, M., Russell, D. W., Mallinckrodt, B., & Zakalik, R. A. (2004). Cultural equivalence of adult attachment across four ethnic groups: Factor structure, structured means, and associations with negative mood. *Journal of Counseling Psychology, 51,* 408–417.

Westen, D., Nakash, O., Thomas, C., & Bradley, R. (2006). Clinical assessment of attachment patterns and personality disorder in adolescents and adults. *Journal of Consulting and Clinical Psychology, 74,* 1065–1085.

Woodhouse, S. S., Schlosser, L. Z., Crook, R. E., Ligiero, D. P., & Gelso, C. J. (2003). Client attachment to therapist: Relations to transference and client recollections of parental caregiving. *Journal of Counseling Psychology, 50,* 395–408.*

Zhang, X., Li, T., & Zhou, X. (2008). Brain responses to facial expressions by adults with different attachment-orientations. *NeuroReport, 19,* 437–441.

19

From Attachment Research to Clinical Practice

Getting It Together

Jeremy Holmes

Asked by the editors for an overview or "capstone" (J. H. Obegi, personal communication, 2007) for this fascinating and outstanding volume, my first reaction after reading it was one of temporary alexithymia. So much here is salient, cogent, consensual, and scholarly that it is difficult to know where to start or what to add. Assuming that I have recovered a degree of narrative competence, I adopt the angle of an attachment-*informed* psychoanalytic clinician (Eagle & Wolitzky, Chapter 14, this volume; Slade, 2008), inevitably with a somewhat Eurocentric slant. I look at what I take to be the key clinical messages to emerge from the book, and point to areas that warrant further development. Among the great strengths of this volume are the ways in which it bridges the gap between the world of adult attachment measures based on self-report in the Hazan–Shaver tradition, and the perspective of the complex and time-consuming rater-based measures that characterize the Ainsworth–Main–Fonagy developmental line.

The key question for the clinician new to attachment theory is how to relate to an alien discourse (research) and theoretical perspective (attachment); this entails a novel internal as well as external dialogue. Depending on the personal and professional security of the participant, reactions may vary among secure welcoming and exploration of similarities and differences (Eagle & Wolitzky, Chapter 14, this volume, are exemplary); avoidance and rejection; collusion (e.g., glossing over of significant differences); and confusion and loss of bearings.

I start with a number of ground-clearing considerations. First, there is in my view an endemic theory–practice gap in psychoanalytic therapy and training (Holmes, Mizen, & Jacob, 2007). Would-be psychoanalytic therapists are confronted by a complex and ramifying body of theory, of varying empirical validity and internal coherence—but with little specific guidance about what and when practically to say and do from moment to moment in the consulting room, and how such interventions relate to theory. (It is usually assumed that these skills will be absorbed into implicit memory via personal analysis and reinforced by supervision.) This contrasts with nonpsychoanalytic therapies, such as cognitive-behavioral, which are comparatively theory-light, and in which theoretical models—confronting dysfunctional depressive beliefs by inviting the client to test them, for example—are closely tied to specific therapeutic interventions.

A second issue concerns the impact of research findings, underpinned by robust theory, in relation to psychoanalytic practice. Adopting new ways of working, whose objective must be better outcomes for clients, may entail painful modifications of well-worn consulting room behaviors. An example, to be discussed below, is the finding that a therapist's nondefensive responses to therapeutic ruptures strengthen the therapeutic alliance (Safran & Muran, 2000). Research is more usually embraced for the clinically peripheral, albeit important, issue of justifying psychoanalytic practice in a political climate in which funding depends on providing empirically validated treatments.

Third, as here brilliantly argued by Mallinckrodt, Daly, and Wang (Chapter 10, this volume), the mindset of the clinician is radically different from that of the researcher. The clinician has to decide, on the balance of probabilities, how best to proceed in the here and now—whether to speak or remain receptively silent, to reveal feelings or to remain opaque, how many sessions to offer and how frequently, whether to make an extratransferential or transferential interpretation. That is not to say that the clinician, essentially a craftsperson, is not also a scientist-practitioner—saying to him- or herself, explicitly or implicitly, for example, "Let's see what happens with this client if I try focusing only on empathic ruptures or only offering supportive reflections," and incorporating the results of such "miniexperiments" into his or her repertoire.

But even the use of the word *decide* fails to capture much of what goes on at a preconscious procedural level in clinical interactions. It would be unusual for a clinician to make conscious decisions at more than one or two key moments in a session, just as a driver may, and with consultation with a passenger, have to choose deliberately which way to go at a crossroad; yet unconscious choice is going on all the time (selecting speeds, directions, etc., at a semiautomatic level).

Thus, fourth, the process of client–therapist engagement in a session is delicate and difficult to study in a way that both does justice to the subtleties of the object of scrutiny and at the same time is amenable to scientific analysis. Bion (1967), half-quoting T. S. Eliot (1986), famously enjoined the clinician to enter a session "beyond memory and desire" (*The Waste Land*: "April is the cruellest month ... mixing memory and desire"). This injunction is not far removed from Dr. Johnson's 18th-century advice to "Clear your mind of cant" (i.e., private, esoteric meanings)—a charge that undoubtedly applies to the various subsects of psychoanalysis. Freud (1914/1958) saw both the overall trajectory of a therapy, and that of a particular session as comparable to a chess game, in which there are standard openings and endings, but whose unpredictability and complexity mean that the "middle game" can only be characterized in terms of such general concepts as *working through*. Paradoxically, it is only when the practitioner has fully internalized the rules and objectives of the psychotherapy game (or dance) that Bionic emptiness and receptiveness can prevail.

The strength and relevance of attachment theory, with its roots in ethology as well as psychoanalysis, are that it has established scientifically valid general principles underlying the minutiae of caregiver–care seeker interactions, applicable equally to parents and children and to therapists and patients. Attachment theory predicates freedom on secure attachment—client to therapist, and therapist to his or her model.

A basic assumption of psychoanalysis is that therapeutic interactions are inevitably colored by transferential unconscious expectations, wishes, fears, and defenses (and countertransferential responses to them). Psychoanalysis tends to see these communications as primarily motivated by sexuality and/or aggression. By highlighting the need for security and the mastery of fear as a motivational system in its own right, attachment theory adds a new principle—and one that may more accurately correspond to clinical reality—available to explain the deep structures underlying client–therapist interactions (Slade, 2008).

Since *meaning making,* as I discuss below, is one of the key components of effective therapy, this new principle is likely to improve the efficacy of the therapist's work. In this sense, *all* psychoanalytic work is "informed" rather than "defined" by specific theoretical perspectives. Thus one might speak of "Kleinian-informed" or "intersubjectively informed" psychoanalysis. Bollas (2007) argues that the greater the variety of theoretical perspectives that practitioners are aware of, the more flexible and apposite they are likely to be; effective practitioners, especially with difficult clients, combine adherence to models with flexibility (Gustafson, 1986).

In what follows, I have, for heuristic purposes (see Castonguay & Beutler, 2006), divided the contribution of attachment concepts and research to psychoanalytic practice under three headings: *the therapeutic relationship, meaning making,* and *promoting change.* The division is somewhat artificial, in that a good therapeutic alliance in itself promotes (and, indeed, some argue is merely a proxy for) change, and no doubt a feeling of positive change strengthens the therapeutic bond. Nevertheless, this tripartite division of the therapeutic symphony into compound time helps identify themes and furthers structural analysis.

THE THERAPEUTIC RELATIONSHIP

Transference and Attachment

Contemporary psychoanalytic theorizing provides an increasingly convergent picture of the therapeutic relationship (Gabbard, 2005). The neo-Kleinian approach emphasizes the *total transferential situation* (Joseph, 1985), extending what the client brings from the past to encompass the here-and-now therapist's reactions evoked by the client and the specific constellation thereby created. Interpersonal psychoanalysis (Wallin, 2007) similarly views the therapeutic relationship as a co-creation involving the unconscious desires, defenses, and enactments of both participants. Benjamin (2004), Aron (2000), and (from a slightly different perspective) Ogden (1989) all write of the *analytic third* as a co-created entity, unique to each therapeutic relationship, with a life of its own that cannot be derived exclusively from either the characteristics of the client or the theoretical models of the therapist.

However, psychoanalysis has struggled to theorize the "real" relationship or the *unobjectionable positive transference* (Gabbard, 2005), which is a sine qua non for maintaining treatment. Attachment theory helps here, in that it provides a common-sense model of the therapist–client relationship. Distress evokes attachment behaviors. Attachment overrides all other motivations (exploratory, playful, sexual, gustatory, etc.). Attachment behaviors involve seeking proximity to an older, wiser figure who is able to assuage distress. Once soothed and safe, and only then, the sufferer is able to resume normal behaviors, which often include *companionable interaction* (Heard & Lake, 1997) with a coparticipant. The architecture of the therapeutic relationship is that of a person in distress, seeking a safe haven and in search of a secure base, and a caregiver with the capacity to offer security, soothing, and exploratory companionship.

This relationship is inevitably colored by transference, in the sense that the client brings to the relationship largely unconscious expectations, schemas, and internal working models, based on (but not identical with) actual experiences of care seeking. Using Shaver and Mikulincer's (Chapter 2, this volume) *hyperactivation–deactivation* dichotomy as a heuristic, we can imagine the defensive styles that shape the relational expectations clients bring into the consulting room. Building on this, Daly and Mallinckrodt's qualitative study (discussed in Mallinckrodt et al., Chapter 10, this volume) brilliantly illustrates how skillful therapists accommodate and gradually modify these transferential expectations. Dozier, Stovall-McClough, and Albus (2008) have shown how the therapist's own attachment style meshes with that of the client in productive or unproductive ways. Therapist–client "fit" can be classified by using Racker's (1968/1982) psychoanalytic analysis of countertransference as either *concordant* or *complementary*. Daly and Mallinckrodt's work suggests that successful therapy requires initial concordance on the part of the therapist. This means partial acceptance of the role allocated—allowing for a degree of intellectualization with deactivating clients, and of boundary flexibility with hyperactivating ones. Later the therapist moves to a noncomplementary, more challenging role, thereby disconfirming the client's maladaptive, transferential expectations and opening the way for psychological reorganisation (see below). This acceptance of initial transference links with Tolmacz's (Chapter 11) interesting suggestion that the very phenomenon of transference itself can be seen in terms of defects in mentalization; when in a transferential state, people are operating in what Fonagy and Target (1997) call *psychic equivalence* mode (i.e., they assume that their perception of the world is identical with the state of the world as it is). As the therapist gradually challenges this, so the client begins to become aware that reality is filtered through the prism of his or her mind and to adopt different styles of thinking and being.

The Lineaments of a Secure Base

It is generally assumed that therapists whose attachment style is secure are likely to be effective in providing a secure base for their clients. Clearly, secure attachment style is a broadly defined category that does not specify what exactly good therapists do, and don't do, in the consulting room. To extrapolate from the mother–infant literature on security, an effective caregiver is responsive (Slade, 2005), reliable and consistent, *mind-minded* (Meins, Fernyhough, Russell, & Clark-Carter, 1998), and able to repair disruptions of parent–infant emotional connectedness (Tronic, 1998).

   Rupture repair, a concept developed by Safran and Muran (2000), is associated with good outcomes in therapy. Given the emphasis in psychoanalytic practice on negative transference, it is to be expected that psychoanalytic therapists would do well in this area, although the evidence suggests that clients hold back negative feelings from their analysts no less than in other modalities of therapy (Safran & Muran, 2000). Relational psychoanalysis emphasizes how therapist *enactments* (e.g., starting a session late, falling asleep, being inattentive or intrusive) need to be nondefensively acknowledged as "real,"—not merely as "transferential," but also as "induced," often outside the awareness of both therapist and client (Wallin, 2007). When the therapist and client together mentalize such ruptures (i.e., reflectively think about them in an interactive way), this not only leads to strengthening of the therapeutic bond but also is a change-promoting maneuver, since it enhances the client's capacity for self-awareness and negotiating skills in intimate relationships.

Goal-Corrected Empathic Attunement

Bowlby (1988) argued that in the course of effective therapy, the therapist assumes some of the properties of a secure base in a client's life. However, this can only be in a virtual or playful way, in that the therapist's availability is usually highly restricted between sessions. How the occupants of a person's secure-base hierarchy are chosen is not entirely clear (I routinely ask clients at assessment, "Who would you contact first if there was a crisis in your life?"). It is also far from clear, and an open research question, what turns a professional relationship into a secure base. Indeed, as Farber and Metzger (Chapter 3, this volume) and Mallinckrodt et al. (Chapter 10, this volume) have shown, we have a better picture of how insecurity *interferes* with forming a secure base than we have of what actually enables one to be formed in psychotherapy. Clinical experience, with some research backing (Farber & Metzger, Chapter 3, this volume), suggests that *care seeker–caregiver emotional connectedness* is a key feature of a secure base. Interactions in which security-providing parents soothe and assuage their children's freely expressed distress in the Strange Situation leads to classification as secure, in contrast to insecure children, whose affects are either restricted (deactivation) or amplified unassuagably (hyperactivation).

Emotional connectedness is thus clearly a feature of psychotherapeutic relationships, and it is possible that this might be one marker of the extent to which the therapeutic relationship is a secure base. But what do we mean by *emotional connectedness*? A number of authors have drawn attention to the importance of *positive interactive sequences* in therapy sessions. Malan (1979) wrote of "leapfrogging" between client and therapist as the therapist responds to the client's material with an apposite intervention, which in turn stimulates further discourse from the client, and so on. His marker for a successful interpretation was an increase *or decrease* in empathy (the latter denoting a defensive reaction to an intervention that might otherwise "hit the spot"), although how this alteration was measured was not specified; Malan relied on retrospective accounts by therapists. These accounts suggested that this empathic shift referred to a change in the "feel" and intensity of the session, together with nonverbal affective markers such as crying, laughter, and/or changes in voice tone or posture on the part of the client.

Gergely and Watson's (1996) landmark paper focuses on affective sequencing between parents and infants. They identified *contingency* and *marking* in the context of intense mutual gaze, in the course of mirroring sequences in which, to use Winnicott's (1971, p. 16) description, the "mother's face is the mirror in which the child first begins to identify himself." *Contingent* responses denote the way in which the caregiver waits for the infant to initiate affective expression; the caregiver's response is *marked* by an exaggerated simulacrum of the infant's expression. The child thereby begins to "see" and "own" his or her feelings: Contingency links the caregiver's responses to the child's own actions and internal feelings, whereas marking enables the child to differentiate the caregiver's mirroring response from the caregiver's own affects. This in turn soothes and regulates affect.

These interactive sequences thus involve (1) *affect expression* by the care seeker; (2) an *empathic resonance* on the part of the caregiver, who puts him- or herself into the shoes of the child; and (3) *affect regulation*, in that the caregiver tends to up-regulate or down-regulate, depending on what emotion is communicated (e.g., stimulating a bored child, soothing a distressed one). The result is (4) *enlivenment*—mutual pleasure and playfulness, or, to use Stern's (1985) phrase, "the evocation of vitality affects." This leads to (5) *exploratory play* or companionable interaction (Heard & Lake, 1997)—in other words, exploring in security. Johnson (Chapter 16, this volume) elegantly illustrates similar processes at work in the interactions between members of a couple. Similar sequences are arguably to be found in therapist–client interactions. McCluskey (2005) describes a series of empirical studies in which she has filmed and rated student therapists and simulated clients. She shows that initial attunement (stage 1), in the sense of an affective response on the part of the therapist, in itself is insufficient to comprise a secure base. Two further steps are needed in order to liberate exploration and companionable interaction. The first (stage 2) is affect regulation that is mainly communicated nonverbally by the therapist's facial expression and tone of voice, often with a marked quality: "You did *what*?!", "That sounds *painful*," "Ouch!!", "It sounds like you might be feeling pretty sad right now," "I wonder if there isn't a lot of rage underneath all this." A historic example comes from Freud's Dora case, in which Freud wrote in a footnote that he took note of the "exact words" that Dora used "because they took me aback" (quoted in Bollas, 2007, p. 31).

The therapist communicates to the client that he or she has heard and felt the feeling, and then reflects this back as an analytic *third* in the room for both to examine. This leads to enlivening on the part of the client and to stage 3, companionable exploration of the content or meaning of the topic under discussion. McCluskey (2005) dubs this sequence *goal-corrected empathic attunement* (GCEA), in which there is a continual process of mutual adjustment or *goal correction* between client and therapist as they attempt emotionally and thematically to entrain or stay on track (both locomotive metaphors).

Empowerment

An important early finding in attachment research (Ainsworth, Blehar, Waters, & Wall, 1978) was that the attachment pattern observed in the Strange Situation was a relational and not a temperamental feature, since at 1 year children could be secure with their mothers and insecure with their fathers or vice versa (by 30 months the maternal pattern tended to dominate; Ainsworth et al., 1978). Nevertheless, the role of fathers in attachment has been relatively neglected (in the case of disorganized attachment, for the obvious reason that many of the children studied come from mother-only families; Lyons-Ruth & Jacobvitz, 2008). The Grossmanns' longitudinal studies (Grossmann, Grossmann, & Kindler, 2005) are an honorable exception: they have shown that the father's paternal contribution in childhood to eventual security in early adulthood is as important as that of the mother, and that combined parental impact is greater than the sum of each alone.

The Grossmanns (Grossmann et al., 2005) delineate the paternal role as somewhat different from the maternal. (The sexist implications of this dichotomy are acknowledged and could perhaps be reframed as *security-providing* and *empowering* parental functions.) When asked to help their children perform a building or sporting task (e.g., teaching a child to swim), successful security-providing fathers offer their offspring a "You can do it" message, creating a zone of protection within which sensory–motor development can proceed. In the Strange Situation, fathers operate nearer the fulcrum of the security–exploration "seesaw" than do mothers (Grossmann et al., 2005), using distraction and activity as a comforting maneuver rather than hugging and gentle soothing. Several authors in the present volume (Farber & Metzger, Chapter 3, and Florsheim & McArthur, Chapter 15) also emphasize this exploratory—as opposed to the merely anxiolytic—aspect of a secure base.

A relevant recent study comes from Slade, Grienenberger, Bernbach, Levy, and Locker (2005), who found that measures of maternal sensitivity alone were insufficient to capture security-providing functions and identified an additional dimension of *mastery*, denoting the presence of an adult in charge of the play space. This spatial metaphor links with the often-cited Vygotskyan notion (see Leiman, 1995) of the *zone of proximal development*—which denotes not just the "cambium" (now a botanical metaphor) in the developmental process, where the child is directed toward tasks that are neither too easy nor too hard, but also the physical "defensible space" surrounding the child whose security the parent is able to guarantee (cf. Leiman, 1995). There are parallels here with the provision of therapeutic space (which is also a "space of time"; cf. Lakoff & Johnson, 1980) and with Freud's (1914/1958) injunction that interpretations should be aimed at clients' emergent thoughts, neither too deep nor too superficial. Relevant here is Mallinckrodt, Porter, and Kivlighan's (2005) finding (summarized here by Mallinckrodt et al. in Chapter 10) that clients who reported feeling secure with their therapists also tended to report that their sessions felt "deeper and smoother," which the authors believed was an indication of exploration, in contrast with the reports of insecure clients. Woodhouse, Schlosser, Crook, Ligiero, and Gelso's (2003) unexpected finding that clients who felt secure with their therapists reported more *negative* countertransference suggests that these clients felt safer to explore troubling content.

In her construct of GCEA, McCluskey (2005), drawing on Heard and Lake (1997), emphasises the *goal*-oriented aspect of exploration, which is perhaps downplayed in much of the attachment literature and which deserves more empirical attention. She sees the outcome of secure attachment through effective assuagement of attachment behaviors as being the

> effective capacity to influence one's environment. ... What is sought by the care-seeker ... is a relationship with someone which puts them in touch with how they might, with or without help, reach their goals for themselves; or if their goals are unrealisable ... the interaction promotes that sense of well-being [cf. Stern's (1985) "evocation of vitality affects"] that comes from being in touch with another person who can stay with and *name* what one is experiencing rather than denying it, changing it, or fleeing from it. (p. 87; emphasis added).

From a Lacanian perspective (Lacan, 1977), language is a paternal function. "*Le no(m) du pere*" encapsulates the paternal Oedipal prohibition that severs the infant's fantasy of merging with the mother, but also the liberating "naming of parts," including the self (which in Western culture includes the family name). Consideration of the goal-directed empowerment (with its paternal resonance), which secure attachment can facilitate, leads us to the question of language and meaning in psychotherapy.

MEANING MAKING

Explanatory Framework

A significant feature of all medical or quasi-medical procedures (including folk remedies and shamanic rituals) is an explanatory framework that brings order to the inchoate experience of illness, whether physical or mental (Holmes & Bateman, 2002). Bateman and Fonagy (2004) argue that a feature of effective therapies for borderline personality disorder (BPD) is a high degree of internal coherence, presumably as a counterbalance to the ever-present threat of chaos and incoherence typical of BPD. An explanatory framework is both anxiety-reducing in itself and provides the scaffolding for mutual exploration that follows, once attachment-related anxiety has been assuaged.

This mutual incompatibility between threat-triggered attachment behavior and exploration is the leitmotiv to which attachment in its clinical guises continually returns. In infants and young children, this is manifested in observable behaviors—pulling in to the secure-base figure when threatened, turning out into the world of play and exploration when secure. Inhibitions and compromises of this pattern are the mark of insecurely attached children. In adults these shifts are usually much more subtle, although most adults will have had the experience of "holding on" to some pain (physical or emotional) while in the public arena until they can let go—usually with physical accompaniments such as hugging, hand holding, and tearfulness—when with a loved one.

Companionable Exploration

In the consulting room, sensitivity to the ebb and flow of attachment and exploration is the hallmark of a skillful therapist. As discussed above, GCEA entails secure-base responses to clients' distress. This is in part a matter of timing and tone of voice, but accurate verbal identification of feelings (i.e., the emergence of shared meanings) is in itself soothing, and the exploration that ensues once feelings have been correctly identified is always a "conversation" (Margison, 2002)—often, as we shall see, a "conversation about a conversation."

Highly specific meanings derived from the minutiae of a person's life are co-created by therapist and client. Elaborating this personal vernacular or *idiolect* (Lear, 1993) is a crucial aspect of psychotherapeutic work. When things are going well, as Bollas (2007) describes, the receptive unconscious of the analyst is tuned in to the expressive unconscious of the client, and the task of the ego or conscious self is, rather like that of the good-enough mother in Winnicott's (1971, p. 76) model of the child playing "alone in the presence of the mother," merely to guard the space in a nonintrusive way. The analyst's explanatory framework comes into play when there are blocks to this free flow of communication, and here ideas about patterns of insecure attachment and how they manifest themselves in narrative, dialogic, and relational style become relevant.

Main (1991) is credited with attachment theory's decisive "move to the level of representation." Clearly *representation* is neither exclusively nor necessarily verbal. The primitive teleological thinking characteristic of pre-mentalizing toddlers (Fonagy, 2006) is both representational and meaningful, in the sense that an infant begins to develop a mental map of the interpersonal world based on "if this, then that" logic. However, the capacity to represent the self, others, and their relationship *verbally* is the next vital developmental step, enabling a child to negotiate the interpersonal world that will be the matrix of all future existence once the physical "matrix" (i.e., the mother) is relinquished. Language gives us a self, which becomes both a center of experience and an object in the world that can be described, discussed, and worked on.

Narrative Styles

Arising out of its overall theoretical framework, attachment theory has arguably contributed three great empirical discoveries to contemporary developmental psychopathology. The first is the establishment of the ubiquity of the hyperactivation–deactivation axis. The second, the protective role of reflective function in the face of developmental difficulty, is discussed later. The third is the establishment of a relationship between childhood attachment patterns and narrative styles in adolescence and young adulthood. *How* we talk about ourselves and our lives, rather than *what* we talk about, probes the inner world (whether conceived as object relations, internal working models, or schemas); it thereby bypasses the problem of the "presentation of self in everyday life" (Goffman, 1959/1968). which ensures that what is directly accessible to the other is a manipulated, censored version of the flux of unconscious feelings and experience. Main's development of the Adult Attachment Interview (AAI) was an inspired, intuitive, and subsequently empirically validated guess in this direction (see Hesse, 2008).

By analogy to the *fluid attentional gaze* (Main, 1999) of the secure infant, who seamlessly negotiates the transitions among secure-base seeking, social referencing, and exploratory play, Main characterizes secure narratives as *fluid* and *autonomous*—neither over- nor underelaborated, with a balance of affect and cognition appropriate to the topic discussed. In the context of therapy, secure narrative styles are "meaningful," in the Wittgensteinian sense, in that they become part of an open-ended language game played by therapist and client. By contrast, insecure styles lead to therapeutic conversations that are under- or oversaturated with meaning, or lacking in meaning, depending on whether they represent deactivating or hyperactivating strategies or unresolved attachments.

A key part of therapeutic work, far removed from an exclusive preoccupation with making "correct interpretations," consists of moving the client toward the elaboration of mutual meanings, or a more secure narrative style: "Can you elaborate on that?", "What exactly do you mean by that?", "I can't quite visualize what you are talking about here. Can you help?", "What did that feel like to you?", "I'm getting a bit confused here; can you slow down a bit?", "There seems to be something missing in what you're saying. I wonder if there some part of the story we haven't quite heard about?" A therapist is probing in this kind of dialogue for specificity, visual imagery, and metaphor, which will enable him or her to conjure up in the mind's eye aspects of a client's experience (cf. Holmes, 2008). This then becomes a shared object or analytic third (Benjamin, 2004; Ogden, 1989), which can be companionably explored (Heard & Lake, 1997) and, in the case of metaphors, played with and elaborated.

There is at least some evidence to support the idea that successful therapy is associated with changes in narrative style (Avdi & Georgaca, 2007; Levy et al., 2006). In Chapter 14, however, Eagle and Wolitzky rightly question whether the notion of *autobiographical competence* (Holmes, 2001) is a valid marker of progress in therapy, since it could merely be a manifestation of compliance and/or intellectualization, or could emerge in the consulting room without necessarily denoting generalization beyond (or true structural change in) the personality. Indeed, Levy and Kelly (Chapter 6, this volume) note that some individuals exhibit a *pseudosecurity,* in which clients may give relatively coherent narrative juxtaposed with grossly insecure behaviors with attachment figures. This may be particularly true of clients in whom unresolved/disorganized attachment on the AAI coexists with other-wise secure-autonomous narratives. On the other hand, Levy and Kelly also point in Chapter 6 to evidence that mentalizing is related to basic cognitive capacities and, by implication, that deficits in these capacities as reflected in poor mentalizing, may underlie behavioral dysregulation.

Main's schema contrasts the fluidity of secure styles with the fixity or incoherence of the insecure. Psychic health is characterized by some psychoanalytic writers in terms of a harmonious and creative collaboration between unconscious and conscious processes (Loewald, 1980; Rycroft, 1971). Secure narrative styles can be seen as infinite (in Matte-Blanco's [1975] sense of the unconscious as an *infinite set*) open-ended systems, always subject to further "vision and revision" (Eliot, 1986), in contrast to the fixed defensive narratives of insecure attachment.

To summarize, attachment theory's contribution to meaning making in psychotherapy underpins a metatheoretical perspective in which specific interpretations do not count as much as the restoration or elaboration of the *capacity to make shared meanings,* regardless of their content. Lyons-Ruth and the Boston Change Process Study Group (2001) have focused on the mutative aspects of *noninterpretive mechanisms* in psychoanalytic work—where therapist and client come together in a meaningful, shared "present moment" (Stern, 2004), which may well emerge from something one or the other has said, but whose impact lies primarily in the mutuality the meaning creates. This leads us to my third theme.

PROMOTING CHANGE

I have already moved to the ways in which attachment-informed therapy may, or may not, produce benefit to its clients—how attachment ideas might help clarify therapeutic action. This has been a source of debate, and not a little heartache, for psychoanalysis. But as Gabbard and Westen (2003, p. 837) perhaps disingenuously put it, the issue for contemporary psychoanalysis of "what is therapeutic ... is an empirical question which can no more be answered by logic and debate than the question of whether one or another treatment for heart disease is more effective." Attachment theory is now tentatively beginning to make an evidence-informed contribution to this issue. Cobb and Davila (Chapter 9, this volume) have put forward a persuasive model in which the interconnecting dimensions of the psychobiological system (cognitive, behavioral, affective) are differentially targeted by varying therapeutic approaches, but nevertheless produce changes in security.

Mentalization

It should be noted, however, that there *are* questions of logic and debate here as well as fact. According to Gustafson (1986), drawing on Bateson (1972, who in turn based his ideas on Bertrand Russell's theory of *logical types*), psychic change invariably entails taking a perspective at a metalevel, or higher logical type, from the problematic behaviors or experience that lead clients to seek help. If mentalization (Jurist & Meehan, Chapter 4, this volume) can be characterized as *thinking about thinking* (Holmes, 2006) or *mind-mindedness* (Meins et al., 1998) this brings us immediately to the current interest in the capacity for *reflectiveness* on one's own and others' mental states as (1) a mark of caregiving behaviors promoting secure attachment; (2) a mark of secure attachment itself; and (3) a focus for therapeutic action in a range of psychotherapies, including psychoanalytic psychotherapy.

Fonagy et al.'s reflective function scales for the AAI heralded the landmark discovery that prospectively measuring reflective function in adults predicted their subsequent children's attachment status (Fonagy, Steele, Steele, & Target, 1997). Van IJzendoorn's (1995) meta-analysis confirmed the predictive power of parental security or insecurity for infants' attachment classifications. A number of different laboratories and investigative tools have shown that children whose mothers can reflect not just on their own mental states but also on those of their offspring are more likely to be secure, despite socioeconomic stress, than those whose mothers' reflective abilities are compromised (Lyons-Ruth & Jacobvitz, 2008).

In parallel with these empirical studies, Allen, Fonagy, and others (Allen & Fonagy, 2006) have developed the theoretical concept of *mentalization* as a unifying psychotherapeutic concept. (I remain narcissistically wedded to my own antinarcissistic definition of *mentalization* as the ability "to see ourselves as others see us, and others as they see themselves.")

A psychotherapy session—of whatever stripe—provides an arena designed to foster mentalization. Cognitive therapy tends to focus on the client's own (and others' presumed) thought processes and the ways in which reality is thereby distorted, thus helping the client to see painful thoughts, and the emotions derived from them, as "just thoughts." Psychoanalytic psychotherapy goes beyond this in two ways. First, it is inter- as well as intrapsychic, working on the unconscious here-and-now interactions between therapist and client as a primary mentalization focus. Second, adopting a developmental perspective, it tries to mentalize the states of mind of both child and caregiver that form the client's developmental history.

There is some evidence (Fonagy et al., 1996) that enhancing reflective function/mentalization is associated with good outcomes in psychotherapy, especially with deactivating clients. As already argued, psychotherapy is a *corrective emotional experience* (Alexander & French, 1946), both in the sense that the client may have for the first time the experience of feeling safe enough to look at his or her feelings (since they are now mutually "regulated" via GCEA), and also in the pedagogic sense that the skill of mentalization can be acquired in the course of therapy, both via modeling (the therapist's mentalizing "out loud" his or her own and the client's joint emotions and enactments) and by trial and error (the therapist's encouraging the client to work on self-understanding at the zone of proximal development).

What is it about mentalization that is associated with psychic health? An evolutionary answer suggests that in a social species such as our own (and all other primates; Suomi, 2008), the ability to read and regulate one's own and understand others' minds enhances social skillfulness; it thereby enables the individual to achieve relationships that are more satisfying and intimate, and less likely to be jeopardized by unmodulated affect. To mentalize is to "know thyself," which has been an underlying ethic of psychotherapy, both traditional and modern. Eagle and Wolitzky's (Chapter 14, this volume) caveats, however, apply equally to mentalization as to narrative competence: (1) The ability to mentalize in a session may not be generalized outside the consulting room; and (2) mentalization can easily be confused with intellectualization (i.e., a defense against, rather than an embracing and regulation of, troubling emotions).

Paradox and Change in Psychotherapy

If, as in classical psychoanalysis, Oedipus lies at the core of psychotherapeutic metapsychology, an inherently *paradoxical* view of psychic life is implied: We are often our own worst enemies; perversely, we bring about the very dangers and disasters we most wish to avoid; what we want is also what we most fear; those we love may also be those we most hate; we are frequently strangers to ourselves. The aim of therapy, in this view, is to replace this tragic vision with an ironic acceptance of our fate and our unruly childlike selves (Schafer, 1983).

Psychoanalysis from its inception to the present day (Caper, 1999), partly no doubt to encourage "brand identity," differentiates itself from therapies based on suggestion. *Suggestion* in its original conception referred to client–therapist positive transference, or placebo effect, but also encompasses behavioral, cognitive-behavioral, and "life coaching" approaches. People tend to turn to the paradoxical promises of psychoanalytic therapy when common-sense solutions to their problems have failed.

Psychoanalysis uses paradox to outwit the inherent paradoxes of psychological disturbance. It is paradoxical in that, other than the "fundamental rule" ("Say anything that comes into your mind, however irrelevant, embarrassing, or trivial it may seem"), no directions are given; the presenting symptom often decreases in salience not as a result of specific therapeutic maneuvers or interpretations, but as the therapeutic relationship itself assumes the central focus of therapeutic work. Paradoxically also, the intensity of the therapeutic relationship is both "real"—the client may develop an intimacy with the therapist greater than any previously experienced in adult life—and yet "unreal" in that it remains encapsulated within the ethical and physical confines of the contract and the consulting room. The therapist remains a quasi-secure base rather than the real thing.

Other therapeutic modalities also implicitly or explicitly use paradox as therapeutic techniques. The Milan school of family therapy (see Gustafson, 1986) offers families a "no-change" message and "prescribes the symptom" (e.g., "We suggest that Caroline go on starving herself, as she cannot be sure the family would not fall apart if she stopped being such a worry and regained normal weight"). This strategy recognizes the power of stasis and defense, as well as subtly making therapeutic "failure" impossible, in that such injunctions either reinforce the influence of the therapist if they are adhered to or stimulate healthy rebelliousness and autonomy. Similarly, dialectical behavior therapy (Linehan, 1993) gives its clients with BPD symptomatology a poised message of a "change versus no change"—simultaneously validating the clients' symptomatic behaviors as a way of coping with intolerable mental pain, while encouraging them to find new, less self-destructive ways of coping.

As described by Jurist and Meehan (Chapter 4, this volume) Fonagy's account of the mentalization-fostering aspects of psychotherapy can also be seen as paradoxical. Bleiberg (2006) sees mentalization as a necessary social skill enabling the mentalizer to read the intentions of the other—from an evolutionary perspective, a vital "friend-or-foe" appraisal as small groups of hominids learned to collaborate and compete. However, once the other is identified as unthreatening, mentalization is inhibited. The appraiser's guard is down, and psychic energy can be put to other uses. The extreme instances of this are seen in intimate relationships between infants and their mothers and between romantic partners. Brain patterns in both are similar, with inhibition of the neuroanatomical pathways subsuming mentalization. This releases psychic energy from the appraisal task, and perhaps explains the necessary idealization ("My baby/lover/mum is the best baby/lover/mum in the whole world") in which the negative features inherent in such relationships are ignored or discounted.

A similar process may occur in psychotherapy, as the client begins to imbue the therapist and therapeutic situation with secure-base properties, and to relax (literally, if lying on the couch) into a comfortable state of held intimacy (Marci, Ham, Moran, & Orr, 2007). However, while encouraging the development of trust, the therapist will also insist that the client direct his attention to the nature of the trusting relationship (i.e., that the client acquire, activate and extend mentalizing pathways). Thus a psychotherapy session is *recursive,* in the sense that it loops back on itself in a way that nontherapeutic relationships tend not to, except perhaps when repair work (i.e., an everyday form of "therapy") is needed. To take a commonplace example, there is often a tussle between therapist and client—especially if the client has a deactivating style—about reactions to breaks. The client may insist that it is perfectly all right for the therapist to have a holiday ("Everyone needs a break, especially in your sort of work"), while the therapist relentlessly probes for signs of disappointment, rejection, and anger, sometimes much to the client's irritation.

This conceptualization of therapeutic action can perhaps be seen as a *positive double bind*. In Bateson's (1972) classic formulation of the double bind, the potentially psychotic adolescent is given an approach–avoidance message from his or her "schizophrenogenic" parent, thereby triggering a psychotic response as the only possible escape from an intolerable bind. Although this etiological model has been almost entirely disproved, it lives on in Main's approach–avoidance model for disorganized attachment (Main, 1995). A positive feedback loop is initiated in which the child feels threatened by the very person (i.e., the parent) to whom he or she would naturally turn for succor when faced with threat. The more the child's attachment behaviors are activated, and the more he or she seeks out a secure base, the more threatened the child feels, and so on. The bizarre dissociative manifestations of disorganized attachment, such as furling into oneself, rocking, and head banging, are seen as attempts to "solve" or escape from this impossible dilemma.

But because it leads inevitably to change of some sort, a double bind can also foster positive developments. Therapy puts the client in a paradoxical bind ("change vs. no change," "inhibit mentalization vs. mentalize") forcing the emergence of new structures and extending the client's range of interpersonal skills and resources. This analysis is at least plausible, given that attachment and mentalization are subsumed under distinct neuroanatomical pathways: (Jurist & Meehan, Chapter 4, this volume): Attachment pathway A involves the middle prefrontal lobes, while B, the *theory-of-mind* route (of which mentalization is an example), relates to the amygdala.

All this remains speculative, but is consistent with *chaos theory* (Gleick, 1987), a mathematical approach appropriate to the unstable and fluid world of interpersonal relationships. Chaos theory suggests that injecting energy into closed but unstable systems—chemical reactants or weather systems, for example—can lead to the emergence of new and more complex chemical or meteorological structures. Change in psychotherapy can be thought of as similarly arising out of the transferential crucible of security and insecurity implicit in intense but rigidly time-restricted intimacy (see Scharff & Scharff, 1998).

A relevant clinical approach comes from Lear's (1993) extension of Strachey's (1934) classic *mutative interpretation* hypothesis. Consistent with Daly and Mallinckrodt's qualitative study of therapists (Mallinckrodt et al., Chapter 10, this volume), Lear sees transformational transference as a three-stage process whereby the therapist first enters the client's preexisting internal world, with its assumptions, preconceptions, and linguistic manifestations (the shared associations and meanings that develop in the course of a therapy, or idiolect). Second, the therapist begins to disconfirm transferential expectations—neither colluding with the client's preconceptions, nor allowing him- or herself to be discounted as alien and irrelevant. The client is thus in a bind: His or her internal world has been colonized by therapy; the therapist will neither conform to it nor accept decolonializing

FUTURE DIRECTIONS

expulsion. Thus, third, the client is forced to revise his or her expectations, assumptions, and schemas. In so doing, as the client's perceptions of self, the therapist, and their relationship become "detransference-ized," he or she becomes more realistic in making appraisals and more skillful in doing so.

Although analyses of adult attachment rely on the deactivation–hyperactivation axis, several authors point to the not uncommon clinical observation that sudden "flips" from one attachment style to another occur. This is perhaps most commonly seen when a previously deactivated client suddenly becomes flooded with panic, anxiety, and demandingness, and becomes temporarily hyperactivating (Eagle & Wolitzky, Chapter 14, this volume). Conversely, from a psychoanalytic perspective, hyperactivation can be seen as a hysterical defense, in which a client, estranged from his or her true feelings displays, not the real thing, but a simulacrum of emotion, often via envious identification with the parental couple (Britton, Feldman, & O'Shaughnessy, 1989). The sudden realization by the client that, despite *Sturm und Drang*, "I actually don't feel *anything*" may mark the beginning of a less self-estranged inner life. In the case of Y, Berant (Chapter 8, this volume) has documented this pattern well, using a novel combination of Rorschach data, a self-report measure of attachment, and clinical observation. Cobb and Davila (Chapter 9) suggest that "flipping" occurs because people hold multiple, and sometimes incompatible, working models.

Deactivation and hyperactivation thus become not immutable traits, but alternative epigenetic pathways in which one or the other predominates; both may, if challenged and reorganized via therapeutic paradox, open up to new and less maladaptive relationships. Mikulincer, Shaver, Cassidy, and Berant (Chapter 12, this volume) outline how each attachment style is associated with particular defensive maneuvers, and convincingly review numerous experimental studies (many of which are their own) supporting their speculations.

DISORGANIZED ATTACHMENT AND BPD

Prospective studies (Grossmann et al., 2005) have established robust links between insecure attachment in childhood and reduced life satisfaction and less satisfying romantic relationships in early adulthood. However, the majority of people with insecure but organized attachment styles are probably not on direct developmental pathways to psychopathology, even if their vulnerability to depression and anxiety (especially when they are faced with untoward life events) is higher than that of persons with more favorable attachment experiences in childhood.

By contrast, disorganized attachment both emerges from and is associated with high levels of social and individual disturbance (Lyons-Ruth & Jacobvitz, 2008), and therefore represents a risk factor for the development of psychiatric disorders. The majority of people suffering from BPD are unresolved or preoccupied in relation to attachment (Westen, Nakash, Thomas, & Bradley, 2006). It is a reasonable, albeit as yet unproven, hypothesis that many of these individuals would have been classified as disorganized in childhood (Holmes, 2003).

In the attachment literature, disorganized attachment, and its adult equivalent of unresolved with respect to trauma, are categories orthogonal to the hyperactivation–deactivation axis. Helping clients with BPD to move toward more organized forms of insecurity, or even to secure attachment styles, is a major therapeutic challenge. Attachment perspectives can help us understand some of the common therapeutic difficulties presented by people suffering from BPD. Using the heuristic of this chapter, we can identify difficulties in each of the three therapeutic arenas discussed earlier.

The Therapeutic Relationship

To apply Main's conceptualization of disorganized attachment to clients with BPD, clients entering treatment find themselves in an irresolvable dilemma, leading to various pathological solutions such as dissociation, bizarre experiences, or self-injurious behavior. They want help, but fear that by exposing themselves to it, they will once again be traumatized.

This analysis goes some way toward explaining some of the difficulties clients with BPD have in forming a therapeutic alliance. Attachment needs in such people are highly aroused but difficult to assuage. They view help with extreme suspicion, leading them either to resist engagement or to become excessively dependent (centrifugal or centripetal patterns). These clients often find it difficult, particularly in the early stages of treatment, to adapt to the rhythms of attachment and separation inherent in the therapeutic process. In the face of these responses, therapists often enact one of the two patterns comparable to those identified in mothers of disorganized infants (Lyons-Ruth & Jacobvitz, 2008): fearful withdrawal ("John keeps missing sessions; he's not really motivated, and it would be a bit of a relief if he were to drop out. To be honest, he scares and confuses me") or self-referential interpretations ("Susan is projecting her own aggression and despair onto me, and insists on extra sessions as a way of controlling me"). Unsurprisingly, therapists are often viewed by their clients with BPD as unconcerned, abandoning, hostile, or intrusive.

Meaning Making

Similar difficulties beset the elucidation of meaning for clients with BPD. Clients are typically invited to think about why they did or felt such and such—"what is going on" in relation to the therapist, the therapeutic situation, or a significant other—and/or to listen to the therapist speculating about these issues and their putative developmental origins. Clients with BPD may experience such questions, however valid, as either persecutory or incomprehensible. The lapses of mentalization identified as characteristic of the caregiver of a disorganized child mean that a client with BPD lacks the experience of "the fundamental need of every infant to find his mind, his intentional state, in the mind of the other" (Fonagy & Target, 1997, p. 187). Being understood, rather than leading to a GCEA-type sense of relief, calming of the attachment system, and triggering of exploration and companionable exploration, is equated with having one's thoughts and feelings invaded, stolen, or dictated. Interpretations may be experienced as "mad," denigrating, or pointless.

Promoting Change

Third, the idea of change itself is far from straightforward in BPD. Linehan (1993) argues that for clients with BPD, invitations to change habitual patterns of behavior, however apparently self-defeating these patterns may be, are likely to be ineffective. Deliberate self-harm, the temporary comforts of substance abuse, the vicissitudes of chaotic relationships, affective oscillations between blissful fusion and feelings of fear and loathing—all these serve a psychological purpose. They attempt to reproduce, albeit in pathological and partial form, some of the physiological aspects of a secure base (warmth, oral comfort, being held; Holmes, 2001), or to blot out feelings of emptiness and despair. Death or oblivion is sought as an all-accepting safe "bourne," albeit one from which no traveler returns. Less self-defeating, healthy alternatives may appear to offer little more than a void or an impossible dream. As noted earlier, Linehan's (1993) dialectical behavior therapy involves offering the client paradoxical messages of "change versus no change." This ensures that self-esteem is maintained by praise for having achieved a modicum of psychological survival, while at the same time inviting clients to consider different methods of affect regulation and the development of the self-awareness needed to learn from experience.

Mentalization-Based Therapy

In view of the difficulties identified above, it is no surprise that conventional psychotherapeutic approaches to BPD are on the whole ineffective, or possibly even iatrogenic, when measured against the natural tendency to remit (Bateman & Fonagy, 2004). The two best-known evidence-based treatments for BPD—dialectical behavior therapy (Linehan, 1993) and mentalization-based therapy (Bateman & Fonagy, 2004)—are stand-alone tailored approaches, based on but markedly different from their parent therapies (behavior therapy and psychoanalytic psychotherapy, respectively). Both, in different ways, attempt to find ways around the difficulties of alliance building and maintenance, of achieving stable meanings, and of promoting change without undermining existing methods of survival.

Bateman and Fonagy's (2004) psychoanalytically informed partial hospitalization program, mentalization-based therapy, has produced impressive results. This approach has been strongly influenced by attachment theory. Initially it was thought that clients with BPD lacked mentalization skills; therapy was focused on the need to foster these, with a strong emphasis on rupture repair work focusing on the therapeutic relationship itself and encouraging clients to think about what might or might not have been happening in their minds and the minds of others in potentially therapeutic "living–learning" incidents (arguments in the day hospital, missing sessions, violent episodes, getting drunk or drugged, risky sexual activity, etc.). However, the evidence suggests that disorganized children do not lack mentalization skills, although their development of these skills is somewhat delayed compared with that of secure children (Gergely, 2007). As Jurist and Meehan point out in Chapter 4, it seems rather that in persons with BPD arousal is often so overwhelming that it inhibits their fragile mentalization capacities, and that this is what underlies much of the relational turbulence so typical of this diagnostic group. Therapeutic strategies therefore need to incorporate not just mentalization skills training, both formal and opportunistic, but also training in self-soothing and other strategies needed to reduce arousal ("pressing the pause button," mindfulness exercises, etc.).

The psychoanalytic notion of *attacks on linking* (Bion, 1967) as a feature of severe psychological disturbance is consistent with these current attachment views on mentalization (Holmes, 2006). Clients with BPD are cut off from their thinking, mentalizing capabilities when they are in a state of arousal. Valuing a move to a more coherent inner life—in which feelings and thinking work in concert, in the context of an enduring link with a caregiving other—is the corrective emotional experience needed for change to be triggered. The link with the therapist offers the possibility of a secure base, albeit one that will inevitably be compromised by often aggressive transference–countertransference enactments, and whose repeated repair will form a vital part of the therapeutic process. Nevertheless, more coherent, organized forms of relating both to oneself and others will emerge through this link.

CONCLUSIONS

This volume testifies to attachment theory's continuing role as a fertile theoretical empirical and clinical resource. It provides descriptive accounts of intimate relationships consistent with the interior narratives that are the essence of psychoanalysis. Attachment theory started from Bowlby's insistence that security is a basic psychobiological force equal to, and in a sense preceding, sexuality and aggression (Holmes, 2007; Slade, 2008). With current interest in mentalization, attachment theory has now moved its focus from security to the very heart of intimate relationships. Evolutionary theory suggests that flying first evolved in birdlike reptiles as a means of evading predators; once established, however, flight opened up the skies as a rich new ecological niche for its possessors. Similarly, attachment may have first evolved as a way of ensuring infants' survival in a hostile savannah, but physical proximity led to emotional closeness, and from that has flowed much of what we value about being human. It is hard to imagine either developmental psychopathology or evidence-informed psychotherapy without the continuing contribution of attachment theory. This volume is both a marker of what has been achieved and an inviting pointer to future developments.

REFERENCES

Ainsworth, M., Blehar, M., Waters, E., & Wall, S. (1978). *Patterns of attachment: A psychological study of the Strange Situation*. Hillsdale, NJ: Erlbaum.

Alexander, F., & French, T. (1946). *Psychoanalytic therapy: Principles and applications*. New York: Ronald Press.

Allen, J., and Fonagy, P. (Eds.). (2006). *Handbook of mentalization-based treatment*. Chichester, UK: Wiley.

Aron, L. (2000). Self-reflexivity and the therapeutic action of psychoanalysis. *Psychoanalytical Psychology, 17*, 7667–7690.

Avdi, E., & Georca, E. (2007). Narrative research in psychotherapy: A critical review. *Psychology and Psychotherapy: Theory, Research and Practice, 80*, 407–419.

Bateman, A., & Fonagy, P. (2004). *Psychotherapy for borderline personality disorder: Mentalization-based treatment*. Oxford: Oxford University Press.

Bateson, G. (1972). *Steps to an ecology of mind*. New York: Ballantine.

Benjamin, J. (2004). Beyond doer and done to: An intersubjective view of thirdness. *Psychoanalytic Quarterly, 73*, 5–46.

Bion, W. (1967). *Second thoughts: Selected papers on psycho-analysis*. New York: Aronson.

Bleiberg, E. (2006). Treating professionals in crisis. In J. Allen & P. Fonagy (Eds.), *Handbook of mentalization-based treatment* (pp. 231–248). Chichester, UK: Wiley.

Bollas, C. (2007). *The Freudian moment*. London: Karnac.

Bowlby, J. (1988). *A secure base: Parent–child attachment and healthy human development*. London: Routledge.

Britton, R., Feldman, M., & O'Shaughnessy, E. (1989). *The Oedipus complex today*. London: Karnac.

Caper, R. (1999). *A mind of one's own*. London: Routledge.

Castonguay, L., & Beutler, L. (2006). *Principles of therapeutic change that work*. Oxford: Oxford University Press.

Dozier, M., Stovall-McClough, K., & Albus, K. (2008). Attachment and psychopathology in adulthood. In J. Cassidy & P. R. Shaver (Eds.), *Handbook of attachment: Theory, research, and clinical applications* (2nd ed., pp.. 718–744). New York: Guilford Press.

Eliot, T. S. (1986). *Collected poems*. London: Faber.

Fonagy, P. (2006). The mentalization-focused approach to social development. In

J. Allen & P. Fonagy (Eds.), *Handbook of mentalization-based treatment* (pp. 53–100). Chichester, UK: Wiley.

Fonagy, P., Leigh, T., Steele, M., Steele, H., Kennedy, R., Mattoon, G., et al. (1996). The relation of attachment status, psychiatric classification and response to psychotherapy. *Journal of Consulting and Clinical Psychology, 64,* 22–31.

Fonagy, P., Steele, M., Steele, H., & Target, M. (1997). *Reflective-functioning manual for application to Adult Attachment Interviews, Version 4.1.* Unpublished manuscript, University College London.

Fonagy, P., & Target, M. (1997). Attachment and reflective function: Their role in self-organization. *Development and Psychopathology, 9,* 679–700.

Freud, S. (1958) Remembering, repeating, and working through. In J. Strachey (Ed. & Trans.), The *standard edition of the complete psychological works of Sigmund Freud* (Vol. 12, pp. 147–156). London: Hogarth Press. (Original work published 1914)

Gabbard, G. (2005). Major modalities: Psychoanalytic/psychodynamic. In G. Gabbard, J. Beck, & J. Holmes (Eds.), *Oxford textbook of psychotherapy* (pp. 3–14). Oxford: Oxford University Press.

Gabbard, G., & Westen, D. (2003). Rethinking therapeutic action. *International Journal of Psycho-Analysis, 84,* 823–841.

Gergely, G. (2007). The social construction of the subjective self. In L. Mayes, P. Fonagy, & M. Target (Eds.), *Developmental science and psychoanalysis: Integration and innovation* (pp. 17–56). London: Karnac.

Gergely, G., & Watson, J. (1996). The social biofeedback model of parental affect-mirroring. *International Journal of Psycho-Analysis, 77,* 1181–1212.

Gleick, J. (1987). *Chaos.* London: Penguin.

Goffman, I. (1968). *The presentation of self in everyday life.* London: Penguin. (Original work published 1959)

Grossmann, K., Grossmann, K. E., & Kindler, H. (2005). Early care and the roots of attachment and partnership representations: The Bielefeld and Regensburg longitudinal studies. In K. E. Grossmann, K. Grossmann, & E. Waters (Eds.), *Attachment from infancy to adulthood: The major longitudinal studies* (pp. 98–136). New York: Guilford Press.

Gustafson, J. P. (1986). *The complex secret of brief psychotherapy.* New York: Norton.

Heard, D., & Lake, B. (1997). *The challenge of attachment for care-giving.* London: Routledge.

Hesse, E. (2008). The Adult Attachment Interview: Protocol, method of analysis, and empirical studies. In J. Cassidy & P. R. Shaver (Eds.), *Handbook of attachment: Theory, research, and clinical applications* (2nd ed., pp. 552–598). New York: Guilford Press.

Holmes, J. (2001). *The search for the secure base: Attachment theory and psychotherapy.* London: Routledge.

Holmes. J. (2003). Borderline personality disorder and the search for meaning: An attachment perspective. *Australian and New Zealand Journal of Psychiatry, 37,* 524–532.

Holmes, J. (2006). Mentalizing from a psychoanalytic perspective: What's new? In J. G. Allen & P. Fonagy (Eds.), *Handbook of mentalization-based treatment* (pp. 31–50). Chichester, UK: Wiley.

Holmes, J. (2007). Sense and sensuality: Hedonic intersubjectivity and the erotic imagination. In D. Diamond, S. J. Blatt, & J. Lichtenberg (Eds.), *Attachment and sexuality* (pp. 137–160). New York: Analytic Press.

Holmes. J. (2008). Mentalization and metaphor in poetry and psychotherapy. *Advances in Psychiatric Treatment, 14,* 163–169.

Holmes, J., & Bateman, A. (2002) *Integration in psychotherapy: Models and methods.* Oxford: Oxford University Press.

Holmes, J., Mizen, S., & Jacob, C. (2007). Psychotherapy training for psychiatrists: UK and global perspectives. *International Review of Psychiatry, 19,* 93–100.

Joseph, B. (1985). Transference: The total situation. *International Journal of Psycho-Analysis, 66,* 447–454.

Lacan, J. (1977). *Ecrits: A selection* (A. Sheridan, Trans.). London: Tavistock.

Lakoff, G., & Johnson, J. (1980). *The metaphors we live by.* Chicago: University of Chicago Press.

Lear, J. (1993). An interpretation of transference. *International Journal of Psycho-Analysis, 74,* 739–755.

Leiman, M. (1995). Early development. In A. Ryle (Ed.), *Cognitive analytic therapy: Developments in theory and practice* (pp. 103–120). Chichester, UK: Wiley.

Linehan, M. (1993). *Cognitive-behavioral treatment of borderline personality disorder.* New York: Guilford Press.

Levy, K. N., Meehan, K. B., Kelly, K. M., Reynoso, J. S., Weber, M., Clarkin, J. F., et al. (2006). Change in attachment patterns and reflective function in a randomized control trial of transference-focused psychotherapy for borderline personality disorder. *Journal of Consulting and Clinical Psychology, 74,* 1027–1040.

Loewald, H. (1980). *Papers on psychoanalysis.* New Haven, CT: Yale University Press.

Lyons-Ruth, K., & the Boston Change Process Study Group. (2001). The emergence of new experiences: Relational improvisation, recognition process and nonlinear change in psychoanalytic psychotherapy. *Psychologist-Psychoanalyst, 21,* 13–17.

Lyons-Ruth, K., & Jacobvitz, D. (2008). Attachment disorganization: Genetic factors, parenting strategies, and developmental transformation from infancy to adulthood. In J. Cassidy & P. R. Shaver (Eds.). *Handbook of attachment: Theory, research, and clinical applications* (2nd ed., pp. 666–697). New York: Guilford Press.

Main, M. (1991). Metacognitive knowledge, metacognitive monitoring, and singular (coherent) vs. multiple (incoherent) models of attachment: Findings and directions for future research. In C. M. Parkes, J. Stevenson-Hinde, & P. Marris (Eds.), *Attachment across the life cycle* (pp. 127–159). London: Tavistock/ Routledge.

Main, M. (1995). Recent studies in attachment: Overview, with selected implications for clinical work. In S. Goldberg, R. Muir, & J. Kerr (Eds.), *Attachment theory: Social, developmental, and clinical perspectives* (pp. 407–474). Hillsdale, NJ: Analytic Press.

Main, M. (1999). Epilogue. In J. Cassidy & P. R. Shaver (Eds.), *Handbook of attachment: Theory, research, and clinical applications* (pp. 845–887). New York: Guilford Press.

Malan, D. (1979). *Individual psychotherapy and the science of psychodynamics.* London: Butterworth.

Mallinckrodt, B., Porter, M. J., & Kivlighan, D. M. J. (2005). Client attachment to therapist, depth of in-session exploration, and object relations in brief psychotherapy. *Psychotherapy: Theory, Research, Practice, Training, 42,* 85–100.

Marci, C. D., Ham, J., Moran, E., & Orr, S. P. (2007). Physiologic correlates of perceived therapist empathy and social-emotional process during psychotherapy. *Journal of Nervous and Mental Disease, 195,* 103–111.

Margison, F. (2002). Psychodynamic interpersonal therapy. In J. Holmes & A. Bateman (Eds.), *Integration in psychotherapy: Models and methods* (pp. 107–124). Oxford: Oxford University Press.

Matte-Blanco, I. (1975). *The unconscious as infinite sets.* London: Routledge.

McCluskey, U. (2005). *To be met as a person: The dynamics of attachment in professional encounters.* London: Karnac.

Meins, E., Fernyhough, C., Russell, J., & Clark-Carter, D. (1998). Security of attachment as a predictor of symbolic and mentalising abilities: A longitudinal study. *Social Development, 7,* 1–24.

Ogden, T. (1989). *The matrix of the mind.* Northvale, NJ: Aronson.

Racker, H. (1982). *Transference and counter-transference.* London: Karnac. (Original work published 1968)

Rycroft, C. (1982). *Critical dictionary of psychoanalysis* (2nd ed.). London: Penguin.

Safran, J., & Muran, J. (2000). *Negotiating the therapeutic alliance: A relational treatment guide.* New York: Guilford Press.

Schafer, R. (1983). *The analytic attitude.* New York: Basic Books.

Scharff, J., & Scharff, D. (1998). *Object relations individual therapy.* Northvale, NJ: Aronson.

Slade, A. (2005). Parental reflective functioning: An introduction. *Attachment & Human Development, 7,* 269–281.

Slade, A. (2008). The implications of attachment theory and research for adult psychotherapy: Research and clinical perspectives. In J. Cassidy & P. R. Shaver (Eds.), *Handbook of attachment: Theory, research, and clinical practice* (2nd ed.). New York: Guilford Press.

Slade, A., Grienenberger, J., Bernbach, E., Levy, D., & Locker, A. (2005). Maternal reflective functioning, attachment, and the transmission gap: A preliminary study. *Attachment & Human Development, 7,* 283–298.

Stern, D. (1985). *The interpersonal world of the infant.* New York: Basic Books.

Stern, D. (2004). *The present moment in psychotherapy and everyday life.* New York: Norton.

Strachey, J. (1934). The nature of the therapeutic action of psycho-analysis. *International Journal of Psycho-Analysis, 50,* 275–292.

Suomi, S. (2008). Attachment in rhesus monkeys. In J. Cassidy & P. R. Shaver (Eds.). *Handbook of attachment: Theory, research, and clinical practice* (2nd ed.). New York: Guilford Press.

Tronic, E. (1998). Dyadically expanded states of consciousness and the process of therapeutic change. *Infant Mental Health Journal, 19,* 290–299.

van IJzendoorn, M. (1995). Adult attachment representations, parental responsiveness, and infant attachment: A meta-analysis on the predictive validity of the Adult Attachment Interview. *Psychological Bulletin, 117,* 387–403

Wallin, D. (2007). *Attachment in psychotherapy.* New York: Guilford Press.

Westen, D., Nakash, O., Thomas, C., & Bradley, R. (2006). Clinical assessment of attachment patterns and personality disorder in adolescents and adults. *Journal of Consulting and Clinical Psychology, 74,* 1065–1085.

Winnicott, D. W. (1971). *Playing and reality.* London: Penguin.

Woodhouse, S. S., Schlosser, L. Z., Crook, R. E., Ligiero, D. P., & Gelso, C. J. (2003). Client attachment to therapist: Relations to transference and client recollections of parental caregiving. *Journal of Counseling Psychology, 50,* 395–408.

Index

Page numbers followed by an *f*, *n*, or *t* indicate figures, notes, or tables.